A Way Recovery

HABET EL BARAKA OIL — NIGELLA SATIVA

A pure natural product, extracted coldly without any additives

Compocition :-

(Black seed oil)

Nigellone, Minerals, Sulphur, Phosphorus, Phosphates, Iron, Calcium, Digestive Enzymes, Carboihydrates, Fat Protein and Vitamins A (Retionl) and E (Tocopherols).

Properties:-

It has a powerfull effect for the protection against diseases and improving the - functions and vitality of the body .

Indications :-

* Strengthening immunity system and increasing body vigor .
* General strengthening and appetizer.
* Cough, branchopneumonia, chest and abdominal diseases
For Strong Hair And For Pid Folling

Dosaqe and Directions for use

Aduits : Full tea spoon Twice daily One Hour Befor Meal
Children : A Half full tea spoon twice daily Before One hour.

Natice Important :

It is preferred to take the oils separately or with honey, fresh juice, warm drinks
(1 hour befor meal)

Package: 120 ML - 60 ML
30 ML - 15 ML
250 ML

To be kept in a dry cool place, away from sun, heat and light.

Registeration No. 94 / 952

El Captain Company
(CAP PHARM)
For Extracting Natural Oils, Herbs and Cosmetics
Tel.: 5118096 - 0106094516 Fax: 5129080
Elabour - Cairo - Egypt
www.elcaptain.com

The Complete German Commission E Monographs

THE COMPLETE GERMAN COMMISSION E MONOGRAPHS

THERAPEUTIC GUIDE TO HERBAL MEDICINES

Developed by a Special Expert Committee of the German Federal Institute for Drugs and Medical Devices

Senior Editor
Mark Blumenthal
Founder and Executive Director
American Botanical Council

Associate Editors
Werner R. Busse, Ph.D., Alicia Goldberg, Joerg Gruenwald, Ph.D.,
Tara Hall, Chance W. Riggins, Robert S. Rister

Primary Translator
Sigrid Klein, Ph.D.

Associate Translator
Robert S. Rister

With a Foreword by
Varro E. Tyler, Ph.D., Sc.D.
Dean and Distinguished Professor of Pharmacognosy Emeritus
School of Pharmacy and Pharmacal Sciences, Purdue University

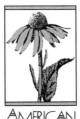

American Botanical Council
Austin, Texas

Published in cooperation with
Integrative Medicine Communications
Boston, Massachusetts
1998

© 1998 American Botanical Council
Published in cooperation with Integrative Medicine Communications.
All Rights Reserved. Neither this book nor any part may be stored, reproduced, or transmitted in any
form or by any means, mechanical or electronic, without prior permission from Permissions Department,
American Botanical Council at 6200 Manor Rd., Austin, Texas 78723, or e-mail address: abc@herbalgram.org.

First edition 1998
Printed in the United States of America
                 5 4 3

ISBN 0-9655555-0-X

Library of Congress Catalog Card Number: 96-78896
Reprinted May 1999
Reprinted September 1999

∞ The paper used in this publication is acid-free and meets the minimum requirements of the American National Standard for Information Sciences — Permanence of Paper for Printed Library Materials, ANSI Z39. 48-1984.

Design by Drew Patterson   *Electronic production by Bonnie Glendinning*

Dedication

This book is respectfully dedicated to the people who have pursued the mastery of their lives with a commitment to the responsible use of herbs and other natural substances. We also dedicate this volume to the American health consumers who have chosen herbs and phytomedicines as a means to enhance their overall health. It is our hope that the availability of the information contained in this book will further encourage the responsible use of the gentle medicines provided by Nature.

Contents

Foreword	ix
Editorial Acknowledgments	xi
General Notice and Disclaimer	xvi
Acknowledgment of Contributors	xv
Members of the Commission E	xvii
How to Use This Book	xix

Part One Introduction — 3

Part Two Monographs

1. Complete List of Monographs by Approval Status	73
2. Approved Herbs	79
3. Approved Component Characteristics	237
4. Approved Fixed Combinations	245
5. Unapproved Herbs	307
6. Unapproved Component Characteristics	385
7. Unapproved Fixed Combinations	403

Part Three Therapeutic Indexes

8. Uses and Indications of Approved Herbs	419
9. Contraindications of Approved Herbs	433
10. Side Effects of Approved Herbs	443
11. Side Effects of Unapproved Herbs	451
12. Pharmacological Actions of Approved Herbs	459
13. Pharmacological Actions of Unapproved Herbs	471
14. Interactions of Herbs with Conventional Drugs	475
15. Duration of Administration for Approved Herbs	483

Part Four   Chemical and Taxonomic Indexes

   16. Chemical Glossary and Index   487

   17. Taxonomic Cross-Reference

       By English Common Name   499

       By Botanical Name   516

       By Pharmacopeial Name   533

Part Five   European Regulatory Literature

   18. Excerpts from the *German Pharmacopoeia*   553
       Hawthorn fluidextract, Hawthorn leaf with flower, Horse Chestnut seed, Horse Chestnut seed standardized extract, Lemon Balm, Milk Thistle fruit

   19. Excerpts from the *European Pharmacopoeia*   567
       Extracts, Powders, Tinctures, Witch Hazel leaf, German Chamomile flower, Senna leaf, Alexandrian Senna Pods, Tinnevelly Senna Pods, Valerian root

   20. European Economic Community (EEC) Standards for Quality of Herbal Remedies   583

Part Six   Appendix

Abbreviations and Symbols   587

Weights and Measures   591

German *Federal Gazette* (*Bundesanzeiger*) Numbers and Publication Dates of Commission E Monographs   593

List of European Scientific Cooperative on Phytotherapy (ESCOP) Monographs   613

List of World Health Organization (WHO) Monographs   615

General Glossary   617

General References   641

General Index   643

Addendum – Contraindications of Unapproved Herbs   681

Errata   685

FOREWORD

The therapeutic use of herbs and phytomedicines has always been very popular in Germany. About 600 - 700 different plant drugs are currently sold there, singly and in combination, in *Apotheken* (pharmacies), *Drogerien* (drugstores), *Reformhaüser* (health food stores), and *Märkte* (markets). In addition to the self-selection of herbal products by consumers, about 70 percent of the physicians in general practice prescribe the thousands of registered herbal remedies, and a significant portion of the $1.7 billion annual sales (a conservative estimate) is paid for by government health insurance. In 1988, 5.4 million prescriptions were written for a single phytomedicine, ginkgo biloba extract, a figure that does not include the substantial over-the-counter sales of the product.

In view of this significant role which phytomedicines play in Germany, it is only natural that the government there would develop a mechanism to assure users of their safety and efficacy. The process is unique. For various reasons, other advanced nations have not yet chosen to emulate it. But it is worthy of imitation, and it is probably only a matter of time before consumers in other countries are able to benefit from the German experience.

This experience began in 1976 when the Federal Republic of Germany defined herbal remedies in the same manner as other drugs–specifically as plants, parts of plants, or preparations of plants, either in the processed or crude state–intended to cure, alleviate, or prevent disease, suffering, physical injury, or symptoms of illness, or to influence the nature, state, or function of the body or mental health conditions. Interestingly, herbal remedies are considered as a single active constituent, even though they may contain many different chemical constituents. Isolated constituents of plant origin–morphine, quinine, digitoxin, etc. — are not legally considered to be herbal remedies.

Then, in 1978, the *Bundesgesundheitsamt* (Federal Health Agency), now called the Federal Institute for Drugs and Medical Devices, established an expert committee on herbal remedies, composed principally of members proposed by associations of the health professions, to evaluate the safety and efficacy of phytomedicines. This so-called "Commission E" included physicians, pharmacists, pharmacologists, toxicologists, representatives of the pharmaceutical industry, and lay persons. Its assessment is independent of the Federal Health Agency, which handles only the organizational details.

Unlike the United States Food and Drug Administration which evaluates drugs only in a passive manner based on data supplied by the manufacturer, Commission E actively checks so-called bibliographic data independently. Such data include information obtained from clinical trials, field studies, collections of single cases, scientific literature including facts published in the standard reference works, and expertise of medical associations. If controlled clinical data are lacking, safety and efficacy can still be determined on the basis of information in the literature, the presence of supplemental data supporting clinical results, and significant experimental studies supporting traditional use.

Application of this kind of evaluation process results in the establishment of "reasonable certainty" of the safety and efficacy of the herb being evaluated. It is not the full equivalent of the "absolute certainty" required by the USFDA for all drugs. However, it is much less costly than the $350 million expenditure required to prove the safety and efficacy of a new chemical entity in the United States. This is an important point. Expenditures of that magnitude will never be made for classic herbal remedies because patent protection is not ordinarily available for them and these exorbitant research costs cannot be recovered. Besides, the German experience has definitely shown that reasonable certainty of safety and efficacy is adequate for long-used remedies.

After Commission E has completed its evaluation, a draft monograph is prepared with a positive or negative assessment regarding suitability for medicinal use, and after allowing a suitable period for comments and their consideration, a monograph is published in the *Bundesanzeiger* (Federal Gazette). Such monographs normally include nomenclature, part used, constituents, range of application, contraindications, side effects, incompatibilities with other medications, dosage, use, and action of the herb.

By 1993, about 300 such monographs had been prepared. Approximately two-thirds of them are positive assessments covering herbs that have been found to be safe and effective; the remainder are negative, usually because use of the drug presents an unsatisfactory risk-benefit ratio. Although critical scientists and clinicians might quibble with a few of the findings in some of the monographs–I do so myself–it is necessary to remember that, taken as a whole, they represent the most accurate information available in the entire world on the safety and efficacy of herbs and phytomedicines. As such, they are worthy of careful study by anyone interested in any type of drug therapy. Ignorance of the Commission E monographs is ignorance of a substantial segment of modern medicine.

Consequently, it is a pleasure to note that the American Botanical Council has sponsored the translation into English and the publication of these significant studies. The information contained in them is now made readily available in the common language of science to a vast audience worldwide. Without question, their ready availability will benefit all of us, consumers and healthcare practitioners alike.

VARRO E. TYLER, PH.D., SC.D.

Dean and Distinguished
Professor of Pharmacognosy Emeritus
School of Pharmacy and Pharmacal Sciences
Purdue University

Editorial Acknowledgments

We are deeply indebted to the many friends and colleagues who have contributed their time and efforts to the numerous editorial and publication tasks needed to make this volume of English translations of the German Commission E monographs a reality.

First, we offer our gratitude and appreciation to Dr. Varro E. Tyler, Dean and Distinguished Professor of Pharmacognosy Emeritus of the School of Pharmacy and Pharmacal Sciences at Purdue University, for his valuable support and editorial advice. Professor Tyler has voiced consistent public statements supporting the idea that the Commission E monographs represent the most rational system in any industrialized nation for assessing the safety and efficacy of herbs when sold as nonprescription medicines. Professor Tyler is an ardent advocate of the reform of regulations dealing with herbs and phytomedicines in the United States. He prefers a system like Commission E which assesses the safety and efficacy of various phytomedicines based on both traditional and historical use as well as on modern scientific data. Also, we are indebted to Professor Tyler for his cogent remarks in the foreword of this volume in which he elaborates the need for a systematic English translation of these monographs. He was also most helpful in reviewing the manuscript and assisting in the fine points of the translations.

We are also grateful to our good friend, botanist, author, and highly acclaimed botanical photographer, Steven Foster, who wrote the first overview about Commission E, thus allowing the American Botanical Council to secure funding to begin the translation and editorial process for these monographs. Steven's superlative botanical photographs grace the book's cover.

An enormous debt of thanks and gratitude goes to Sigrid Klein, Ph.D., a pharmaceutical chemist formerly associated with Murdock-Madaus-Schwabe (Nature's Way) in Utah, who painstakingly translated the vast majority of these monographs from the original German. As much as anyone else associated with this project, Dr. Klein deserves the acknowledgment and the appreciation of the botanical and phytomedicine community.

Much of the detail work of this volume was produced with the assistance of our associate editors. We received invaluable assistance from Dr. Werner Busse of the W. Schwabe Company in Karlsruhe, Germany, who not only provided meticulously detailed editorial assistance of the monographs and the Introduction, but also provided us some of the original German documents of the monographs published in 1994 and 1995 as well as original versions of *German Pharmacopoeia* monographs and related regulatory materials. Tara Hall managed the project at its inception and the end. Without her devotion, clarity, patience, and persistence, this book would not exist. Dr. Joerg Gruenwald of PhytoPharm Consulting in Berlin provided editorial and translation expertise based on his experience in the German phytomedicine industry. Chance Riggins, an ABC intern with a passion for plants, provided much editorial checking plus development of some of the indexes.

We are also indebted to Robert Rister who joined the project at a critical time, contributing his skills as a chemist, German translator, and editor. Robert is responsible for creating some of the indexes associated with this volume. Alicia Goldberg of PhytoMed International in Santa Cruz, California, came to us toward the end of the project to help complete all the various sections, re-review them, and prepare them for final publication. Her contribution in getting the work finished is immeasurable.

Many of our colleagues in Germany provided their expertise and familiarity with the Commission E process to assist this work. We extend our heartfelt appreciation to Barbara Steinhoff, Ph.D., of the *Bundesfachverband der Arzneimittel-Hersteller* (BAH), the German Pharmaceutical Manufacturers' Association in Bonn, Germany. Dr. Steinhoff was extremely generous with her time, providing valuable detailed editorial review of draft translations of all of the monographs and the Introduction. Additionally, she supplied us with critical information and miscellaneous articles from German pharmaceutical journals and provided us the original German versions of the Commission E monographs upon which some of our translations are based.

Members of the Commission E also reviewed some of the text and provided supplemental documents. Dr. Konstantin Keller, of the German Federal Institute for Drugs and Medical Devices and the referee of the Commission E, provided us a checklist of all monographs published by the commission, which we have included in the indexes section. Dr. Keller also contributed his time and expertise in editing our introduction to this volume. We appreciate the time and effort of Prof. Dr. Heinz Schilcher of the Institute of Pharmaceutical Biology at Berlin Independent University for his peer review of the Introduction. Prof. Schilcher has been a member of Commission E since it was formed in 1978, making him the longest-serving member of that body and, thus, someone with considerable expertise on this subject. He is also Vice President of the Commission. Prof. Schilcher contributed a considerable amount of his time providing detailed editing of the introduction, as well as sending us additional references. We are also grateful to Prof. Dr. Gerhard Franz, of the Institute of Pharmacy at the University of Regensburg in Regensburg, Germany, for his peer review insights. Prof. Franz is also a member of Commission E.

Dr. Rudolf Bauer of the Heinrich Heine University, Institute for Pharmaceutical Biology in Dusseldorf, Germany, reviewed our four monographs on various echinacea species and parts. Melville K. Eaves and Dr. U. Mathes of the Willmar Schwabe Co. provided some original German monographs on *Ginkgo biloba* extract plus information on the pathological stages of benign prostatic hypertrophy. Dr. Georg Seidel of Madaus AG in Cologne reviewed the monographs on echinacea and milk thistle as well as others. Dr. Götz. Harnischfeger of Schaper and Brümmer of Salzgitter, Germany, helped to clarify fine points regarding the black cohosh monograph. Dr. Helmut Wiedenfeld of the University of Bonn Pharmaceutical Institute gave us valuable information on the policy regarding plants with pyrrolizidine alkaloids (e.g., coltsfoot herb and comfrey leaf and root).

We are indebted to Fr. Sabine Koerner of the *Deutscher Apotheker Verlag* (German Pharmaceutical Publishers) in Stuttgart for kind permission to reprint selected monographs from the *German Pharmacopoeia*. We also extend our gratitude to Dr. Agnes Artiges of the European Pharmacopoeia Commission of the Council of Europe in Strasbourg, France, for graciously allowing us to reprint selected monographs from the *European Pharmacopoeia*. We also acknowledge our colleague, Dr. Hubertus Cranz of the European Proprietary Medicines Manufacturer's Association (AESGP) in Brussels, who assisted us in the matter of obtaining these reprint permissions.

EDITORIAL ACKNOWLEDGMENTS

Many friends and colleagues in the academic community in the U.S. and Canada also assisted us in editing and reviewing the material in this book. Dr. James A. Duke, formerly of the U.S. Department of Agriculture for 30 years, was a constant champion of this project. We are grateful for his editorial contributions, particularly in the areas of taxonomy and nomenclature. Our appreciation goes to Professor Norman R. Farnsworth of the Program for Collaborative Research in the Pharmaceutical Sciences at the University of Illinois at Chicago for his valuable assistance on matters related to key points on *Eleutherococcus* and other botanicals. We are most grateful to Arthur O. Tucker, Ph.D., of Delaware State University, who contributed his valuable time and expertise in editing and correcting the taxonomic and nomenclature aspects of this work. Appreciation and gratitude are extended to Dennis V. C. Awang, Ph.D., former head of the Natural Products Testing Branch of the Bureau of Drug Research at the Health Protection Branch in Ottawa, Canada, current president of Medi-Plant Consulting Services in Ottawa. Dr. Awang's many years of expertise in natural products and their chemistry have been an invaluable editorial resource for the development of this book.

We extend special thanks for the production of the Glossary and Therapeutic Indexes to Sue Crow, RN, MSN,CIC, Louisiana State University, School of Medicine in Shreveport. We also received assistance on the Glossary and Therapeutic Indexes from Andrew T. Weil, M.D., author and director of the Program for Integrative Medicine at the University of Arizona. Tom Carlson, M.D., vice-president of Field Ethnobiology at Shaman Pharmaceuticals in South San Francisco, California and Peter Goldman, M.D. of the Harvard University School of Public Health assisted with the review of the Therapeutic Indexes and the Glossary. Ted L. Edwards, Jr., M.D., a physician in Austin, Texas, provided us information on heart disease for the Hawthorn flower and leaf monograph. We are also grateful to Wayne B. Katz, M.D. of the Scripps Institute of La Jolla, California, for his editorial contributions and William Straub, M.D., of Middleton, Massachusetts, who also assisted us in reviewing sections of the manuscript.

There are a number of people on the staff of the American Botanical Council (ABC) who provided invaluable editorial and project management services to make this volume possible. Dr. Wayne Silverman, Chief Administrative Officer, was responsible for much of the fund-raising efforts to help finance the translations, editing and publication of this book. Julie Weismann helped guide the project through the second third of the editorial and formatting process. Her assistance and focus were extremely valuable. Karen Newton transcribed and re-entered various sections, particularly the glossary. Meredith Barad, an ABC intern and premedical student, helped compile much of the glossary of terms. Wali Stopher, our resident *HerbalGram* copy editor, reviewed the entire manuscript on several occasions and provided detailed copy and grammatical edits. Gayle Engels has assisted in various areas regarding planning for the printing and handling our many advance pre-publication orders. Cecelia Thompson and Margaret Wright provided invaluable accounting services. Additional acknowledgments are extended to Barbara Johnston, Ginger Hudson-Maffei, Ginger Webb, Dawnelle Malone, Betsy Levy, Linda Prudhomme, Lauren Holmans, Lisa Larousse, Lisa Newton, Vicki Adams, Susan McFarland, Lavinia Baumhoff, George Solis and Joni McClain — all staff members of ABC who have contributed to this publication project.

Imre Eifert and Pia Bauer of the University of Texas assisted in translation questions.

The book design and the cover were the work of Drew Patterson. The various edits and re-edits in the main text and the many indexes were patiently and skillfully entered into computers by Layne Jackson and Bonnie Glendinning. Thanks also go to Steve Indig at

Insty Prints and the gang at Kinko's in Westlake Hills. Terry Raines of Raines Graphics assisted in the planning and design of the book.

Finally, we are most grateful to the various foundations, corporations, and individuals whose financial contributions funded this project and publication. We acknowledge their contributions on the following page.

MARK BLUMENTHAL

Austin, Texas
April 1998

Acknowledgment of Contributors

This important work could not have been made possible without the dedicated financial assistance of supporting foundations, organizations, businesses and individuals. The American Botanical Council and those who will utilize this valuable resource are indebted to them for their foresight in recognizing the part this book will play in changing health care in the United States.

The printing of Commission E Monographs was made possible through a major grant from the **Moody Foundation of Galveston, Texas**.

Major Corporate Partners to the project include:

Amway Corporation
Canadian Health
  Food Association
Capsugel
Celestial Seasonings
Enzymatic Therapy
ExtractsPlus
Emil Flachsmann AG
Frontier Natural
  Products Co-op
General Nutrition Centers

Henkel Corporation
Herb Pharm
Herbalife
Leiner Health Products
Monsanto Company
MW International
NaturaLife
Nature's Bounty
Nature's Herbs
Nature's Resource
  Premium Herbs

Nature's Way
New Visions International
Pharmacist's Ultimate
  Health
Pharmaton Natural
  Health Products
Shaperite
Solaray, Inc.
Stryka Botanics Co., Inc.
Triarco

Corporate Friends to the project include:

Bio-Botanica, Inc.
Botanicals International
Carter-Wallace, Inc.
Doctor's Nutriceuticals®,
  DR Rx, Inc.
Finzelberg
Gaia Herbs
Indena
Indiana Botanic Gardens

Lichtwer Pharma
Müggenburg Extrakt
Nature's Apothecary
Nature's Sunshine
  Products, Inc.
Odwalla Juice Company
Pharmline
Plantation Medicinals
QBI - Quality Botanical
  Ingredients, Inc.

R. P. Scherer
Schiff-Weider Nutrition
  International
Swiss Caps
Traditional Medicinals
Wakunaga of America
  Co., Ltd.
Whole Herb Company

General Notice and Disclaimer

The editors have attempted to exercise the utmost care in providing accurate translations of the monographs as published by Commission E of the German Institute for Drugs and Medical Products in the *Bundesanzeiger*, the German equivalent of the U.S. *Federal Register*. As is the case with any work that is based on translations, there may be some latitude in choosing English terminology for German words, either common or technical. Also, the editors have made every possible attempt to verify the accuracy of the indexes, cross-references, and other materials presented in this volume.

It should be noted by the reader that constant changes in information resulting from ongoing research and clinical experience, differences in opinions among authorities, unique individual circumstances, and the possibility of human error in compiling this publication require that the reader use judgment and other resources when making decisions based on this material.

The information contained in the monographs was originally intended as package insert information for physicians, pharmacists, other health professionals, and consumers in Germany. Accordingly, the publication of this material in English is intended primarily to help provide English-speaking health professionals with much-needed therapeutic information on botanicals.

However, this book is not intended as a guide to self medication by consumers. The lay reader is advised to discuss the information contained herein with a doctor, pharmacist, nurse or other authorized health care practitioner. Neither the editors nor the publisher accepts any responsibility for the accuracy of the information itself or the consequences from the use or misuse of the information in this book.

Members of Commission E

This list includes all active members of Commission E and their deputies. For more information on the composition of the Commission, please see page 28 of the Introduction.

Distinguished physicians and scientists serving on the Commission include:

Toxicology/Pharmacology

Member: Prof. Dr. rer. nat. Hilke Winterhof
University of Münster
Institute of Pharmacology and Toxicology

Clinical Pharmacology

Member: Prof. Dr. med. Dieter Loew
Wiesbaden

Deputy: Prof. Dr. med. I. Roots
Director of the Institute for Clinical Pharmacology
University Clinic Charité, Berlin

Medical Statistics

Member: Prof. Dr. phil. Wilhelm Gaus
University of Ulm, Department of Biometry and Medical Documentation

Deputy: Prof. Dr. phil. nat. Berthold Schneider
University of Hanover
Institute for Biometry of Medicine

Pharmacy

Member: Prof. Dr. phil. Franz-C. Czygan
University of Würzburg
Chair of Department of Pharmaceutical Biology

Deputy: Prof. Dr. rer. nat. G. Franz
University of Regensburg,
Chair of Department of Pharmaceutical Biology

Medical Practice

Members: Dr. med. Fritz Oelze
Hamburg

Dr. Manfred Bocksch
Doctor of General Medicine
Eurasburg

Priv. Doz. Dr. med. Karin Kraft
University of Bonn

Univ. Prof. Dr. rer. nat. Heinz Schilcher
Marx-Zentrum Pharmacy
Munich

Dr. med. Egon Frölich
Chief Physician of the Rheintal Clinic
Bad Krozingen

Dr. med. Waltraut Weigel
Ortenburg-Dorfbach

Univ. Prof. Dr. med. habil. Hartwig Wilhelm Bauer
Munich

Natural Practitioner Josef Karl
Munich

Deputies: Dr. med. Christian Hentschel
Chief Physician of the Blankenstein Clinic
University of Hattingen

Prof. Dr. med. Heribert Frotz
Chief Physician of the Internal Section
of the Marienkrankenhaus
Bergisch-Gladbach

Prof. Dr. med. Günther Faust
Doctor of General Medicine
Mainz

Prof. Dr. rer. nat. habil. Ulrike Lindequist
Ernst-Moritz-Arndt University
Institute for Pharmaceutical Biology
Greifswald

Dr. med. Markus Wiesenauer
Weinstadt

Dr. med. Gerd Hennig
Bad Wörishofen

Dr. med. Klaus Mohr
Staufenberg

Dr. rer. nat. Wolfgang Widmaier
Stuttgart

How to Use This Book

This outline is designed to help the reader find information in the various sections of the book. The book is made up of the following sections:

Part One: Introduction and Overview

The Introduction discusses the monographs in relation to the regulatory situations in the U.S and Germany, including analysis of the German phytomedicinal market and Commission E. The Introduction also discusses the criteria by which herbs were evaluated, distinguishes between types of monographs, and explains the subsections of the monographs. A summary and a detailed outline of the contents of the Introduction are provided on (pages 5 - 7). References are included on (pages 67 - 70).

Part Two: Monographs (page 73)

The monographs are usually titled by the generally accepted English common name and are separated into Approved and Unapproved Herbs. Single herbs, component characteristics, and fixed combinations are divided into different sections. For quick reference, the page number for each herb monograph is provided in the beginning of Part One in the Complete List of Monographs by Approval Status (pages 73 - 78).

Part Three: Therapeutic Indexes (page 419)

This section provides a guide to the therapeutic use of Commission E herbs and contains an index on each of the following:
  - Uses and Indications of Approved Herbs
  - Contraindications of Approved Herbs
  - Side Effects of Approved and Unapproved Herbs (2 sections)
  - Pharmacological Actions of Approved and Unapproved herbs (2 sections)
  - Interactions of Herbs with Conventional Drugs
  - Duration of Use for Approved Herbs

An explanatory paragraph in each index explains how to use the appropriate therapeutic information contained in this section. The monographs should be consulted for additional relevant data before any therapeutic or clinical decisions are made.

Part Four: Chemical and Taxonomic Indexes (page 487)

Chemical Glossary and Index

This section consists of an alphabetical listing of the various chemical compounds and classes of chemical compounds included in the monographs. The Commission E focused on producing therapeutic use monographs and, therefore, most monographs and the index contain only key active chemical components, i.e. compounds that are known to contribute to the overall efficacy of the herbal drug.

Taxonomic Cross-Reference

This section contains the nomenclature and taxonomy of the plants: English common name, Latin binomial, plant family, pharmacopeial name, and German name. This information is organized into three tables by the English, Latin and pharmacopeial names. The German name can be found in the General Index that also includes the English common names, Latin binomials, and pharmacopeial names found throughout the text.

Part Five: European Regulatory Literature (page 553)

The *German Pharmacopoeia* section contains six analytical monographs which describe the quality control procedures required for German manufacturers. The following herbs are included: Hawthorn fluidextract, Hawthorn leaf with flower, Horse Chestnut seed, Standardized Horse Chestnut seed extract, Lemon Balm, and Milk Thistle fruit.

The excerpts from the *European Pharmacopoeia* represent quality and identity standards and test methods for the following herbs: Witch Hazel leaf, German Chamomile flower, Senna leaf, Alexandrian Senna pods, Tinnevelly Senna pods, and Valerian root. This section also provides definitions and formulation methods for extracts, powders, and tinctures.

The **European Economic Community (EEC) Standards** section includes guidelines for detailed qualitative and quantitative labeling parameters, description of the methods of preparation, and quality control tests.

Part Six: Appendix

The Appendix includes the following sections: **Abbreviations and Symbols** (page 587) used in the text of the Monographs and in the supplemental European Regulatory Literature in Part Five.

Weights and Measures (page 591) used in the text of the Monographs and in the supplemental European Regulatory Literature in Part Four.

German *Federal Gazette* Numbers and Publication Dates of Commission E Monographs (page 593). This section contains a complete list of monographs with the date of original publication, revision date and *Bundesanzeiger* (German *Federal Gazette*) number. The date and number allows the reader to access the original German monographs.

European Scientific Cooperative on Phytotherapy (ESCOP) Monographs (page 613). This section provides an overview of the 50 herbs that were evaluated in therapeutic monographs by ESCOP, a scientific organization assisting in the harmonization of therapeutic data on herbal drug products sold in the European Union.

World Health Organization (WHO) Monographs (page 615). This section provides an overview of the 28 herb monographs produced by the WHO to assist regulatory agencies in the evaluation of the quality, safety and efficacy of herbal medicines.

General Glossary (page 617). This section includes a comprehensive glossary of Anatomical, Botanical, Medical, Pharmaceutical, and Physiological terms to assist the reader in understanding technical terminology.

General References (page 641). The references listed were used to provide additional information in the translation and expansion of the original German monographs.

General Index (page 643). The general index contains the following information: English common name, Latin binomial, Pharmacopeial name, German name, therapeutic classification (uses, contraindications, side effects), chemical names, and other relevant data from the text of the book. The page numbers of the complete monographs are printed in bold type.

Quick Guide to Finding Information

A. By the Name of the Herb. Readers who know the name of a particular herb have three ways to find relevant information from the monographs:

- The **Complete List of Monographs by Approval Status** (page 73), provides a listing of all the monographs, arranged alphabetically by English common name. This list is divided based on monograph type and approval status.

- The **General Index** (page 643) lists all herb names with their page numbers. Thus, if the reader knows the botanical name, pharmacopeial name, or German name, the herb can be found alphabetically in the General Index.

- The **Taxonomic Cross-Reference** (page 499) provides plant synonyms according to approximately 530 correlations of English Common Names, Latin binomials, Plant Families, Pharmacopeial names, and German names. If reader has the name of an herb that does not correspond to a monograph title, many synonyms can be found in the Taxonomic Cross-Reference.

B. By Therapeutic Use. If the reader wishes to find information on the safe and effective treatment using herbs and phytomedicines, the therapeutic indexes listed below provide information from the monographs, indexed by medical indications and related therapeutic parameters.

List of **Uses and Indications** (page 419): This section provides an alphabetical list of conditions with the relevant approved herbs indicated for that condition. (For example, St. John's Wort would be found under the headings Anxiety and Depression.) For more information about a particular herb, the General Index (page 643) lists in bold the page number of the complete herb monograph.

List of **Contraindications** (page 433): This section alphabetically lists the conditions when particular herbs should not be used. (For example, Kava Kava should not be used for cases of endogenous depression and is, therefore, listed under that heading.) For more information about a particular herb, the General Index lists in bold the page number of the complete herb monograph.

List of **Side Effects** (page 443): There are two indexes, each listing the Side Effects of Approved and Unapproved Herbs, respectively. These indexes, found on pages 443 and 451, alphabetically list the potential side effects from using certain herbs. (For example, sensitive individuals may experience an allergic skin reaction after using Anise seed. Anise seed would be listed under the heading Allergic Reactions, Skin.) For more information on using the herb, the General Index lists in bold the page number of the complete herb monograph. If the reader is researching a side effect and would like to investigate a different herb to treat a condition, the Uses and Indications section (page 419) provides an alphabetical list of conditions and relevant herbs.

Pharmacological Actions of Approved Herbs (page 459) and Unapproved Herbs (page 471) are listed alphabetically. For example, if a health professional or consumer is looking for herbs with documented antispasmodic activity (documented by experimental or clinical research), they can find 30 herbs listed under the heading Antispasmodic on page 463 of the chapter.

List of **Herb-Drug Interactions** (page 475): This section outlines potential interactions between herbs and conventional drugs. These interactions are shown in two tables, first by the herb and then by the drug.

Duration of Administration (page 483). Herbs that are generally limited to a specified period of time are listed in this section.

By Page Headers. The top of each page contains the chapter title and the name of the specific monograph or other item (e.g., a definition in the Glossary) that begins on the particular page. This allows the reader to determine where he or she is with respect to the sections of the book.

The Complete German Commission E Monographs

Part One

Introduction

INTRODUCTION

MARK BLUMENTHAL
Founder and Executive Director
American Botanical Council
Editor, *HerbalGram*

INTRODUCTION CONTENTS

List of Tables in Introduction	8
Summary	8
Market Conditions and Regulatory Climate for Herbs in the United States	10
Consumer Use of Herbs	10
Market Statistics	11
Dietary Supplement Health and Education Act of 1994 (DSHEA)	12
OTC Drugs	13
European-American Phytomedicines Coalition Petitions to FDA	14
Commission on Dietary Supplement Labels	15
World Health Organization Guidelines for the Assessment of Herbal Medicines	16
Herbs and Phytomedicines in the European Community	17
Definitions	17
European Scientific Cooperative on Phytotherapy (ESCOP)	18
Herbs and Phytomedicines in Germany	18
Education of Health Professionals and Phytomedicine Research	18
Basic Rules for Rational Phytotherapy	19
Scientific Research and Medical Use of Phytomedicines	19
The Market for Herbs and Phytomedicines in Germany	20
Demographics	20
Retail Outlets	22
Physician Prescriptions and Reimbursement	22
Number of Products	23
Market Statistics	23
Leading Phytomedicines	25
The German Legal and Regulatory Environment and the History and Background of Commission E	27
Legal History	27
Composition of Commission E	28
Traditional Medicines	29

Commission E Evaluation Methods and Criteria	29
Bibliographic Review	29
References	30
Evaluation of Safety and Efficacy: Positive and Negative Monographs	32
Positive (Approved) Monographs	33
Negative (Unapproved) Monographs	34
Negative-Null (Unapproved) Monographs	36
Quality Standards and Phytoequivalence	37
Overview of Commission E Monographs	37
Quantity of Monographs	37
Quantity of Plants in the Monographs	38
Monograph Format	40
Explanation of Monograph Sections	41
Monograph Title	41
Revisions and Corrections	41
Common Names	41
Publication Date	42
Name of Drug	42
Pharmacopeial Names	42
Composition of Drug	43
Botanical Name	43
Plant Family	44
Chemical Constituents	44
Uses	44
Contraindications	45
Side Effects	46
Interactions with Other Drugs	47
Dosage	47
Mode of Administration	48
Duration of Administration	49
Risks	49
Evaluation	50
Actions	50
Types of Monographs	50
Single Herbs – Monopreparations	50
Fixed Combinations	50
Evaluation Criteria for Fixed Combinations Established by Commission E in 1989	51
Component Characteristics	52
Bath Additives	53
Indexes and Cross References	53
Uses and Indications of Approved Herbs Index	53
Contraindications of Approved Herbs Index	53

Side Effects of Approved and Unapproved Herbs Indexes	54
Interactions with Conventional Drugs Index	54
Pharmacological Actions of Approved and Unapproved Herbs Indexes	54
Duration of Administration for Approved Herbs Index	54
Taxonomic Cross-Reference	55
Chemical Glossary and Index	55
Glossary of Anatomical, Botanical, Medical, Pharmaceutical, and Physiological Terms	55
European Regulatory Literature	55
Excerpts from the *German Pharmacopoeia*	55
Excerpts from the *European Pharmacopoeia*	56
EEC Standards for Quality of Herbal Remedies	56
Translation of the Monographs	57
Archaic Language	57
Brightening or Coloring Agent	57
Comminuted	57
Drug vs. Herb	57
Evaluation	58
Flavor Corrigent	58
Irrigation Therapy	58
Name of Drug	58
None Known	58
Pharmacopeia/Pharmacopoeia	59
Revision vs. Correction	59
Seed vs. Fruit	59
Teas or Infusions	59
References to Other Compendia	59
German *Federal Gazette* Numbers	60
Comments on Specific Monographs	60
Editor's Notes	60
Chamomile	60
Echinacea	61
Eleuthero (Siberian Ginseng)	61
Ginger	62
Ginkgo	62
Hawthorn	63
Horse Chestnut Seed	63
Sarsaparilla	64
Valerian	64
Recent Changes at Commission E	64
Other Books with Commission E Monographs and Related Data	65
Conclusion	66
References	67

List of Tables in Introduction

Table 1:	Herb Supplement Sales in Food, Drug, and Mass Market Retail Outlets in U.S. — 1997	11
Table 2:	Herb Supplement Sales in Natural Food Stores in U.S. — 1997	12
Table 3:	Sales of OTC Herbal Remedies in the European Union — 1996	17
Table 4:	Therapeutic Categories of Phytomedicine Sales in the European Union	18
Table 5:	Conditions Treated with Phytomedicines by General Practitioners in Germany	20
Table 6:	Conditions for which German Consumers Use Phytomedicines	21
Table 7a:	The Market for Phytomedicines Sold in German Pharmacies — 1996	24
Table 7b:	Retail Sales of Herbal Medicines in German Pharmacies by Indication — 1996	24
Table 8:	Indications for the 100 Most Commonly Prescribed Herbal Medications in Germany, listed in order of Gross Sales in Pharmacies — 1995	24
Table 9:	Most Frequently Prescribed Monopreparation Phytomedicines in Germany, According to Sales — 1996	25
Table 10a:	Leading Proprietary Monopreparation Phytomedicines in Germany	26
Table 10b:	Selected Leading Proprietary Combination Phytomedicines in Germany	26
Table 11:	The Commissions of the German Federal Institute for Drugs and Medical Devices (BfArM)	28
Table 12:	Clinical Studies on Leading European Phytomedicines	32
Table 13:	Unapproved Monographs with Documented or Suspected Risk	35
Table 14:	Unapproved Monographs with No Documented Risk	36
Table 15:	Overview by Monograph Category	38
Table 16:	Therapeutic Overview of Monographs	38
Table 17a:	Original Format for Approved Monographs (pre-1992)	40
Table 17b:	Revised Format for Approved Monographs (1992 - 1995)	40
Table 17c:	Original Format for Unapproved Monographs (pre-1992)	40
Table 17d:	Revised Format for Unapproved Monographs (1992 - 1995)	41

Summary

Increased use of herbal medicines in the United States requires a thorough review of appropriate methods to evaluate them for safety and therapeutic benefits. Some experts have called for reformed regulations to ensure that these products be labeled with adequate directions for use and reasonable information regarding their benefits and potential risks.

This Introduction covers aspects of the market for herbal products in the U.S., including consumer attitudes and market statistics. A review of the current regulatory situation is also presented, with focus on the Dietary Supplement Health and Education Act of 1994 (DSHEA) and the difficulty in obtaining over-the-counter (OTC) drug status for well-researched herbs and phytomedicines. Considerable coverage is made of the market situation for herbs and phytomedicines and the strong proactive consumer demand for and acceptance of natural products, especially those perceived to benefit health, from simple herbal teas for treatment of minor illnesses to tonics that are believed to enhance wellness in the present and to prevent serious illnesses.

Herbs and phytomedicines are experiencing explosive growth in pharmacies and other mass-market retail outlets. An estimated 30 percent of American adults — 60 million — are reported to be using herbs and phytomedicinal products, spending an estimated $3.24 billion in 1996. These high rates of sales growth and the potential profits have drawn the interest of the investment banking community, where it is said that the herb sector of the dietary supplement market represents one of the biggest financial investment opportunities since the advent of the high-technology industry.

The change in social attitudes toward natural medicine ensures continued growth in herb use well into the future. As these products become a more integral part of American culture, increased efforts will be required in evaluating the quality, overall safety, potential benefits and effectiveness, and appropriate therapeutic and clinical guidelines for their responsible use.

The current regulatory system under DSHEA allows products to be labeled to communicate to consumers the potential safety problems that may be associated with the product. The new law now permits manufacturers to publish potential side effects, contraindications appropriate for some users and, if needed, additional special warnings. Section 6 of the law allows "statements of nutritional support" and statements about how the product affects the "structure and function" of the body. However, a product cannot make a statement that is deemed "therapeutic" or imply that it is useful to diagnose, treat, cure, or prevent any disease. Herbal products are not permitted labeling that contains a drug claim, except for a few herb products that are approved for over-the-counter drug use. A recent report by the President's Commission for Dietary Supplement Labels has suggested that the U.S. Food and Drug Administration (FDA) establish an expert panel to review herbs for potential OTC approval. A petition by European and American phytomedicine manufacturers has requested that FDA allow well-researched European phytomedicines the status of old drugs so they would not have to be evaluated by the prohibitively costly new drug application process. FDA has not responded to this petition, partly due to its discomfort with herbs and the lack of an appropriate mechanism to deal with herbs.

Feasible models for regulatory reform can be found in Europe, particularly Germany, where herbs and phytomedicines are accepted and integrated into medicine and pharmacy. In 1978 the German Ministry of Health established Commission E, a panel of experts charged with evaluating the safety and efficacy of the herbs available in pharmacies for general use. The Commission (*Kommission* in German) reviewed over 300 herbal drugs. Results were published by the German Federal Health Agency (now Federal Institute for Drugs and Medical Devices) in the form of monographs in the *Bundesanzeiger*, the German *Federal Gazette*. A total of 380 monographs were published (254 approved; 126 unapproved), plus 81 revisions. These monographs provide guidelines for the general public, health practitioners, and companies applying for registration of herbal drugs. In general, they do not contain standards for assaying the quality and purity of herbal drugs found in either the *European Pharmacopoeia* or the *German Pharmacopoeia* (*Deutsches Arzneibuch*). The process followed by Commission E resulted in what has been called by Prof. Varro E. Tyler "the most accurate information available in the entire world on the safety and efficacy of herbs and phytomedicines."

This book contains all monographs published by Commission E between 1983 and 1995, including all revisions (incorporated into the monographs). It also includes extensive indexes of therapeutic data (uses, contraindications, side effects, drug interactions, etc.), plus chemical and taxonomic cross-references (English, Latin, German, and pharmacopeial names), excerpts from European regulatory literature, glossary of terms, and general index.

Market Conditions and Regulatory Climate for Herbs in the United States

Consumer use of herbs and medicinal plant products in the United States over the past two decades has become a mainstream phenomenon. No longer relegated primarily to health food stores, mail order houses, and multilevel marketing organizations, herbs and phytomedicines (advanced medicinal preparations made of herbs) have become one of the fastest growing segments in retail pharmacies, supermarkets, and other mass market outlets. In addition, major health insurance companies are beginning to include herbs as covered modalities of "alternative therapies" and herb products are being considered for use by some managed care organizations.

Consumer Use of Herbs

In general, consumers use herbal products as therapeutic agents for treatment and cure of diseases and pathological conditions, as prophylactic agents to prevent disease over the long term, and as proactive agents to maintain health and wellness. Additionally, herbs and phytomedicinals can be used as adjunct therapy, to support conventional pharmaceutical therapies. This last use is usually found in societies where phytotherapy (the use of herbal medicines in clinical practice) is considerably more integrated with conventional medicine, as in Germany.

Many herbal products are used to treat minor conditions and illnesses (coughs, colds, upset stomach) in much the same manner as conventional FDA-approved over-the-counter (OTC) nonprescription drugs are used. Additionally, a growing number of health consumers often use herbs and other dietary supplements as preventive measures and to increase the body's general wellness and strengthen the immune system (e.g., reduction of cardiovascular risk factors, increase in liver and immune system functions, increase in feelings of wellness). In the former case, consumers often substitute herbs and phytomedicines for conventional OTC nonprescription medications for relatively minor, self-diagnosable, self-treatable, self-limiting illnesses. Unfortunately, there is no appropriate regulatory mechanism to address the safety and efficacy of herbal products as OTC drugs in the U.S., for reasons explained below.

One study of consumer preferences attempted to measure potential use of herbal products by consumers who claimed that they were not yet users of herbs but would consider using them within the next five years. The study, conducted in 1996, indicated that 63 percent of the 1,008 people surveyed said that herbal supplements will be "the answer to many common ailments" or "part of our daily regimen" within five years. The study revealed that consumers would consider taking an herbal remedy for increasing energy (60 percent), preventing colds (56 percent), boosting the immune system (54 percent), and improving sleep (43 percent). Of the 505 men included in the survey, 18 percent would consider taking an herbal supplement to help with prostate problems. When asked what factors would make them decide to use herbs, the respondents cited recommendations by a physician (66 percent), "Because it can't hurt and might help" (41 percent), "Because nothing else has helped my condition" (34 percent), news coverage on herb benefits (26 percent), and friends using herbs (15 percent). Only four percent of respondents said they would never consider using herbs (Anon., 1996).

Market Statistics

The size of the herb market in the U.S. was estimated at about $1.6 billion in 1994 (Brevoort, 1996), with some projections reaching around $2 billion in 1996. However, a survey published in early 1997 by *Prevention* magazine/NBC News estimated that 60 million adult Americans — one-third of all adults — had used herbal medicines in 1996, spending an average of $54 per person annually. This brings the estimated total retail value of herbs sold in the United States to $3.24 billion in 1996 (Johnston, 1997).

The difficulty in determining the actual size of the market for herbs and phytomedicinal products in the U.S. has persisted because these products were formerly sold mostly through channels of distribution normally not subject to econometric tracking services (health food stores, mail order, multi-level marketing organizations). However, with increased sales of herbs in mainstream retail outlets, more accurate statistics are becoming available. As Table 1 shows, the total of herbs sold in the mass-market outlets (grocery stores, pharmacies, and mass merchandiser retail stores) was $441.5 million in 1997. This is a dramatic 79.5 percent increase over total 1996 sales of $246 million (Glovsky, 1998).

An excellent example of the mainstream acceptance of well-researched herbs and phytomedicines can be seen in the huge increase in sales of St. John's Wort, an herb that has made moderate increases in the health food market for the past 10 years but was virtually unknown outside health food stores. Sales for St. John's Wort climbed from relative obscurity in the mass market to fifth place with an impressive $47.8 million for the calendar year, with about 90 percent of those sales being generated during the six-month period after June 27, when the television show *20/20* profiled the herb. The program reported that St. John's Wort was extensively used in Germany and that a meta-analysis of 23 clinical studies published in the *British Medical Journal* had concluded that St. John's Wort was more effective than placebo in treating cases of mild to moderate depression (Linde et al., 1996). An editorial in the *BMJ* stated that the phytomedicine produced fewer adverse side effects than conventional prescription drugs, thereby ensuring better patient compliance (DeSmet and Nolen, 1996).

Of the 14 herbs listed as top sellers in Table 1, all but one (Goldenseal root, *Hydrastis canadensis*) are the subject of some degree of pharmacological or clinical research, especially in Western Europe. Ten of these herbs are the subjects of positive monographs produced by Commission E as approved nonprescription medications.

Table 1: Herb Supplement Sales in Food, Drug, and Mass Market Retail Outlets in U.S. — 1997

Total Herbal Supplements	$441,502,560	Grapeseed extract	$9,965,772
Ginkgo	90,197,288	Evening Primrose oil	7,299,353
Ginseng	86,048,080	Cranberry	6,182,210
Garlic	71,474,288	Valerian	6,104,450
Echinacea/Goldenseal[1]	49,189,576	Bilberry	4,555,723
St. John's Wort[2]	47,774,792	Milk Thistle	3,037,672
Saw Palmetto	18,381,592	Kava Kava	2,950,132

[1] Reflects sales of echinacea and goldenseal as individual products as well as the combination.
[2] St. John's Wort sales reflect the May 5 *Newsweek* article and June 27 ABC News *20/20* program that featured the herb as a treatment for depression.
Source: IRI Scanner Data, FDM (Food, Drug, Mass Market combined), Total U.S., 52 weeks ending 12/28/97.

Table 2 shows the herbs with top sales status in the health food market, according to an annual survey conducted by *Whole Foods*, a leading trade magazine for the natural food and dietary supplements industry. These figures represent sales in health food stores only and are based on survey questionnaires with only about 100 stores responding, out of over 9,000 stores in the industry. The survey was based on sales for calendar year 1996 projected on the first two months of 1997, and was published in October 1997 (Richman and Witkowski, 1997). Therefore, this survey does not reflect the full year's sales and, consequently, the huge increase in sales in St. John's Wort in the second half of the year in response to the national media coverage is only partially reflected in this ranking.

Table 2: Herb Supplement Sales in Natural Food Stores in U.S. — 1997

1997		1996	1997		1996
1.	Echinacea	1	10.	Siberian Ginseng	7
2.	Garlic	2	11.	Bilberry	23
3.	Ginkgo biloba	4	12.	Cranberry	18
4.	Goldenseal	5	13.	Dong quai	17
5.	Saw Palmetto	9	14.	Grapeseed extract	15
6.	(tie) Aloe	12	15.	Cascara Sagrada	10
6.	(tie) Asian Ginseng	3	16.	St. John's Wort	n/a
7.	Cat's Claw	14	17.	Valerian	13
8.	Astragalus	27	18.	Ginger	18
9.	Cayenne	11	19.	Feverfew	23

Five herbs (cat's claw, saw palmetto, ginkgo biloba, echinacea, and kava kava) have been on the list all three years that the study has been conducted. The top 10 herbs comprise 56.98 percent of sales.
Source: Richman and Witkowski, 1997.

Dietary Supplement Health and Education Act of 1994 (DSHEA)

Additional evidence of widespread consumer interest in herbs and other natural products, now legally classified as "dietary supplements" in the United States, can be found in the estimated two million letters, faxes, and phone calls by Americans to members of Congress during 1993 and 1994 in support of legislation that would protect and increase access to the products themselves and information on their responsible use. The Dietary Supplement Health and Education Act of 1994 (DSHEA) created a new legal definition for dietary supplements: vitamins, minerals, herbs or other botanicals, amino acids, and any other "dietary substance for use by man to supplement the diet by increasing total dietary intake," including "a concentrate, metabolite, constituent, extract, or combination" of these ingredients (103d Congress, 1994).

Granting herbs some legal protection as "dietary supplements" in the U.S. was clarified in the Report from the Senate Committee on Labor and Human Resources that accompanied Senate Bill 784, the Hatch-Harkin bill in the Senate, eventually passed as DSHEA. The report said, "Unlike many drugs, the role of herbal dietary supplements is to enhance the diet by adding safe and natural plants and their constituents to support and protect bodily functions and processes. Containing combinations of numerous naturally-occurring plant chemicals, herbs generally act in a wider, more general, less specific way than most single-ingredient pharmaceutical drugs. Their actions are more 'gentle' than conventional medicines and work usually in more long-term situations." (U.S. Senate, 1994.) The report attributed this information to the now-classic textbook by the late German physician Rudolf F. Weiss, *Lehrbuch der Phytotherapie* (the sixth edition has been translated into English as *Herbal Medicine*), one of the most important textbooks for training physicians in Germany on the clinical uses of herbs and phytomedicines.

Despite some of the regulatory advances heralded by proponents of DSHEA, there are some significant limitations. Section 6 of DSHEA deals only with herbs as dietary supplements, i.e., as foods. Although a limited amount of information regarding an herb's physiological effects can be conveyed on a product label, therapeutic or drug claims are not permitted. That is, DSHEA allows for "statements of nutritional support" or so-called "structure and function claims" (statements indicating how a product will affect the structure or function of the body). However, "health claims" (allowed for conventional foods and dietary supplements in the Nutrition Labeling and Education Act of 1990, (NLEA) are statements that characterize the relationship between a nutrient or food component and a specific disease or health-related condition. The subject of health claims was considered by the seven-member Presidential Commission on Dietary Supplement Labels (CDSL), who proposed criteria and procedures to review and evaluate such claims to the President, Congress, and the Secretary of Health and Human Services. The CDSL has recommended that a standard of "significant scientific agreement" — the standard set for health claims for conventional foods — be applied to dietary supplements, insofar as manufacturers may wish to file for approval of a health claim for a dietary supplement under NLEA. However, this more strict criterion is not relevant to a structure/function claim under DSHEA (CDSL, 1997).

OTC Drugs

The current OTC drug monograph system in the U.S. has limited ability to review herbs for their potential to increase the body's wellness, to promote resistance to disease, and to act in a proactive manner not directly associated with a pathology. There are few regulatory options for drugs or herbs that have preventive actions. For example, in recent years garlic was one of the best-selling nonprescription medicines in German pharmacies, because the government (i.e., Commission E) recognized the value of garlic preparations as an adjunct therapy when dietary measures have failed to deal with "age related vascular changes." The Commission reviewed numerous clinical studies on garlic preparations that confirmed low-density lipoprotein-lowering activity of the bulb and its preparations, as well as its related ability to lower other cardiovascular risk factors. An indication such as cardiovascular risk is often not amenable to self-diagnosis and self-treatment, is not self-limiting (the condition does not abate within a reasonable period — usually a few days) and, therefore, is currently not subject to consideration under the OTC Drug Review in the U.S.

There are additional limitations of the current OTC drug system in the U.S. with respect to reviewing herbs and phytomedicines. Under FDA policy, novel ingredients that require evaluation for safety and efficacy are *new drugs* and thus must go through a New Drug Application (NDA). This process is time consuming (average 15 years) and extremely costly; one study in 1996 reported an average cost of $500 million per new drug (PhRMA, 1998). Proponents of rational use of herbs and phytomedicines are quick to point out that without patent protection to ensure market exclusivity, most herbal, phytomedicinal, and pharmaceutical companies are not willing to invest the millions of dollars required for an NDA (Tyler, 1994).

A premise of the OTC Monograph Review process in 1972 was that all ingredients included in the review process be regarded as "old" drugs. Old drugs were treated more leniently than a new drug, which would require an NDA, because old drugs had been on the market in the U.S. "for a material time" (at least five years) and "to a material extent" (at least 10 million doses).

European-American Phytomedicines Coalition Petitions to FDA

Since the 1970s FDA has taken the position that old drug status extends only to ingredients sold in the U.S. For certain key European phytomedicines to participate in the OTC review process, a group of European and American companies working through the European-American Phytomedicines Coalition (EAPC) filed a petition with the FDA to open the OTC review to old drugs from Europe that have been sold for a material time and to a material extent. The EAPC petition sought to extend this policy to phytomedicines sold for a material time and to a material extent in selected Western countries that have a well developed system of pharmacovigilance (adverse reaction reporting system). Thus, the safety of these European phytomedicines has been well established by common use in countries where reliable epidemiological data is available (Pinco and Israelsen, 1992).

The EAPC petition was filed July 24, 1992. By spring 1998, almost six years after the filing, the FDA had not yet responded directly to the petition. This lack of timely response has given some herbal advocates the impression that the agency (at least those in the Center for Drug Evaluation and Research) is not interested in developing a reasonable mechanism for evaluating herbs as nonprescription drugs. Critics point to statements from FDA that herbs sold for health purposes are essentially drugs. In June 1993 the agency wrote in a proposed rule on NLEA in the *Federal Register*: "When herbs are consumed primarily for their taste, aroma, or nutritive value, they are foods. If the herbs are intended to be consumed for their medicinal effects, however, they are drugs." (FDA, 1992.) Without the ability for industry to submit herbs for review as *old drugs* under the OTC Review system, as proposed by the EAPC petition, industry would have no other option but submit them as *new drugs*, an impossible prospect in light of the high costs associated with new drug approvals.

In 1994 and 1995, in order to add some substance to its 1992 petition, the EAPC filed petitions to amend the nighttime sleep-aid monograph to include valerian root (Pinco and Israelsen, 1994) and the anti-emetic monograph to include the popular herb and spice ginger (Pinco and Israelsen, 1995). Both petitions cited the widespread safe and effective use of these common botanical products in Europe as OTC medications, with no evidence of adverse reaction reports in countries where the reporting of such events (pharmacovigilance) is routine. Both petitions documented the safety and efficacy of the two ingredients as determined by human clinical trials and registrations as medicines in various Western European countries. To date (spring 1998) FDA has not responded to these two petitions. This lack of response has given additional impetus among some members of the herb industry and some scientists with interests in herbal research and education to support the concept of herbs as dietary supplements under DSHEA. Prospects appear uncertain for obtaining OTC drug status for herbs whose safety and efficacy to treat minor, self-limiting conditions has been reasonably established by both scientific data and empirical use.

In October 1996 the FDA issued an advance notice of proposed rulemaking (ANPR) proposing conditions for consideration of OTC drug review that would virtually preclude qualification of European phytomedicines (FDA, 1996). Before the publication of the ANPR the message that members of the herb industry and a number of scientific authorities interpreted from the lack of FDA response to the EAPC petition was that the agency was not really serious in dealing with herbs *as drugs*. That is, despite previous FDA statements that herbs were really drugs and not foods or dietary supplements, when given an opportunity to evaluate and consider the approval of a few select herbs according to the procedures appropriate for OTC drugs, the agency appeared unable or unwilling to act. With the provisions of the ANPR, the agency proposed regulations consistent with its previous narrow policies regarding herbs. Thus, the potential in the short term for the approval of select herbs and phytomedicines as OTC drugs remains unclear.

Commission on Dietary Supplement Labels

With the OTC drug route currently blocked for a subset of herbal products, the herb industry has only one option — to market these products as "dietary supplements" under the terms of DSHEA. In November 1997 the Commission on Dietary Supplement Labels (CDSL), created by DSHEA and appointed by President Clinton in 1995, presented its report to the President, the Congress, and the Secretary of the Department of Health and Human Services. The report recommended that the FDA "give special attention to the feasibility of approving botanical remedies for OTC uses in cases in which sufficient evidence is available. The Commission [CDSL] recommended that FDA convene a botanical products review panel to evaluate petitions concerning such products. Such a panel should include experts with an appropriate scientific background in pharmacognosy as well as experts in other applicable disciplines. In its deliberations this panel should give priority to botanical remedies having the strongest supporting evidence." (CDSL, 1997.) Cited as examples of remedies to consider are the botanicals currently being reviewed by the United States Pharmacopeial Convention (USP) and the extensive monographs by the World Health Organization. The report recommended that FDA "put a high priority on expediting such a review panel." The CDSL report also acknowledged that it did not have any authority in the area of drugs; its recommendations are in the domain of herbs as dietary supplements (CDSL, 1997). As part of public testimony to the CDSL, several herb leaders from various groups presented documentation that herbs were rationally regulated as medicines in leading European countries, particularly Germany, in which the Commission E expert panel process was emphasized (Bayne et al., 1996).

The growing consumer use of these products and increased professional interest in their therapeutic potential require that new regulatory models be considered for evaluating the safety and efficacy of herbs and phytomedicines as drugs. There has never been a greater need for authoritative, reliable information on the use of botanicals. Much of the information on the clinical or pharmacological studies of herbs and phytomedicines is still not being incorporated into curricula at medical and pharmacy schools in the U.S., although a growing number of schools are beginning to offer courses in herbs and phytomedicines, either as the entire course, or as part of a course on "alternative," "unconventional," or the now increasingly preferred "integrative" medicine. Such a course will inevitably attempt to cover the entire range of the sciences and disciplines that encompasses herbal medicine: anthropology and ethnobotany, medical botany, pharmacognosy, phytochemistry, natural products research, pharmacology, plant ecology, and whole systems theory.

In general, health professionals have three basic methods of obtaining scientific information on using these natural products: independent study, including books, articles, and so-called "third party literature" of varying degrees of quality and authority; continuing education courses; and the directions for use and label claims on the products themselves. However, until a regulatory system in the U.S. is developed to review and evaluate the safe and responsible therapeutic uses of herbs and phytomedicines, health professionals will not be able to obtain adequate therapeutic information from product labels. Instead, they will seek guidance from the authoritative information found in the official herbal monographs produced by Commission E and the World Health Organization (WHO), as well as unofficial monographs from professional organizations such as the European Scientific Cooperative on Phytotherapy — ESCOP, the American Herbal Pharmacopoeia — AHP, and the United States Pharmacopeia — USP.

WORLD HEALTH ORGANIZATION GUIDELINES FOR THE ASSESSMENT OF HERBAL MEDICINES

In some of the industrialized nations, regulators and health professionals have already come to terms with the challenge of evaluating and regulating herbs and phytomedicines (Akerele, 1992; Blumenthal, 1994). In 1991 WHO published its "Guidelines for the Assessment of Herbal Medicines" in recognition of the worldwide growth in the use of herbs in both official and unofficial medicine. The main purpose was to aid member nations in establishing appropriate regulatory criteria and procedures to evaluate the quality, safety, and efficacy of herbal medicines.

The guidelines call for the recognition that long-term historical use of a botanical in traditional medicine constitutes a presumption of safety unless contradicted by modern scientific research:

> A guiding principle should be that if the product has been traditionally used without demonstrated harm, no specific regulatory action should be undertaken unless new evidence demands a revised risk-assessment....As a basic rule, documentation of a long period of use should be taken into consideration when safety is being assessed. This means that, when there are no detailed toxicological studies, documented experience on long-term use without evidence of safety problems should form the basis of the risk assessment. However, even in cases of long-used drugs, chronic toxicological risks may have occurred, but may not have been recognized. If available, the period of use, the health disorders treated, the number of users, and the countries with experience should be specified. If a toxicological risk is known, toxicity data have to be submitted. Risk assessment, whether it is independent of dose (e.g., special danger of allergies), or whether it is a function of dose, should be documented. In the second instance the dosage specification must be an important part of the risk assessment. An explanation of the risks should be given, if possible. The potential for misuse, abuse, or dependence has to be documented. If long-term traditional use cannot be documented, or doubts on safety exist, toxicity data should be submitted (WHO, 1991).

Regarding establishing efficacy, WHO guidelines state:

> The indication(s) for the use of the medicine should be specified. In the case of traditional medicines, the requirements for proof of efficacy shall depend on the kind of indication. *For treatment of minor disorders and for nonspecific indications, some relaxation is justified in the requirements for proof of efficacy, taking into account the extent of traditional use; the same considerations apply to prophylactic use.* [Emphasis added.] Experience with individual cases recorded in reports from physicians, traditional health practitioners, or treated patients should be taken into account. Where traditional use has not been established, appropriate clinical evidence should be taken into account (WHO, 1991).

WHO guidelines also called for the establishment of monographs to determine the identity, quality, and therapeutic information on herbal medicines (Akerele, 1992). WHO monographs contain standards for determining the identity and purity of herbal drugs as well as detailed information on the therapeutic aspects of the herbs. The first set of 28 WHO monographs covering 41 species is to be published in 1998 (Blumenthal, 1997).

Herbs and Phytomedicines in the European Community

In Western Europe, the professional use of herbs and phytomedicines enjoys relatively strong integration with conventional medicine. In the countries of the European Union (formerly European Economic Community, EEC), herbal medicines are generally sold in pharmacies as licensed nonprescription or prescription medicines. According to EU directive 65/65/EEC, all phytomedicines are treated as drugs. Registrations based on quality, safety, and efficacy are required (Keller, 1994; Schilcher, 1991). Exceptions include the Netherlands and the United Kingdom, where botanicals are still sold as food supplements or dietary supplements (Gruenwald, 1998).

Definitions

According to European Union definitions, herbal medicinal products (medicines) are "medicinal products containing as active ingredients exclusively plant material and/or vegetable drug preparations." Vegetable drugs are "plant material used for a medicinal purpose. An herbal drug or a preparation thereof is regarded as one active ingredient in its entirety whether or not the constituents with therapeutic activity are known." Herbal medicinal preparations are "comminuted or powdered vegetable drugs, extracts, tinctures, fatty or essential oils, expressed plant juices, etc. prepared from herbal drugs, and preparations whose production involves a purification or concentration process. However, chemically defined isolated constituents or their mixtures are not considered herbal medicinal products. Other substances such as solvents, diluents, preservatives [or] may form part of vegetable drug preparations. These substances must be indicated." Constituents with known therapeutic activity "are chemically defined substances or groups of substances which are known to contribute to the therapeutic activity of a vegetable drug or of a preparation." (Commission of European Communities, 1989.) (This definition formerly contained the term "vegetable drug" when first published; however, this term was replaced by "herbal medicinal product" by EU in November 1997 [Busse, 1997c]). Some scientists consider isolated plant substances used as conventional drugs in pharmacy and medicine (e.g., digitoxin, atropine, escin, etc.) as phytomedicines, but these are not regulated as phytomedicines under German or EU drug laws (Schilcher, 1997b).

Table 3: Sales of OTC Herbal Remedies in the European Union — 1996

Nation	Annual Retail Sales in millions (US $)	%	Per capita
Germany	$3,500	50.0	$42.9
France	1,800	25.7	31.2
Italy	700	10.0	12.2
United Kingdom	400	5.7	6.9
Spain	300	4.3	7.6
Netherlands	100	1.4	6.4
All others	130	2.9	4.5
Total	$7,000	100.0	$19.1 (mean)

Estimation based on Institute for Medical Statistics (IMS) market analysis of 1994 plus average growth rates. Source: PhytoPharm Consulting, Berlin (Gruenwald, 1998).

Table 4: Therapeutic Categories of Phytomedicine Sales in the European Union

Cardiovascular	27.2%
Respiratory	15.3
Digestive	14.4
Tonic	14.4
Hypnotic/Sedative	9.3
Topical	7.4
Others	12.0

Source: Gruenwald, 1995.

European Scientific Cooperative on Phytotherapy (ESCOP)

The European market for herbs and phytomedicines is characterized by the availability of a fairly large number of products. A report conducted in 1991 of the Member States (nations) indicated that about 1,400 herbal drugs were available in the EEC. When this study focused on herbs used in five of the 10 Member States, 145 herbal drugs were noted (Keller, 1996). According to Dr. Konstantin Keller of the German Federal Institute for Drugs and Medical Devices (BfArM), "this shows that herbal drugs are indeed a major problem for harmonization in the EU." (Keller, 1996).

One important initiative in the development of herbal monographs in Western Europe is ESCOP (European Scientific Cooperative on Phytotherapy), an affiliation of 15 national associations of phytotherapy, mostly from Western Europe, that formed in 1989 as a result of the European harmonization process. Since June 1997 ESCOP has produced a series of 50 herbal monographs to respond to the increasing integration of the European Union (EU). The need for harmonized drug monographs for herbs was recognized so that there could be standards for botanicals popularly used in medicine and pharmacy in Europe.

The ESCOP monographs were published in volumes ("fascicules") of 10 monographs each. They were published in the form of standardized drug dossiers of European drug licensing, known as specific product characteristics (SPCs). Unlike a pharmacopeial monograph that focuses on standards for identity and quality, ESCOP monographs, like those of Commission E, deal with therapeutic aspects of each phytomedicine. Thus, ESCOP monographs include approved therapeutic uses and contain the format much like recent Commission E monographs, including recommended dosage, side effects and contraindications (if any), and other specific instructions for health professionals, industry, regulators, and patients (Blumenthal, 1997).

ESCOP monographs do not deal directly with qualitative standards for herbal drugs; this area is covered in other pharmacopeial monographs. For example, the *European Pharmacopoeia* includes 60 monographs on herbal drugs. An additional 45 draft monographs have been published for comments. According to Keller, "This cooperative approach will greatly facilitate harmonization of herbal remedies." (Keller, 1996).

HERBS AND PHYTOMEDICINES IN GERMANY

Education of Health Professionals and Phytomedicine Research

One of the driving forces that has resulted in mainstream acceptance of phytomedicine in Germany is the inclusion of phytotherapy in the medical and pharmacy school curricula. In the opinion of several medical groups, "modern phytotherapy is not perceived as alternative medicine, but as a part of so-called traditional medicine" [i.e., conventional medicine] (Schilcher, 1997c). Since 1993 all medical school students in Germany must successfully complete a portion of their board examinations in the area of phytotherapy as a precondition for practicing medicine (Schilcher, 1991). Medical education on medicinal plants and phytomedicines includes regular lectures in universities and medical schools, four one-week courses with 26 hours of lectures in phytotherapy in *Weiterbildung* (continuing education), lectures and courses in *Fortbildung* (postgraduate education), the publication of scientific literature (papers and books), the Commission E Monographs, and directions on product uses according to section 11 of the Second Medicines Act (AMG 76) (Schilcher, 1991, 1997c).

Basic Rules for Rational Phytotherapy

According to Prof. H. Schilcher, Vice President of Commission E, "rational phytotherapy" in Germany is based on four basic rules for phytomedicines (also known as phytopharmaca):

1. Dose-response relationship. Phytomedicines in the therapeutic arena can be applied in a dose-effectiveness manner. Possible dosage-dependent reversals of effects should not be interpreted as "homeopathic effects" — a reference to the observation that homeopathic medicines produce symptoms at higher potencies in healthy individuals. That is, sometimes a variation in the dosage of a phytomedicine can produce a different effect than a higher or lower dosage of the same herbal drug and this cannot be dismissed as homeopathic. For example, in phytotherapy extracts of Goldenrod (*Solidago virgaurea*) in low doses have no diuretic (aquaretic) effect. However, in therapeutically adequate doses (6 - 12 gram dried herb daily dose per the monograph) they do produce aquaretic effects; however, in very high doses (in animal experiments) they have shown diuretic-inhibiting effects (Schilcher, 1998c).

2. Efficacy-constituent relationship. Efficacy (experimentally demonstrated from clinical studies) or effectiveness (observed in a patient in a clinical setting) can be deduced, in most cases, from the specific ingredients. They are co-determined for the effectiveness; that is, in most cases, not one but two or three different plant constituents are known to be responsible for the observed effectiveness. For example, the activity of the herb St. John's Wort in the treatment of mild to moderate cases of depression is now believed to be attributable to at least three types of substances found in the flowers and leaves: hypericins, hyperforin, and flavonoids.

3. Total extracts vs. isolated constituents. Typically, phytomedicines that are standardized extracts consisting of primary active components, secondary components, and accompanying compounds (coeffectors) manifest better effects and a greater therapeutic range of activity than individual isolated compounds (i.e., conventional drugs).

4. Pharmaceutical quality. Phytomedicines with a high level of pharmaceutical and medical quality are the basic requirement for successful phytotherapy. For example, some reports of herbal medicines that produced negative outcomes can be attributed to the administration of unsuitable materials, which, after close expert examination, were deemed of poor quality (Schilcher, 1997c).

Scientific Research and Medical Use of Phytomedicines

Because of the high level of professional interest in herbs and phytomedicines in Germany, there is a considerable amount of scientific research conducted. Pharmacological and experimental studies are available mainly for the most important herbs and herbal preparations on the market, such as Valerian root, Echinacea herb and root, Ginkgo leaf special extract, St. John's Wort, Chamomile flowers, Milk Thistle fruit extract, and Hawthorn leaf and flower extracts. However, the concentration of research on these botanicals should not be misinterpreted to mean that other herbs are ineffective. The lack of pharmacological and experimental studies on other botanicals can be attributed to the fact that, since the end of World War II, testing of phytopharmaca (phytomedicines) was no longer included in the research programs of the schools of pharmacology. Phytopharmacology was pursued in the laboratories of only a few commercial companies specializing in plant medicines. However, at that time there was not a pressing need for phytopharmacological research because the effectiveness and safety of the drug, not the mechanisms of action, were of greater interest, because of the special status of phytomedicines under the first German drug law. Also, herbal medicines were not as widely employed in medical specialties; most previous practitioners of phytotherapy had been doctors of naturopathy and general practitioners. More recent testing, however, has revealed mechanisms of action of some phytomedicines that yield greater effectiveness. This can reveal parameters for standardization of a given phytomedicine and its correct dosage, thereby making it more suitable for specialized branches of clinical medicine (Schilcher, 1997c).

Table 5 shows various health problems general practitioners in Germany treat on a daily basis that can be effectively treated with phytomedicines, usually at a reasonable cost. (See also Table 6 for consumer use patterns and Table 12 for an overview of clinical studies on leading phytomedicines.)

Table 5: Conditions Treated with Phytomedicines by General Practitioners in Germany

Condition	% Treated With Phytomedicines
Psychovegetative syndrome	25
Diseases of:	
respiratory tract (esp. types of bronchitis)	16
heart and circulation (esp. arterial, venous, cerebral)	13
digestive organs (gastritis to Crohn's)	9
locomotor apparatus (movement of limbs)	6
urogenital tract (dysuria in women or BPH in men)	8

Source: Schilcher, 1997c based on Härter, Klimm and Salz.

The Market for Herbs and Phytomedicines in Germany

Demographics

As noted in Table 3, the use of herbs and phytomedicines in the European Union totaled about $7 billion in retail sales in 1996, with about half ($3.5 billion) being sold in Germany (Gruenwald, 1998). In 1970 an estimated 52 percent of the general public in Germany used herbal remedies. That number had grown in 1993 to about 62 percent as reported in a major survey conducted by the Institute for Demoscopy (IfD) in Allensbach (IfD, 1997) and to 65 percent in 1997 (Steinhoff, 1997b).

In general, self-medication with medicinal plants and related products in Germany is as follows: 66 percent of herb users utilize herb products for colds; 38 percent for flu; 25 percent for digestive upsets, headaches, and insomnia (see Table 6). The demographics of herb use reveal that 72 percent are people with at least some college education. The survey also noted a decrease in the number of phytomedicines being dispensed by prescription due to a corresponding increase in self-medication (IfD, 1997; Steinhoff, 1997b).

The Institute for Demoscopy survey also noted other interesting aspects of popular uses of herbs in Germany. "According to the study, significant importance is given to medicines used for prevention. About 39 percent of the polled individuals use the remedies exclusively for prevention, while an additional 45 percent also use other natural medicines. Furthermore, natural remedies are increasingly used in combination with other drugs. For an acute disease, only 3 percent of consumers using natural remedies would take these exclusively, while 64 percent would take natural remedies with other drugs." (Steinhoff, 1997b.) The survey indicated that natural remedies are used mostly for cold and flu symptoms, indigestion, headaches, insomnia, gastric discomforts, nervousness, cardiovascular disorders, exhaustion, and fatigue (Steinhoff, 1997b).

Gender plays an important role in the use of herbal medicines. According to the IfD survey, in 1970 55 percent of women used herbs; this increased to 74 percent in 1997. The use by men has increased as well, from 49 percent in 1970 to 55 percent in 1997. Regarding age, the use of phytomedicines increased in the 16 to 29 age group from 36 percent to 54 percent from 1970 to 1997 (Schilcher, 1998b).

Surprisingly, a poll published in July 1997 by the Cologne Institute of Social Psychology in conjunction with the Institute for Pharmaceutical Biology at the University of Tubingen revealed that, in some cases, German consumers still prefer conventional (synthetic) medications. In 310 interviews laypeople were asked about their perceptions of botanical and conventional medicines. About 80 percent could differentiate between the two types and could name specific examples of each. While 70 percent could correlate correctly a phytomedicine and its proper use, 83.9 percent were able to correctly identify the uses of synthetic medicines. Those questioned in the poll indicated a preference for phytomedicines for the following uses: common cold, digestive or intestinal upset, nervousness, and kidney-bladder illness. However, they preferred to treat liver and gallbladder diseases and cardiovascular disorders with synthetic drugs (Schilcher, 1998b).

Table 6: Conditions for which German Consumers Use Phytomedicines

Condition	1970 Poll	1997 Poll
Common cold	41%	66%
Flu	31	38
Digestive or Intestinal Complaints	24	25
Headache	13	25
Insomnia	13	25
Stomach Ulcer	21	24
Nervousness	12	21
Circulatory disorders	15	17
Bronchitis	12	15
Skin diseases	8	12
Fatigue & exhaustion	8	12

Statistics are derived from consumer polls conducted by the Institute for Demoscopy in Allensbach, Germany.
Source: IfD, 1997; Schilcher, 1998c.

Retail Outlets

In Germany herbal products of various classes are sold in a variety of retail outlets. An *Apotheke* (pharmacy) has registered pharmacists who recommend and dispense nonprescription drugs (within limits), as well as drugs prescribed by physicians. In *Drogerien* (drugstores) one can find preparations for minor illnesses, such as colds, strains, and pains from overexertion. The type of preparations sold in *Drogerien* is defined by law. *Reformhäusern* (health food stores) and *Märkte* (markets, including *Supermärkte*, supermarkets) tend to offer products that boost health, as contrasted to products that fight disease. They also offer herbal teas and products that do not meet the pharmaceutical standards of phytomedicines (often chemically standardized) and are thus not approved as drugs. These products are sold outside pharmacies as "Traditional Medicines" under provisions of Article 109a of the Second Medicines Act. (See below.)

In Germany, approved herbs have nonprescription drug status; this is not the same as OTC status. Many herbal drugs are available only from a licensed pharmacist (*Apothekenpflicht*, a word that implies ethical drugs from pharmacies), but are not available from drugstores or health food stores. Article 42 of the Second Medicines Act (AMG 76) lists medicinal plants that are not allowed to be sold outside pharmacies (a so-called "negative list"). These include Henbane (Approved by Commission E), Foxglove leaf (*Digitalis purpurea*) — not reviewed by the Commission, and, interestingly, the common laxative, Senna leaf (Approved) (Shilcher, 1997b.)

Articles 44 and 45 of the Second Medicines Act regulate the "exceptions to the obligation to supply drugs (conventional and herbal) in pharmacies only" by the creation of three categories of drugs: prescription only (new drugs and drugs with risks), pharmacy only, and outside pharmacy. The first two classes may be prescribed by a physician and reimbursed by the health insurance system, but the third is never reimbursed by medical insurance (Keller, 1998b). This class consists of "drugs which are intended by the pharmaceutical entrepreneur solely to serve purposes other than the curing or alleviation of diseases, suffering, bodily injuries or sickness symptoms shall be released for trade outside pharmacies." (Keller, 1998b.) Such products include natural curative waters, their salts, therapeutic clays and muds, bath oils, plants and parts of plants, mixtures of whole or cut plants or parts of plants as finished drugs, distillates of plants and plant parts (essential oils), and juices pressed from fresh plants if they are made without the use of solvents other than water (from Article 44 of the Second Medicines Act) (Keller, 1998b).

Physician Prescriptions and Reimbursement

All phytomedicines prescribed by a physician must be supplied by pharmacists. According to some estimates, in addition to the 25,000 doctors conducting a natural medical practice, up to 80 percent of German physicians (particularly general practitioners) routinely prescribe phytomedicines as part of clinical therapy (Gruenwald, 1995; Shilcher, 1998b). Prescribed phytomedicines are also known as "semi-ethical" drugs. In 1996 semi-ethical phytomedicine sales constituted 17 percent of total nonprescription drug sales in Germany and 54 percent of all nonprescription phytomedicines (see Table 7). According to the 5th Social Act, phytomedicines that conform to the Commission E positive monographs (approved) are financed by the national health insurance system (Schilcher, 1998c).

In some cases, phytomedicines are preferred to conventional drugs. For drugs prescribed for benign prostatic hyperplasia (BPH), for example, almost 90 percent are phytomedicines, owing mainly to their lower rates of adverse side effects. In the area of physician prescriptions of psychoactive herbal drugs (e.g., St. John's Wort and Kava Kava), the strong increase in medical use is not a result of increased demands from patients but more from "scientific assurances in the form of convincing clinical and pharmacological studies." (Schilcher, 1998b.)

Number of Products
In 1978 when the Second Medicines Act became law, new regulations covering medicinal products included items sold in pharmacies, drug stores, health food stores, and other retail outlets. Because of the broad coverage and due to the fact that differing forms of administration and dosage sizes were considered separate products, herbal drug products in 1990 numbered about 60,000, compared to 126,000 registered finished drugs (including conventional medications). Of the 60,000 herbal products, about 40,000 are herbal teas. These herbal products are based on about 1,400 medicinal plant parts (flowers, leaves, herbs, roots, etc.) derived from 600 to 700 plant species (Keller, 1991). (For example, three different parts from one plant can be sold as three different products.) Another source notes that only about 100 of these medicinal plants are significant from a clinical and economic perspective (Schilcher, 1998b).

For comparison, in 1978 there were about 78,000 herbal products on the German market (Schilcher, 1997b) that "were produced by about 180 medium-sized and smaller pharmaceutical operations." (Schilcher, 1998b.) Thus, the Commission's work helped to remove unsafe and questionable products from the market.

Market Statistics
The primary market for medicinal herbs and phytomedicinal products in Germany is expressed via sales in licensed pharmacies where these products have the status of drugs approved by the Ministry of Health. The total market for such products in relation to conventional nonprescription medicines sold in pharmacies is shown in Table 7a.

Phytomedicines comprise about 30 percent of all drugs sold in German pharmacies. Prescribed phytomedicines (i.e., semi-ethical) constitute approximately 17 percent of the total drug market, while nonprescription phytomedicines comprise about 13 percent of the total market. These statistics can be viewed another way: about 30 percent of all phytomedicines sold in Germany are prescribed by physicians, with the balance (70 percent) being sold as nonprescription medicines (Fresenius, Niklas, and Schilcher, 1997). Despite widespread acceptance and recommendation by health professionals, in Germany, as in other developed countries, the trend toward self-medication has increased. In 1978, 44 percent of the public chose not to see a physician for minor conditions but to self-medicate instead; that figure rose to 58 percent in early 1997, according to the survey conducted by the Institute for Demoscopy in Allensbach (IfD, 1997). However, despite the increase in the rate of self-medication, the survey also noted, "For many consumers, it is important that natural remedies can be prescribed by the physician and that they are paid for by their health insurance. Consumers are prepared to provide a co-payment for drugs up to approximately 30 percent of the total costs." (Steinhoff, 1997b.)

Table 7a: The Market for Phytomedicines Sold in German Pharmacies — 1996

	Sales in millions (US $)[1]	Market Share (%)	Change From 1995 (%)
Total OTC market	8,654	100	+2
Non-herbal drugs	6,011	70	+2
All herbal drugs	2,644	30	+3
Prescribed herbal drugs (semi-ethical)	1,437	17	+1
Self-medication with herbal drugs	1,207	13	+5

[1]based on US$ to DM exchange rate of $1 = 1.80 DM (0.55 DM per $) on Jan. 26, 1998.
Source: Institute for Medical Statistics (IMS); courtesy PhytoPharm Consulting, Berlin (Gruenwald, 1998).

Table 7b: Retail Sales of Herbal Medicines in German Pharmacies by Indication — 1996

Indication/Use	Sales in millions (US$)[1]
Tonics & geriatric	$ 240.9
Cough & cold	196.4
Stomach & digestion	156.2
Heart & circulation	152.9
Sedation & sleep	112.8
All others	336.1
Total	$1,195.2

[1]based on US$ to DM exchange rate of $1 = 1.80 DM (0.55 DM per $) on Jan. 26, 1998.
Source: Institute for Medical Statistics (IMS), per Steinhoff, 1997b.

Table 8: Indications for the 100 Most Commonly Prescribed Herbal Medications in Germany, Listed in Order of Gross Sales in Pharmacies — 1995

Indication	Number of Products	Sales in millions (US$)[1]
Central nervous system disorders	19	$345.38
Respiratory disorders	29	143.27
Urinary tract disorders	11	118.26
Cardiovascular disorders	10	115.76
Stomach, Bowel, Liver, or biliary tract disorders	10	82.03
Promoting resistance to diseases	6	50.75
Skin and connective tissue disorders	11	44.21
Gynecological disorders	4	17.34

[1]based on US$ to DM exchange rate of $1 = 1.80 DM (0.55 DM per $) on Jan. 26, 1998.
Source: German Public Health Insurance Drug Index as published in the *Arzneiverordnungsreport* — 1996 (Prescription Drug Report) (Schwabe and Pfaffrath, 1996), in Schulz, Hänsel, and Tyler, 1997.

It should be noted that the market for urologic agents from phytomedicines in Germany is quite healthy. According to Prof. Dr. H. Schilcher of Commission E, over 80 percent of the products used for benign prostatic hyperplasia (BPH) are phytomedicines. BPH medicines thus constitute one of the leading categories of phytomedicines; no other indication has such a high rate of phytomedicinal use (Schilcher, 1997b).

Leading Phytomedicines

A review of the best-selling phytomedicines composed of single herbs can be instructive in understanding the extent of their use, both as nonprescription and prescription medications. According to the *Arzneiverordnungsreport* (*Prescription Drug Report*) published in 1997 by Schwabe, the following sales were recorded for the most frequently prescribed herbal monopreparations in 1996 (Schwabe, 1997). These figures reflect sales for semi-ethical phytomedicines, i.e., herbal drugs with nonprescription status prescribed by physicians.

Table 9: Most Frequently Prescribed Monopreparation Phytomedicines in Germany, According to Sales — 1996

Herb/Phytomedicine (Number of Products)	Therapeutic Category	Retail Sales in millions(US$)[1]	Change From 1995 (%)
1. Ginkgo Biloba Leaf Extract (5)	circulatory preparations	211.938	-8.7
2. St. John's Wort (7)	antidepressant	71.039	+31.1
3. Horse Chestnut seed (3)	vein preparations	51.195	+10.8
4. Yeast (2)	antidiarrheal, acne	33.049	+2.4
5. Hawthorn flower and leaf	cardiac preparations	29.057	-6.8
6. Myrtle (*Myrtus communis*) (1)	cough remedy	27.098	+0.6
7. Saw Palmetto	urologic	24.400	+31.8
8. Stinging Nettle root (1)	urologic	20.187	-4.4
9. Ivy (3)	cough remedy	19.074	+8.0
10. Mistletoe (1)	cancer treatment	18.060	+3.9
11. Milk Thistle (1)	hepatoprotectant	16.867	+0.9
12. Bromelain — pineapple enzyme (2)	antiinflammatory	13.219	+71.2
13. Echinacea (2)	immunostimulant	10.799	-20.2
14. Chamomile	dermatological	8.278	-7.3
15. Chaste Tree (Vitex) (2)	gynecological	7.987	+83.9
16. Greater Celandine (1)	gastrointestinal agent	6.342	-9.9
17. Black Cohosh (1)	gynecological	6.302	+1.5
18. Kava Kava (1)	tranquilizer	5.819	-38.8
19. Artichoke (1)	hypocholesteremic	5.242	
20. Comfrey (1)	dermatological	4.880	-11.4

[1]Currency in US$ based on 1.80 German marks (DM) (0.55 DM per $) on Jan. 26, 1998.
Sources: Schwabe, U. *Arzneiverordnungsreport* (Prescription Drug Report) — 1997. Courtesy PhytoPharm Consulting GmbH, Berlin (Gruenwald, 1998).

Table 10a: Leading Proprietary Monopreparation Phytomedicines in Germany

Herb	Trade Name	Manufacturer	Application
Black Cohosh	Remifemin	Schaper & Brümmer	menopause
Chaste Tree	Agnolyt	Madaus	premenstrual syndrome
Echinacea	Echinacin	Madaus	immunostimulant
Garlic	Kwai	Lichtwer Pharma	cardiovascular
Ginger	Zintona	Herbalist & Doc	motion sickness
Ginkgo	Tebonin	Schwabe	circulatory/cognitive
	Rokan	Intersan/Schwabe	circulatory/cognitive
Ginseng	Ginsana	Pharmaton	tonic
Hawthorn	Crataegutt	Schwabe	cardiotonic
	Faros	Lichtwer	cardiotonic
Horse Chestnut Seed Extract	Venostasin	Klinge Pharma	venous tonic
	Venoplant	Schwabe	venous tonic
Kava Kava	Antares	Krewel	anxiety
	Laitan	Schwabe	anxiety
Milk Thistle	Legalon	Madaus	hepatoprotection
Saw Palmetto	Prostagutt	Schwabe	prostate (BPH)
	Talso	Sanofi/Winthrop	prostate (BPH)
St. John's Wort	Jarsin	Lichtwer Pharma	depression
	Kira	Lichtwer Pharma	depression
	Remotiv	Bayer	depression

Products are listed in alphabetical order by common name of herb, not by ranking in market status. Tebonin is the top-selling monopreparation phytomedicine in total sales value, ranking 3rd in all phytomedicine prescriptions written (both monopreparations and combinations) and 29th in all prescriptions written for all drugs (including conventional drugs). Although all these products are available nonprescription, this ranking does not include additional sales generated by self-medication purchases.

Table 10b: Selected Leading Proprietary Combination Phytomedicines in Germany

Herb	Ingredients	Manufacturer	Application
Esberitox	Echinacea purpurea root, Wild Indigo root (*Baptisia tinctoria*), Arbor vitae tips (*Thuja occidentalis*)	Schaper & Brümmer	immunostimulation colds and flu
Iberogast	Wild candytuft (*Iberis amara*), Angelica root, Chamomile flowers, Caraway, Milk Thistle fruits, Lemon Balm, Peppermint, Greater Celandine	Steigerwald	stomach disorders
Kytta Sedativum F	Valerian root, Hops, Passionflower	Kytta-Siegfried	sedative

(continued on next page)

Table 10b: Selected Leading Proprietary Combination Phytomedicines in Germany (cont'd)

Herb	Ingredients	Manufacturer	Application
Prostagutt Forte	Saw Palmetto, Stinging Nettle root	Schwabe	prostate (BPH)
Sinupret	Gentian root, Primrose flowers, Sorrel, Elder flowers, Vervain	Bionorica	sinus
Sedariston Konzentrat	Valerian root, St. John's Wort	Steiner	sedative

Products are listed in alphabetical order, not by ranking in market status. Sinupret is the most frequently prescribed phytomedicine (both in monopreparations and combinations) and is ranked 10th in all prescriptions written for all drugs in 1995 (Schulz, Hänsel and Tyler, 1998). Although all these products are available nonprescription, this ranking is based on number of prescriptions written and does not include additional sales generated by self-medication purchases.

THE GERMAN LEGAL AND REGULATORY ENVIRONMENT AND THE HISTORY AND BACKGROUND OF COMMISSION E

Legal History

In contrast to other countries in Europe, herbal medicines have a special status in Germany, beginning with the Imperial Decree of 1901 that permitted the trade of many botanical drugs outside pharmacies. This was incorporated into Articles 29 - 31 of the First Medicines Act (AMG) of 1961 (Schilcher, 1998b).

The legal basis for modern drug laws in Germany is based on European Community Directives 65/65/EEC issued in 1965, plus Directives 75/318/EEC and 75/319/EEC, issued in 1975. Under the terms of these directives all member states of the European Community pledged to establish a formal review of all medicinal products on the market at that time and to assure that they met appropriate standards for quality and purity. Products were to be reviewed for safety and efficacy and re-registered by 1990 in Germany.

Consequently, on August 24, 1976, Germany passed the Second Medicines Act (*Arzneimittelgesetz* 1976, or AMG 76), which went into effect January 1, 1978, and required that the entire range of medicines in the pharmaceutical market (including conventional drugs, as well as medicinal plants and phytomedicines) be reviewed by scientific committees. AMG 76 includes special sections on phytomedicines: Article 22 Abs. 2 Nr.2, Section Article 25 Abs., Article 36, Article 44, and Article 45.

In 1978 the Minister of Health established a series of commissions to review various categories of drugs, including an expert committee for herbal drugs and preparations from medicinal plants, Commission E. These commissions were situated at the *Bundesgesundheitsamt* (BGA), the Federal Health Agency, charged with reviewing and approving the safety and efficacy of all drugs. In 1994 the BGA became the *Bundesinstitut für Arzneimittel und Medizinprodukte* (BfArM), the Federal Institute for Drugs and Medical Devices.

According to the AMG 76, for preparations that were already on the market at that time, a transition period of 12 years was allowed, following European guidelines. During this time, the products remained on the market, but evidence of quality, safety, and effectiveness still required validation. The regulations were designed so that the manufacturer had to provide proof of pharmaceutical quality for traditional herbal ingredients, whereas evaluations of safety and effectiveness were relegated to the monographs to be published by Commission E (Steinhoff, 1997b).

However, all drugs that came into the market after the law went into effect (1978) had to be evaluated according to the procedures for new drug approvals. This applied to herbal and conventional drugs alike. The manufacturer must apply every five years for an extension of the drug registration. Proof of quality, safety, and effectiveness applied equally; however, for safety and effectiveness, reference to bibliographic evidence was allowed for herbal drugs (Steinhoff, 1997b).

Table 11: The Commissions of the German Federal Institute for Drugs and Medical Devices (BfArM)

Commission	Area of Expertise
B1	Angiology, cardiology, nephrology
B2	Rheumatology
B3	Neurology
B4	Endocrinology
B5	Gastroenterology, metabolism, urology
B6	Infectious diseases, oncology, immunology, pulmonology
B7	Dermatology, hematology
B8	Balneology
B9	Dentistry, odontology
B10	Infusion and transfusion medicine
B11	Radiology and nuclear medicine
C	Anthroposophic therapy and substances
D	Homeopathic therapy and substances
E	Phytotherapy and herbal substances
F	Veterinary medicine
109a AMG 76	Traditional Medicines

These commissions scientifically evaluated the following number of medicines: from 1978 until September 1994: 1,369 conventional drugs, 360 herbal drugs, and 187 veterinary drugs (Busse, 1997a). By the end of 1995, the total number of herbs evaluated by Commission E was 360, whereas the number of herb parts reviewed as preparations was at least 391. This seeming discrepancy is because in some cases there is a monograph for each of several parts from the same plant (e.g., Senna fruit and Senna leaf; Hawthorn leaf with flower, Hawthorn fruit, leaf, or flower respectively).

Composition of Commission E
According to the Second Medicines Act the members of the scientific committees must have experience in the respective therapeutic area. Commission E was composed of 24 members proposed by associations of the health professionals (physicians, pharmacists, non-medical practitioners (*Heilpraktiker*), pharmacologists, toxicologists, and biostatisticians) and by representatives of the pharmaceutical industry (Keller, 1992). Fifty percent are experts from the clinical or therapeutic field (Busse, 1996). Scientists and physicians serving on the Commission have authored over 1,000 scientific publications, not only in phytotherapy, but also in medicine, pharmacology, dentistry, health care delivery, and medical ethics. One longstanding member has written that the interdisciplinary nature of the Commission is unique in the entire world (Schilcher, 1997b). The Commission will be appointed every three years by the Minister of Health. The Commission is headed

by a Chairman (Dr. Oelze) and a Vice President (Prof. Dr. H. Schilcher). The contact to the BfArM is Dr. K. Keller, who is considered the "Referee" (*Berichterstatter*). For a list of the current members of the Commission, please see page xvii.

Traditional Medicines

For old herbal products already on the market that could not meet Commission E standards, a Traditional Medicine status was introduced in January 1992 that permitted the re-registration of traditional medicines without requiring rigorous studies and scientific data on a specific product (Steinhoff, 1993/4b). According to Article 109a of the AMG 76, these traditional products must be safe and meet standards for quality. The challenge of proving efficacy can be overcome by using traditional use as a criterion for effectiveness "for drugs that have proven useful for many years." (Steinhoff, 1997b.)

These "traditionally used preparations" also must pass the review and control of the new Commission to 109a AMG 76, established in August 1996. This commission makes lists for traditional medicines (not limited to herb-based products) to include specific products mentioned in Article 44(1) AMG 76. Medicinal claims must be limited to minor conditions and preventive statements, and the phrase "traditionally used in" must be on the label. They can be intended only for indications such as strengthening, invigorating, or supporting the body (possibly not unlike a structure-function claim under DSHEA in the U.S.), but they cannot be intended to cure or treat a disease. Phytomedicines approved by this commission do not qualify for reimbursement from medical health plans (Shilcher, 1998c). This commission is also composed of an interdisciplinary group of experts. Prof. H. Schilcher is Vice President of both this commission and Commission E (Schilcher, 1997b).

In sum, although these products must still meet standards for quality manufacture, their historical uses are not documented by plausible scientific data. Thus, there is a distinction between the standards for the approval of Traditional Medicines and the scientific standards for herbal drugs approved by Commission E (Busse, 1997; Steinhoff, 1993/4b, Schilcher 1998).

Regarding the standards for quality, the pharmaceutical quality of Traditional Medicines must be documented. As of the fall of 1997 the Commission to 109a AMG 76 has listed over 800 substances (many herbal) that the manufacturers have petitioned for inclusion. The BfArM does not inspect the manufacture of these medicines, but the pharmaceutical manufacturer must provide a statutory declaration for the herb ingredient, dosage form, and intended use. (Steinhoff, 1997b).

COMMISSION E EVALUATION METHODS AND CRITERIA

Bibliographic Review

According to Section 26 of the Second Medicines Act, in accordance with applicable European drug law, bibliographic data were used to assess the safety and efficacy of medicines evaluated by Commission E. Members used 100-200 references from around the world to evaluate each herb (Schilcher, 1997b).

Unlike FDA drug reviews in which data is passively submitted to the agency by the manufacturer, the members of Commission E actively collected bibliographic data on the herbal drugs being reviewed. This work has been supported since 1992 by the industry and scientific coalition *Kooperation Phytopharmaka* (Steinhoff, 1997a). The following are examples of the data collected and reviewed:

1. Traditional use. Literature can reveal the long-term use of a botanical substance and can indicate relative safety and presumed efficacy.

2. Chemical data. Herbal drugs have been analyzed to determine their chemical composition, especially the main constituents. Knowledge of these chemical constituents can indicate the potential activity and/or toxicity of a botanical, depending on the known range of compounds and their relative quantities.

3. Experimental, pharmacological, and toxicological studies. Laboratory/experimental (in vitro) and pharmacological/toxicological (in vivo) studies are published worldwide on whole plant extracts or constituents of medicinal plants. These studies provide documentation of the historical or traditional uses of a plant, even though clinical studies may be lacking.

4. Clinical studies. In many European countries, clinical studies on leading medicinal plants and phytomedicines are conducted routinely, according to strict scientific controls. These studies can suggest and often confirm the safety and efficacy of herbs and their preparations. Many clinical studies conducted recently correspond to Good Clinical Practice (GCP) guidelines.

5. Field and epidemiological studies. The use of a medicinal plant by a particular population over time is also useful when evaluating safety and efficacy. The Commission reviewed such studies, if they were available.

6. Patient case records submitted from physicians' files. Case reports from individual patients in clinical practice, although not considered as important as controlled clinical studies, are nevertheless useful in obtaining information from the experiences of attending physicians using herbs and phytomedicines.

7. Additional studies, including unpublished proprietary data submitted by manufacturers. On occasion, a particular herb may have extensive chemical, toxicological, pharmacological, and clinical testing conducted by a manufacturer. The Commission was able to review such data, while maintaining the confidentiality of the information. Commission referee Dr. K. Keller of BfArM writes, "Due to the great number of individual drugs, the work of the committee was concentrated on the evaluation of active constituents. The evaluation is based on bibliographic data presented by manufacturers or organizations of manufacturers of herbal medicinal products. These documents are completed by data obtained from literature search, for example online research in EMBASE, MEDLARS, and TOXALL, and other data available to our office." (Keller, 1992.)

The proposed monograph format was published and reviewed in about three months by all Commission members, other scientists, scientific associations, universities, and other experts, who could make comments to the proposed monograph. All comments were then considered by the Commission in its final monograph (Schilcher, 1997b).

References

Readers will quickly notice that the Commission E monographs do not include any references to the literature used by the Commission members in assessing the safety and efficacy of the herbal drugs under review. This is unlike the format for the monographs published in 1990 and subsequently by ESCOP. Commission E and ESCOP monographs are similar insofar as they are therapeutic monographs and do not detail standards for quality as are found in a pharmacopeial monograph.

According to Prof. Schilcher every monograph has a *Begrundung*, an unpublished justification with most of the relevant references. This material is stored at the BfArM in Berlin and only in conflicts or cases of disputes to the Medical Act can an attorney or a scientific organization view these references. The references were originally included in data reviewed by members of the Commission in determining monograph evaluations (Schilcher, 1998a).

The Commission E monographs were developed to inform the consumer and to facilitate the companies' applications for registration of the herbs as licensed drugs. The monographs were created as official government documents. Although the monographs cannot serve as a guide to additional information, they are based on extensive review of the scientific and historical data as well as the interdisciplinary expertise of the members of the Commission. Also, some of the materials upon which the monographs were based were unpublished studies of proprietary products from manufacturers in Germany; thus, these references could not be published. The background material for these monographs, produced by *Kooperation Phytopharmaka* (KP), did contain references but these longer documents have not been published (Steinhoff, 1997). Thus, for these reasons, references are not included in Commission E's monographs.

In 1992 *Kooperation Phytopharmaka* was established as an umbrella organization of about 150 pharmaceutical manufacturers particularly active in the field of phytomedicine. *Kooperation Phytopharmaka* is advised by three associations of the pharmaceutical industry, *Bundesfachverband der Arzneimittel-Hersteller* e.V. (BAH, the Federal Association of Pharmaceutical Manufacturers), *Bundesverband der Pharmazeuthischen Industrie* e.V. (BPI, the Federal Association of the Pharmaceutical Industry), and the *Verband der Reformwaren-Hersteller* e.V. (VRH, the Association of Manufacturers of Health Foods), as well as the *Deutsche Gessellschaft für Phytotherapie* e.V. (GPhy, the German Society of Phytotherapy), a scientific organization. One of the main objectives of KP since its beginning has been the collection and preparation of scientific material on medicinal plants, evaluation of this material by experts in the field of phytomedicine, and submission of this prepared material (comparable to an expert report) to Commission E (Steinhoff, 1997). These summaries consist of exhaustive literature reviews on chemistry, toxicology, pharmacology, and clinical experience (some exceeding 100 pages). No positive or negative recommendation is included in these summaries (Busse, 1997c). Many of the Commission E monographs are based on material prepared by KP, but the KP monographs served as only one basis for the development of the Commission E monographs. In the past few years KP has taken on the task of revising the "old" material, i.e., collecting information, (e.g., clinical studies) published since the publication of the Commission E monograph. This updated material is now being used by manufacturers to lend support to substantiation of individual therapeutic indications and efficacy of herbal drug products during the process of re-registration for drug status with the BfArM (Steinhoff, 1997).

Table 12: Clinical Studies on Leading European Phytomedicines

This table lists leading phytomedicines in Germany and the number of clinical studies cited in *Rational Phytotherapy* (Schulz, Hänsel, and Tyler, 1998). In some cases, all studies were conducted on one proprietary product such as Horse Chestnut seed extract where in other categories, for example, ginkgo, the studies were based on two standardized extracts. In yet others, different types of galenical preparations were used in different studies. For example, some valerian studies were based on aqueous extracts while others used a hydro-alcoholic extract; 12 clinical trials are referenced using alcoholic extracts of St. John's Wort (some also containing valerian extract) and 10 based on a leading standardized extract.

Phytomedicine	Years	Number of Studies	Total Persons
Garlic	1986-92	18	2,920
Ginkgo	1975-96	36[1]	2,326
Hawthorn	1981-96	13	791
Horse Chestnut seed	1973-96	8	798
Kava Kava	1989-95	6	469
St. John's Wort	1979-97	22	1,851
Valerian	1977-96	8	560

[1] These refer to studies dealing only with cognitive effects of Ginkgo Biloba extract. Other studies have measured effects on peripheral circulation and other actions of Ginkgo.
Source: Schulz, Hänsel, and Tyler, 1998.

Evaluation of Safety and Efficacy: Positive and Negative Monographs

The Commission E review process is only slightly comparable to the OTC review process of old drugs conducted by the U.S. Food and Drug Administration since 1972. The results of field studies and single cases were only eligible when evaluated according to scientific standards. When lacking controlled studies, safety and efficacy for known substances still can be determined on the basis of other information, such as well documented review articles, older clinical trials, and well documented knowledge on traditional use (Busse, 1996). However, experience from long-term therapeutic or traditional use without supplementary data cannot be accepted as sufficient evidence of safety (Busse, 1997c).

In comparing the German legal and regulatory situation with that of the U.S., Commission E member M. Wiesenauer notes that plant drugs were equated with synthetic drugs in Germany by legislative fiat. Then the Commission set about the task of determining the safety and effectiveness of each preparation (Wiesenauer, 1989). Approved and unapproved herbs are divided into separate sections of this book. There are several ways to distinguish between a positive and negative monograph. Positive monographs always show the approved use and dosage. If no approved uses are given in a monograph, if there is no dosage listed, and if the efficacy of the plant has not been sufficiently proven, or there are risks that outweigh the documented benefits (e.g., Monkshood, Male Fern), the assessment will be a negative one (Steinhoff, 1994a).

Several of the herbs approved by Commission E are relatively powerful, pharmacologically active, and also potentially toxic herbs. "It is important to realise that Commission E does not restrict its activities to mildly acting products, but also prepares monographs on potent herbal remedies, such as *Hyoscyamus niger* [Henbane], *Rauvolfia serpentina* [Indian Snakeroot] and *Urginea maritima* [Squill], all of which should be treated as prescription only drugs. In other words, the existence of a positive Commission E monograph does not imply that the herbal drug is sufficiently harmless to be treated as an over-the-counter product. However, as each monograph outlines the accepted uses and health risks of the herb in question, the work of the Commission E provides useful information if one has to assess the safety of individual source plants." (Gericke, 1995.)

In a few cases new data necessitated the change of an herbal drug from approved status to unapproved as in the case of Bishop's Weed fruit, originally published as an approved monograph in 1986. However, in 1994, as a result of a new risk-benefit assessment based on toxicological data and case reports of adverse reactions, the original monograph was replaced (not revised) with a new negative monograph that noted the risks of this herb (Keller, 1998; Steinhoff, 1997b). The same process also occurred with Madder root, granted a positive monograph for treatment of kidney stones in 1986, but replaced in 1992 with a negative monograph, due to new pharmacological research on rats indicating that the compound lucidin may be mutagenic and carcinogenic. Reclassification of both Bishop's Weed fruit and Madder root to negative monograph status (Unapproved) because of new data indicating potential risks that outweigh possible benefits attests to the rationality of the Commission E process. This constant vigilance by Commission members regarding what has been termed the "doctrine of absolute proof" to assess safety is a significant characteristic of the Commission E evaluation process.

Positive (Approved) Monographs
As is true for any body of scientists evaluating the benefits and marketability of medicines, Commission E was concerned about the safety of the herbs and phytomedicines it reviewed. According to Professor Varro E. Tyler, Dean and Distinguished Professor of Pharmacognosy Emeritus at Purdue University, the Commission reviewed safety data according to a "doctrine of absolute proof" for safety (Tyler, 1994). The Commission attempted to ensure that these medicines were reasonably safe when used according to the dosage, contraindications, and other warnings and provisions specified in the monographs.

Regarding efficacy, the Commission was guided by what Professor Tyler has termed the "doctrine of reasonable certainty." (Tyler, 1994.) That is, as long as the scientific data provided reasonable verification of particular historical use, the Commission would grant a positive evaluation. Accordingly, some of the early work of the Commission (1978 - 1989) was characterized by positive evaluations for some herbs for which a significant body of clinical studies did not exist. Most positively evaluated monographs are based on open clinical studies or data derived from field studies, patient case records, and pharmacological research or proprietary data submitted by individual companies (Schilcher, 1997b). Numerous negative evaluations also were made during this period.

However, after 1990 the Commission began to focus more on good clinical practices (GCP) clinical studies to document the uses. In some cases, monographs for herbs that previously were granted approval for several uses were amended to a more restricted indication. A good example is the monograph for Hawthorn, originally published in 1984. The Hawthorn monograph initially contained a range of cardiovascular indications that included applications between stages I and II of the New York Heart Association's functional classification for heart disease. The approved indications formerly read as follows: "sensation of pressure and anxiety in the heart area," "geriatric heart condition that does not yet require digitalis," and "mild forms of bradycardia." However, in July 1994 the Commission published four separate monographs for various parts of the hawthorn plant. Only Hawthorn leaf with flower was approved for the more limited indication "for decreasing cardiac performance as described in functional Stage II of NYHA." This approval was based on clinical studies published for proprietary medicines made of both hawthorn parts and based on observations by physicians from clinical experience. Other hawthorn preparations made individually from berry (fruit), leaf, or flower were negatively evaluated due to the lack of evidence in clinical trials. However, they are still sold as "traditionally used Hawthorn preparations" only to support general heart function, according to provisions of Article 109a of the AMG (Schilcher, 1997b). (See Traditional Medicines above.)

This process of negative evaluations of the older dosage forms was challenged by the BAH. BAH suggested that because hawthorn preparations "form an important part of the German phytomedicines market with respect to self-medication," therefore, "when new clinical studies become available, it is important to check, and possibly amend, the older monographs, because the status of scientific knowledge represented by them may change owing to new research results. This, however, must under no circumstances automatically mean that the older results published in a monograph are no longer valid, and, unless there is a direct conflict, those results must maintain their status as scientific documentation and be included in a monograph as before, perhaps with a slightly modified indication claim." Unfortunately, Commission E did not agree with this proposition, and the final monographs on Crataegus [Hawthorn] were published on 19 July 1994 without the same indications published in the 1984 monograph (Steinhoff, 1997). (For more on Hawthorn, please see pages 39 and 63.)

Negative (Unapproved) Monographs

Negative assessments (i.e., Unapproved monographs) were made by Commission E in cases where "no plausible evidence of efficacy" was available or when safety concerns outweighed the potential benefits. The objective of the Commission was to "eliminate drugs with even minor risks, because these risks are not tolerable if they are not balanced by an acceptable benefit." (Keller, 1992.) Also, the Commission published negative monographs for medicinal plants which had no clinical or pharmacological studies or no plausible evidence of efficacy reported in traditional medicine or empirical medicine (Schilcher, 1997b). Herbs that were evaluated negatively are published in the Unapproved Herbs section of this book. Monographs on these herbal drugs and their phytomedicinal preparations are published without dosage recommendations. "Herbs which pose a risk have to be withdrawn immediately." (Busse, 1997c.) Unapproved Herbs that do not pose a health risk can be sold in the German market only until the year 2004.

According to Prof. Schilcher, the fact that by 1995 the Commission had negatively evaluated at least 115 herbal drugs is evidence that in Germany "scientifically oriented criteria for assessment apply for plant medicines." (Schilcher, 1997b.)

Interestingly, the 126 unapproved monographs, although they constitute only 33 percent of the total monographs published, produce 97 of the total number of categories of adverse side effects. This is consistent with the fact that 45 herbs were negatively evaluated precisely due to documentation or reasonable suspicion of these types of risks. By comparison, the 254 positive monographs contain only 75 types of side effects (mostly adverse; not all side effects listed are adverse). This constitutes 29 percent more side effects noted for Unapproved herbs than for Approved herbs. (This data is found in Table 13.)

Table 13: Unapproved Monographs with Documented or Suspected Risk

The herbs in this table were evaluated negatively by Commission E due to the presence of actual risk or concern about potential risks. In some cases, documentation of benefit also may be inadequate. For complete information on some risks, the monograph should be consulted.

Herb	Risk
Angelica seed and herb	Photosensitivity caused by coumarins
Basil	Mutagenic effect of estragole
Bilberry leaf	High or chronic dose can cause intoxication
Bishop's Weed fruit	Allergic reactions; photosensitivity due to khellin
Bladderwrack	Hyperthyroidism due to daily dose over 150 mcg iodine
Borage	Hepatotoxic pyrrolizidine alkaloids
Bryonia	Numerous risks cited
Celery	Allergic skin reactions; can contain large amounts of phototoxic furanocoumarin
Chamomile, Roman	Rare allergic reactions
Cinnamon flower	Allergic reactions to skin and mucosa
Cocoa	Allergic skin reactions and migraine headaches
Colocynth	G.i. irritation and possible hemorrhagic diarrhea due to curcurbitacin; kidney damage, cystitis
Coltsfoot	Hepatotoxic pyrrolizidine alkaloids
Delphinium flower	Alkaloids can cause bradycardia, hypotension, cardiac arrest, central paralyzing and curare-like effect on respiratory system
Elecampane	Irritation of mucosa and allergic contact dermatitis due to alantolactone
Ergot	Wide spectrum of activity
Goat's Rue	Hypoglycemic effect of galegin
Hound's Tongue	Hepatotoxic pyrrolizidine alkaloids
Kelp	Hyperthyroidism due to daily dose over 150 mcg iodine
Lemongrass, Citronella oil	Toxic alveolitis associated with inhaling undetermined amount of oil
Liverwort herb	Irritation of skin and mucous membranes associated with protoanemonin in fresh plants
Madder root	Mutagenic and carcinogenic potential of lucidin content
Male Fern	Wide spectrum of adverse reactions
Marjoram	Potential unclear risks of arbutin and hydroxyquinone content
Marsh Tea	Poisoning associated with abusive dosing, e.g., abortions
Monkshood	Serious, varied spectrum of effects possible within therapeutic dose
Mugwort	Abortifacient action reported.
Nutmeg	Psychoactive, abortifacient effect of large doses
Nux Vomica	Spastic CNS action of strychnine
Oleander leaf	Poisoning, sometimes fatal, due to oleandrin
Papain	Increased tendency to bleed for someone with clotting disorders
Parsley seed	Large doses of apiol in essential oil produce vascular congestion and contraction of smooth muscles in bladder, intestines, and uterus
Pasque flower	Fresh plants and preparations with protoanemonin produce severe irritation of skin and mucosa
Periwinkle	Suppressed immune system in animal experiments

(continued on next page)

Table 13: Unapproved Monographs with Documented or Suspected Risk (cont'd)

Herb	Risk
Petasites leaf	Hepatotoxic pyrrolizidine alkaloids
Rhododendron, Rusty-leaved	Poisoning due to grayanotoxine content
Rue	Phototoxic and mutagenic effects, liver and kidney damage associated with furanocoumarins
Saffron	Adverse effects noted in doses over 10 g used for abortion
Sarsaparilla root	Gastric irritation and temporary kidney impairment suspected
Scotch Broom flower	Contraindicated in MAOI therapy and hypertension
Senecio herb	Hepatotoxic pyrrolizidine alkaloids
Soapwort herb, Red	Mucous membrane irritation with high levels of saponins
Tansy flower and herb	Poisoning due to abuse of large doses of herb with possible thujone content of oil
Walnut hull	Potential mutagenic effect of juglone
Yohimbe bark	Nervousness, tremor, sleeplessness, anxiety, hypertension, and tachycardia, nausea, vomiting associated with therapeutic administration of yohimbine; interaction with psychopharmacological herbs

Negative-Null (Unapproved) Monographs

If there is neither a risk nor sufficiently documented efficacy, the monograph is termed *null* by Commission E. The term *neutral* is preferred by the German manufacturers. Null (neutral) monographs do not note any risk associated with the use of the herbs (Steinhoff, 1997). Nevertheless, despite the fact that the industry uses the term *neutral*, "the official position [of BfArM] is that they are negative monographs because there is a negative vote on individual claims promoted by industry." (Keller, 1998a, b.) The term "null" is used internally by the Commission to refer to these so-called "neutral" monographs, but they are published as "negative" in the *Bundesanzeiger* (Schilcher, 1997b). Because they have received a negative evaluation due to lack of scientific documentation, they are included in the Unapproved Herbs section of this book. As seen in Table 14, many of these 46 herbs are common foods (Figs and Spinach leaf), spices (Dill weed and Oregano), and tea ingredients (Hibiscus, Raspberry leaf, and Rose Hip), which, despite lack of documentation, are relatively safe in normal use. Prof. Schilcher notes that if the industry is able to provide new studies to document efficacy, they may be able to achieve positive status as drugs, but no new monographs will be produced (Schilcher, 1998a). Table 14 provides a complete list of negative monographs without documented risk.

Table 14: Unapproved Monographs with No Documented Risk

The following 55 botanical drugs were negatively evaluated by Commission E because they lacked scientific documentation of the uses claimed by industry. They are considered relatively safe since no documentation was made of risks; they are considered "neutral" by the German phytomedicine industry.

Ash	Damiana leaf and herb	Hawthorn flower
Alpine Lady's Mantle	Dill weed	Hawthorn leaf
Blackberry root	Echinacea angustifolia herb & root/Pallida herb	Heather herb and flower
Burdock root		Hibiscus
Calendula herb	Eyebright	Hollyhock flower
Cat's Foot flower	Figs	Horse Chestnut leaf
Chestnut leaf	Ginkgo Biloba leaf	Hyssop
Cornflower	Hawthorn berry	Jambolan seed

(continued on next page)

Table 14: Unapproved Monographs with No Documented Risk (cont'd)

Linden Charcoal	Oat herb	Rose Hip seed
Linden flower, Silver	Olive leaf	Rupturewort
Linden leaf	Olive oil	Red Sandalwood
Linden wood	Oregano	Spinach leaf
Loofa	Orris root	Strawberry leaf
Lungwort	Papaya leaf	Sweet Woodruff
Mentzelia	Peony	Verbena herb
Milk Thistle herb	Pimpinella	Veronica herb
Mountain Ash berry	Raspberry leaf	White Dead Nettle herb
Muira Puama	Rose Hip	Zedoary rhizome
Night-blooming Cereus	Rose Hip and seed	

QUALITY STANDARDS AND PHYTOEQUIVALENCE

In addition to the therapeutic parameters noted in each of the monographs, every monograph includes implied standards for quality, according to the current issue of the *German Pharmacopoeia* (*DAB*). However, a few of the more recently published Commission E monographs contain specific standards for assessing the quality of the herbal drug (Busse, 1996). These include the monographs for Ginkgo Biloba leaf dry extract, Horse Chestnut seed extract, and Lecithin. Since the early 1990s Commission E has issued an increasing number of monographs on specifically defined plant preparations. "This was due to further improvements in the analytical procedures applied for quality control of plant preparations (e.g., extracts). It was shown that differing methods of manufacturing (e.g., the use of different solvents for extraction, purification steps) resulted in extracts of different quality. The results from pharmacological and clinical trials with one extract could thus not automatically be transferred to another preparation." (Busse, 1996). A good example of this process is the Commission E monograph on Ginkgo Biloba leaf dry extract, based on several patented, standardized extracts of a 50 to 1 average concentration, with chemically defined standardization for ginkgolides (6 percent) and ginkgo flavonglycosides (24 percent), and a maximum level of ginkgolic acid (max. 5 ppm). In spring of 1997, the BfArM sent a letter to manufacturers of phytomedicines requiring proof that all ginkgo extracts have less than 5 ppm ginkgolic acid in order for products to receive license renewals, due to concerns about the potential allergenic effects of ginkgolic acid (Thiele, 1997).

Regarding research conducted on proprietary preparations like the ginkgo extracts described above, if a manufacturer is able to document the same bioequivalence (or *phytoequivalence*, as it is often called for plant medicines) in addition to the chemical profile, then these results may be transferable to a claim for a preparation (Schilcher, 1997b). No new pharmacological or clinical studies are required; however, the documentation must demonstrate phytoequivalence via in vitro pharmacokinetic studies (Schilcher, 1998a).

OVERVIEW OF COMMISSION E MONOGRAPHS

Quantity of Monographs

Commission E published a total of 462 monographs. This includes 81 revisions to monographs, which sometimes were revised two or three times. In some cases, new monographs were published to replace earlier versions (e.g., Hawthorn, noted above). Rather than show the revision as an addendum to a monograph, we have incorporated revisions directly into the body of the text. Thus, for example, if a monograph was published in 1988 and subsequently revised with a new warning or modified dosage, we have added the warning or new dosage in the text, noting the original date of publication and any subsequent revisions at the top of each monograph.

Quantity of Plants in the Monographs

The original mission of Commission E was to evaluate approximately 1,400 herbal drug preparations made from 600 to 700 plant species (Keller, 1991). A total of 380 monographs are published in this book, representing about 360 plant species. According to the BfArM's *Liste der Monographien der E-Kommission (Phytotherapie)*, supplied to the American Botanical Council by Dr. Konstantin Keller, Referee of Commission E, as of January 23, 1996, there were 254 positively evaluated herbs, component characteristics, and fixed combinations plus 129 negatively (including "neutral") evaluated herbs, components, and fixed combinations (i.e., Unapproved). The number of monographs published is 472, including 81 revisions.

Table 15: Overview by Monograph Category

	Number of Monographs
Approved Monopreparations	186
Approved Component Characteristics	2
Approved Fixed Combinations	66
Total Approved Monographs	**254**
Unapproved Monopreparations (including "neutral")	110
Unapproved – Documented or Suspected Risk (45)	
Unapproved – No Documentation of Efficacy (57)	
Unapproved Component Characteristics	10
Unapproved Fixed Combinations	6
Total Unapproved Monographs	**126**
Total Monographs published in this book	380

(exclusive of 81 revisions incorporated into text)

Table 16: Therapeutic Overview of Monographs

Therapeutic Condition/Aspect	Quantity
Uses/Indications – Approved monographs	161
Contraindications – Approved monographs	69
Side Effects – Approved monographs	74
Side Effects – Unapproved monographs	96
Duration of Use Limits – Approved monographs	42
Pharmacological Actions – Approved monographs	127
Pharmacological Actions – Unapproved monographs	42

The figures in this chart refer to the actual number of conditions in each category. That is, there are 74 types of side effects noted for Approved herbs, with varying numbers of herbal drugs listed as producing each effect.

Regarding total numbers of species mentioned in the monographs, a count reveals the following statistics: There are approximately 360 species of plants referred to in the 308 single monographs (i.e., all monographs on single preparations, and component characteristics, excluding fixed combinations). Numerous monographs list two or more species in the same genus that contain suitable botanical material for the herbal drug. In some cases, a synonym is also included (we have added some where we deemed appropriate); in all, 45 synonyms are named. Thus, the total number of taxa mentioned in the monographs is about 405.

Most of the monographs deal with one specific plant part. In a few cases different parts of the same plant are monographed separately, e.g., Buckthorn berry and Buckthorn bark, Senna leaf and Senna pod. In at least 15 monographs more than one plant part is included in the monograph, e.g., Parsley herb and root, Witch Hazel leaf and bark, Yarrow flower and herb, Angelica seed and herb, and Echinacea Angustifolia herb and root with Echinacea Pallida herb.

The count of approved versus unapproved is skewed somewhat toward the negative because, in some instances, multiple parts of one single plant received negative evaluations. For example, as previously noted, there are three negative monographs for Hawthorn, unofficially considered "neutral." These evaluations were made on the basis that the clinical efficacy of preparations of leaf only, flower only, or fruit (berry) only were not sufficiently known; only field studies and patient case records were available for preparations made from either fruits or flowers only. The best research data available to the Commission members pertained to a standardized extract made of both leaf and flower having a range of minimum and maximum content of flavonoids or procyanidins. Hence, the extract received a positive evaluation while the three other types of preparations based solely on one plant part did not. Similarly, preparations made of dried Ginkgo leaf plus five distinct types of dry extracts or fluidextracts are negatively evaluated in one unapproved monograph but a standardized acetone-water extract does receive a positive evaluation.

Unapproved herb monographs contain a "Uses" section that refers to observations of historical or current use in Germany not documented by the available scientific literature. Thus, the Uses section in an unapproved monograph does not connote approved use by Commission E.

The Unapproved herbs with no risks are being allowed on the market until the end of 2004, after which they will cease to be available as licensed phytomedicines produced by a pharmaceutical company. Since January 1992 new regulations have allowed that they can be sold as Traditional Medicines, with the label noting that the product is "traditionally used for..." (*traditionell angewendet*). This exempts the product from having to undergo scientific evaluation and proving efficacy if it can be shown that the product has been marketed continuously since 1978 (the date of the Second Medicines Act) and that the herbal drug is safe. A new commission (Commission 109a AMG 76) was established to review traditional use claims, limited to terms such as "mild medicine" or "used within a traditional context" and with no pathologies listed. A revision now requires these products to be on the market continuously since 1978, if the monograph has a "low" or mild indication. If new clinical data is available, the traditional medicine can be registered (at least theoretically) without a "traditional" labeling (Keller, 1998; Steinhoff, 1997). "It should be noted that medicinal products that conform to Commission E monographs are not listed as *traditionell angewendet*." (Keller, 1998.) Finally, a physician may continue to prescribe an unapproved herb after 2004 (Schilcher, 1997b).

Monograph Format

The monographs were published in two formats. From 1983 to 1992 the information was presented in the original format of a package insert of an herb on a generic basis. Much of the input for the development of these monographs was provided by major German phytomedicine manufacturers. The dosage forms and specific parameters of the preparation types were not defined in every monograph in detail although they were in some. This resulted in monographs that manufacturers used as product inserts and in some cases as the basis for marketing authorization applications.

After 1992, the format was modified based on newer scientific research, often conducted on product-specific materials, and on the EU Directive 65/65/EEC. In these new monographs all therapeutic information has been subsumed under "Clinical Data." The new format corresponds to the information sheet for health professionals, or summary of product characteristics (SPCs) (Keller, 1998).

Table 17a: Original Format for Approved Monographs (pre-1992)

Name of Drug
Composition of Drug
Uses
Contraindications
Side Effects
Interaction with Other Drugs
Dosage
Mode of Administration
Duration of Administration
Action(s)

Table 17b: Revised Format for Approved Monographs (1992 - 1995)

Name of Drug
Composition of Drug
Pharmacological Properties, Pharmacokinetics, Toxicology
Clinical Data
    1. Uses
    2. Contraindications
    3. Side Effects
    4. Interaction with Other Drugs
    5. Dosage
    6. Mode of Administration
    7. Risks
Evaluation

Table 17c: Original Format for Unapproved Monographs (pre-1992)

Name of Drug
Composition of Drug
Uses
Risks
Evaluation

In some monographs, e.g., Pasque flower and Saffron, the negative assessment is mentioned in the Risks section and there is no Evaluation section. The Pharmacological Actions are noted in only a few unapproved monographs, e.g., Asparagus herb, Celery, Cocoa, and Pasque flower.

Table 17d: Revised Format for Unapproved Monographs (1992 - 1995)

Name of Drug
Composition of Drug
Pharmacological Properties, Pharmacokinetics, Toxicology
Clinical Data
    1. Uses
    2. Risks
Evaluation

EXPLANATION OF MONOGRAPH SECTIONS

Monograph Title

In most monographs we have chosen the preferred English common name for the monograph title. Whenever possible, we also list the plant part or parts covered by the monograph. In some cases, an herbal drug used in Germany has no accepted English common name. When this has occurred, we have titled the monograph by the designation of the genus, from which it is derived, which may become the accepted common name. An example is Mentzelia for *Mentzelia cordifolia*. Listed below the English title are the Latin pharmacopeial and German names. The official title of each monograph published in the original German version of the *Bundesanzeiger* was the pharmacopeial name for the herbal drug. Although pharmacopeial names are normally used in Europe and should be well-known to scientists the world over, in order to simplify matters for the English reader, we have employed the preferred English common name for the monograph title.

Revisions and Corrections

The Commission published a total of 81 revisions to the monographs. These reflect the relatively fluid nature of the available data on herbs and phytomedicines; as new information was reviewed, some changes in the monograph were justified. Revisions include changes in dosage, changes in warning, side effects, contraindications, and even approved uses. In some cases, an entire monograph was replaced with a new monograph, or, as is the case with Hawthorn, three monographs (see below).

Common Names

We have chosen the common name most widely used in the U.S. For most of the herbs we relied on *Herbs of Commerce*, a listing of the appropriate common names as compiled and published by the American Herbal Products Association, the leading herb industry trade association (Foster et al., 1992). *Herbs of Commerce* is a self-regulatory initiative which establishes uniform common names for the most popular herbs sold in the U.S. The book lists approximately 550 herbs in U.S. commerce, including their proper Latin binomials. In the frequent situation where an herb has more than one commonly used name, or when an herb name is spelled several ways, we have made our choice based on the term preferred by the AHPA, if it is listed. As examples, we have used the term "stinging nettle" instead of "nettle" for nettle herb and nettle root and we have spelled "passionflower" as one word instead of the also commonly used two words.

In most cases we have also listed the plant part on which the monograph is based in the monograph title. This is particularly important in cases where one plant part is approved (e.g., Echinacea purpurea herb; Hawthorn leaf and flower) while another part of the same plant is not approved (e.g., Echinacea purpurea root; Hawthorn berry, leaf, or flower). In a few monographs, only the name of the herb is used for the monograph title (e.g., Hibiscus, Hyssop). This is also true where more than one plant part is included. For example, for Borage, the monograph includes both the flower and the herb; however, rather than title the monograph "Borage flower and herb" we chose to call it Borage.

The common names of some herbs presented problems not only with nomenclature but also with proper alphabetization. For example, should Red Clover be in the C's or R's? Similarly, should Red Sandalwood be listed under R or S? With respect to herbs like Red Clover where "Red" is an integral part of the herb's name, we have included it as the first word of the herb, in the R section. However, there are monographs for both Red Sandalwood and White Sandalwood (two different plants); we have put both in the S section, as "Sandalwood, Red" and "Sandalwood, White." Similarly, "Blonde Psyllium Seed" is found as "Psyllium Seed, Blonde" in the P's with Psyllium Seed, Black. "German Chamomile" is found under "Chamomile, German" since Chamomile is the primary name. In general, the naming of other herbs follows this policy in this publication.

The German name of each preparation, listed in italics, includes the name of the plant and the plant part used, in the compound nature of the German language. For example, Purple Coneflower *herb* (*Echinacea purpurea*) is called *Purpursonnenhutkraut* while Purple Coneflower *root* is *Purpursonnenhutwurzel*. Some German names actually include the type of preparation, such as Peppermint oil, *Pfefferminzöl*.

Publication Date

The original date of the publication of each monograph is provided with the date of any revision or replacement. Many monographs were revised more than once; this is noted with multiple revision dates. The *Bundesanzeiger* numbers for the publications are provided in the section, List of All Commission E Monographs Published in the German *Federal Gazette* (*Bundesanzeiger*) on page 593.

Name of Drug

This section provides the pharmacopeial name or names of the plant parts. In the original German monograph, the German common name also was provided. We have thus added the English name in this section.

Pharmacopeial Names

For several hundred years pharmacopeial (aka pharmaceutical) names have provided a convenient system for pharmacists, physicians, and botanists to identify a substance used as materia medica by referring to its Latin name plus the plant part or type of preparation being used. Pharmacopeial names are not to be confused with Latin binomials, which consist of the genus and species of the plant according to taxonomic rules of botanical classification initially established by the 18th century Swedish botanist Carl von Linné (Linnaeus).

For example, peppermint is known technically by its Latin binomial *Mentha* x *piperita* (always italicized) where *Mentha* is the genus for various mints, x refers to a hybrid and *piperita* refers to that particular species, peppermint. This allows peppermint to be distinguished from other related mints such as spearmint (*M. spicata*) or field or common mint (*M. arvensis*). Thus, the pharmacopeial name for peppermint leaf would be Menthae piperitae folium (non-italicized) where folium refers to leaf. The pharmacopeial name for peppermint herb (the entire aerial or aboveground part of the plant) would be Menthae piperitae herba. Similarly, the pharmacopeial name for the distilled oil of peppermint is

Menthae piperitae aetheroleum, where aetheroleum refers to the volatile or essential oil. Accordingly, a preparation made from the plant's root is called radix, rhizome is rhizoma, flower is flos, fruit is fructus, seed is semen, seed husk is testa, bark is cortex, and so on. (These Latin names are written in the singular form; some national pharmacopeias use the plural form.)

It is a common practice in botany for scientists who study plant classification to reclassify or rename a plant. For example, the popular European herb milk thistle, sometimes called Marian thistle or Mary's thistle, is currently written as *Silybum marianum* in its Latin binomial form; however, an earlier name for this plant was *Carduus marianus*. Consequently, the pharmacopeial name for milk thistle is Cardui marianum, based on the archaic Latin binomial. Accordingly, the approved monograph for drug preparations made from the fruits (seeds) of milk thistle is described as Cardui mariae fructus, whereas the separate unapproved monograph for the herb (i.e., the aerial parts, particularly the leaves) is Cardui mariae herba. Similarly, the pharmacopeial name for Burdock root is Bardanae radix, referring to previous nomenclature for this botanical.

In some monographs, pharmacopeial names were not used as the official title by Commission E. This is particularly the case where two plant parts are described in the same monograph. An example would be Mugwort (Unapproved) where the monograph covers both the herb and root (Artemisiae vulgaris herba and Artemisiae vulgaris radix); the original monograph title was Artemisia vulgaris, the Latin binomial for the herb. In such cases, we use the most appropriate common name and list the Latin binomial in the second line. Another example of this type is the monograph for Belladonna (Approved) where both the belladonna leaf (Belladonnae folium) and the Belladonna root (Belladonnae radix) are included in the monograph. In this example, the official title of the monograph was *Atropa belladonna*, the Latin binomial. We have chosen the English common name Belladonna as the monograph title; however, we also might have used Deadly Nightshade, another common term for this herb. Both common names are listed in *Herbs of Commerce*, although Belladonna is preferred (Foster, 1992).

Composition of Drug

This section includes the plant part, botanical name, plant family, required time of harvest, and, in some cases, some of the primary chemical constituents. We have attempted to preserve the integrity of the monographs by retaining the original nomenclature. However, in some monographs we have added in brackets taxonomic revisions, synonyms, and notes on species actually found in trade, when we thought such an addition was warranted.

Botanical Name
In the body of the monograph we have reprinted the precise Latin names published by Commission E, including parenthetical synonyms. In some instances we have inserted revised synonyms in brackets after the Latin binomial published by Commission E. These synonyms are based on taxonomic revisions supplied by Professor Arthur O. Tucker of Delaware State University. In some instances, we have adopted the *International Code of Botanical Nomenclature* (Greuter et al., 1988) and *Herbs of Commerce* (Foster, 1992) as the basic criteria for publishing synonyms of the Latin binomials used in the monographs.

Latin names in the Composition of Drug section: In the original German versions of the monographs multiple mentions of a genus are written with the genus name spelled in full each time. For example, in Black Psyllium, the genus *Plantago* is mentioned four times: two taxa are represented as being suitable for use as the drug (*P. psyllium* and *P. indica*), with a botanical synonym listed for each taxon (*P. afra* and *P. arenaria* respectively). In accordance with conventional botanical notation, we have abbreviated subsequent mention of the names in the style used above.

As with some *Plantago* species, several species of plants are sometimes found in the same monograph. Another example is the monograph for Goldenrod which includes the species *Solidago virgaurea*, *S. gigantea*, and *S. canadensis*.

A stylistic note: When Latin names are used for the title of the monograph, we have taken the editorial liberty of capitalizing both the genus and species names. Plant parts (e.g., leaf, root, flower) are not capitalized in the monograph title heading. We have repeated this style when referring to the particular monograph anywhere else in the text. Accordingly, the title for the monograph for the leaf of *Echinacea purpurea* is written "Echinacea Purpurea leaf" where the specific name "Purpurea" is being capitalized to denote its being the title of a monograph. The same is true for our treatment of "Ginkgo Biloba Leaf Extract." Nowhere else would we write Ginkgo biloba with a capital "B" — the term usually being italicized to denote its use as a Latin binomial. We hope this does not cause any confusion for our readers.

Plant Family
The original monographs usually do not mention the family name for the plant drug in the "Composition" section. However, we have inserted the family name in brackets after the Latin binomial because knowledge of a plant's botanical relationships can increase general awareness of the plant, its potential chemical profile, and possible similarities of pharmacological actions.

Botanists sometimes use more than one name for a plant family. For example, for members of the composite family, such as the genera *Arnica* (Arnica), *Matricaria* (Chamomile), *Echinacea* (Echinacea, Purple Coneflower), and *Inula* (Elecampane), we have used the newer synonym Asteraceae, although Commission E sometimes uses the term Compositae, the older term and the one still widely employed both in Europe and the U.S. Both names are acceptable. Similarly, we have used Apiaceae instead of Umbelliferae for members of the carrot family, although both terms are accepted by taxonomists. Commission E published the latter name in its monographs. Modern botanical nomenclature requires all plant family names to end in "-aceae."

Chemical Constituents
The Commission E monographs do not include the complete chemistry of herbal drugs. Some of the monographs mention a specific main compound or compounds that are important in contributing to the plant's effectiveness; however, in most cases, a general class of compounds is usually listed, e.g., bitter principles,tannins, essential oil.

Uses

We have chosen the word "Uses" as the section heading, although "Indication" is also an appropriate translation of *Anwendungsgebiete*. The Uses in the Approved Herbs monographs include only those indications approved by the Commission based on the evaluation of the relevant literature. However, this does not represent the total possible range of applications of the herbal drug in folk medicine or in clinical practice.

Phytomedicines licensed in Germany are allowed to be labeled for the approved Commission E use only. Thus, this section becomes one of the most significant sections of the monograph, particularly in Germany where it is an official guide for patients and healthcare practitioners, but also for those outside Germany who are viewing the Commission E process as a potential model for the rational evaluation and regulation of the therapeutic uses of herbs. Where both external and internal uses are given, they are listed separately.

Most of the Uses can be divided into 11 general medical categories: Cardiovascular; Dermatological; Endocrinology, Reproductive System, Obstetrics/Gynecology, and Prostate; Gastrointestinal; Hematology, Lymphatic, and Cancer; Immunology, AIDS, and Infectious Diseases; Liver and Gallbladder; Neurology and Psychiatry; Ophthalmology; Respiratory (lower and upper respiratory tract including ears, nose, throat, sinuses); and Urinary Tract System (kidney, ureter, bladder). A key indicating these categories is given in the Uses Index on page 419.

Contraindications

The Commission reviewed literature to establish conditions or diseases that should be contraindicated with the use of a particular herb. A total of 67 separate contraindications are mentioned in the monographs. They are classified into the same medical categories as noted in Uses above, with the addition of Ophthalmology.

The range of contraindications includes allergy to particular constituents, children and infants, diabetes, pregnancy and lactation, and specific conventional medications (e.g., cardiac glycosides, as is the case for some strong botanicals used clinically in Germany but not widely available in the U.S., i.e., Lily-of-the-valley, Pheasant's Eye herb, and Squill).

In the case of allergies and hypersensitivities (23 herbs and three combinations are noted) the Commission took the conservative view that cross-sensitivities were possible. However, "If [a patient] is not allergic towards these drugs [of a particular plant family] or towards the plant family, there is no reason why he should not use the herbal remedy if it is indicated. *But still he must be informed on it.*" [emphasis added] (Keller, 1992.)

Pregnancy was included as a contraindication if there were bibliographic data that the herbal preparation had been successfully used for self-induced abortion, or if there were experimental data proving a genotoxic risk for some constituents present in the drug in significant amounts. The Commission used a 100-fold safety factor in considerations of genetic risk (Wiedenfeld, 1996). In total, 26 herbs are contraindicated in pregnancy, plus 25 fixed combinations of these herbs (mainly combinations containing either Anise oil or Fennel oil, not the simple fruits/seeds). One herb in injectable form (Echinacea Purpurea herb) is also contraindicated, but this does not apply to oral doses.

For lactation 11 herbs are contraindicated, plus one combination containing Senna leaf. Of these 11, six are anthraquinone-containing stimulant laxatives. (There are actually five herbs; Buckthorn bark and Buckthorn berry are listed in individual monographs.)

Some herbs are contraindicated for conditions involving the liver and gallbladder. A total of eight herbs, plus combinations containing some of these herbs, are contraindicated for various liver disorders. The best known example is Licorice: in cholestatic liver disorders (Licorice plus six combinations containing Licorice) and cirrhosis (Licorice plus five combinations with Licorice). Seven herbs plus 10 combinations are contraindicated for "Liver Disease." Fourteen herbs and 19 fixed combinations are contraindicated in gallstones. For bile duct obstruction, 13 herbs plus 13 combinations containing these herbs are contraindicated.

If the Commission was aware that the diuretic (aka aquaretic) effect of an herb was due to essential oils irritating the kidney, not only was the indication eliminated, but a warning was included to ensure the herb not be used by persons suffering kidney disease. This contraindication appears in at least six monographs (Asparagus root, Juniper berry, Lovage root, Parsley herb and root, Watercress, and White Sandalwood).

Many of the contraindications are based on theoretical considerations, not on case studies. "In most cases the contraindications are not seen as concretely associated with the mentioned herbs, but they were listed as general considerations." (Schilcher, 1997b.)

Finally, the Commission was concerned about the issue of the safety of pregnant and lactating women and children under 12 years of age. As noted above, some of the monographs deal specifically with contraindications for pregnant and nursing women. According to the Medicines Testing Guidelines (1994) and the Fifth Amendment to the Second Medicines Act (2 AMG 76), physicians' observation studies for these groups must be conducted to determine proper dose levels and safety. Since such studies on crude herbs or advanced phytomedicines have been conducted in only a few cases, the following terms apply to the herbal drugs approved by Commission E: "Due to the absence of physician's observational studies this phytomedicine should not be used by pregnant or nursing women or by children under the age of 12." (Schilcher, 1998b).

An index of all contraindications for approved herbs can be found on page 433. As with the Uses section, there is a key in the Contraindications cross-reference showing the groupings of the various conditions by physiological system. An index of contraindications for unapproved herbs can be found on page 681.

Side Effects

As Referee Dr. K. Keller notes, "the consumer probably does not expect...side effects from natural remedies." (Keller, 1992). The Commission took pains to point out possible adverse effects. The monographs also note 74 adverse side effects that may be produced as a result of ingestion of the 186 Approved Herbs. Not surprisingly, there are 96 side effects mentioned for Unapproved Herbs, almost 30 percent more for 108 Unapproved Herbs compared to the Approved. One would expect to see more adverse side effects noted for the Unapproved Herbs — their relative toxicity is often the basis for a negative evaluation.

As with the contraindications, side effects are arranged in a separate index according to 11 medical categories. Side effects of approved herbs include the following examples: ocular accommodation disturbances, albuminuria, allergies, cramps, diarrhea, fever, gastrointestinal disturbance, headache, hematuria, intestinal sluggishness associated with stimulant laxatives, nausea, photosensitization, and vomiting. These include 44 monographs (31 single herbs and 13 Fixed Combinations) listing gastrointestinal disorders (e.g., those associated with ingestion of various saponins) and eight monographs (4 single, 4 combinations) listing photosensitizing properties.

Many of the side effects sections state that in "rare cases" or in "sensitive individuals" the effect may occur, particularly when discussing a possible adverse effect that is not typical of the herb but either has been documented from the literature or is based on theoretical presumptions.

As with the Contraindications section, many monographs do not list adverse side effects, but include the statement "None known." For these herbal drugs for which there is documentation of potential or actual side effects, we have developed two indexes: one each for Approved (page 443) and Unapproved herbal drugs (page 451). In both indexes we have grouped into a key the reported side effects by physiological systems.

Interactions with Other Drugs

One of the benefits the Commission E monographs offer to health professionals and consumers is information on the potential adverse or synergistic reactions associated with the simultaneous use of herbs and conventional drugs. Both well-documented and proposed interactions are listed in a total of 53 monographs. These interactions are described in 38 monographs on single preparations (37 Approved and one Unapproved, Sarsaparilla) plus 15 Fixed Combinations of the Approved herbs. The 38 single herb monographs consist of a total of 32 plants, occasionally with two or more monographs for different parts of the same plant. For example, Buckthorn bark and berry are two monographs as are Eucalyptus leaf and essential oil, Senna leaf and pod, etc. The herbs are shown to interact with substances such as alcohol, conventional drugs (by type or specific drug), caffeine-containing beverages, common nutrients (calcium), and constituents in other herbal drugs.

Not all the interaction data is derived from studies and case histories. Curiously, "Most interactions mentioned in the positive monographs are based on theoretical grounds." (Schilcher, 1997b.) For example, some herbs like Marshmallow root and combinations in which it is included and Flaxseed contain mucilaginous constituents. Thus, at least seven monographs mention that an herbal drug containing mucilage can delay the absorption of other drugs taken simultaneously. These are typical examples of interactions inferred from a theoretical basis (Schilcher, 1997b).

Five of the monographs on herbs with stimulant laxative action (e.g., Aloe, Buckthorn, Senna) contain the following cautionary statement:

> Drug preparations [i.e., herbal laxative drugs] have a higher general toxicity than the pure glycosides, presumably due to the content of aglycones. Experiments pertaining to the genotoxicity of [name of herb] and its preparations are not available. Some positive data were obtained for aloe-emodin, emodin, physcion and chrysophanol. No data are available for their carcinogenicity.

The Commission's concern about this issue probably was based on a single case of cancer in a young woman, allegedly due to danthrone, an anthraquinone laxative that is not present in any Commission E herb, approved or unapproved. There are data from the Salmonella Ames assay and mammalian cell cultures that the laxative constituents lucidin, emodin, and aloe-emodin (three compounds found in four Approved herbs, as far as data from the monograph reveals) could have genotoxic effects, but there are no indications of this from in vitro or in vivo studies or human studies (Tyler, 1996; Steinhoff, 1997a).

An index of herb-drug interactions organized by herb begins on page 475. An index of interactions by conventional pharmaceutical drugs and other substances is found on page 479.

Dosage

The dosage for each herbal drug or herbal combination is shown only in the Approved monographs. Dosage information was gleaned from results of clinical studies, clinical experience by physicians who routinely use herbal drugs in Germany, experience drawn from self-medication, or calculations of a specified active ingredient. For example, for Cascara Sagrada, the dosage range is listed as 20 - 30 mg hydroxyanthracene derivatives daily; this is based on known safe and effective dosage levels for such active ingredients in stimulant laxatives.

The phrase "calculated as..." is frequently used in the dosage sections. This refers to the dosage of an herbal drug based on the calculation of a particular active or marker compound in the herb or extract. In the case of St. John's Wort, for example, the daily dose is 2 - 4 g of the crude herb or the equivalent of 0.2 - 1 mg of total hypericin, usually in the form of a standardized dry extract.

Although most dosages listed in the monographs appear reasonable based on the available literature, a few monographs include what appear to be either excessive or inadequate doses. For example, in the monograph for Rosemary, the internal dose for rosemary essential oil is stated at between 10 to 20 drops. This level appears to be excessive by a factor of 5 to 10. When Rosemary oil was official in the *United States Pharmacopeia* (from 1840 - 1955) the internal dose was specified as 0.1 ml, equivalent to 2 drops. Some authorities say that internal use of rosemary oil may produce abortifacient action, according to Tyler citing Pahlow (Tyler, 1996). However, Schilcher writes that the old USP dosage is inadequate and that adverse reactions to Rosemary oil are not noted in the dosage level recommended in the Commission E monograph (Schilcher, 1997b).

In another example, a dose of 40 mg of crude powdered root of Black Cohosh appears on the surface to be inadequate to produce the intended estrogenic effect for menstrual and menopausal applications. Forty mg is less than 10 percent of the net weight of the average size of a "0" size gelatin capsule of Black Cohosh root powder as it is customarily sold in the U.S. Much of the clinical research upon which the monograph is based refers to 40 mg of powdered root extract equivalent to 40 mg of dried root (1:1 ratio). We have been assured by Dr. Götz Harnischfeger of the phytomedicine manufacturer Schaper and Brümmer that the monograph indeed does stipulate 40 mg of the crude dried root or rhizome (Harnischfeger, 1996).

Prof. Schilcher prefers the term "Posology" for this section but we have translated *Dosierung* as Dosage. Posology is the pharmaceutical term which can suggest both dosage (amount and frequency of administration) and mode of administration, or the galenical form in which the dosage is given, such as tea, tincture, or external ointment (Schilcher, 1997).

Mode of Administration

The mode of administration refers to the method of preparation and form of taking the herb. The earlier monograph format contains a Mode of Administration section. The later format includes Mode of Administration either with the Dosage section or in a separate section.

Various types of pharmaceutical products made from medicinal plants are often referred to as galenical preparations. Preparations are noted for both internal and external uses. They include comminuted or powdered herbs for teas (either as infusions or decoctions), essential oils for inhalation or for addition to salves and ointments (often referred to as semi-solid preparations), pressed juice from the fresh plant, liquid extracts in the form of tinctures and fluidextracts, dry extracts, and solid forms for internal use (tablets and capsules containing powdered herb or dry extract).

In some of the monographs the mode of administration can be quite specific, e.g., in the stipulation of the range of alcohol required in an aqueous-alcoholic extract (for example, 50 - 70 percent in Chaste Tree fruit).

Sometimes the mode of administration will correspond to particular approved uses and plant constituents. For example, Iceland Moss is approved for two uses: "(a) Irritation of the oral and pharyngeal mucous membranes and accompanying dry cough. (b) Loss of appetite." The mode of administration for use (a) is comminuted herb for infusions and other galenical formulations for internal use, based on the mucilage content of the herb; however, a different preparation is stipulated for use (b): "Comminuted herb, preferably for cold macerates and other bitter-tasting preparations for internal use," based on the second main constituent, the bitter principle.

Duration of Administration

The amount of time that a person consumes any medicine, natural or synthetic, is of considerable therapeutic relevance. Accordingly, Commission E has limited the period of use of 45 approved herbal drugs. The old monograph format contains a Duration of Use section after the Mode of Administration section; the new format contains this information in the Special Cautions for Use section found under the Clinical Data heading.

The Commission stipulated either specific ranges of use or a maximum period of use for the approved remedy. This was done for two reasons. First, there were safety concerns; second, in several of the monographs, duration of use was specified as either a minimum or optimum period required for the botanical to provide effective beneficial action. Examples include Ginkgo Biloba Leaf Extract (six to eight weeks minimum use, depending on the indication), Ginseng root (up to three months with a repeated regimen being "feasible"), and Hawthorn leaf with flower (six weeks minimum).

Regarding issues of safety, of particular note is the limitation of the use of stimulant laxatives (Aloe, Buckthorn bark and berry, Cascara Sagrada, Senna leaf and pod, and Rhubarb root) for a period not to exceed one to two weeks. With respect to herbal drugs used for diarrhea (Bilberry fruit, Blackberry leaf, Jambolan bark, Lady's Mantle, Psyllium seed and husk, etc.), the monographs suggest that if the diarrhea persists more than three to four days, a physician must be consulted. Licorice root preparations with a content of 300 mg glycyrrhizin should not exceed four to six weeks. With respect to the popular herb Uva Ursi, used as a urinary tract antiseptic, Commission E stipulates that medicines containing the chemical arbutin should not be taken more than one week or more than five times per year.

For herbs containing hepatotoxic pyrrolizidine alkaloids (PA) (Comfrey leaf and herb, Comfrey root, Petasites root) a duration not to exceed four to six weeks is advised. In both Comfrey monographs the PA level is required to be no more than 100 micrograms per dose; the Comfrey preparations are approved for external use only. In the German market there are specially cultivated varieties (cultivars) of Comfrey that do not contain PAs (Schilcher, 1997b). At any rate, the 100 micrograms PA in the Comfrey monographs is limited to external use only, whereas the monograph for Petasites root is limited to only 1 microgram PA, due to its approval for internal use. Chapter 15 consists of a table listing all the limitations of Duration of Administration for Approved Herbs. See page 483.

Risks

The risks associated with the use of a particular botanical are enumerated in the Unapproved Herbs monographs. In many cases, the risks cited constitute concern by the Commission of the potential of the herb to produce adverse effects. In cases where the assessment of known or potential risks was deemed relatively high and without adequate documentation of benefit for the preparation (high risk to benefit ratio), the Commission chose a negative evaluation. In such cases the negatively evaluated medicinal plant should be taken from the market soon and not in 2004. Nearly all products for internal use made from Comfrey root were removed from the market in 1992 in accordance with section 8 of the Second Medicines Act of 1976 (Schilcher, 1997b).

Evaluation

For all herbs in the Unapproved Herbs section the Commission has published a justification for its negative assessment. In most cases, the available literature did not adequately document the historical and current popular use of the herbal drug. This does not mean that the particular medicinal plant is not effective, just that when the Commission was making its evaluation, the scientific material was inadequate in "a natural science sense." (Schilcher, 1997b.) Also, for many of the Unapproved herbs, in light of the potential risks involved, a positive assessment could not be allowed. Where no clear benefit is present, the potential risks are given more weight than similar risks applied to an Approved Herb with a better documented benefit.

Actions

In almost all of the Approved Monographs and in some of the Unapproved Monographs, the Actions (*Wirkungen*) section refers to pharmacological actions carried out in laboratory conditions, either experimentally in vitro, or in vivo in test animals, and in animal organs. These actions usually do not refer to observations based on human clinical trials and are meant to help describe the potential activity of the herbal drug. Prof. Schilcher has translated this section as "Medicinal Actions," a term that implies (to us) medicinal applications, which we are not sure we are ready to accept. Hence, we use only the word Actions, qualifying it here as pharmacological.

TYPES OF MONOGRAPHS

Single Herbs — Monopreparations

The vast majority of monographs pertain to single herbs, that is, herb sold as drug products generally referred to as monopreparations, as distinguished from more complex formulas containing multiple herbs in combination. As noted in table 15, there are 296 monographs dealing with single herbs: 186 approved and 110 unapproved.

Fixed Combinations

Fixed combinations refer to formulas containing multiple herbal ingredients. In phytotherapy the use of fixed combinations is quite typical (Schilcher, 1997b). Until 1990 the majority of herbs used in German phytotherapy were combinations. The Commission reviewed a total of only 72 combinations of herbs. Of these, 66 were approved and 6 were not approved. Unlike some of the classic herbal formulas described in systems of traditional medicine in Asia (e.g., Traditional Chinese Medicine and Ayurvedic medicine of India) where formulas routinely contain up to a dozen or more botanicals, the herbal formulas reviewed by Commission E generally contain two to three herbs, sometimes four, or occasionally five. According to German drug regulations in the AMG for the registration of combinations, a manufacturer must prove that "every medicinally active component contributes to the positive evaluation of the medicine." (Steinhoff, 1997b.)

A review of the approved combinations indicates that the largest single category of use is for digestive complaints (35 combinations). These contain most possible combinations of the following herbs (or their essential oils): Anise seed, Angelica root, Bitter Orange peel, Caraway seed, German Chamomile flower, Fennel seed, Gentian root, Peppermint leaf, and Wormwood. Some formulas also include Artichoke leaf or Dandelion root to help increase bile production.

The next largest category of fixed combinations consists of herb formulas approved for colds, flus and catarrhal conditions of the upper respiratory tract with or without viscous phlegm, dry or spastic cough, and related conditions (21 combinations). In general, these formulas include Camphor, Eucalyptus essential oil, or Purified Turpentine oil, combined with other herbs, such as Ivy leaf and Primrose root.

The third largest category of indications for which fixed combinations are approved is unrest and insomnia due to nervousness. The herbs in these combinations are Hops, Lemon Balm, Passionflower, and Valerian root.

In at least one instance, an Unapproved herb is included in an Approved Fixed Combination based on the effective action of the herb with the other Approved herbs. Oleander leaf powdered extract (unapproved by itself), with its positively inotropic and negatively chronotropic actions, is combined with Pheasant's Eye fluidextract, Lily-of-the-valley powdered extract, and Squill powdered extract for "Mild, limited heart action and circulatory instability." The Oleander leaf monograph (Unapproved) reads, "Since the effectiveness of oleander leaf preparations is not yet adequately documented, and in considering that there is no correlation between the content of individual glycosides and the efficacy of the herb, a therapeutic administration of oleander leaf is not justifiable." This was the case in 1990, when the Oleander monograph was written. By 1993, when the Fixed Combination containing Oleander powdered leaf extract was approved, however, the pharmacokinetics of oleandrin were better known. "For oleandrin, an absorption rate of 86 percent is given." This rate is similar to that of digoxin (Schilcher, 1997b). This is in keeping with the general trend of the Commission after 1993 to approve plant extracts rather than whole plants.

Evaluation Criteria for Fixed Combinations Established by Commission E in 1989

The following was published by the German Federal Health Agency (BGA)

Fixed drug combinations are traditionally used in phytotherapy. Commission E evaluates fixed drug combinations exclusively from plants, plant parts, and preparations thereof, which are not prepared according to homeopathic processes or are used under aspects of homeopathic or anthroposophic therapy. In this pursuit, Commission E is guided by the following criteria:

Each medicinally effective component must contribute to the positive evaluation of effectiveness and safety. The monographs of Commission E and other scientific findings must be considered. For the evaluation of combinations in regard to benefit/risk the following considerations are to be observed:
  – basic idea
  – effectiveness of the combination
  – safety of the combination

I. Basic Idea:
The medicinally active components each must make a positive contribution to the evaluation of the total preparation; they must contribute to its effectiveness and safety. Proof of effectiveness may be established through clinical or pharmacological documentation for each component, or through documentation for the whole preparation. The components must be at a dosage appropriate for effectiveness.

II. Effectiveness of the Fixed Combination
A positive evaluation is given when the medicinally active component contributes to therapeutic effectiveness. Medicinally active components may also be present, whose contribution to the effectiveness of the whole combination can be explained on the basis of its effects. The combination must specifically indicate therapy or prophylaxis. An indication is a condition of illness, a functional disturbance, a syndrome, or a pathological unit of a known type. It is conceivable that the single components of a fixed combination can, at the same time, bring relief for various symptoms of such a condition or illness. Yet, it would not be correct to consider each symptom as an indication for a fixed combination, since this symptom may also occur with other diseases, and the other components may be irrelevant for this symptom. A combination with components acting in the same way is possible.

Fixed combinations can be considered positive if:
1. additive synergistic effects of the components

(continued on next page)

Evaluation Criteria for Fixed Combinations Established by Commission E in 1989 (cont'd)

with equal or various targets exist, and/or
2. a more than additive effect of the fixed combination occurs compared to the single components, and/or
3. side effects of a single component are lessened or negated (e.g., dosage reduction of components acting in the same direction), and/or
4. the combination instigates a therapy simplification or improvement in therapy safety. This can be the case if:
   an improvement of compliance (by reduction of the medication frequency and/or simplification of dosage administration), and/or an improvement in absorption, and/or an avoidance of galenic incompatibilities is obtained, and/or
5. one of the medicinally active components lessens or negates one or more of the side effects of another component, if the side effect normally occurs.

III. Safety of the Fixed Combination
1. Considerable pharmacokinetic and/or pharmacodynamic interactions exist that do not improve the benefit/risk ratio, or even worsen it.
2. The half-life and/or the duration of the actions of the medicinally active components differ widely. However, this is not necessarily correct, if it can be demonstrated that the combination is clinically of benefit, despite this time-related difference.
3. The combination contains a component which is intended to effect an unpleasant reaction, in order to prevent abuse.

The safety of all fixed combinations is to be tested with suitable methods. However, this is not necessary for fixed combinations with components known to be medicinally active, if the safety is determined from the formulation, dosage, form of administration, and range of indications based on scientific data. (Federal Health Agency, 1989)

Component Characteristics

Component characteristics refer to herbal materials added to various combinations of herbs and other substances for which the efficacy of the formula may depend on the safety and efficacy of a particular ingredient. For example, in the case of Cajeput oil, the Commission decided that there was adequate evidence to approve the combination of this essential oil with other botanical ingredients in 43 formulas corresponding to 43 claimed uses found in the German market. Similarly, the Commission approved Nasturtium herb and leaf as an ingredient in 12 botanical formulas and their 12 corresponding uses found in the market.

The Commission found 10 herbs for which it did not approve combinations with the herb as a component, including Aspen bark, Basil oil, California Poppy, Purple Coneflower root (*Echinacea purpurea*), and Mistletoe berry and stem. Interestingly, in the same year that the Commission published the monograph on Echinacea purpurea root as an Unapproved Component Characteristic (1992), a clinical study was published in which an extract of *E. purpurea* root was found to be effective in shortening the severity and duration of colds and flus (Bräunig et al., 1992).

Many of the Unapproved Component Characteristics are combined with homeopathic drugs, vitamins and other nutritional components (e.g., alpha-tocopherol acetate), phytochemicals (e.g., cineole, globulin from pumpkin seed flower, beta-sitosterol, esculin), and Unapproved Herbs (e.g., Night-blooming Cereus flowers, Sassafras root bark). Many herbs that are combined with the primary component herb are listed by common name only in the Approved and Unapproved Component Characteristics sections. Because of the number of botanicals listed and their minor importance, we have not included the Latin binomial for each herb listed.

Bath Additives

Therapeutic baths containing herbs are a popular method of treatment in Europe, where this practice is known as *balneology*. By putting crude herbs or herbal extracts and essential oils into hot bath water, the body is able to gradually absorb some of the active phytochemicals from the herbs, as the pores open in the hot water. Although some herbs are approved for use in baths (e.g., Chamomile, Valerian), the Commission did not review herbs to be used in this manner. In 1988 Commission B8 was established to assess the safety and efficacy of all bath additives, thereby removing such review from the scope of Commission E (Busse, 1997b).

INDEXES AND CROSS-REFERENCES

In order to make this publication as useful as possible, particularly to health professionals and researchers, we have attempted to provide as much information as possible in the form of indexes and cross-references. This allows for a "user-friendly" method of accessing information by looking up a particular use, side effect, contraindication, or drug interaction and then referring to a specific monograph. When these indexes are being used as a quick reference, the reader is encouraged to refer to the monograph for more complete information. The indexes and cross-references are not intended to be used as the sole mechanism in making therapeutic decisions but instead as a skeletal reference to the monographs — a database for research. Similarly, to help the reader with the taxonomy and nomenclature, cross-references of English, German, Latin, and pharmacopeial names are provided, as well as a column showing the herbs by botanical family.

Uses and Indications of Approved Herbs Index

This section, condensed from the monographs, provides information on the appropriate use of herbs. It links medical indications and uses cited in the text and the Approved Herbs found effective in their treatment. However, some of the herbs listed here may have been found effective for treatment of minor symptoms or for prevention of a condition or disease, or in some cases as adjuvant (secondary) therapy. For example, Blonde Psyllium seed husk is used as an adjuvant therapy for anal fissures — a mild laxative to soften the stool but not directly beneficial to the anal fissures themselves. Herbs in approved fixed combinations are abbreviated "F.C."

The information is prepared as a guide for health professionals, researchers, and consumers but should not be considered a suggestion for self-medication. It is essential that the reader refer to the complete monograph in order to view the role the herb may provide for each indication as well as any contraindications and side effects. A guide of indications by medical category is included to help identify the types of indications listed in this section. Immediately following this guide, the herbs are listed alphabetically under each indication.

Contraindications of Approved Herbs Index

This chapter, condensed from the monographs, provides contraindications cited in the text with the herbs that should be avoided with particular conditions or diseases. It is essential that the reader refer to the complete monograph before making any therapeutic judgements. For example, the contraindication listed in the Anise seed monograph is "allergy to anise and anethole" but this section lists Anise seed under "Allergy/ Hypersensitivity" without specifying an allergy to a particular constituent of the herb. A guide of contraindications by medical category is included to help identify the types of contraindications listed in this section. Immediately following this guide, the herbs are listed alphabetically under each contraindication.

Side Effects of Approved and Unapproved Herbs Indexes

There are two indexes, both condensed from the monographs, that list potential adverse side effects of Approved Herbs and Unapproved Herbs. These are listed in an index format. The listing of a particular herb to a corresponding side effect does not necessarily constitute a clear correlation of the herb with the effect; it means that it may be produced under certain conditions in some individuals. It is essential that the reader refer to the complete monograph for the available data included by the Commission before making any therapeutic judgments. Side effects are sometimes only observed "in rare cases" and/or "in sensitive individuals." For example, nausea and vomiting are listed here as possible side effects of Uva Ursi. However, the monograph clarifies that "nausea and vomiting may occur in persons with sensitive stomachs." Thus, inclusion of a particular herb under a corresponding side effect should not be interpreted as an inevitable result of using the herb.

A guide of side effects by medical category is included to help identify the types of side effects listed in this section. Immediately following this guide, the herbs are listed alphabetically under each side effect.

Interactions with Conventional Drugs Index

This section, condensed from the monographs, summarizes all the possible antagonistic or synergistic interactions an herb may have with conventional pharmaceutical medicines, as determined by the literature available to the Commission. The interactions are divided into two sub-indexes: by the herb with the corresponding drugs and by drug and other substance with the corresponding herbs. It is essential that the reader refer to the complete herb monograph before making any therapeutic judgments.

Pharmacological Actions of Approved and Unapproved Herbs Indexes

There are two indexes, both condensed from the monographs, that provide a list of pharmacological actions of Approved and Unapproved Herbs. In some cases, the pharmacological actions listed were demonstrated in in vitro experiments or in vivo studies (on animals) but may not have been confirmed in human clinical trials. Thus, they are not necessarily correlated to the activity observed in human clinical trials and/or clinical experience. Their inclusion is intended to help health professionals understand the potential activity, risks, or benefits of the herb. It is essential that the reader refer to the complete herb monograph before making any therapeutic judgments.

A guide of pharmacological actions by medical category is included to help identify the types of actions listed in this chapter. Immediately following this guide, the herbs are listed alphabetically under each pharmacological action.

Duration of Administration for Approved Herbs Index

This section consists of a table listing 42 Approved Herbs for which the monographs note some time limitation of administration. In general, most of the Approved Herbs are relatively safe to take without limiting the duration of use. However, responsible therapeutic use of some herbs may require that they be used for only a set period of time. This is due to several factors, including concern regarding laxative dependence and potential intestinal sluggishness for stimulant laxatives. Nine herbs listed in this section are approved to treat diarrhea; in cases where the diarrhea persists for more than 3 to 4 days, the monograph instructs the patient to seek medical advice. The rationale for the limitation of administration of other herbs is not explained in some of the monographs.

Taxonomic Cross-Reference

The taxonomic cross-reference provides a means of accessing the monographs using different types of nomenclature. Five separate indexes are provided: English common name, Latin binomial, family name, pharmacopeial name, and German common name.

Chemical Glossary and Index

We have provided a comprehensive chemical index so the reader may locate those herbs that contain a compound or class of compounds, included in each herb's monograph. This index presents definitions of the chemical classifications listed in the monographs and an index of herbs by compound.

Despite the wealth of information available on the chemical constituents of most of the herbs reviewed by Commission E and because the monographs are intended as therapeutic guides, the Commission chose to mention only compounds or the general classes of naturally occurring phytochemicals (tannins, flavonoids, saponins, etc.) believed to contribute to the plant drug's efficacy. The chemical index lists only those compounds and classes of chemicals mentioned in the monographs.

In some cases only one main compound is mentioned, due to safety concerns. An example is the monograph for Nutmeg (Unapproved), which lists the safrole content but does not mention myristicin, a chemical whose name is derived from Nutmeg's genus (generic) name, *Myristica*, and that has known hallucinogenic effects when taken in excessive dosage (Hocking, 1997). Consequently, in the chemical tables, myristicin is mentioned only with Parsley seed, not Nutmeg.

Within each monograph chemical constituents are found generally in the Composition of Drug section. However, they are sometimes mentioned in other sections. For example, in the Cinchona bark monograph quinidine and quinine are mentioned in the Contraindications and Side Effects sections.

GLOSSARY OF ANATOMICAL, BOTANICAL, MEDICAL, PHARMACEUTICAL, AND PHYSIOLOGICAL TERMS

To help the general reader with the various technical terms used in the translations of the monographs, we have provided definitions for most of the technical or uncommon terms found in the monographs. These include terms from botany, medicine, pharmacy, and human anatomy and physiology. Chemical and biochemical terms are not defined in this glossary but can be found in the Chemical Glossary and Index (see above).

EUROPEAN REGULATORY LITERATURE

Excerpts from the *German Pharmacopoeia*

The *German Pharmacopoiea* (*Deutsches Arzneibuch*, or *DAB*) contains monographs on the quality and standards of many herbal drugs, medicinal plant preparations, and natural substances (e.g., essential oils) sold in Germany. As is customary in pharmacopoeial standards monographs, the approved medicinal uses of the herb are not listed, but instead they contain the standards for assuring the proper identity and purity of the herbal drug. This section contains six monographs as examples of the level of quality control measures required for manufacturers of phytomedicines in Germany. Included are monographs taken from *DAB* 8, *DAB* 9, and *DAB* 10: Hawthorn fluidextract *DAB* 10 (Crataegi extractum fluidum), Hawthorn leaf with flower (Crataegi folium cum flore), Horse Chestnut seed (Hippocastani semen), Standardized Horse Chestnut seed extract (Hippocastani semen extractum siccum normatum), Lemon Balm *DAB* 10 (Melissae folium), and Milk Thistle fruit (Cardui mariae fructus). When the work of Commission E was terminated in 1994, *DAB* 10 was valid; currently *DAB* 1997 is valid (Schilcher, 1997b). ABC received permission to reprint translations of these monographs from the publisher, *Deutscher Apotheker Verlag* in Stuttgart, Germany. Consistent with European harmonization efforts, current work on updating the monographs for the *DAB* is being conducted in concert with the *European Pharmacopoeia* (Koerner, 1997).

Excerpts from the *European Pharmacopoeia*

We are grateful to Dr. A. Artiges of the *European Pharmacopoeia* Commission of the European Department for the Quality of Medicines, the Council of Europe, Strasbourg, France, for permission to include several samples of the monographs for herbal drugs. These monographs represent quality and identity standards and test methods for many herbal drugs sold in Europe and are included in this book as examples of monographs produced to help ensure proper identity and quality of herbal drugs. Monographs for the *European Pharmacopoeia* are produced by a joint effort of scientists and health professionals from many countries in Western Europe.

We have included sections explaining methods for formulation of leading dosage forms: Extracta (extracts), Pulveres (powders), and Tincturae (tinctures). These sections include definitions of the dosage forms and instructions in their preparation. We also include the following six monographs on herbal drugs: Hamamelidis Folium (Witch Hazel leaf), Matricariae Flos (German Chamomile flower), Sennae Folium (Senna leaf), Sennae Fructus Acutifoliae (Alexandrian Senna pods), Sennae Fructus Angustifoliae (Tinnevelly Senna pods), and Valerianae Radix (Valerian root). These monographs do not include therapeutic information found in those produced by Commission E; they include only pharmaceutical quality parameters and methods, including methods to determine identity, and descriptions of tests and assay methods to determine purity, including the types of reagents and related chemicals required.

EEC Standards for Quality of Herbal Remedies

In 1975 the European Economic Community (EEC) published Directive 75/318/EEC dealing with the special problems associated with herbal medicines (e.g., multiple chemical compounds and the variability of these compounds). In particular, the directive attempts to clarify distinctions between herbs and conventional drugs ("chemically defined active ingredients"). The directive notes, "Consistent quality for products of vegetable origin can only be assured if the starting materials are defined in a rigorous and detailed manner, including the specific botanical identification of the plant material used. It is also important to know the geographical source and conditions under which the vegetable drug is obtained in order to ensure material of a consistent quality." (EEC, 1975.) This section includes guidelines for qualitative and quantitative details of the constituents, descriptions of the method of preparation, quality control of the herbal preparations (if different from the dried herb, e.g., analysis of the starting material, tests for microbiological quality, detection of pesticide residues, fumigants, solvents, radioactivity, heavy metals, etc.), and other control tests that must be conducted during the manufacturing process.

Translation of the Monographs

Archaic Language

In some of the original German text, archaic or out-of-date medical terms were used, some of which do not translate easily into English. An example is the German word *Sympathalgie*, meaning facial neuralgia (*Gesichtsneuralgie*), a term found in the Nux Vomica monograph. Other terms include antiphlogistic (*antiphlogistisch*), an old term for antiinflammatory, and secretolytic (*sekretolytisch*) for anti-secretory, to describe the action of Verbena.

Brightening or Coloring Agent

Schmuckdroge in the Evaluation section of some Unapproved Herbs has been translated as "brightening agent" in reference to the addition of color to a tea mixture. "Coloring agent" is also used in some of the translations. With Unapproved herbs that are allowed as brightening agents or flavor corrigents (see below), the herbs did not receive a positive evaluation because they either lacked adequate scientific documentation of historical use or they may pose some toxicity when used in normal doses. However, their use in small amounts with other ingredients does not constitute a problem regarding safety. Thus, the Commission approved their uses for color but not for any added therapeutic benefits. Examples of herbs that were negatively evaluated for therapeutic use but were allowed as brightening agents include Roman Chamomile (safe, efficacy undocumented), Cornflower (safe, efficacy undocumented), and Delphinium flower (unsafe alkaloids at normal dose constitutes risk but safe as a coloring agent at one percent level).

Comminuted

In many of the monographs in the section on Mode of Administration the word *Zerkleinerte* has been translated as *comminuted*, a term meaning to reduce to small particles or powder by crushing, grinding, or powdering. Originally, we considered using the word *ground* to denote the physical action of crushing the herbal material into an almost powdered form. However, since "comminuted" can refer to both a coarse as well as a fine powder form and thus has a wider range of meaning than either *ground* or *powdered*, we chose this somewhat archaic but more precise term.

Drug vs. Herb

In most cases in the monographs, the word herb refers to the aerial or aboveground portion of a plant. The word *droge* refers to whatever part or parts of the plant are officially listed in the monograph and therefore could refer to any plant parts. In this sense, the term drug is used in its pharmaceutical meaning of crude drug, a term formerly used in pharmacy to refer to herbs and other medicinal plant materials in their dried (from Old Dutch *droog*, to dry) whole, cut, or powdered forms, before they have undergone any additional pharmaceutical processing, i.e., been made into a tincture, fluidextract, standardized extract, etc. It should also be noted that in Germany, herbs are approved as legitimate drugs and, therefore, the term drug also takes on a legal/regulatory connotation as part of an approved system of medicine.

Evaluation

The section at the end of each Unapproved monograph is called *Beurteilung*. It can be translated Assessment, Evaluation, Judgment, or Recommendation. We have chosen Evaluation for the section where Commission E explains why the herb was not approved.

Flavor Corrigent

The Evaluation section of some of the monographs of Unapproved Herbs cites the use of an herb as a "flavor corrigent" (*Geschmackskorrigenz*) — a term used to denote an agent added to others to modify or correct the actions of other ingredients, in this case, to make a positive contribution to flavor. For example, the monographs for Basil leaf, Buchu leaf, Hyssop herb, Orris root, and Rose Hip and seed are unapproved for drug use, but each are approved as a "corrigent" to add to the taste of teas. The herbs did not receive a positive evaluation because they lacked adequate scientific documentation of historical use; however, there is no problem regarding safety. Thus, the Commission approved their uses for flavor purposes when added to other herbs in a tea mixture — they do not contribute any documented therapeutic benefits.

Irrigation Therapy

We have translated *Flüssigkeitszufuhr* as "irrigation therapy," denoting either the washing out of a cavity or area with fluids or, literally, the introduction of liquids, referring to "more than average intake of liquid, aquaresis." (Franz, 1997.) Schilcher notes that enough liquids must be drunk to reduce microorganisms in the lower urinary tract and kidneys to pass liquids freely, without electrolyte content. This process is aquaresis, but is not a classic diuretic effect (Schilcher, 1998a). Irrigation therapy is noted in monographs for Asparagus root, Goldenrod, Parsley herb and root, and others.

Name of Drug

We have translated *Bestandteile des Arzneimittels* as "Name of Drug" for the initial section of most monographs. It could also be translated "Part of Drug," "Constituents of Drug," or as "Description of Drug." However, "description" might be misinterpreted as a botanical description of the plant itself. Professor Schilcher in his English translations in *Phytotherapy in Paediatrics* has used "Official Name" in reference to the fact that the pharmacopeial name for the monograph was found in this first section. However, since we included the preferred English common name for the benefit of English readers, we could not use "Official Name" as the designation in this section.

None Known

In many of the monographs the term *Keine bekannt* was used, which we have translated as "None known." This phrase often appears under the Contraindications, Side Effects, and Interactions with Other Drugs sections and refers to the fact that the Commission was unable to find any reports in the literature to justify comments under these respective sections. Prof. Schilcher has translated this as "None reported," which he says more accurately reflects the Commission's meaning.

Pharmacopeia/Pharmacopoeia

We prefer the more modern spelling of pharmacopeia when using this word in a generic sense. However, some pharmacopeias still use the older spelling (with the "o") and whenever the official title of a volume is used, we defer to the publisher.

Revision vs. Correction

As noted previously, the Commission published at least 83 revisions to previous monographs. These revisions include changed dosage, altered or added warnings, side effects, and so on. These revisions were known as *Berichtigung*, which also means "correction" or "amendment."

Seed vs. Fruit

In common English usage in the U.S. for some herbs, the word "seed" is often used to refer to plant parts that are, from a strictly botanical view, actually fruits. Examples include Milk Thistle "seed," Anise and Fennel "seeds," and Parsley "seed" — all fruits. In botany a fruit is the matured pistil or ovary of the flower with or without accessory structures; a seed is a fertilized or ripened ovule containing an embryo, with one or two seed coats and with or without endosperm (albumin) (Hocking, 1968). Another authoritative text notes that seeds consist of a kernel surrounded by one, two, or three seed coats and that "care must be taken to distinguish seeds from fruits or parts of fruits containing a single seed, e.g., cereals and the mericarps of the Umbelliferae." (Trease and Evans, 1966.) In the case of Milk Thistle, we have designated the plant part as fruit in keeping with the official pharmacopeial name of the monograph, Cardui mariani fructus. However, with Anise, Fennel, and Parsley we have used the term seed as stylistic preference due to common usage.

Teas or Infusions

In the Mode of Administration section we have translated *Aufgüsse* as "infusions" rather than "teas." This refers to the act of pouring boiling water over some chopped herbs and allowing the mixture to steep for several minutes. A tea that is made by adding boiling water and continuing to add more heat to the mixture is called a decoction, and is usually reserved for making water extracts of heavy, dense plant materials, such as roots, barks, and sometimes seeds. The precise methods of preparation for infusions and decoctions is presented in the eighth edition of the *German Pharmacopoeia* (*DAB 8*).

REFERENCES TO OTHER COMPENDIA

Some of the Commission E monographs cite drug standards in the *German Pharmacopoeia* (*Deutsches Arzneibuch*), the *Swiss Pharmacopoeia* (*Pharmacopoea Helvetica*), or the *Austrian Pharmacopoeia* (*Osterreichisches Arzneibuch*). When a reference to such a compendium is made, the Commission is citing that pharmacopeia as the standard for identity and purity of the drug material for which Commission E is providing therapeutic guidance. For example, in the Commission E monograph for Condurango bark the Dosage section refers to the sixth edition of the *Swiss Pharmacopoeia* (*Pharmacopoea Helvetica VI*) in citing the standard for the liquid extract; water extract, hydroalcoholic extract, and tincture are all referenced to the *Erg. B 6.* (*Ergänzungsbuch zum Deutsche Arzneibuch, Sechste Ausgabe, Supplement to the German Pharmacopoeia, Sixth Edition*). The *Erg. B 6* contains many additional herbal monographs (Schilcher, 1997b).

German Federal Gazette Numbers

At the top of each monograph we have provided the original date of publication and the date(s) of any revision(s) or replacement. However, we have not included the actual *Federal Gazette* (*Bundesanzeiger*) issue number, as originally cited in each German monograph. We have provided a complete list of all monographs published by Commission E, including the date of publication and *Bundesanzeiger* issue number for each monograph, listed alphabetically by official monograph title (usually the Latin pharmacopeial name). This list is found in an appendix on page 593. Researchers interested in obtaining the original German version of a monograph are referred to this section.

Comments on Specific Monographs

Editor's Notes

Although the Commission E monographs are considered authoritative in their review of safety and efficacy criteria, we have included an "editor's note" in brackets when we want to clarify a statement in the monograph, or when we may question a statement or conclusion of the Commission, or if we wish to direct the reader to another monograph on a plant in the same genus. For example, some herbs that are Approved are also found in the Unapproved section, according to the species or plant part used. Examples include two types of Echinacea in each section, two monographs for Ginkgo biloba, four for Hawthorn, and two for Horse Chestnut. However, insofar as we have made such comments on a case-by-case basis, our review and possible challenge of such statements by Commission E have not been carried out in a comprehensive manner; we have commented in areas that we considered worthy of mention. The following specific comments provide additional information on commonly used herbs. Also we have included editor's notes in brackets in numerous monographs where we have chosen to provide additional information to help explain the text (e.g., the four stages of heart disease in the Hawthorn leaf with flower monograph and the stages of benign prostatic hyperplasia in Saw Palmetto).

Chamomile

German Chamomile is approved for both internal use (digestive) and external use. However, there is no approval for chamomile internally for its reputed mild sedative effects. This is presumably because no scientific literature supported any central nervous system effects of chamomile when the Commission published the monograph in 1984 or when it was revised in 1990. However, in 1994 and 1996 two pharmacological studies on apigenin, a constituent in the extract of chamomile, found that the compound binds at benzodiazepine receptor sites in the human brain (Viola et al., 1996). This research, although still preliminary, offers for the first time a molecular-pharmacological rationale for understanding a potential sedative action for chamomile. Therefore, if the Commission were still evaluating herbs — which it is not — German Chamomile flowers could be reviewed in light of this new data; however, chamomile still would not be approved for mild sedative purposes because the experimental data cannot be transferred to human experience without clinical confirmation (Schilcher, 1997b).

Echinacea

Of the four Echinacea monographs, two are positive (*Echinacea pallida* root and *E. purpurea* leaf) and two are negative (*E. purpurea* root and *E. angustifolia* root). Echinacea expert Steven Foster has noted that based on a historical confusion of plant identity and the persistence of adulterated commercial supplies of *E. purpurea* root with *Parthenium integrifolium*, the assumption was made by some observers that the Commission decided to place *E. purpurea* root in a negative category. Work on the chemistry of vouchered *Echinacea* species from 1988 onward by R. Bauer and H. Wagner at the Institute for Pharmaceutical Biology in Munich revealed clear chemical profiles for *E. angustifolia* and *E. pallida* (Bauer and Wagner, 1991). As a result, it became obvious that earlier pharmacological studies on *E. angustifolia* actually involved *E. pallida*. Historically, *E. pallida* and *E. angustifolia* have been offered to the trade in mixed lots under the name "Kansas Snake root." Therefore, lack of current pharmacological and clinical studies on *E. angustifolia* root and *E. angustifolia/E. pallida* aerial (above-ground) parts resulted in the issuance of a negative monograph until further scientific information becomes available (Foster, 1996).

However, despite previous problems concerning the botanical identity of *Echinacea* species in commercial preparations and research materials, the true reason for the disparity in approvals is based on the availability of the research on the respective species. According to Prof. Schilcher, experimental and clinical studies are available on the flowering tops (herb) and roots of *E. purpurea*, roots of *E. pallida*, and roots of *E. angustifolia*. The Commission decided that only the results from the research conducted on the fresh plant juice from the flowering herb of *E. purpurea* and from the water-alcohol extract of *E. pallida* roots are adequate for a positive monograph. In the meantime there have been additional studies based on the alcoholic extract of the roots of *E. purpurea*, that in Schilcher's personal opinion should become a positive monograph (Schilcher, 1997b). Clinical research was carried out in 1992 on an extract of the root of *E. purpurea*, suggesting clinical benefits in patients with colds and flus (Bräunig et al., 1992). The same year Commission E published a monograph on *E. purpurea* root as an Unapproved Component Characteristic, although not all members of the Commission supported this decision (Schilcher, 1997b).

The monograph on Echinacea Pallida root is an example of a case where specifications based on a proprietary extract of an herb were approved. This preparation consists of a "tincture (1:5) with 50 percent (v/v) ethanol prepared from a native dry extract (50 percent ethanol, 7 to 11:1) corresponding to 900 mg of the dried plant."

It should also be noted that in Germany, physicians previously had access to injectable drug products made from either a monopreparation of *E. purpurea* herb juice or a fixed combination that contained *E. pallida*. Thus, the monographs for *E. purpurea* herb and *E. pallida* root both note that there are adverse side effects associated with intraperitoneal (injectable) forms of these echinacea products. There are no contraindications or adverse effects reported for echinacea products taken orally.

Eleuthero (Siberian Ginseng)

The Commission notes an interesting contraindication for the drug made from the roots and rhizomes of the herb Eleuthero (Siberian ginseng, *Eleutherococcus senticosus*, sometimes still referred to in the Chinese literature by its former Latin binomial, *Acanthopanax senticosus*). The monograph states that it is contraindicated for hypertension. Eleuthero is generally considered by most herbalists in the U.S. to be milder in activity than the more stimulating root of Asian Ginseng (*Panax ginseng*). However, there is documentation in the literature of at least two studies in which it was recommended that Eleuthero not be given to persons with a blood pressure in excess of 180/90 mm Hg (Farnsworth, 1985). Presumably, this information prompted the Commission to note this possible adverse effect in some people and thus the contraindication.

Ginger

An example of a warning about which we have taken issue can be found in the monograph on Ginger root. Commission E contraindicates the common spice as a remedy for morning sickness during pregnancy. However, there is no evidence that the therapeutic dosage for antinauseant activity cited by Commission E (1 gram of dried root) produces any harm to either the fetus or the mother. The Commission presumably based its caution on two studies published in the 1980s in Japan on 6-gingerol, one of the compounds isolated from ginger rhizome. In vitro tests indicated that the gingerol had mutagenic activity in vitro at high doses (Namakura and Tamamoto, 1982; Nagabhushan et al., 1987). However, other compounds in ginger have been found to exhibit anti-mutagenic activity (Kada et al., 1978). Ginger is also widely used in Traditional Chinese Medicine (TCM), but without contraindications in pregnancy. "On the contrary, ginger has been traditionally used for nausea and vomiting in pregnancy, though as in typical TCM usage, rarely by itself. There is no lack of remedies for these conditions using ginger. Also, there is no contraindication of ginger in any of the recent issues of the *Pharmacopoeia of the People's Republic of China* (newest edition, 1995); the dosage is 3-9 grams for both fresh and dried ginger." (Leung, 1998). A literature review of all available clinical studies on ginger could find no scientific or medical evidence for Commission E's contraindication during pregnancy (Fulder and Tenne, 1996). Prof. Schilcher agrees with this assessment of ginger's presumed safety during pregnancy (Schilcher, 1997b).

Using the fact that ginger is approved by Commission E as a nonprescription remedy for motion sickness in Germany, in 1995 the European-American Phytomedicine Coalition (EAPC) filed a citizens petition with the FDA for ginger to be reviewed as an OTC drug for anti-nausea and motion sickness (Pinco and Israelsen, 1995). The petition included clinical studies on ginger in experimental conditions as well as in situ (e.g., with first-time sailors at sea). It also contained extensive market data in Europe and other countries where ginger is employed as a medicine. The totality of the materials support the safety and efficacy of ginger as a medicine. By spring 1998 the FDA had not yet responded to this petition.

Ginkgo

A monograph for ginkgo leaf and various types of extracts from Ginkgo leaf is listed as unapproved; a standardized dry extract of *Ginkgo biloba* leaf is listed in the approved section. The 1993 and 1994 monographs on *Ginkgo biloba* clearly focus on specific extracts or preparations rather than on the plant as a whole. For instance, the approved Ginkgo extract is the extract on which almost all the scientific and clinical studies on the effectiveness of Ginkgo biloba extract have been carried out (Foster, 1996). Thus, only the acetone-water extract of Ginkgo would be approved. The Commission's evaluation on ginkgo was based on the review of a 210-page monograph on ginkgo research submitted by the *Kooperation Phytopharmaka* in which no effects were documented for dried ginkgo leaf (Schilcher, 1997b).

In May 1997, the BfArM sent a letter to manufacturers of ginkgo extracts and other preparations regarding the levels of ginkgolic acid in these products (Thiele, 1997). The letter stated that, based on the present level of knowledge, the BfArM considered it necessary to reduce the content of ginkgolic acid in finished ginkgo preparations to a maximum level of 5 ppm (parts per million). If proof of this level cannot be documented, "the registration for these pharmaceuticals will be canceled since in this case, there is the well-founded suspicion that the pharmaceuticals — when used in accordance with the instructions [in the monographs] — produce damaging effects which exceed a justifiable degree according to the knowledge of medical science." (Thiele, 1997.) The discussion on this issue had not yet been finalized by the end of 1997. Numerous responses from members of industry (both pro and con the 5 ppm proposal) were submitted to the BfArM (Steinhoff, 1997). However, according to Prof. Schilcher, the Commission did discuss the maximum 5 ppm level and agreed to the requirement (Schilcher, 1997b).

Hawthorn

In January 1984 all the preparations of Hawthorn berry, leaf, and flower were approved in one monograph on the basis of historical experience, many pharmacological studies, about 20 open clinical studies, and many patient case reports (Schilcher, 1997b). The originally approved monograph indications were for functional stages I and II of NYHA (New York Heart Association assessment of the four stages of heart disease). This earlier monograph also included sensation of pressure in the chest, cardiac degeneration not yet requiring digitalis (*Altesherz*), and slight forms of bradycardic arrhythmias (Steinhoff, 1997).

Later, however, the pharmacodynamics (the effects of a substance on the physiological processes) of a 45 percent ethanol extract or 70 percent methanol extract of flowering leaf tops with defined content of flavonoids and proanthocyanidins were elaborated. The other three Hawthorn preparations were reevaluated: "the flowers, leaves, and fruits as single compounds received a negative assessment because there no longer seemed to be sufficient scientific evidence to justify their inclusion." (Steinhoff, 1993/1994a.)

Commenting on the Hawthorn monograph changes, Prof. Schilcher has written that in 1984 the Commission had an abundance of scientific material, although none were studies carried out according to GCP (good clinical practices). The studies (both experimental and clinical) in the past six years confirmed the previous knowledge of Hawthorn's activity and resulted in a more precise indication for the approved monograph, i.e., NYHA Stage II only (Schilcher, 1997b). This brought the monographs in line with the 10th edition of the *French Pharmacopeia*, which specifies "dried flowering tops" of *Crataegus monogyna*. For this reason, there are four Hawthorn monographs: the Approved flower with leaves, and the three Unapproved for berry, flower, and leaf individually. These four monographs were published in July 1994 and replaced the original monograph. Presently, the only approved indication (in the leaf with flower monograph) is limited to "decreasing cardiac output according to functional stage II of the NYHA." The approval of the one Hawthorn preparation based on the extract of leaf with flower is another example of the trend by the Commission not only to rely on new scientific data for evaluations, but also to reassess and approve specific, well-defined extract preparations, often ones that are proprietary. (See pages 34 and 39 for related information.)

Horse Chestnut Seed

The 1994 revision of the Horse Chestnut seed monograph includes a detailed description of the pharmacokinetics (the absorption/resorption of substances in the human body) of the approved herb. The 1993 monograph on Horse Chestnut leaf and flower was written without benefit of detailed pharmacokinetic findings, and thus the herb was not approved. Also, the approved formulation for Horse Chestnut was much more stringently defined than earlier. The old monograph (December 5, 1984) defined the drug as Horse Chestnut seed with 3 percent triterpene glycosides calculated as aescin, and indicated a daily dose corresponding to 30-150 mg aescin. The new monograph (April 15, 1994) allows only a defined extract with an aescin content of 16-21 percent in a slow-release dosage form.

Sarsaparilla

Sarsaparilla (Unapproved) has been a commonly used botanical in herbal teas as well as a flavoring for soft drinks in the U.S. for over a century. Oral ingestion has produced few reports of adverse reactions. It is thus curious that the Commission would note the "risk" that "Taking sarsaparilla preparations leads to gastric irritation and temporary kidney impairment." However, per our note in this monograph, "Contrary to the undocumented claims of gastric irritation due to saponin content of sarsaparilla root, we can find nothing in the scientific literature that substantiates this assertion. It is well known that many commonly consumed vegetables contain saponins and sarsaparilla root is a common ingredient in soft drinks, e.g., root beer and many herbal teas. Therefore, we disagree with the Commission that potential gastric irritation is a problem associated with the ingestion of this plant in normal quantities."

Prof. Schilcher of the Commission agrees with our assessment; he notes that the Commission's cautions were based on "a theoretical standpoint and we have in Germany little experience with sarsaparilla"; he also conjectures that any gastrointestinal problems potentially attributable to saponins in sarsaparilla may be a function of dosage (Schilcher, 1997b).

Valerian

In 1994 the EAPC filed a citizens petition to amend the OTC drug monograph for nighttime sleep-aid drug products to include preparations made from the root of valerian (Pinco and Israelsen, 1994). The petition included clinical studies documenting the activity of valerian as a non-habit-forming sedative, plus extensive market data in Europe and other countries where valerian is employed as a medicine — both supporting the safety and efficacy of valerian as a medicine. By spring 1998 the FDA had not yet responded to this petition.

Recent Changes at Commission E

Since 1995 Commission E has not issued any new monographs. The new role of the Commission is to act as a Commission for Registration for phytomedicines to be sold on a prescription basis and also to participate in making decisions concerning the extension of registrations of nonprescription phytomedicines, (such as post-registration approvals (Schulte, 1995).

With no new monographs being produced, the *Kooperation Phytopharmaka* is collecting new studies published subsequent to the approval of the Commission E monographs. The new data are being submitted for consideration in the preparation of ESCOP monographs and are also being considered by BfArM in determining the licensing and registration of phytomedicinal drug products. The licensing requirements stipulate that scientific material on phytomedicines undergoing license review must be up-to-date (Schilcher, 1998c).

INTRODUCTION

The purpose of Commission E now is to act mainly as a highly authoritative advisory board to the BfArM to review individual applications for phytomedicines seeking market authorization in Germany. The status of a phytomedicine's having a positive monograph is no longer sufficient to constitute registration of an herbal drug. The Commission will continue to consider if the documentation based on a positive monograph is sufficient for the registration of an herbal drug in Germany. If external experts and the Commission agree that the data in a product registration is up-to-date and accurate, then the BfArM has the choice of approving the registration. If the BfArM does not agree with the Commission's evaluation, then it must justify its position in a public report. To date, this situation has not occurred; the BfArM has always agreed with the Commission's assessments so far (Schilcher, 1998a).

Of the phytomedicines registered according to the Second Medicines Act since 1994, 610 of these are based on a positive Commission E monograph (Schilcher, 1998a). Thus, even in the view of external experts, the positive monographs are still up-to-date (Schilcher, 1997b).

There is additional interest in development of therapeutic monographs outside Germany by ESCOP even though the ESCOP monographs are scientific but not official government publications. With no new monographs being produced or revised by Commission E, and with the eventual expansion of the European Union's efforts to harmonize drug regulations throughout Western (and perhaps Eastern) Europe, the Commission E monographs will become a matter of historical documentation and a basis for the scientific documentation of herbs and phytomedicine in the future.

OTHER BOOKS WITH COMMISSION E MONOGRAPHS AND RELATED DATA

This volume is the only publication in English of the complete work of Commission E. Other authors and editors have included complete monographs or fragments of Commission E monographs in some publications or have alluded to them throughout the text of their work. Most notable of the latter in the U.S. is Professor Varro E. Tyler's best-selling book, *Herbs of Choice: The Therapeutic Use of Phytomedicinals* (1994), the first book in English in relatively widespread circulation that draws extensively from the Commission E monographs. Using his facility with the German language and his intimate knowledge of pharmacognosy, Prof. Tyler includes the recommended Commission E dosages for approved uses for numerous herbs and phytomedicines discussed in this useful volume. He also includes relevant safety data from the Contraindications and Side Effects sections, as well as other special warnings as needed.

In 1992, the British Herbal Medicine Association published the *British Herbal Compendium Volume I*, a companion volume to the *British Herbal Pharmacopoeia* (1990). The BHC contains monographs on 84 herbs that are described in the BHP. Forty-nine of the BHC monographs include sections containing translations of monographs from Commission E. In 1994, CRC Press and MedPharm Publishers printed the English translation of the excellent German work *Teedrogen* (Tea Drugs) by Professor Dr. Max Wichtl. The new volume was translated and edited by Norman G. Bissett as *Herbal Drugs and Phytopharmaceuticals* and included excerpts from 116 Commission E monographs.

Two recent books from Germany published in English are intended for health professionals: *Phytotherapy in Paediatrics*, by Commission E member Professor Heinz Schilcher, contains English translations of 100 Commission E monographs as well as 15 monographs published by ESCOP, the herbs in the monographs having been mentioned in the text (Schilcher, 1997). Prof. Schilcher and leading pediatricians have selected the 100 most important medicinal plants and this "handbook for physicians and pharmacists" has now been translated into six languages.

Another recently published book for health professionals is *Rational Phytotherapy: A Physician's Guide to Herbal Medicine*, by Volker Schulz, Rudolf Hänsel, and Varro E. Tyler (1997). This book often comments on early findings versus the later, more clinically oriented findings of Commission E. However, it also includes considerable review of the clinical studies supporting the safe and effective (rational) use of a number of leading phytomedicines used in Germany, as well as summaries of therapeutic categories for which some herbs have been approved by Commission E.

There have been several reference books published recently that have included data from the Commission E monographs. These include the extensive *Encyclopedia of Common Ingredients Used in Foods, Drugs and Cosmetics 2nd edition*, by Albert Y. Leung and Steven Foster (1996). Of the 500-plus herbs monographed in this useful volume, many refer to the herb's approved uses according to Commission E. The authors based their references to Commission E on a previous draft version of this book. Similarly, the *American Herbal Products Association's Botanical Safety Handbook* (1997), edited by Michael McGuffin, Christopher Hobbs, Roy Upton, and Alicia Goldberg, used an earlier draft of this work as one of the 30 general references upon which it relied in assessing the relative safety of some 600 herbs sold in the U.S. herbal market.

Further, the 1998 - 1999 edition of *Poisoning & Toxicology Compendium*, by Jerrold B. Leikin, M.D., and Frank P. Paloucek, Pharm.D., published by Lexi-Comp Inc. and the American Pharmaceutical Association, contains a section on the safety and toxicological aspects of herbal medicines, with tables on herb-drug interactions and herbs contraindicated in pregnancy and lactation based on this translation of the Commission E monographs (Blumenthal, 1997).

In the area of popular literature, two herbal best sellers were published in summer 1997 that contain data based on this book. In *Green Pharmacy* (Duke, 1997), renowned economic botanist James A. Duke, Ph.D., alludes to the Commission E approvals of numerous herbs contained in his book. Consumer health author Jean Carper's *Miracle Cures* (HarperCollins, 1997) also refers to the government-approved status of the therapeutic benefits of many of the herbs and phytomedicines covered in her book. Both authors were provided early drafts of these translations.

Incidentally, Prof. H. Schilcher, Vice President of Commission E, was the first author to publish Commission E monographs in the German literature with the publication of his book, *Phytotherapy in Paediatrics*, originally published in 1988. His German book *Little Handbook for the Most Important Herbs in Self-Medication*, based principally on the Commission E work of which he has played an integral part, will be published in 1998. Prof. Schilcher's *Little Medicinal Plant Dictionary* has sold over 96,000 copies and contains two chapters based on uses and dosages of herbs approved by Commission E.

Conclusion

One of the benefits of the Commission E system is that it can provide an excellent model for regulatory reform, in the United States and possibly other countries, by providing a rational process for reviewing herbs and phytomedicines for their safety and efficacy. One of the unique features of Commission E is the interdisciplinary composition of its membership: approximately half of the members have theoretical expertise with herbs and phytomedicines and half of the members have practical experience with phytotherapy.

The reader is cautioned that a potential drawback may be a narrow interpretation that these monographs represent the only reasonable uses or indications of the herbs described in the monographs. There is ample room for new research to document and confirm heretofore scientifically unproven uses for herbs. In this sense, the Commission E monographs may constitute a good focal point for the development of rational regulations that accommodate the need to provide health practitioners and consumers with reliable, authoritative information on the therapeutic benefits and risks of herbal medicines. However, the Commission E model should not be viewed as an endpoint of herbal regulations; instead, it can be seen as a point of departure, a baseline upon which new data can be reviewed in the much larger field of herbs used in the U.S. today. Using an expert panel system similar to Commission E to review herbal literature could provide substantial benefits for healthcare and self-care in the U.S. in the near future.

REFERENCES

AESGP. 1995. Economic and Legal Framework for Non-Prescription Medicines in Europe. Brussels: European Proprietary Medicines Manufacturer's Association (AESGP), Jun., 36-43.

Akerele, O. 1992. Summary of WHO Guidelines for the Assessment of Herbal Medicines. In *HerbalGram* 28: 13-16.

Anonymous. 1996. Survey Indicates Increasing Herb Use. *HerbalGram* 37: 56.

Bauer, R. and H. Wagner. 1991. Echinacea species as potential immunostimulatory drugs. In *Economic and Medicinal Plant Research* Vol. 5. H. Wagner and N.R. Farnsworth (eds.). New York: Academic Press: 253-351.

Bayne, H., M. Blumenthal, L.D. Israelsen. 1966. A Survey of Regulations of Herbal Medicines in Six Industrialized Nations: Executive Summary. Austin, Texas: American Botanical Council.

Bergner, P. 1994. German Evaluation of Herbal Medicines. *HerbalGram* 30: 17,64.

Bisset, N.G. (trans.) and Wichtl, M. 1994. *Herbal Drugs and Phytopharmaceuticals*. Boca Raton, Florida: CRC Press.

Blumenthal, M. 1998. Perspectives on the Safety of Herbal Medicines. In Leikin, J.B. and Paloucek, F.P. *Poisoning & Toxicology Compendium*. Hudson, Ohio: Lexi-Comp Inc.

Blumenthal, M. 1997. Herbal Monographs Initiated by Numerous Groups. *HerbalGram* 40: 30-35, 37-38.

Blumenthal, M. 1995. Herb Sales Up 35 Percent in Mass Market. *HerbalGram* 34: 66.

Blumenthal, M. 1994. Regulatory Models for Approval of Botanicals as Traditional Medicines. Presentation at "Botanicals: Role in U.S. Healthcare?" conference sponsored by the Office of Alternative Medicine, National Institutes of Health, Washington, D.C. Dec. 14.

Bradley, P. 1992. *The British Herbal Compendium*. Bournemouth, England: British Herbal Medicine Association.

Braunig, B., M. Dorn, E. Limburg, E. Knick. 1992. *Echinacea purpurea* root for strengthening the immune response in flu-like infections. *Zeitschrift fur Phytotherapie* 13: 7-13.

Brevoort, P. 1996. The U.S. Botanical Market — An Overview. *HerbalGram* 36: 49-57.

Busse, W. 1997a. How Can Lessons Learned (and Unlearned) from Non-U.S. Markets Be Applied to the U.S. Market? Presentation at Third Drug Information Association Workshop on Botanicals: Botanical Testing: Developing the Scientific and Clinical Evidence to Support the Clinical Use of Heterogeneous Botanical Products. Washington, D.C., Jan. 27.

Busse, W. 1997b. Personal communication, Aug. 14.

Busse, W. 1997c. Personal communication, Dec. 19.

Busse, W. 1996. Personal communication, Mar. 28.

Carper, Jean. 1997. *Miracle Cures.* New York: Harper Collins.

Commission of European Communities. 1989. Notice to Applicants for Marketing Authorization for Medicinal Products for Human Use in the Member States of the European Community. Vol. III. Guidelines on the Quality, Safety and Efficacy of the Medicinal Products for Human Use. Jan., 1989. (Note for guidance relating to Part 1 of the Annex to Directive 75/318 EEC, as amended.)

Commission on Dietary Supplement Labels. 1997. *Report to the President, the Congress, and the Secretary of Health and Human Services.* Nov. 24.

Deutsches Arzneibuch. Amtlich Eausgabe. Stuttgart, Germany: Deutscher Apotheker Verlag.

Duke, J.A. 1997. *The Green Pharmacy.* Emmaus, Penn. Rodale Press.

De Smet, P.A.G.M. 1993. Legislatory Outlook on the Safety of Herbal Medicines. In De Smet, P.A.G.M., K. Keller, R. Hänsel, and R.F. Chandler. *Adverse Effects of Herbal Drugs* Vol. 2, Berlin: Springer-Verlag.

De Smet, P.A.G.M. and W.A. Nolen. 1996. St. John's Wort as an antidepressant. *British Medical Journal* 313: 241-247.

European Economic Community. 1975. Directive 75/318/EEC. Standards for Quality of Herbal Remedies.

Farnsworth, N.R. 1985. Siberian Ginseng (*Eleutherococcus senticosus*): Current Status as an Adaptogen. In *Economic and Medicinal Plant Research, Vol. I.* Wagner, H., H. Hikino, and N.R. Farnsworth (eds.). London: Academic Press.

Federal Health Agency. 1989. Evaluation Criteria for Fixed Drug Combinations. *Natur- und Ganzheitsmedizin (Complementary and Wholistic Medicine)* 6:159-160.

Food and Drug Administration. 1996. Eligibility Criteria for Considering Additional Conditions in the Over-the-Counter Drug Monograph System; Request for Information and Comments. Advance Notice of Proposed Rulemaking. *Federal Register* Vol. 61, No. 193, Oct. 3: 51625-31.

Food and Drug Administration. 1993. Food Labeling: General Requirements for Health Claims for Dietary Supplements. Proposed Rule. *Federal Register* Vol. 58, No. 116, Jun. 18: 33700-14.

Foster, S. 1996. Personal communication, March 3.

Foster, S. (ed.) 1992. *Herbs of Commerce.* Austin, Texas: American Herbal Products Association.

Foster, S. 1990. Ginkgo, *Ginkgo biloba.* Botanical Series No. 304. American Botanical Council, Austin, Texas. p. 7.

Franz, G. 1997. Personal communication, Dec. 15.

Fresenius, W., H. Niklas and H. Schilcher. 1997. *Nonprescription Medicines (Freiverkäufliche Arzneimittel.* 3rd ed. Stuttgart: Wissenschaft Verlagsgesellschaft.

Fulder, S. and M. Tenne. 1996. Ginger as an Anti-nausea Remedy in Pregnancy: The Issue of Safety. *HerbalGram* 38: 47-50.

Gericke, N. 1995. The Regulation and Control of Traditional Herbal Medicines. Cape Town, South Africa: Traditional Medicines Programme at the University of Cape Town.

Glovsky, S. 1998. Personal communication, Mar. 4.

Greuter, W. et al. (eds.) 1988. *International Code of Botanical Nomenclature* (Adopted by the 14th International Botanical Congress, Berlin, July-August, 1987). Koenigstein, Germany: Koeltz Scientific Books.

Gruenwald, J. 1998. Personal communication, Jan. 25.

Gruenwald, J. 1997. Most frequently prescribed herbal monopreparations in Germany, listed according to active ingredient and sales. *HerbalGram* 39: 68.

Gruenwald, G. 1995. The European Phytomedicines Market: Figures, Trends, Analyses. *HerbalGram* 34: 60-66.

Harnischfeger, G. 1996. Personal communication to Mark Blumenthal, Jun. 27.

Hocking, G.M. 1955. *A Dictionary of Terms In Pharmacognosy and Other Divisions of Economic Botany.* Springfield, IL: Charles C. Thomas.

IfD survey 6039. 1997. Institute for Demoscopy in Allensbach, Germany. Report on Natural Medicines — Mar. 1997.

Johnston, B. 1997. One-Third of Nation's Adults Use Herbal Remedies: Market Estimated at $3.24 Billion. *HerbalGram* 40: 49.

Kada, T., K. Morita, and T. Inoue. 1978. Anti-mutagenic action of vegetable factors on the mutagenic principle of tryptophan pyrolysate. *Mutation Research* 53: 351-353.

Keller, K. 1998a. Personal communication, Jan. 2.

Keller, K. 1998b. Personal communication, Jan. 6.

Keller, K. 1996. Herbal Medicinal Products in Germany and Europe: Experiences with National and European Assessment. *Drug Information Journal*, Vol. 30: 993-948.

Keller, K. 1994. Phytotherapy at a European level. *European Phytotelegram*, ESCOP, Aug.: 40-45.

Keller, K. 1992. Results of the revision of herbal drugs in the Federal Republic of Germany with a special focus on risk aspects. *Zeitschrift für Phytotherapie* 13: 116-120.

Keller, K. 1991. Legal Requirements for the use of phytopharmaceutical drugs in the Federal Republic of Germany. *Journal of Ethnopharmacology* 32: 225-229.

Koerner, S. 1997. Personal communication from Deutscher Apotheker Verlag to M. Blumenthal, Nov. 25.

Leung, A.Y. 1998. Personal communication, Mar. 2.

Linde, K., G. Ramirez, C.D. Mulrow, A. Pauls, W. Weidenhammer, D. Melchart. 1996. St. John's Wort for depression — an overview and meta-analysis of randomized clinical trials. *British Medical Journal* 313: 253-258.

Nagabhushan, M. et al. 1987. Mutagenicity of gingerol and shogaol and antimutagenicity of zingerone in Salmonella/microsome assay. *Cancer Letters* 36: 221-223.

Namakura, H. and T. Yamamoto. 1982. Mutagen and antimutagen in ginger, *Zingiber officinale*. *Mutation Research* 103: 119-126.

Pinco, R.G. and L.D. Israelsen. 1995. European-American Phytomedicines Coalition Citizen Petition to Amend FDA's Monograph on Antiemetic Drug Products for Over-the-Counter ("OTC") Human Use to Include Ginger. May 26.

Pinco, R.G. and L.D. Israelsen. 1994. European-American Phytomedicines Coalition Citizen Petition to Amend FDA's Monograph on Nighttime Sleep-aid Drug Products for Over-the Counter ("OTC") Human Use to Include Valerian. Jun. 7.

Pinco, R.G. and L.D. Israelsen. 1992. European-American Phytomedicines Coalition Citizen Petition to Amend FDA's OTC Drug Review Policy Regarding Foreign Ingredients. Jul. 24.

PhRMA (Pharmaceutical Research and Manufacturers of America). 1998. Information from worldwide website at http://www.phrma.org/, Mar. 19.

Richman, A. and J.P. Witkowski. 1997. Herbs by the Numbers: Whole Foods' Third Annual Natural Herbal Product Sales Survey. *Whole Foods* Oct.: 20-28.

Schilcher, H. 1998a. Personal communication, Feb. 9.

Schilcher, H. 1998b. The Present State of Phytotherapy in Germany. *Deutsche Apotheker Zeitung* 138 Jahrgang, No. 3, Jan. 15: 144-149.

Schilcher, H. 1998c. The Phytotherapy Situation in the Republic of Germany. *Münchner Medizinische Wochenschrift.* Feb. (in press).

Schilcher, H. 1998d. Personal communication, Apr. 1.

Schilcher, H. 1997a. *Phytotherapie in Paediatrics: Handbook for Physicians and Pharmacists.* Stuttgart: Medpharm Scientific Publishers.

Schilcher, H. 1997b. Personal communication, Dec. 30.

Schilcher, H. 1997c. Standards for the Discipline of Phytotherapy in Postgraduate and Continuing Education. *Ärztezeitschrift für Naturheilverfahren* 38: 336-341

Schilcher, H. 1996. The Status of Phytotherapy Within Specific Therapeutic Trends and Traditional Medicine. *Ärztezeitschrift für Naturheilvarfarhen* 37(1), Jan.: 23-34.

Schilcher, H. 1991. The Importance of Phytotherapy in Medical Schools. *Zeitschrift für Phytotherapie* (*Journal of Phytotherapy*), Vol. 3.

Schulte, G. 1995. Letter to H. Schilcher, August 25.

Schulz, T.K., R. Hänsel, V.E. Tyler. 1997. *Rational Phytotherapy: A Physician's Guide to Herbal Medicine.* Berlin: Springer-Verlag.

Schwabe, U. 1997. Arzneiverordnungsreport (Prescription Drug Report) – 1997. Stuttgart: Gustav Fischer Verlag.

Steinhoff, B. 1997a. Personal communication, Dec. 12.

Steinhoff, B. 1997b. Herbal Medicines – Increasingly Preferred. *Pharmazeutische Zeitung* 142(49), Dec. 4: 38-43 (4412-4417).

Steinhoff, B. 1994a. Personal communication, Apr. 11.

Steinhoff, B. 1993/1994a. New Developments regarding Phytomedicines in Germany. *British Journal of Phytotherapy*, Vol.3, No. 4: 190-193.

Steinhoff, B. 1993/1994b. The Legal Situation of Phytomedicines in Germany. *British Journal of Phytotherapy*, Vol. 3, No. 2: 76-80.

Thiele, A. 1997. Averting of drug-induced risks, grade II: pharmaceuticals containing Ginkgo biloba leaves. Communication to Dr. Willmar Schwabe GmbH & Co., May 27.

Trease, G.E. and W.C. Evans. 1996. *A Textbook of Pharmacognosy.* London: Bailliere, Tindall and Cassell.

Tyler, V.E. 1997. "When Will There Come a Savior...?" *HerbalGram* 41:27,28,56.

Tyler, V.E. 1996. Personal communication, Dec. 31.

Tyler, V.E. 1994. *Herbs of Choice: The Therapeutic Use of Phytomedicinals.* Binghampton, NY: Pharmaceutical Products Press.

Tyler, V.E. 1992. Phytomedicines in Western Europe: Their Potential Impact on Herbal Medicine in the United States. In Kinghorn, D.I. and Balandrin, M.F. *Human Medicinal Agents from Plants.* Washington, D.C. American Chemical Society. Reprinted in *HerbalGram* 30: 24-30, 67, 68, 77.

United States Congress. Dietary Supplement Health and Education Act of 1994. Public Law 103-417, 108 Stat. 4325-4333. Oct. 25, 1994.

United States Senate Committee on Labor and Human Resources. Report on the Dietary Supplement Health and Education Act of 1994. 103-410. Oct. 8, 1994.

United States Congress. Nutrition Labeling and Education Act of 1990. Public Law 101-535. 104 Stat. 2353-2364. Nov. 8, 1990.

Viola, H., M.L. de Stein, C. Wolfman, et al. 1996. Apigenin, a component of *Matricaria recutita* flowers, is a central benzodiazepine receptor-ligand with anxiolytic effects. *Planta Medica* 61:213-6.

Weidenfeld, H. 1996. Personal communication to R. Rister, Mar. 6.

Wiesenauer, M. 1989. Drugs for special therapies. (In German) Review. *Fortschritte der Medizin*, 107 (35): 741-2, 752, Dec. 10.

World Health Organization. 1991. Guidelines for the Assessment of Herbal Medicines. Geneva: WHO, in *HerbalGram* 28 (1993): 17-20.

103d Congress. Public Law 103-417 – Oct. 25, 1994. Dietary Supplement Health and Education Act of 1994.

Part Two

Monographs

1. Complete List of Monographs by Approval Status   73

2. Approved Herbs   79

3. Approved Component Characteristics   237

4. Approved Fixed Combinations   245

5. Unapproved Herbs   307

6. Unapproved Component Characteristics   385

7. Unapproved Fixed Combinations   403

Chapter 1

Complete List of Monographs by Approval Status

This chapter lists the monographs by the English common names used in this book under headings corresponding to their approval status and monograph type. The original monographs were published using the pharmacopeial name.

Approved Herbs
1. Agrimony
2. Aloe
3. Angelica root
4. Anise seed
5. Arnica flower
6. Artichoke leaf
7. Asparagus root
8. Autumn Crocus
9. Belladonna
10. Bilberry fruit
11. Birch leaf
12. Bitter Orange peel
13. Black Cohosh root
14. Blackberry leaf
15. Blackthorn berry
16. Blessed Thistle herb
17. Bogbean leaf
18. Boldo leaf
19. Bromelain
20. Buckthorn bark
21. Buckthorn berry
22. Bugleweed
23. Butcher's Broom
24. Calendula flower
25. Camphor
26. Caraway oil
27. Caraway seed
28. Cardamom seed
29. Cascara Sagrada bark
30. Celandine herb
31. Centaury herb
32. Chamomile flower, German
33. Chaste Tree fruit
34. Chicory
35. Cinchona bark
36. Cinnamon bark
37. Cinnamon bark, Chinese
38. Cloves
39. Coffee Charcoal
40. Cola nut
41. Coltsfoot leaf
42. Comfrey herb and leaf
43. Comfrey root
44. Condurango bark
45. Coriander seed
46. Couch Grass
47. Dandelion herb
48. Dandelion root with herb
49. Devil's Claw root
50. Dill seed
51. Echinacea Pallida root
52. Echinacea Purpurea herb
53. Elder flower
54. Eleuthero (Siberian Ginseng) root
55. Ephedra
56. Eucalyptus leaf
57. Eucalyptus oil
58. Fennel oil
59. Fennel seed
60. Fenugreek seed
61. Fir Needle oil
62. Fir Shoots, Fresh
63. Flaxseed
64. Fumitory
65. Galangal
66. Garlic
67. Gentian root
68. Ginger root
69. Ginkgo Biloba Leaf Extract

Approved Herbs (cont'd)

70. Ginseng root
71. Goldenrod
72. Guaiac wood
73. Gumweed herb
74. Haronga bark and leaf
75. Hawthorn leaf with flower
76. Hay flower
77. Heart's Ease herb
78. Hempnettle herb
79. Henbane leaf
80. Hops
81. Horehound herb
82. Horse Chestnut seed
83. Horseradish
84. Horsetail herb
85. Iceland Moss
86. Indian Snakeroot
87. Ivy leaf
88. Jambolan bark
89. Java tea
90. Juniper berry
91. Kava Kava
92. Kidney Bean pods (without seeds)
93. Knotweed herb
94. Lady's Mantle
95. Larch Turpentine
96. Lavender flower
97. Lemon Balm
98. Licorice root
99. Lily-of-the-valley herb
100. Linden flower
101. Lovage root
102. Mallow flower
103. Mallow leaf
104. Manna
105. Marshmallow leaf
106. Marshmallow root
107. Maté
108. Mayapple root and resin
109. Meadowsweet
110. Milk Thistle fruit
111. Mint oil
112. Mistletoe herb
113. Motherwort herb
114. Mullein flower
115. Myrrh
116. Niauli oil
117. Oak bark
118. Oat straw
119. Onion
120. Orange peel
121. Paprika (Cayenne)
122. Parsley herb and root
123. Passionflower herb
124. Peppermint leaf
125. Peppermint oil
126. Peruvian Balsam
127. Petasites root
128. Pheasant's Eye herb
129. Pimpinella root
130. Pine Needle oil
131. Pine Sprouts
132. Plantain
133. Pollen
134. Poplar bud
135. Potentilla
136. Primrose flower
137. Primrose root
138. Psyllium seed husk, Blonde
139. Psyllium seed, Black
140. Psyllium seed, Blonde
141. Pumpkin seed
142. Radish
143. Rhatany root
144. Rhubarb root
145. Rose flower
146. Rosemary leaf
147. Sage leaf
148. Sandalwood, White
149. Sandy Everlasting
150. Sanicle herb
151. Saw Palmetto berry
152. Scopolia root
153. Scotch Broom herb
154. Senega Snakeroot
155. Senna leaf
156. Senna pod
157. Shepherd's Purse
158. Soapwort root, Red
159. Soapwort root, White
160. Soy Lecithin
161. Soy Phospholipid
162. Spiny Restharrow root
163. Squill
164. St. John's Wort
165. Star Anise seed
166. Stinging Nettle herb and leaf

167. Stinging Nettle root
168. Sundew
169. Sweet Clover
170. Thyme
171. Thyme, Wild
172. Tolu Balsam
173. Tormentil root
174. Turmeric root
175. Turmeric root, Javanese
176. Turpentine oil, Purified
177. Usnea
178. Uva Ursi leaf
179. Uzara root
180. Valerian root
181. Walnut leaf
182. Watercress
183. White Dead Nettle flower
184. White Mustard seed
185. White Willow bark
186. Witch Hazel leaf and bark
187. Woody Nightshade stem
188. Wormwood
189. Yarrow
190. Yeast, Brewer's
191. Yeast, Brewer's/ Hansen CBS 5926

Approved Component Characteristics

1. Cajeput oil
2. Nasturtium

Approved Fixed Combinations

1. F.C. of Angelica root, Gentian root, and Bitter Orange peel
2. F.C. of Angelica root, Gentian root, and Caraway seed
3. F.C. of Angelica root, Gentian root, and Fennel
4. F.C. of Angelica root, Gentian root, and Wormwood
5. F.C. of Angelica root, Gentian root, Wormwood, and Peppermint oil
6. F.C. of Anise oil and Iceland Moss
7. F.C. of Anise oil, Fennel oil, and Caraway oil
8. F.C. of Anise oil, Fennel oil, Licorice root, and Thyme
9. F.C. of Anise oil, Primrose root, and Thyme
10. F.C. of Anise seed, Fennel seed, and Caraway seed
11. F.C. of Anise seed, Ivy leaf, Fennel seed, and Licorice root
12. F.C. of Anise seed, Linden flower, and Thyme
13. F.C. of Anise seed, Marshmallow root, Eucalyptus oil, and Licorice root
14. F.C. of Anise seed, Marshmallow root, Iceland Moss, and Licorice root
15. F.C. of Anise seed, Marshmallow root, Primrose root, and Sundew
16. F.C. of Birch leaf, Goldenrod, and Java tea
17. F.C. of Camphor, Eucalyptus oil, and Purified Turpentine oil
18. F.C. of Caraway oil and Fennel oil
19. F.C. of Caraway oil, Fennel oil, and Chamomile flower
20. F.C. of Caraway seed and Fennel seed
21. F.C. of Caraway seed, Fennel seed, and Chamomile flower
22. F.C. of Dandelion root with herb, Celandine herb, and Artichoke leaf
23. F.C. of Dandelion root with herb, Celandine herb, and Wormwood
24. F.C. of Dandelion root with herb, Celandine herb, and Wormwood
25. F.C. of Dandelion root with herb, Peppermint leaf, and Artichoke leaf
26. F.C. of Eucalyptus oil and Pine Needle oil
27. F.C. of Eucalyptus oil, Primrose root, and Thyme
28. F.C. of Ginger root, Gentian root, and Wormwood
29. F.C. of Gumweed herb, Primrose root, and Thyme
30. F.C. of Ivy leaf, Licorice root, and Thyme
31. F.C. of Javanese Turmeric root, Celandine herb, and Wormwood
32. F.C. of Javanese Turmeric root, Peppermint leaf, and Wormwood

Approved Fixed Combinations (cont'd)

33. F.C. of Licorice root and German Chamomile flower
34. F.C. of Licorice root, Peppermint leaf, and German Chamomile flower
35. F.C. of Licorice root, Primrose root, Marshmallow root, and Anise seed
36. F.C. of Marshmallow root, Fennel seed, Iceland Moss, and Thyme
37. F.C. of Marshmallow root, Primrose root, Licorice root, and Thyme oil
38. F.C. of Milk Thistle fruit, Peppermint leaf, and Wormwood
39. F.C. of Passionflower herb, Valerian root, and Lemon Balm
40. F.C. of Peppermint leaf and Caraway seed
41. F.C. of Peppermint leaf and Fennel seed
42. F.C. of Peppermint leaf, Caraway seed, and Chamomile flower
43. F.C. of Peppermint leaf, Caraway seed, and Fennel seed
44. F.C. of Peppermint leaf, Caraway seed, Chamomile flower, and Bitter Orange peel
45. F.C. of Peppermint leaf, Caraway seed, Fennel seed, and Chamomile flower
46. F.C. of Peppermint leaf, Fennel seed, and Chamomile flower
47. F.C. of Peppermint leaf, German Chamomile flower, and Caraway seed
48. F.C. of Peppermint oil and Caraway oil
49. F.C. of Peppermint oil and Fennel oil
50. F.C. of Peppermint oil, Caraway oil, and Chamomile flower
51. F.C. of Peppermint oil, Caraway oil, and Fennel oil
52. F.C. of Peppermint oil, Caraway oil, Fennel oil, and Chamomile flower
53. F.C. of Peppermint oil, Fennel oil, and Chamomile flower
54. F.C. of Pheasant's Eye fluidextract, Lily-of-the-valley powdered extract, Squill powdered extract, and Oleander leaf powdered extract
55. F.C. of Primrose root and Thyme
56. F.C. of Primrose root, Marshmallow root, and Anise seed
57. F.C. of Primrose root, Sundew, and Thyme
58. F.C. of Senna leaf and Blonde Psyllium seed husk
59. F.C. of Senna leaf, Peppermint oil, and Caraway oil
60. F.C. of Star Anise seed and Thyme
61. F.C. of Sundew and Thyme
62. F.C. of Thyme and White Soapwort root
63. F.C. of Turmeric root and Celandine herb
64. F.C. of Uva Ursi leaf, Goldenrod, and Java Tea
65. F.C. of Valerian root and Hops
66. F.C. of Valerian root, Hops, and Lemon Balm
67. F.C. of Valerian root, Hops, and Passionflower herb

Unapproved Herbs

1. Alpine Lady's Mantle herb
2. Angelica seed and herb
3. Ash bark and leaf
4. Asparagus herb
5. Barberry
6. Basil herb
7. Bilberry leaf
8. Bishop's Weed fruit
9. Bitter Orange flower
10. Blackberry root
11. Blackthorn flower
12. Bladderwrack
13. Borage
14. Bryonia root
15. Buchu leaf
16. Burdock root
17. Calendula herb
18. Cat's Foot flower
19. Celery

Unapproved Herbs (cont'd)

20. Chamomile, Roman
21. Chestnut leaf
22. Cinnamon flower
23. Cocoa
24. Coltsfoot
25. Corn Poppy
26. Cornflower
27. Damiana leaf and herb
28. Delphinium flower
29. Dill weed
30. Echinacea Angustifolia herb and root/Pallida herb
31. Elecampane root
32. Ergot
33. Eyebright
34. Figs
35. Ginkgo Biloba leaf
36. Goat's Rue herb
37. Hawthorn berry
38. Hawthorn flower
39. Hawthorn leaf
40. Heather herb and flower
41. Hibiscus
42. Hollyhock flower
43. Horse Chestnut leaf
44. Hound's Tongue
45. Hyssop
46. Jambolan seed
47. Jimsonweed leaf and seed
48. Kelp
49. Lemongrass, Citronella
50. Linden Charcoal
51. Linden flower, Silver
52. Linden leaf
53. Linden wood
54. Liverwort herb
55. Loofa
56. Lungwort
57. Madder root
58. Male Fern
59. Marjoram
60. Marsh Tea
61. Mentzelia
62. Milk Thistle herb
63. Monkshood
64. Mountain Ash berry
65. Mugwort
66. Muira Puama
67. Night-blooming Cereus
68. Nutmeg
69. Nux Vomica
70. Oat herb
71. Oats
72. Oleander leaf
73. Olive leaf
74. Olive oil
75. Oregano
76. Orris root
77. Papain
78. Papaya leaf
79. Paprika (Cayenne) species low in capsaicin
80. Parsley seed
81. Pasque flower (Pulsatilla)
82. Peony flower and root
83. Periwinkle
84. Petasites leaf
85. Pimpinella herb
86. Raspberry leaf
87. Rhododendron, Rusty-leaved
88. Rose Hip
89. Rose Hip and seed
90. Rose Hip seed
91. Rue
92. Rupturewort
93. Saffron
94. Sandalwood, Red
95. Sarsaparilla root
96. Sarsaparilla, German
97. Senecio herb
98. Soapwort herb, Red
99. Spinach leaf
100. Strawberry leaf
101. Sweet Woodruff
102. Tansy
103. Verbena herb
104. Veronica
105. Walnut hull
106. White Dead Nettle herb
107. Yohimbe bark
108. Zedoary rhizome

Unapproved Component Characteristics

1. Aspen bark and leaf
2. Basil oil
3. California Poppy

4. Cocoa seed
5. Colocynth
6. Echinacea Purpurea root
7. Horse Chestnut bark and flower
8. Mistletoe berry
9. Mistletoe stem
10. Scotch Broom flower
11. Sweet Violet flower
12. Sweet Violet root and herb
13. Yellow Jessamine root

Unapproved Fixed Combinations

1. F.C. of Belladonna with drugs in homeopathic preparations
2. F.C. of Belladonna with other drugs
3. F.C. of Lily-of-the-valley herb and Squill
4. F.C. of Pheasant's Eye herb and Lily-of-the-valley herb
5. F.C. of Pheasant's Eye herb and/or Lily-of-the-valley herb and/or Squill and/or Oleander leaf with herbs that do not contain cardiac glycosides
6. F.C. of Pheasant's Eye herb and/or Lily-of-the-valley herb and/or Squill and/or Oleander leaf with chemically defined drugs

Chapter 2

Approved Herbs

The herbs in this section received positive evaluations by Commission E. Their approved uses are officially recognized by the German government primarily for nonprescription and clinical applications.

Agrimony
Agrimoniae herba
Odermennigkraut
Published March 13, 1986; Revised March 13, 1990

Name of Drug
Agrimoniae herba, agrimony, cocklebur.

Composition of Drug
Agrimony herb consists of the dried, above-ground parts of *Agrimonia eupatoria* L. and/or *A. procera* Wallroth [Fam. Rosaceae], harvested shortly before or during flowering, or equivalent preparations in effective dosage.

The herb contains tannins and flavonoids.

Uses
Internal:
  Mild, nonspecific, acute diarrhea; inflammation of oral and pharyngeal mucosa.
External:
  Mild, superficial inflammation of the skin.

Contraindications
None known.

Side Effects
None known.

Interactions with Other Drugs
None known.

Dosage
Unless otherwise prescribed:
For internal application:
Average daily dosage:
  3 g of herb;
  equivalent preparations.

Mode of Administration
Comminuted herb or herb powder for teas; other galenical preparations for external and internal use.

Action
Astringent

Aloe
Aloe barbadensis, Aloe capensis
Aloe
Published August 21, 1985; Replaced July 21, 1993

Name of Drug
Aloe barbadensis, Curaçao aloe.
Aloe capensis, Cape aloe.

Composition of Drug
Curaçao aloe consists of the dried latex of the leaves of *Aloe barbadensis* Miller [syn. A. vera (L.) N. L. Burm.] [Fam. Liliaceae], as well as its preparations in effective dosage.

Cape aloe consists of the dried latex of the leaves of several species of the genus Aloe, especially *A. ferox* Miller and its hybrids, as well as their preparations in effective dosage.

Aloe contains anthranoids, mainly of the aloe-emodin type. These drugs must conform to the currently valid pharmacopeia.

Pharmacological Properties, Pharmacokinetics, Toxicology
1,8-dihydroxy-anthracene derivatives have a laxative effect. This effect is primarily caused by the influence on the motility of the colon, an inhibition of stationary and stimulation of propulsive contractions. This results in an accelerated intestinal passage and, because of the shortened contraction time, a reduction in liquid absorption. In addition, stimulation of the active chloride secretion increases the water and electrolyte content.

Systematic studies pertaining to the kinetics of aloe preparations are not available; however, it must be supposed that the aglycones contained in the drug are already absorbed in the upper small intestine. The ß-glycosides are prodrugs which are neither absorbed nor cleaved in the upper gastrointestinal tract. They are degraded in the colon by bacterial enzymes to aloe-emodin anthrones.

Aloe-emodin anthrone is the laxative metabolite. In humans, rhein was demonstrated in the urine after consumption of 86 and 200 mg of aloe powder.

Active metabolites, such as rhein, infiltrate in small amounts into the milk ducts. A laxative effect on nursing infants has not been observed. The placental permeability for rhein is very small.

Drug preparations [i.e., herbal stimulant laxative drugs] have a higher general toxicity than the pure glycosides, presumably due to the content of aglycones. An aloe extract containing 23 percent aloin and less than 0.07 percent aloe-emodin, as well as aloin, produced no mutagenic effects in bacterial and mammalian test systems. For aloe-emodin, emodin and chrysophanol, partially positive results have been obtained. There are no available data regarding carcinogenicity.

Clinical Data

1. Uses
Constipation.

2. Contraindications
Intestinal obstruction, acutely inflamed intestinal diseases, e.g., Crohn's disease, ulcerative colitis, appendicitis, abdominal pain of unknown origin. Not to be prescribed to children under 12 years of age or during pregnancy.

3. Side Effects
In single incidents, cramp-like discomforts of the gastrointestinal tract. These cases require a dosage reduction.

Long-term use/abuse: disturbances of electrolyte balance, especially potassium deficiency, albuminuria and hematuria. Pigment implantation into the intestinal mucosa (*pseudomelanosis coli*), is harmless and usually reverses upon discontinuation of the drug. The potassium deficiency can lead to disorders of heart function and muscular weakness, especially with concurrent use of cardiac glycosides, diuretics and corticosteroids.

4. Special Caution for Use
Stimulant laxatives must not be used over an extended period of time (1 - 2 weeks) without medical advice.

5. Use During Pregnancy
Because of insufficient toxicological investigation, this drug should not be used during pregnancy and lactation.

6. Interactions with Other Drugs
With chronic use/abuse, due to loss in potassium, an increase in effectiveness of cardiac glycosides is possible, as well as an effect on antiarrhythmic agents. Potassium deficiency can be increased by simultaneous application of thiazide diuretics, cortico-adrenal steroids, and licorice root.

7. Dosage
Aloe powder, aqueous and aqueous-alcoholic extracts in powdered or liquid form, for oral use.
Unless otherwise prescribed:
   20 - 30 mg hydroxyanthracene derivatives/day, calculated as anhydrous aloin.

The individually correct dosage is the smallest dosage necessary to maintain a soft stool.
Note: The form of administration should be smaller than the normal daily dosage.

8. Overdosage
Electrolyte and fluid imbalance.

9. Special Warnings
Usage of a stimulating laxative for longer than the recommended short-term application can cause an increase in intestinal sluggishness.

The preparation should be used only if no effects can be obtained through change of diet or usage of bulk-forming products.

10. Effects on Operators of Vehicles and Machinery
None known.
Note: During the course of treatment, a harmless red color may occur in the urine.

Angelica root
Angelicae radix
Angelikawurzel
Published June 1, 1990

Name of Drug
Angelicae radix, angelica root.

Composition of Drug
Angelica root consists of the dried root and rhizome of *Angelica archangelica* L. [Fam. Apiaceae], as well as their preparations in effective dosage.

The drug contains essential oil, coumarin, and coumarin derivatives.

Uses
Loss of appetite, peptic discomforts such as mild spasms of the gastrointestinal tract, feeling of fullness, flatulence.

Contraindications
None known.

Side Effects
The furanocoumarins present in angelica root sensitize the skin to light. Subsequent exposure to UV radiation can lead to inflammation of the skin. During treatment with the drug or its preparations, prolonged sun-bathing and exposure to intense UV radiation should be avoided.

Interactions with Other Drugs
None known.

Dosage
Unless otherwise prescribed:
Daily dosage:
    4.5 g of drug;
    1.5 - 3 g fluidextract (1:1);
    1.5 g tincture (1:5);
    equivalent preparations;
    10 - 20 drops of essential oil.

Mode of Administration
Comminuted herb and other oral galenical preparations.

Actions
Antispasmodic
Cholagogue
Stimulates the secretion of gastric juices

Anise seed
Anisi fructus
Anis
Published July 6, 1988

Name of Drug
Anisi fructus, anise.

Composition of Drug
Anise consists of the dried fruits of *Pimpinella anisum* L. [Fam. Apiaceae], as well as its preparations in effective dosage.
    The drug contains essential oil.

Uses
Internal:
    Dyspeptic complaints.
Internal and external use:
    Catarrhs of the respiratory tract.

Contraindications
Allergy to anise and anethole.

Side Effects
Occasional allergic reactions of skin, respiratory tract, and gastrointestinal tract.

Interactions with Other Drugs
None known.

Dosage
Unless otherwise prescribed:
Internal:
Average daily dosage:
    3 g of drug;
    Essential oil 0.3 g;
    equivalent preparations.
External:
    Preparations containing 5 - 10 percent essential oil.

Mode of Administration
Comminuted drug for infusions and other galenical preparations for internal use or for inhalation.

Note: The purpose of an external application of an anise preparation is the inhalation of essential oil.

Actions
Expectorant
Mildly antispasmodic
Antibacterial

Arnica flower
Arnicae flos
Arnikablüten
Published December 5, 1984

Name of Drug
Arnicae flos, arnica flower.

Composition of Drug
Arnica flower consists of the fresh or dried inflorescence of *Arnica montana* L. or *A. chamissonis* Less. subsp. *foliosa* (Nutt.) Maguiere [Fam. Asteraceae], as well as its preparations in effective dosage.

It contains sesquiterpene lactones of the helenanolid type, predominantly ester derivatives of helenalin and 11,13-dihydrohelenalin. Additionally, the herb contains flavonoids (e.g., isoquercitrin, luteolin-7-glucoside, and astragalin), volatile oil (with thymol and its derivatives), phenol carbonic acid (chlorogenic acid, cynarin, caffeic acid), and coumarins (umbelliferone, scopoletin).

Uses
For external use in injury and for consequences of accidents, e.g., hematoma, dislocations, contusions, edema due to fracture, rheumatic muscle and joint problems. Inflammation of the oral and throat region, furunculosis, inflammation caused by insect bites, superficial phlebitis.

Contraindications
Arnica allergy.

Side Effects
Prolonged treatment of damaged skin, e.g., use for injuries or ulcus cruris (indolent leg ulcers), often causes edematous dermatitis with the formation of pustules. Long use can also give rise to eczema. In treatment involving higher concentrations of the drug, primary toxic skin reactions with formation of vesicles or even necroses may occur.

Interactions with Other Drugs
None known.

Dosage
Unless otherwise prescribed:
Infusion:
    2 g of herb per 100 ml of water.
Tincture for cataplasm:
    Tincture in 3 - 10 times dilution.
For mouth rinses:
    Tincture in 10 times dilution.
As ointment:
    Not more than 20 - 25 percent tincture.
"Arnica oil":
    Extract of 1 part herb and 5 parts fatty oil.
    Ointments with not more than 15 percent "Arnica oil."

Mode of Administration
Whole herb, cut herb, herb powder for infusions, liquid and semi-solid forms of medication for external application.

Actions
Especially when applied topically, arnica preparations have antiphlogistic activity. In cases of inflammation, arnica preparations also show analgesic and antiseptic activity.

Monograph Comments
[**Ed. note:** The following is additional information on Arnica flower that was not part of the Commission E Monograph. It is added for clarification.]

From the *Bundesanzeiger*. Published December 5, 1984.

Arnica Flower
Oral administration of arnica is often accompanied by severe side effects. For this reason the monograph refers to the herb's external use only, in contrast to the comment section in *DAB* 8 (*German Pharmacopoeia*, No. 8), which refers to the internal use of a tea infusion of arnica for circulatory disorders of the heart and brain. (From Comments in *DAB* 8, 2nd Edition (1983), page 167.)

The identity testing of *DAB* 8 is inadequate; for example, a tincture produced from "Mexican arnica" (*Heterotheca inuloides* Cass.) did not contain detectable quantities of arnica. For reliable identification, thin layer chromatographic detection of flavonoids[1] and/or the sesquiterpene lactones[2] may be used.

In contrast to the possibility of internal use, occasionally practiced in folk medicine, (20 - 30 drops up to three times a day), mentioned in the *DAB* 8 comments, this monograph, correctly, contains information on external use only; oral use is considered potentially unsafe from the toxicological viewpoint.

1. H. Wagner, S. Bladt, and E. M. Zgainski: *Drogenanalyse (Plant Drug Analysis)* (Berlin: Springer-Verlag, 1983), p. 176.
2. G. Willuhn and H. D. Herrman, *Pharm. Ztg.* 123, 1803 (1978).

Artichoke leaf
Cynarae folium
Artischockenblätter
Published July 6, 1988; Revised September 1, 1990

Name of Drug
Cynarae folium, artichoke leaf.

Composition of Drug
Artichoke leaf consists of the fresh or dried leaf of *Cynara scolymus* L. [Fam. Asteraceae], and its preparations in effective dosage.

The drug contains caffeoylquinic acid derivatives such as cynarin and bitter principles.

Uses
Dyspeptic problems.

Contraindications
Known allergies to artichokes and other composites.
Obstruction of bile ducts.
In case of gallstones, use only after consultations with a physician.

Side Effects
None known.

Interactions with Other Drugs
None known.

Dosage
Unless otherwise prescribed:
Average daily dosage:
>Drug, 6 g;
>equivalent preparations.

Mode of Administration
Dried, cut leaves, pressed juice of fresh plant, and other galenical preparations for internal use.

Action
Choleretic

Asparagus root
Asparagi rhizoma
Spargelwurzelstock
Published July 12, 1991

Name of Drug
Asparagi rhizoma, asparagus root.

Composition of Drug
Asparagus root consists of the rhizome of *Asparagus officinalis* L. [Fam. Liliaceae], as well as its preparations in effective dosage. The rhizome contains saponins.

Uses
Irrigation therapy for inflammatory diseases of the urinary tract and for prevention of kidney stones.

Contraindications
Inflammatory kidney diseases.
Note: No irrigation therapy if edema exists because of functional heart or kidney disorders.

Side Effects
In rare cases, allergic skin reactions.

Interactions with Other Drugs
None known.

Dosage
Unless otherwise prescribed:
Daily dosage:
>45 - 60 g of rhizome;
>equivalent preparations.

Mode of Administration
Cut rhizome for teas, as well as other galenical preparations for internal use.
Note: Irrigation therapy:
>Be sure to provide adequate fluids.

Actions
Animal experiments indicate a diuretic effect.

Autumn Crocus
Colchicum autumnale
Herbstzeitlose
Published September 18, 1986

Name of Drug
Colchici semen, autumn crocus (meadow saffron) seed.
Colchici tuber, autumn crocus (meadow saffron) tuber.
Colchici flos, autumn crocus (meadow saffron) flower.

Composition of Drug
The drug consists of the dried seeds harvested in June or July, or the cut and dried tubers harvested in July or August, or the fresh flowers harvested in late summer and autumn of *Colchicum autumnale* L. [Fam. Liliaceae], as well as their preparations in effective dosage. *Colchicum autumnale* contains colchicine as active ingredient: at least 0.4 percent in seeds (*DAC* 1979, standard delivery).

Uses
Acute gout attack, familial Mediterranean fever.

Contraindications
Pregnancy.
Note: Care must be observed with old and weakened patients, as well as with those who suffer from heart, kidney or gastrointestinal conditions.

Side Effects
Diarrhea, nausea, vomiting, abdominal pain, leukopenia; with extended use, skin alterations, agranulocytosis, aplastic anemia, myopathy and alopecia.

Interactions with Other Drugs
None known.

Dosage
Unless otherwise prescribed:
   For an acute attack, an initial oral dose corresponding to 1 mg colchicine, followed by 0.5 - 1.5 mg every 1 - 2 hours until pain subsides.
   Total daily dosage must not surpass 8 mg of colchicine.
   For familial Mediterranean fever, prophylactic and therapeutic purposes, dosage corresponding to 0.5 - 1.5 mg of colchicine.

Mode of Administration
Comminuted drug, freshly pressed juice and other galenical preparations taken orally.

Duration of Administration
No repetition of treatment for gout within 3 days.

Actions
Anti-chemotactic
Antiphlogistic
Inhibitor of mitosis

Belladonna
Atropa belladonna
Tollkirsche
Published November 30, 1985

Name of Drug
Belladonnae folium, belladonna leaf, deadly nightshade leaf.
Belladonnae radix, belladonna root, deadly nightshade root.

Composition of Drug
Belladonna leaf consists of the dried leaves, or the dried leaves together with the flowering branch tips, of *Atropa belladonna* L. [Fam. Solanaceae], as well as its preparations in effective dosage.

Belladonna root consists of the dried roots and rhizomes of *A. belladonna* L., as well as its preparations in effective dosage.

The drug contains alkaloids, such as L-hyoscyamine, atropine, and scopolamine, with a total alkaloid content of at least 0.3 percent in the leaves and 0.5 percent in the roots, calculated as hyoscyamine and related to the dried herb.

Uses
Spasms and colic-like pain in the areas of the gastrointestinal tract and bile ducts.

Contraindications
Tachycardiac arrhythmias, prostate adenoma with residual urine formation, narrow-angle glaucoma, acute edema of the lungs, mechanical stenoses of the gastrointestinal tract, megacolon.

Side Effects
Dryness of mouth, decrease in secretion by the perspiration glands, accommodation disturbances, reddening and dryness of skin, hyperthermia, tachycardia, difficulty in micturition (urination), hallucination and spasms (especially with overdosing).

Interactions with Other Drugs
Increase of anticholinergic effect by tricyclic antidepressants, amantadine and quinidine.

Dosage
Unless otherwise prescribed:
Belladonna leaf powder (belladonnae pulvis normatus):
Average single dosage:
  0.05 - 0.1 g;
Maximum single dosage:
  0.2 g equivalent to 0.6 mg total alkaloids, calculated as hyoscyamine;
Maximum daily dosage:
  0.6 g, equivalent to 1.8 mg total alkaloids, calculated as hyoscyamine.
Belladonna root (belladonnae radix):
Average single dosage:
  0.05 g;
Maximum single dosage:
  0.1 g equivalent to 0.5 mg total alkaloids, calculated as hyoscyamine;
Maximum daily dosage:
  0.3 g equivalent to 1.5 mg total alkaloids, calculated as hyoscyamine.
Belladonna extract:
Average single dosage:
  0.01 g;
Maximum single dosage:
  0.05 g, equivalent to 0.73 mg total alkaloids, calculated as hyoscyamine;
Maximum daily dosage:
  0.15 g, equivalent to 2.2 mg total alkaloids, calculated as hyoscyamine.

Mode of Administration
As liquid or solid forms of medication for internal use.

Actions

Belladonna preparations act as a parasympatholytic or anticholinergic via a competitive antagonism of the neuromuscular transmitter acetylcholine. This antagonism concerns mainly the muscarine-like effects of acetylcholine and less the nicotine-like effects on the ganglions and the neuromuscular end plate. Belladonna preparations unfold peripheral effects targeted on the vegetative nervous system and the smooth muscle system, as well as the central nervous system. Because of the parasympatholytic properties, the drug can cause relaxation of organs with smooth muscles and relieve spastic conditions, especially in the gastrointestinal tract and bile ducts. Additionally, Belladonna use may result in muscular tremor or rigidity due to effects on the central nervous system. Belladonna preparations have a positive dromotropic as well as a positive chronotropic effect on the heart.

Bilberry fruit
Myrtilli fructus
Heidelbeeren
Published April 23, 1987; Revised March 13, 1990

Name of Drug
Myrtilli fructus, bilberry, blueberry.

Composition of Drug
Bilberry consists of the dried, ripe fruit of *Vaccinium myrtillus* L. [Fam. Ericaceae], as well as its preparations in effective dosage.

The drug contains tannins, anthocyanins, and flavonoid glycosides.

Uses
Nonspecific, acute diarrhea.
Local therapy of mild inflammation of the mucous membranes of mouth and throat.

Contraindications
None known.

Side Effects
None known.

Interactions with Other Drugs
None known.

Dosage
Internal:
    Daily dosage 20 - 60 g.
External:
    10 percent decoction;
    equivalent preparations.

Mode of Administration
Dried drug for infusions, as well as other galenical preparations for internal use and local application.

Duration of Administration
If diarrhea persists for more than 3 - 4 days, consult a physician.

Action
Astringent

Birch leaf
Betulae folium
Birkenblätter
Published March 13, 1986

Name of Drug
Betulae folium, birch leaf.

Composition of Drug
Birch leaf consists of the fresh or dried leaf of *Betula pendula* Roth (syn. *B. verrucosa* Ehrhart), or *B. pubescens* Ehrhart [Fam. Betulaceae], or of both species, as well as its preparations in effective dosage.

The leaves contain at least 1.5 percent flavonoids, calculated as hyperoside and expressed in terms of the dried herb. In addition to flavonoids, the herb contains saponin, tannins and essential oil.

Uses
Irrigation therapy for bacterial and inflammatory diseases of the urinary tract and for kidney gravel; supportive therapy for rheumatic ailments.

Contraindications
None known.
Note: No irrigation therapy if edema exists due to impaired heart and kidney function.

Side Effects
None known.

Interactions with Other Drugs
None known.

Dosage
Unless otherwise prescribed:
Average daily dosage:
    2 - 3 g of herb several times daily; equivalent preparations.

Mode of Administration
Comminuted herb or dry extracts for teas, as well as other galenical preparations and freshly pressed plant juices for oral use.
Note: For irrigation therapy, observe copious fluid intake.

Action
Diuretic

Bitter Orange peel
Aurantii pericarpium
Pomeranzenschale
Published October 15, 1987; Revised March 13, 1990

Name of Drug
Aurantii pericarpium, bitter orange peel.

Composition of Drug
Bitter orange peel consists of the dried outer peel of ripe fruits of *Citrus aurantium* L. subspecies *aurantium* (synonym *C. aurantium* L. subspecies *amara* Engler) [Fam. Rutaceae], freed from the white pulp layer, as well as its preparations in effective dosage.

The drug contains essential oil and bitter principles.

Uses
Loss of appetite, dyspeptic ailments.

Contraindications
None known.

Side Effects
Photosensitization is possible, especially in fair-skinned individuals.

Interactions with Other Drugs
None known.

Dosage
Unless otherwise prescribed:
Daily dosage:
  Drug:
    4 - 6 g;
  Tincture (according to *DAB* 7):
    2 - 3 g;
  Extract (according to *Erg. B. 6*):
    1 - 2 g.

Mode of Administration
Comminuted drug for teas, other bitter-tasting galenical preparations for oral application.

Black Cohosh root
Cimicifugae racemosae rhizoma
Cimicifugawurzelstock
Published March 2, 1989

Name of Drug
Cimicifugae racemosae rhizoma, black cohosh root.

Composition of Drug
Preparations of black cohosh consist of the fresh or dried rhizome with attached roots of *Cimicifuga racemosa* (L.) Nutt. [Fam. Ranunculaceae] in effective dosage.
  The drug contains triterpene glycosides.

Uses
Premenstrual discomfort, dysmenorrhea or climacteric [menopausal] neurovegetative ailments.

Contraindications
None known.

Side Effects
Occasionally, gastric discomfort.

Interactions with Other Drugs
None known.

Dosage
Unless otherwise prescribed:
Daily dosage:
  Extracts with alcohol 40 - 60 percent (v/v) corresponding to 40 mg of drug.

Mode of Administration
Galenical preparations for internal use.

Duration of Administration
Not longer than 6 months.

Actions
Estrogen-like action
Luteinizing hormone suppression
Binding to estrogen receptors

Blackberry leaf
Rubi fruticosi folium
Brombeerblätter
Published February 1, 1990

Name of Drug
Rubi fruticosi folium, blackberry leaf.

Composition of Drug
Blackberry leaf consists of the dried leaf, fermented or unfermented, gathered during the flowering period, of *Rubus fruticosus* L. [Fam. Rosaceae], as well as its preparations in effective dosage.
　　Blackberry leaf contains tannins.

Uses
Nonspecific, acute diarrhea, mild inflammation of the mucosa of the oral cavity and throat.

Contraindications
None known.

Side Effects
None known.

Interactions with Other Drugs
None known.

Dosage
Unless otherwise prescribed:
Daily dose:
　　4.5 g of leaf;
　　equivalent preparations.

Mode of Administration
Comminuted drug for teas, and other preparations for internal use, as well as for mouth washes.

Duration of Administration
If diarrhea persists for longer than 3 - 4 days, consult with a physician.

Action
Astringent

Blackthorn berry
Pruni spinosae fructus
Schlehdornfrüchte
Published June 1, 1990

Name of Drug
Pruni spinosae fructus, blackthorn fruit, sloe berry.

Composition of Drug
Blackthorn fruit consists of the fresh or dried, ripe fruit of *Prunus spinosa* L. [Fam. Rosaceae], as well as its preparations in effective dosage.
　　The drug contains tannins.

Uses
Mild inflammations of the oral and pharyngeal mucosa.

Contraindications
None known.

Side Effects
None known.

Interactions with Other Drugs
None known.

Dosage
Unless otherwise prescribed:
Daily dosage:
   2 - 4 g drug;
   equivalent preparations.

Mode of Administration
Comminuted herb for teas and other galenical preparations for mouth rinses.

Action
Astringent

Blessed Thistle herb
Cnici benedicti herba
Benediktenkraut
Published October 15, 1987

Name of Drug
Cnici benedicti herba, blessed thistle herb, holy thistle herb.

Composition of Drug
Blessed thistle herb consists of the dried leaves and upper stems, including inflorescence, of *Cnicus benedictus* L. [Fam. Asteraceae], as well as preparations thereof in effective dosage.

The herb contains bitter principles, such as cnicin.

Uses
Loss of appetite, dyspepsia.

Contraindications
Allergies to blessed thistle and other composites.

Side Effects
Allergic reactions are possible.

Interactions with Other Drugs
None known.

Dosage
Unless otherwise prescribed:
Mean daily dosage:
   4 - 6 g of herb;
   equivalent preparations accordingly.

Mode of Administration
Comminuted herb and dried extracts for teas; bitter-tasting galenical preparations for internal use.

Action
Stimulation of the secretion of saliva and gastric juices

Bogbean leaf
Menyanthis folium
Bitterkleeblätter
Published February 1, 1990

Name of Drug
Menyanthis folium, bogbean leaf.

Composition of Drug
Bogbean leaf consists of the leaf of *Menyanthes trifoliata* L. [Fam. Menyanthaceae], as well as its preparations in effective dosage.

The drug contains bitter principles.

Uses
Loss of appetite, peptic discomforts.

Contraindications
None known.

Side Effects
None known.

Interactions with Other Drugs
None known.

Dosage
Unless otherwise prescribed:
Daily dosage:
   1.5 - 3 g of drug;
   Preparations with equivalent bitter
   value.

Mode of Administration
Comminuted herb for teas and other bitter-tasting preparations for internal use.

Action
Stimulation of the secretion of saliva and gastric juices

Boldo leaf
Boldo folium
Boldoblätter
Published April 23, 1987; Revised September 1, 1990

Name of Drug
Boldo folium, boldo leaf.

Composition of Drug
Boldo leaf consists of the dried leaves of *Peumus boldus* Molina [Fam. Monimiaceae], as well as its preparations in effective dosage.

The leaves contain at least 0.1 percent alkaloids, calculated as boldine, and flavonoids.

Uses
Mild spastic complaints of the gastrointestinal tract, dyspepsia.

Contraindications
Obstruction of bile ducts, severe liver diseases. In case of gallstones, to be used only after consultation with a physician.

Side Effects
None known.

Interactions with Other Drugs
None known.

Dosage
Unless otherwise prescribed:
Average daily dosage:
  3 g of herb;
  equivalent preparations.

Mode of Administration
Comminuted herb for infusions and other, virtually ascaridol-free preparations for internal application.

Note: Because of the ascaridol content, essential oil and distillates of boldo leaf should not be used.

Actions
Antispasmodic
Choleretic
Increase in gastric secretions

Bromelain
Bromelainum
Bromelain
Published March 10, 1994

Name of Drug
Bromelainum, bromelain.

Composition of Drug
Bromelain (EC 3.4.22.4) is the genuine mixture of bromelin A and B, the proteolytic enzymes of pineapple fruit, *Ananas comosus* (L.) Merrill [Fam. Bromeliaceae], in effective dosage.

Pharmacological Properties, Pharmacokinetics, Toxicology
In various animal experiments (egg white-, carrageen-, dextran-, and yeast-induced edemas, traumatic edema, adrenalin-caused edema of the lungs), an edema-inhibiting effect was demonstrated with high dosages of bromelain upon oral and intraperitoneal administration. Upon oral intake, bromelain can prolong prothrombin and bleeding time, as well as inhibit the aggregation of thrombocytes. There is no information available on the absorption of the compound in humans after oral ingestion.

Only older data are known regarding acute and chronic toxicity of the compound. The LD^{50} after parenteral application is 85.2 mg/kg for rats, 30 - 35 mg/kg for mice, and for rabbits greater than 20 mg/kg of body weight. There are no data for mutagenicity and carcinogenicity.

With rats and rabbits, there were no indications of embryotoxic or teratogenic effects.

Clinical Data

1. Uses
Acute postoperative and post-traumatic conditions of swelling, especially of the nasal and paranasal sinuses.

2. Contraindications
Hypersensitivity to bromelain.

3. Side Effects
Occasionally gastric disturbances or diarrhea. Sometimes allergic reactions.

4. Special Cautions for Use
None known.

5. Use During Pregnancy and Lactation
No data available.

6. Interactions with Other Drugs
An increased tendency for bleeding in the case of simultaneous administration of anticoagulants and inhibitors of thrombocytic aggregation cannot be excluded. The levels of tetracyclines in plasma and urine are increased by simultaneous intake of bromelain.

7. Dosage
Unless otherwise prescribed:
Daily dosage:
    80 - 320 mg of bromelain (200 - 800 FIP units) in 2 or 3 doses.

Mode of Administration
Solid preparations for oral use.

Duration of Administration
8 - 10 days. If necessary, administration may be prolonged.

8. Overdosage
None known.

9. Special Warnings
None.

10. Effects on Operators of Vehicles and Machinery
None.

Buckthorn bark
Frangulae cortex
Faulbaumrinde
Published November 1, 1984; Replaced July 21, 1993

Name of Drug
Frangulae cortex, buckthorn bark, frangula.

Composition of Drug
Buckthorn bark consists of the dried bark of the trunks and branches of *Rhamnus frangula* L. (syn. *Frangula alnus* Miller) [Fam. Rhamnaceae], as well as its preparations in effective dosage.

The bark contains anthranoids, mainly of the emodin-physcion and chrysophanol type.

These drugs must conform to the currently valid pharmacopeia.

Pharmacological Properties, Pharmacokinetics, Toxicology
1,8-dihydroxy-anthracene derivatives have a laxative effect. These compounds increase the motility of the colon by inhibiting stationary and stimulating propulsive contractions. This results in accelerated intestinal passage and, because of the shortened contraction time, a reduction in liquid absorption through the lumen. In addition, stimulation of active chloride secretion increases the water and electrolyte content of intestinal contents.

Systematic studies pertaining to the kinetics of buckthorn bark preparations are not available; however, it must be supposed that the aglycones contained in the drug are already absorbed in the upper small intestine. The ß-glycosides are pro-drugs which are neither absorbed nor cleaved in the upper gastrointestinal tract. They are degraded in the colon by bacterial enzymes to anthrones. Anthrones are the laxative metabolites.

Active metabolites of other anthronoids, such as rhein, infiltrate in small amounts into the milk ducts. A laxative effect on nursing infants has not been observed. The placental permeability for rhein is very small.

Drug preparations [i.e., herbal stimulant laxatives] have a higher general toxicity than the pure glycosides, presumably due to the content of aglycones. Experiments pertaining to the genotoxicity of buckthorn and its preparations are not available. Some positive data were obtained for aloe-emodin, emodin, physcion and chrysophanol. No data are available for their carcinogenicity.

The fresh bark contains free anthrone and must be stored for one year or artificially aged by heat and aeration. The use of illegally processed buckthorn bark, e.g., fresh bark, will cause severe vomiting, possibly with spasms.

Clinical Data

1. Uses
Constipation.

2. Contraindications
Intestinal obstruction, acute intestinal inflammation, e.g., Crohn's disease, colitis ulcerosa, appendicitis, abdominal pain of unknown origin. Children under 12 years of age; pregnancy.

3. Side Effects
In single incidents, cramp-like discomforts of the gastrointestinal tract. These incidents require a dosage reduction.

With long-term use/abuse: disturbances of electrolyte balance, especially potassium deficiency, albuminuria and hematuria. Pigment implantation into the intestinal mucosa (*pseudomelanosis coli*) is harmless and usually reverses upon discontinuation of the drug. The potassium deficiency can lead to disorders of heart function and muscular weakness, especially with concurrent use of cardiac glycosides, diuretics and corticosteroids.

4. Special Caution for Use
Stimulating laxatives should not be used over an extended period (1 - 2 weeks) without medical advice.

5. Use During Pregnancy and Lactation
Because of insufficient toxicological investigation, this drug should not be used during pregnancy or lactation.

6. Interactions with Other Drugs
With chronic use or in cases of abuse of the drug, a potentiation of cardiac glycosides due to a loss of serum potassium is possible. Also possible is an effect on antiarrhythmic agents. Potassium deficiency can be increased by simultaneous application of thiazide diuretics, corticosteroids, or licorice root.

7. Dosage
Cut bark, powder or dried extracts for teas, decoction, cold maceration or elixir. Liquid or solid forms of medication exclusively for oral use.
Unless otherwise prescribed:
20 - 30 mg hydroxyanthracene derivatives daily, calculated as glycofrangulin A.

The individually correct dosage is the smallest dosage necessary to maintain a soft stool.
Note: The form of administration should be smaller than the normal daily dose.

8. Overdosage
Electrolyte and fluid-regulating measures.

9. Special Warnings
Use of a stimulating laxative for longer than the recommended application can cause intestinal sluggishness.

The preparation should be used only if no effect can be obtained through change of diet or use of bulk-forming products.

10. Effects on Operators of Vehicles and Machinery
None known.

Buckthorn berry
Rhamni cathartici fructus
Kreuzdornbeeren
Published March 16, 1990; Replaced November 25, 1993

Name of Drug
Rhamni cathartici fructus, buckthorn berry.

Composition of Drug
Buckthorn, consisting of the dried ripe berries of *Rhamnus catharticus* L. [Fam. Rhamnaceae] as well as its preparations in effective dosage.

The drug contains anthranoids, mainly of the emodin type.

Pharmacological Properties, Pharmacokinetics, Toxicology
1,8-dihydroxyanthracene derivatives have a laxative effect. This works mainly through its effect on colon motility by inhibiting the stationary and stimulating the propulsive contractions. This results in faster bowel movements and a reduction of fluid absorption due to the shortened contact time. In addition, because of the stimulation of active chloride secretions, water and electrolytes are discharged.

Systematic research on the kinetics of buckthorn berry preparations are not available at present. However, it is assumed that the aglycones contained in the drug are absorbed in the small intestine. The ß-glycosides are prodrugs which are neither absorbed nor cleaved in the upper gastrointestinal tract. They are broken down into anthrones by enzymes in the colon. Anthrones are the laxative metabolites.

Active metabolites of other anthranoids such as cassic acid pass in small amounts into the milk of nursing mothers. A laxative effect on breast-fed babies has, however, not been observed. In animal experiments only a minimal level of absorption through the placenta has been observed.

Drug preparations [i.e., herbal stimulant laxatives] contain a higher level of general toxicity than the pure glycosides, probably due to the high level of aglycones. Research on the genotoxicity of the drug or of drug preparation are not available at present. Some positive results are available for aloe-emodin, emodin, parietin and chrysophanic acid. No research has been done on carcinogenicity.

Clinical Data

1. Uses
Constipation.

2. Contraindications
Obstruction of the bowel or intestines, acute inflammatory conditions of the bowels such as Crohn's disease, colitis, appendicitis; abdominal pains of unknown origin; children under 12 years; pregnancy.

3. Side Effects
Some patients may suffer from gastrointestinal cramps. If this occurs, the dose should be reduced.

In the case of chronic use/overuse: loss of electrolytes, especially loss of potassium, albuminuria, hematuria. Pigment implantation into the intestinal mucosa (*pseudomelanosis coli*) is harmless and usually reverses upon discontinuation of the drug. The potassium deficiency can lead to disorders of heart function and muscular weakness, especially with concurrent use of cardiac glycosides, diuretics and corticoadrenal steroids.

4. Warning
Stimulating laxatives should not be used over an extended period (1 - 2 weeks) without medical advice.

5. Use During Pregnancy and Lactation
Not to be taken during pregnancy or lactation because of the lack of toxicological research.

6. Interactions with Other Drugs and Substances
With chronic use or in cases of abuse of the drug, a potentiation of cardiac glycosides due to a loss of serum potassium is possible. Also possible is an effect on antiarrhythmic agents. Potassium deficiency can be increased by simultaneous application of thiazide diuretics, corticosteroids, or licorice root.

7. Dosage and Mode of Administration
20 - 30 mg hydroxyanthracene derivative per day calculated as glucofrangulin A. The individual dose is the minimum required to produce a soft stool.

The crushed drug for infusions, boiling, cold macerations or elixirs. Liquid or solid form solely for oral administration.
Note: The method of dosing facilitates a smaller than average daily dose.

8. Overdosing
Electrolyte and fluid-regulating measures.

9. Special Precautions
Taking stimulating laxatives for longer than the recommended period can lead to intestinal sluggishness.

The treatment should be used only if a therapeutic effect has not been achieved through change of diet or use of a swelling agent [i.e., bulk laxative].

10. Effects on Operators of Vehicles and Machinery
None known.

Bugleweed
Lycopi herba
Wolfstrappkraut
Published February 1, 1990

Name of Drug
Lycopi herba, bugleweed, gypsywort.

Composition of Drug
Bugleweed consists of the fresh or dried, above-ground parts of *Lycopus europaeus* L. and/or *L. virginicus* L. [Fam. Lamiaceae], as well as their preparations in effective dosage.

The drug contains hydrocinnamic and caffeic acid derivatives, lithospermic acid and flavonoids.

Uses
Mild thyroid hyperfunction with disturbances of the vegetative nervous system. Tension and pain in the breast (mastodynia).

Contraindications
Thyroid hypofunction, enlargement of the thyroid without functional disorders.

Side Effects
In rare cases, extended therapy and high dosages of bugleweed preparations have resulted in an enlargement of the thyroid. Sudden discontinuation of bugleweed preparations can cause increased symptoms of the disease complex.

Interactions with Other Drugs
None known.
 No simultaneous administration of thyroid preparations.
Note: Administration of bugleweed preparations interferes with the administration of diagnostic procedures using radioactive isotopes.

Dosage
The dosage lies between a daily dosage of 1 - 2 g of drug for teas and water-ethanol extracts equivalent of 20 mg of drug.
Note: Each patient has his own individual optimal level of thyroid hormone. Only rough estimations of dosage are possible for thyroid disorders, in which age and weight must be considered.

Mode of Administration
Comminuted herb, freshly pressed juice and other galenical preparations for internal use.

Actions
Antigonadotropic
Antithyrotropic
Inhibition of the peripheral deiodination of T4
Lowering of the prolactin level

Butcher's Broom
Rusci aculeati rhizoma
Mäusedornwurzelstock
Published July 12, 1991

Name of Drug
Rusci aculeati rhizoma, butcher's broom.

Composition of Drug
Butcher's broom consists of the dried rhizome and root of *Ruscus aculeatus* L. [Fam. Liliaceae], as well as its preparations in effective dosage. The drug contains the steroid saponins ruscin and ruscoside.

Uses
Supportive therapy for discomforts of chronic venous insufficiency, such as pain and heaviness, as well as cramps in the legs, itching, and swelling. Supportive therapy for complaints of hemorrhoids, such as itching and burning.

Contraindications
None known.

Side Effects
In rare cases, gastric disorders or nausea may occur.

Interactions with Other Drugs
None known.

Dosage
Unless otherwise prescribed:
Daily dosage:
> Raw extract, equivalent to 7 - 11 mg total ruscogenin (determined as the sum of neoruscogenin and ruscogenin obtained after fermentation or acid hydrolysis).

Mode of Administration
Extracts and their preparations for internal use.

Actions
In animal experiments:
> Increase in venous tone
> Electrolyte-like reaction on the cell wall of capillaries
> Antiphlogistic
> Diuretic

Calendula flower
Calendulae flos
Ringelblumenblüten
Published March 13, 1986

Name of Drug
Calendulae flos, calendula flower.

Composition of Drug
Calendula flower consists of the dried flower heads or the dried ligulate flowers (ray florets) of *Calendula officinalis* L. [Fam. Asteraceae], as well as its preparations in effective dosage.

The drug contains triterpene glycosides and aglycones, as well as carotenoids and essential oils.

Uses
Internal and topical use:
> Inflammation of the oral and pharyngeal mucosa.

External:
> Poorly healing wounds.
> Ulcus cruris.

Contraindications
None known.

Side Effects
None known.

Interactions with Other Drugs
None known.

Dosage
Unless otherwise prescribed:
> 1 - 2 g per cup of water (150 ml) or 1 - 2 teaspoons (2 - 4 ml) tincture per ¼ - ½ l water, or prepared in ointments equivalent to 2 - 5 g crude drug in 100 g ointment.

Mode of Administration
Powdered herb for infusions and other galenical preparations for local application.

Actions
Promotes wound healing.
Antiinflammatory and granulatory action in topical application have been described.

Camphor
Camphora
Campher
Published December 5, 1984; Revised March 13, 1990

Name of Drug
Camphora, camphor.

Composition of Drug
Purified D (+) camphor obtained from the wood of the camphor tree, *Cinnamomum camphora* (L.) Siebold [Fam. Lauraceae], by steam distillation followed by sublimation, synthetic camphor or a mixture of both. It contains not less than 96 and not more than 101 percent 2-bornanone, of which at least 50 percent should be present as the (1R)-isomer.

Uses
External:
  Muscular rheumatism, catarrhal diseases of the respiratory tract, cardiac symptoms.
Internal:
  Hypotonic circulatory regulation disorders, catarrhal diseases of the respiratory tract.

Contraindications
External:
  Injured skin, e.g., burns.
Camphor preparations should not be used in the facial regions of infants and small children, especially in the nasal area.

Side Effects
Contact eczema possible.

Interactions with Other Drugs
None known.

Dosage
Unless otherwise prescribed:
External:
  10 - 20 percent in semisolid preparations
  1 - 10 percent in camphor spirits
Internal:
  Average daily dosage: 30 - 300 mg.

Mode of Administration
Locally or for inhalation:
  in liquid or semi-solid form.
Internal:
  in liquid or solid preparations.

Actions
External:
  Bronchial secretagogue
  Hyperemic
Internal:
  Circulatory tonic
  Respiratory analeptic
  Bronchoantispasmodic

Caraway oil
Carvi aetheroleum
Kümmelöl
Published February 1, 1990

Name of Drug
Carvi aetheroleum, caraway oil.

Composition of Drug
Caraway oil consists of the essential oil obtained from the dried, ripe fruits of *Carum carvi* L. [Fam. Apiaceae], as well as its preparations in effective dosage. The main ingredient of caraway oil is d-carvone.

Uses
Dyspeptic problems, such as mild, spastic condition of the gastrointestinal tract, flatulence and fullness.

Contraindications
None known.

Side Effects
None known.

Interactions with Other Drugs
None.

Dosage
Unless otherwise prescribed:
Daily dosage:
    3 - 6 drops.

Mode of Administration
Essential oil and its galenical preparations for internal use.

Actions
Antispasmodic
Antimicrobial

Caraway seed
Carvi fructus
Kümmel
Published February 1, 1990

Name of Drug
Carvi fructus, caraway seed.

Composition of Drug
Caraway consists of the dried, ripe fruit of *Carum carvi* L. [Fam. Apiaceae], as well as its preparations in effective dosage. The drug contains essential oil.

Uses
Dyspeptic problems such as mild, spastic conditions of the gastrointestinal tract, bloating, and fullness.

Contraindications
None known.

Side Effects
None known.

Interactions with Other Drugs
None known.

Dosage
Unless otherwise prescribed:
Daily dosage:
    1.5 - 6 g of seeds;
    equivalent preparations.

Mode of Administration
Freshly crushed seeds for infusions as well as for other galenical preparations for internal use.

Actions
Antispasmodic
Antimicrobial

Cardamom seed
Cardamomi fructus
Kardamomen
Published November 30, 1985; Revised March 13, 1990, and September 1, 1990

Name of Drug
Cardamomi fructus, cardamom seed.

Composition of Drug
Cardamom consists of the dried, almost ripe, greenish to yellow-gray fruit of *Elettaria cardamomum* (L.) Maton [Fam. Zingiberaceae]. Medicinal use is made only of the seed removed from its fruit capsule, and preparations thereof. The seeds contain essential oil with mainly terpinyl acetate, α-terpineol and 1,8-cineol.

Uses
Dyspepsia.

Contraindications
In case of gallstones, use only after consultation with a physician.

Side Effects
None known.

Interactions with Other Drugs
None known.

Dosage
Unless otherwise prescribed:
Average daily dosage:
    1.5 g of drug;
    equivalent preparations.
Tincture (according to *Erg. B. 6*):
Daily dosage:
    1 - 2 g.

Mode of Administration
Ground seeds, as well as galenical preparations thereof for internal use.

Actions
Cholagogue
Virustatic

Cascara Sagrada bark
Rhamni purshianae cortex
Amerikanische Faulbaumrinde
Published November 1, 1984; Replaced July 21, 1993

Name of Drug
Rhamni purshianae cortex, cascara sagrada bark.

Composition of Drug
Cascara sagrada bark consists of the dried bark of *Rhamnus purshiana* D.C. (syn. *Frangula purshiana* (D.C.) A. Gray ex J.C. Cooper) [Fam. Rhamnaceae], as well as its preparations in effective dosage.

The bark contains anthranoids, mainly of the aloe-emodin type, in addition to those of the chrysophanol and physcion type.

The drug must conform to the currently valid pharmacopeia.

Pharmacological Properties, Pharmacokinetics, Toxicology
1,8-dihydroxy-anthracene derivatives have a laxative effect. This effect is primarily due to the influence of the herb on the motility of the colon, inhibiting stationary and stimulating propulsive contractions. This results in an accelerated intestinal passage and, because of the shortened contact time, a reduction in liquid absorption. In addition, stimulation of the active chloride secretion increases water and electrolyte content.

Systematic studies pertaining to the kinetics of cascara sagrada bark preparations are not available. However, it must be concluded that the aglycones contained in the drug are already absorbed in the upper small intestine. The ß-glycosides are prodrugs which are neither absorbed nor cleaved in the upper gastrointestinal tract. They are degraded in the colon by bacterial enzymes to anthrones. The anthrones are the laxative metabolites.

Active metabolites of other anthronoids, such as rhein, infiltrate in small amounts into the milk ducts. A laxative effect on nursing infants has not been observed. The placental permeability for rhein is very small.

Drug preparations [i.e., herbal stimulant laxatives] have a higher general toxicity than the pure glycosides, presumably due to the content of aglycones. Experiments pertaining to the genotoxicity of cascara sagrada and its preparations are not available. Some positive data were obtained for aloe-emodin, emodin, physcion and chrysophanol. No data are available for carcinogenicity.

The fresh bark contains free anthrone and must be stored for one year or artificially aged by heat and aeration. The use of illegally processed cascara sagrada bark, e.g., fresh bark, will cause severe vomiting, possibly spasms.

Clinical Data

1. Uses
Constipation.

2. Contraindications
Intestinal obstruction, acute intestinal inflammation, e.g., Crohn's disease, colitis ulcerosa, appendicitis, abdominal pain of unknown origin. Children under 12 years of age, pregnancy.

3. Side Effects
In single incidents, cramp-like discomforts of the gastrointestinal tract. These cases require a dosage reduction.

Long-time use/abuse:
> Disturbances of electrolyte balance, especially potassium deficiency, albuminuria, and hematuria. Pigment implantation into the intestinal mucosa (*pseudomelanosis coli*) is harmless and usually reverses upon discontinuation of the drug. Potassium deficiency can lead to disorders of heart function and muscular weakness, especially with concurrent use of heart glycosides, diuretics, or corticosteroids.

4. Special Caution for Use
Stimulating laxatives must not be used over an extended period of time (1 - 2 weeks) without medical advice.

5. Use During Pregnancy and Lactation
Because of insufficient toxicological investigation, this drug should not be used during pregnancy and lactation.

6. Interactions with Other Drugs
With chronic use/abuse, loss in potassium may cause an increase in effectiveness of cardiac glycosides. An effect on antiarrhythmics is possible. Potassium deficiency can be increased by simultaneous application of thiazide diuretics, corticosteroids, and licorice root.

7. Dosage
Cut bark, powder or dry extracts for teas, decoction, cold maceration or elixir. Liquid or solid forms of medication exclusively for oral use.
Unless otherwise prescribed:
> 20 - 30 mg hydroxyanthracene derivatives daily, calculated as cascaroside A.

The individually correct dosage is the smallest dosage necessary to maintain a soft stool.
Note: The form of administration should be smaller than the normal daily dosage.

8. Overdosage
Electrolyte and fluid imbalance.

9. Special Warnings
Use of a stimulating laxative longer than recommended can cause intestinal sluggishness.
The preparation should be used only if no effects can be obtained through change of diet or use of bulk-forming products.

10. Effects on Operators of Vehicles and Machinery
None known.

Celandine herb
Chelidonii herba
Schöllkraut
Published May 15, 1985

Name of Drug
Chelidonii herba, celandine herb.

Composition of Drug
Celandine herb consists of the dried, above-ground parts of *Chelidonium majus* L. [Fam. Papaveraceae], gathered during flowering season, as well as its preparations in effective dosage.

The herb contains at least 0.6 percent total alkaloids, calculated as chelidonine and based on the dried herb.

Uses
Spastic discomfort of the bile ducts and gastrointestinal tract.

Contraindications
None known.

Side Effects
None known.

Interactions with Other Drugs
None known.

Dosage
Unless otherwise prescribed:
Average daily dosage 2 - 5 g of herb, equivalent to 12 - 30 mg total alkaloids calculated as chelidonine.

Mode of Administration
Cut herb, herb powder or dried extracts for liquid and solid medicinal forms for internal use.

Actions
There is evidence of a mildly antispasmodic, papaverine-like action on the upper digestive tract.
In animal experiments:
cytostatic, nonspecific immune stimulation.
Note: The blood pressure-lowering effects and the therapeutic effectiveness for mild forms of hypertonia (borderline hypertonia) need further investigation.

Centaury herb
Centaurii herba
Tausendgüldenkraut
Published July 6, 1988; Revised March 13, 1990

Name of Drug
Centaurii herba, centaury herb.

Composition of Drug
Centaury consists of the dried, aboveground parts of *Centaurium minus* Moench (syn. *C. umbellatum* Gilbert; *Erythraea centaurium* (L.) Persoon) [Fam. Gentianaceae], as well as their preparations in effective dosage.
The drug has a bitter value of minimum 2000.

Uses
Loss of appetite, peptic discomfort.

Contraindications
None known.

Side Effects
None known.

Interactions with Other Drugs
None known.

Dosage
Unless otherwise prescribed:
Average daily dosage:
6 g of drug;
equivalent preparations.
Extract (according to *Erg. B. 6*):
Daily dosage:
1 - 2 g.

Mode of Administration
Ground herb for teas and other bitter-tasting preparations for internal use.

Action
Increase in gastric juice secretion

Chamomile flower, German
Matricariae flos
Kamillenblüten
Published December 5, 1984; Revised March 13, 1990

Name of Drug
Matricariae flos, chamomile.

Composition of Drug
Chamomile, consisting of fresh or dried flower heads of *Matricaria recutita* L. (syn. *Chamomilla recutita* (L.) Rauschert) [Fam. Asteraceae], and preparations thereof at effective dosage. The flowers contain at least 0.4 percent (v/w) essential oil. Main ingredients of the essential oil are α-bisabolol or bisabolol oxide A and B.

The flowers also contain matricin and flavone derivatives such as apigenin and apigenin-7-glucoside.

Uses
External:
Skin and mucous membrane inflammations, as well as bacterial skin diseases, including those of the oral cavity and gums. Inflammations and irritations of the respiratory tract (inhalations).
Ano-genital inflammation (baths and irrigation).
Internal:
Gastrointestinal spasms and inflammatory diseases of the gastrointestinal tract.

Contraindications
None known.

Side Effects
None known.

Interactions with Other Drugs
None known.

Dosage
Boiling water (ca. 150 ml) is poured over a heaping tablespoon of chamomile (ca. 3 g), covered, and after 5 - 10 minutes passed through a tea strainer.

Unless otherwise prescribed, for gastrointestinal complaints a cup of the freshly prepared tea is drunk three or four times a day between meals. For inflammation of the mucous membranes of the mouth and throat, the freshly prepared tea is used as a wash or gargle.
External:
For poultices and rinses, 3 - 10 percent infusions;
As a bath additive, 50 g - 10 liters (approximately 2-½ gallons) water;
Semi-solid formulations with preparations corresponding to 3 - 10 percent herb.

Mode of Administration
Liquid and solid preparations for external and internal application.

Actions
Antiphlogistic
Musculotropic
Antispasmodic
Promotes wound healing
Deodorant
Antibacterial
Bacteriostatic
Stimulates skin metabolism

Chaste Tree fruit

Agni casti fructus
Keuschlammfrüchte
Published May 15, 1985; Replaced December 2, 1992

Name of Drug
Agni casti fructus; chaste tree fruit, vitex fruit.

Composition of Drug
Chaste tree fruit composed of the ripe, dried fruits of *Vitex agnus castus* L. [Fam. Verbenaceae], as well as their preparations in effective dosage.

Pharmacological Properties, Pharmacokinetics, Toxicology
There is evidence that aqueous-alcoholic extracts of chaste tree fruit inhibit secretion of prolactin in vitro. In human pharmacology there are no data about the lowering of prolactin levels. There is no knowledge regarding pharmacokinetics. Systematic studies about toxicology are unknown.

Clinical Data

1. Uses
Irregularities of the menstrual cycle. Premenstrual complaints. Mastodynia.
Note: In case of feeling of tension and swelling of the breasts and at disturbances of menstruation, a physician should be consulted for diagnosis.

2. Contraindications
None known.

3. Side Effects
Occasional occurrence of itching, urticarial exanthemas.

4. Special Cautions for Use
None known.

5. Use During Pregnancy and Lactation
No application during pregnancy.
In animal experiments an influence on the nursing performance was observed.

6. Interactions with Other Drugs
Interactions are unknown. In animal experiments there is evidence of a dopaminergic effect of the drug; therefore, a reciprocal weakening of the effect can occur in case of ingestion of dopamine-receptor antagonists.

7. Dosage
Unless otherwise prescribed:
Daily dosage:
    aqueous-alcoholic extracts corresponding to 30 - 40 mg of the drug.

8. Mode of Administration
Aqueous-alcoholic extracts (50 - 70 percent v/v) from the crushed fruits taken as liquid or dry extract.

9. Overdosage
None known.

10. Special Warnings
None known.

11. Effects on Operators of Vehicles and Machinery
None known.

Chicory
Cichorium intybus
Wegwarte
Published April 23, 1987; Revised September 1, 1990

Name of Drug
Cichorii herba, chicory herb.
Cichorii radix, chicory root.

Composition of Drug
The dried, above-ground parts and/or roots, collected in autumn, of *Cichorium intybus* L. var. *intybus* (syn. *C. intybus* L. var. *sylvestre* Visiani) [Fam. Asteraceae], as well as its preparations in effective dosage. The herb contains bitter principles, inulin, and pentosans.

Uses
Loss of appetite, dyspepsia.

Contraindications
Allergies to chicory and other composites. In case of gallstones, use only after consultation with a physician.

Side Effects
In rare cases, allergic skin reactions.

Interactions with Other Drugs
None known.

Dosage
Unless otherwise prescribed:
Average daily dosage:
   3 g of herb;
   equivalent preparations.

Mode of Administration
Cut herb for teas, as well as other bitter-tasting preparations for internal uses.

Action
Mildly choleretic

Cinchona bark
Cinchonae cortex
Chinarinde
Published February 1, 1990

Name of Drug
Cinchonae cortex, cinchona bark.

Composition of Drug
Cinchona bark consists of the dried bark of *Cinchona pubescens* Vahl (syn. *Cinchona succirubra* Pavon ex Klotzsch) [Fam. Rubiaceae], or of their variations and hybrids, as well as preparations of cinchona bark in effective dosage.

Uses
Loss of appetite, peptic discomforts such as bloating and fullness.

Contraindications
Pregnancy, allergy to cinchona alkaloids, such as quinine and quinidine.

Side Effects
Occasionally, after taking medicines con-

taining quinine, allergic reactions such as skin allergy or fever may occur. In rare cases, there is an increased tendency to bleeding because of a reduction in the blood platelets (thrombocytopenia). If this happens, a doctor must be consulted immediately.

Warning: A sensitization for quinine or quinidine is possible.

Interactions with Other Drugs
If given simultaneously, increases the effect of anticoagulants.

Dosage
Unless otherwise prescribed:
Daily dosage:
    1 - 3 g of drug;
    0.6 - 3 g of cinchona liquid extract with 4 - 5 percent total alkaloids;
    0.15 - 0.6 g cinchona extract with 15 - 20 percent total alkaloids;
Preparations with equivalent bitterness value.

Mode of Administration
Comminuted drug and other bitter-tasting galenical preparations to be taken orally.

Action
Stimulation of the secretion of saliva and gastric juice.

Cinnamon bark
Cinnamomi ceylanici cortex
Zimtrinde
Published February 1, 1990

Name of Drug
Cinnamomi ceylanici cortex, cinnamon.

Composition of Drug
Cinnamon consists of the dried bark, separated from cork and the underlying parenchyma, of young branches and shoots of *Cinnamomum verum* J.S. Presl (syn. *C. zeylanicum* Blume) [Fam. Lauraceae], as well as its preparations in effective dosage.

The bark contains essential oil.

Uses
For loss of appetite, dyspeptic complaints such as mild, spastic condition of the gastrointestinal tract, bloating, flatulence.

Contraindications
Allergy to cinnamon and Peruvian balsam. Pregnancy.

Side Effects
Frequently, allergic reactions of skin and mucosa.

Interactions with Other Drugs
None known.

Dosage
Unless otherwise prescribed:
Daily dosage:
    2 - 4 g of bark;
    0.05 - 0.2 g of essential oil;
    equivalent preparations.

Cinnamon bark, Chinese

Cinnamomi cassiae cortex
Chinesischer Zimt
Published February 1, 1990

Name of Drug
Cinnamomi cassiae cortex, Chinese cinnamon.

Composition of Drug
Chinese cinnamon consists of the dried branch bark and occasionally stem bark, separated from the cork, of *Cinnamomum aromaticum* Nees (syn. *C. cassia* Blume) [Fam. Lauraceae], as well as preparations thereof in effective dosage.

The bark contains essential oil.

Uses
Loss of appetite, dyspeptic complaints such as mild spasms of the gastrointestinal tract, bloating, flatulence.

Contraindications
Allergy to cinnamon or Peruvian balsam.

Side Effects
Frequently, allergic reaction of the skin and mucosa.

Interactions with Other Drugs
None known.

Dosage
Unless otherwise prescribed:
Daily dosage:
　2 - 4 g of bark;
　0.05 - 0.2 g of essential oil;
　equivalent preparations.

Mode of Administration
Cut or ground bark for teas, essential oil, as well as other galenical preparations for internal use.

Actions
Antibacterial
Fungistatic
Promotes motility

Cloves
Caryophylli flos
Gewürznelken
Published November 30, 1985

Name of Drug
Caryophylli flos, cloves.

Composition of Drug
Cloves consist of the hand-picked and dried flower buds of *Syzygium aromaticum* (L.) Merrill et L.M. Perry (syn. *Jambosa caryophyllus* (Sprengel) Niedenzu, *Eugenia caryophyllata* Thunberg) [Fam. Myrtaceae], as well as their preparations in effective dosage.

The drug contains at least 14 percent (v/w) essential oil, in reference to the dried drug.

Uses
Inflammatory changes of the oral and pharyngeal mucosa.

In dentistry, for topical anesthesia.

Contraindications
None known.

Side Effects
In concentrated form, oil of cloves may be irritating to mucosal tissues.

Interactions with Other Drugs
None known.

Dosage
Unless otherwise prescribed:
> For mouth washes corresponding to 1 - 5 percent essential oil.
> In dentistry, undiluted essential oil.

Mode of Administration
Powdered, ground, or whole herb to obtain the essential oil, and other galenical preparations for topical use.

Actions
Antiseptic
Antibacterial
Antifungal
Antiviral
Topical anesthetic
Antispasmodic

Coffee Charcoal
Coffeae carbo
Kaffeekohle
Published May 5, 1988

Name of Drug
Coffeae carbo, coffee charcoal.

Composition of Drug
Coffee charcoal consists of milled, roasted to blackening and carbonizing of the outer seed parts of green, dried fruit of *Coffea arabica* L., *C. liberica* Bull ex Hiern, *C. canephora* Pierre ex Fröhner and other *Coffea* species [Fam. Rubiaceae], as well as

preparations of coffee charcoal in effective dosage.

Uses
Nonspecific, acute diarrhea, local therapy of mild inflammation of the oral and pharyngeal mucosa.

Contraindications
None known.

Side Effects
None known.

Interactions with Other Drugs
None known.
Note: Due to the high adsorption capacity of coffee charcoal, the absorption of other, simultaneously administered drugs can be influenced.

Dosage
Unless otherwise prescribed:
Average daily dosage:
   9 g;
   equivalent preparations.

Duration of Use
If diarrhea persists for more than 3 - 4 days, consult a physician.

Mode of Administration
Powdered coffee charcoal and its preparations intended for internal consumption or local application.

Actions
Absorbent
Astringent

Cola nut
Colae semen
Kolasamen
Published July 12, 1991

Name of Drug
Colae semen, cola nut.

Composition of Drug
Cola nut consists of the endosperm freed from the testa of various *Cola* species Schott et Endlicher, particularly *C. nitida* (Ventenat) Schott et Endlicher [Fam. Sterculiaceae], as well as its preparations in effective dosage.
   The drug contains at least 1.5 percent methylxanthine (caffeine, theobromine).

Uses
Mental and physical fatigue.

Contraindications
Gastric and duodenal ulcers.

Side Effects
Sleep disorders, over-excitability, nervous restlessness, and gastric irritations may occur.

Interactions with Other Drugs
Strengthening of the action of psychoanaleptic drugs and caffeine-containing beverages.

Dosage
Unless otherwise prescribed:
Daily dosage:
   2 - 6 g cola nut (*Erg. B. 6*);

0.25 - 0.75 g cola extract (*Erg. B. 6*);
2.5 - 7.5 g cola liquid extract (*Erg. B. 6*);
10 -30 g cola tincture (*Erg. B. 6*);
60 - 180 g cola wine (*Erg. B. 6*).

Mode of Administration
Powdered drug and other galenical preparations for internal use.

Actions
From animal experiments:
  Analeptic
  Stimulates production of gastric acid
  Lipolytic
  Increases motility
In humans:
  Compared to methylxanthine, caffeine is a weaker diuretic and positively chronotropic.

Coltsfoot leaf
Farfarae folium
Huflattichblätter
Published July 27, 1990

Name of Drug
Farfarae folium, coltsfoot leaf.

Composition of Drug
Coltsfoot leaf consists of the fresh or dried leaves of *Tussilago farfara* L. [Fam. Asteraceae], as well as its preparations in effective dosage.

The drug contains mucilage and tannins. Coltsfoot leaf also contains varying amounts of pyrrolizidine alkaloids with a 1,2-unsaturated necine structure and their N-oxides.

Uses
Acute catarrh of the respiratory tract with cough and hoarseness, acute, mild inflammation of the oral and pharyngeal mucosa.

Contraindications
Pregnancy, nursing.

Side Effects
None known.

Interactions with Other Drugs
None known.

Dosage
Unless otherwise prescribed:
Daily dosage:
  4.5 - 6 g of drug;
  equivalent preparations.

The daily dosage of coltsfoot tea (drug) and of tea mixtures must not exceed 10 μg pyrrolizidine alkaloids with 1,2 unsaturated necine structure, including their N-oxides.

The daily dosage for extracts and pressed juice from fresh plants must not be more than 1 μg of total pyrrolizidine alkaloids with 1,2 unsaturated necine structure, including their N-oxides.

Mode of Administration
Comminuted drug for infusions, pressed plant juice or other galenical preparations for internal use.

Duration of Administration
Not longer than 4 - 6 weeks per year.
Unless otherwise stipulated:
  Ointments or other preparations for external use are made up with 5 - 20 percent of the drug and prepared accordingly.

The daily dose should not exceed more than 100 µg pyrrolizidine alkaloids with 1, 2-unsaturated necine structure including their N-oxides.

Actions
Inhibits inflammation
Furthers the formation of callus
Antimitotic

Comfrey herb and leaf
Symphyti herba/-folium
Beinwellkraut/-blätter
Published July 27, 1990

Name of Drug
Symphyti herba, comfrey herb.
Symphyti folium, comfrey leaf.

Composition of Drug
Comfrey herb consists of the fresh or dried above-ground parts of *Symphytum officinale* L. [Fam. Boraginaceae], as well as their preparations in effective dosage.

Comfrey leaf consists of the fresh or dried leaf of *S. officinale* L., as well as its preparations in effective dosage.

The drug contains allantoin and rosmarinic acid.

Uses
External:
Bruises, sprains.

Contraindications
None known.
Note: Application should only occur on intact skin. During pregnancy use only after consultation with a physician.

Side Effects
None known.

Interactions with Other Drugs
None known.

Dosage
Unless otherwise prescribed:
Ointments and other preparations for external application with 5 - 20 percent dried drug; equivalent preparations.

The daily applied dosage should not exceed 100 µg (mcg) of pyrrolizidine alkaloids with 1,2-unsaturated necine structure, including their N-oxides.

Mode of Administration
Comminuted herb and other galenical preparations for external use.

Duration of Administration
Not more than 4 - 6 weeks per year.

Action
Antiinflammatory

Comfrey root
Symphyti radix
Beinwellwurzel
Published July 27, 1990

Name of Drug
Symphyti radix; comfrey root.

Composition of Drug
Comfrey, consisting of the fresh or dried root section of *Symphytum officinale* L. [Fam. Boraginaceae], and effective pharmaceutical preparations thereof.

The drug contains allantoin and mucopolysaccharides. Comfrey also contains various amounts of pyrrolizidine (senecio) alkaloids with 1,2-unsaturated necine ring structure and their N-oxides.

Uses
External:
Bruising, pulled muscles and ligaments, sprains.

Contraindications
None known.
Note: Application should only occur on intact skin; during pregnancy use only after consulting a physician.

Side Effects
None known.

Interaction with Other Drugs
None known.

Dosage
Unless otherwise prescribed:
Ointments or other preparations for external use are made up with 5 - 20 percent of the drug and prepared accordingly.

The daily dose should not exceed more than 100 µg (mcg) pyrrolizidine alkaloids with 1,2-unsaturated necine structure, including its N-oxides.

Mode of Administration
Crushed root, extracts, the pressed juice of the fresh plant for semi-solid preparations and poultices for external use.

Duration of Treatment
Not longer than 4 - 6 weeks per year.

Actions
Antiinflammatory
Furthers the formation of callus
Antimitotic

Condurango bark
Condurango cortex
Condurangorinde
Published October 15, 1987; Revised March 13, 1990

Name of Drug
Condurango cortex, condurango bark.

Composition of Drug
Condurango bark consists of the dried bark of the branches and trunk of *Marsdenia condurango* Reichenbach fil.

[Fam. Asclepiadaceae], as well as its preparations in effective dosage.

The bark contains bitter principles, such as condurangin.

Uses
Loss of appetite.

Contraindications
None known.

Side Effects
None known.

Interactions with Other Drugs
None known.

Dosage
Unless otherwise prescribed:
Daily dosage:
  Water extract (according to Erg. B. 6):
    0.2 - 0.5 g;
  Extract (according to Erg. B. 6):
    0.2 - 0.5 g;
  Tincture (according to Erg. B. 6):
    2 - 5 g;
  Liquid extract (according to Helv. VI):
    2 - 4 g;
  Bark:
    2 - 4 g.

Mode of Administration
Comminuted bark for teas and other bitter-tasting preparations for oral use.

Action
Stimulation of the secretion of saliva and gastric juices.

Coriander seed
Coriandri fructus
Koriander
Published September 18, 1986

Name of Drug
Coriandri fructus, coriander seed.

Composition of Drug
Coriander consists of the ripe, dried, spherical fruit of *Coriandrum sativum* L. var. *vulgare* (synonym var. *macrocarpum*) Alefeld and/or *C. sativum* L. var. *microcarpum* de Candolle [Fam. Apiaceae], as well as its preparations in effective dosage.

The drug contains at least 0.5 percent (v/w) essential oil.

Uses
Dyspeptic complaints, loss of appetite.

Contraindications
None known.

Side Effects
None known.

Interactions with Other Drugs
None known.

Dosage
Unless otherwise prescribed:
Average daily dosage:
  3 g of drug;
  equivalent preparations.

Mode of Administration
Crushed and powdered drug, as well as other galenical preparations for internal uses.

Powder, dry extracts and other galenical preparations for internal and external use.

Couch Grass
Graminis rhizoma
Queckenwurzelstock
Published February 1, 1990

Name of Drug
Graminis rhizoma, couch grass (Triticum).

Composition of Drug
Couch grass consists of the rhizome, roots and short stems of *Agropyron repens* (L.) P. de Beauvois [Fam. Poaceae], as well as its preparations in effective dosage.

The drug contains essential oil and saponins.

Uses
Irrigation therapy for inflammatory diseases of the urinary tract and for the prevention of kidney gravel.

Contraindications
None known.
Warning: No irrigation therapy if edema exists due to cardiac or renal insufficiency.

Side Effects
None known.

Interactions with Other Drugs
None known.

Dosage
Unless otherwise prescribed:
Daily dosage:
  6 - 9 g of drug;
  equivalent preparations.

Mode of Administration
Comminuted herb decoctions and other galenical preparations for internal use.
Note: For irrigation therapy, observe copious fluid intake.

Action
The essential oil has an antimicrobial activity.

Dandelion herb
Taraxaci herba
Löwenzahnkraut
Published August 29, 1992

Name of Drug
Taraxaci herba, dandelion herb.

Composition of Drug
Dandelion herb, consisting of the fresh or dried above-ground parts of *Taraxacum officinale* G. H. Weber ex Wiggers s.l. [Fam. Asteraceae], as well as their preparations in

effective dosage. The leaf contains bitter principles.

Pharmacological Properties, Pharmacokinetics, Toxicology
Not known.

Clinical Data

1. Uses
Loss of appetite and dyspepsia, such as feeling of fullness and flatulence.

2. Contraindications
Obstruction of the bile ducts, gall bladder empyema, ileus. In case of gallstones, use only after consultation with a physician. Contact allergies caused by sesquiterpene-lactones in the latex have been only rarely observed. Experiments and observations concerning preparations are not available.

3. Side Effects
None known.

4. Special Precautions for Use
None.

5. Use During Pregnancy and Lactation
None known.

6. Interactions with Other Drugs
None known.

7. Dosage
Unless otherwise prescribed:
    4 - 10 g of herb 3 times daily;
    4 - 10 ml liquid extract 1:1 in
      25 percent alcohol 3 times daily.

8. Mode of Administration
Cut herb for infusions, as well as for liquid preparations for internal use.

9. Duration of Administration
Unlimited.

10. Overdosage
None known.

11. Special Warnings
None.

12. Effects on Operators of Vehicles and Machinery
None.

Dandelion root with herb
Taraxaci radix cum herba
Löwenzahnwurzel mit-kraut
Published December 5, 1984; Revised September 1, 1990

Name of Drug
Taraxaci radix cum herba, dandelion root with herb.

Composition of Drug
Dandelion root with herb consists of the entire plant *Taraxacum officinale* G. H. Weber ex Wiggers s.l. [Fam. Asteraceae], gathered while flowering, as well as its preparations in effective dosage.

Ingredients include the bitter principles lactucopicrin (taraxacin), triterpenoids, and phytosterol.

Uses
Disturbances in bile flow, stimulation of diuresis, loss of appetite, and dyspepsia.

Contraindications
Obstruction of bile ducts, gallbladder empyema, ileus. In case of gallstones, use only after consultation with a physician.

Side Effects
As with all drugs containing bitter substances, discomfort due to gastric hyperacidity may occur.

Interactions with Other Drugs
None known.

Dosage
Unless otherwise prescribed:
As tea:
  1 tablespoon of cut drug per cup of water.
As decoction:
  3 - 4 g of cut or powdered drug per cup of water.
As tincture:
  10 - 15 drops 3 times daily.

Mode of Administration
Liquid and solid preparations for oral use.

Actions
Choleretic
Diuretic
Appetite-stimulating

Devil's Claw root
Harpagophyti radix
Südafrikanische Teufelskrallenwurzel
Published March 2, 1989; Revised September 1, 1990

Name of Drug
Harpagophyti radix, devil's claw root.

Composition of Drug
Devil's Claw root consists of the dried, secondary tubers of *Harpagophytum procumbens* (Burchell) de Candolle [Fam. Pedaliaceae], as well as their preparations in effective dosage.
  The drug contains bitter substances.

Uses
Loss of appetite, dyspepsia, supportive therapy of degenerative disorders of the locomotor system.

Contraindications
Gastric and duodenal ulcers. With gallstones, use only after consultation with a physician.

Side Effects
None known.

Interactions with Other Drugs
None known.

Dosage
Unless otherwise prescribed:
Daily dosage:
  For loss of appetite:
    1.5 g of drug;
      preparations of equivalent bitter value;
  Otherwise:
    4.5 g drug;
      equivalent preparations.

Mode of Administration
Comminuted drug for teas and other preparations for internal use.

Actions
Appetite-stimulating
Choleretic
Antiphlogistic
Mildly analgesic

Dill seed
Anethi fructus
Dillfrüchte
Published October 15, 1987; Revised March 13, 1990

Name of Drug
Anethi fructus, dill seed.

Composition of Drug
Dill seed consists of the dried fruit of *Anethum graveolens* L. s.l. [Fam. Apiaceae], as well as its preparations in effective dosage.

The drug contains essential oil rich in carvone.

Uses
Dyspepsia.

Contraindications
None known.

Side Effects
None known.

Interactions with Other Drugs
None known.

Dosage
Unless otherwise prescribed:
Average daily dosage:
    Seed, 3 g;
    essential oil, 0.1 - 0.3 g;
    equivalent preparations.

Mode of Administration
Whole seeds for teas and other galenical preparations for internal application.

Actions
Antispasmodic
Bacteriostatic

Echinacea Pallida root
Echinaceae pallidae radix
Echinacea-pallida-Wurzel
Published August 29, 1992

Name of Drug
Echinaceae pallidae radix, echinacea pallida root.

Composition of Drug
Echinacea pallida root, consisting of fresh or dried root of *Echinacea pallida* (Nutt.) Nutt. [Fam. Asteraceae], as well as its preparations in effective dosage.

Pharmacological Properties, Pharmacokinetics, Toxicology

Animal experiment: In a carbon clearance test, alcohol root extracts show an increase in the elimination of carbon particles by a factor of 2.2.

In vitro:
> Alcohol root extracts show an increase in phagocytic elements by 23 percent when tested in granulocyte smears at a concentration of $10^{-4} - 10^{-2}$ mg/ml.

Clinical Data

1. Uses
Supportive therapy for influenza-like infections.

2. Contraindications
Not to be used when progressive systemic diseases such as the following exist:
> Tuberculosis, leukosis, collagenosis, multiple sclerosis, AIDS, HIV infection, and other autoimmune diseases.

3. Side Effects
None known.

4. Precautions
None.

5. Effects on Pregnancy and Lactation
None.

6. Interactions with Other Drugs
None known.

7. Dosage
Unless otherwise indicated:
Daily dosage:
> Tincture (1:5) with 50 percent (v/v) ethanol from native dry extract (50 percent ethanol, 7 - 11:1), corresponding to 900 mg herb.

Information for children's dosage is not available.

8. Mode of Administration
Liquid forms for oral administration.

9. Duration of Administration
Not longer than 8 weeks.

10. Overdosage
None known.

11. Special Precautions
None known.

12. Effects on Operators of Vehicles and Machinery
None known.

Echinacea Purpurea herb
Echinaceae purpureae herba
Purpursonnenhutkraut
Published March 2, 1989

Name of Drug
Echinaceae purpureae herba, purple coneflower herb.

Composition of Drug
Purple coneflower herb consists of fresh, above-ground parts, harvested at flowering time, of *Echinacea purpurea* (L.) Moench

[Fam. Asteraceae], as well as its preparations in effective dosage.

Use

Internal:
Supportive therapy for colds and chronic infections of the respiratory tract and lower urinary tract.

External use:
Poorly healing wounds and chronic ulcerations.

Contraindications

External:
None known.

Internal:
Progressive systemic diseases, such as tuberculosis, leucosis, collagenosis, multiple sclerosis.

No parenteral administration in case of tendencies to allergies, especially allergies to members of the composite family (Asteraceae), as well as in pregnancy.

Warning: The metabolic condition in diabetics can decline upon parenteral application.

Side Effects

Internal and external application:
None known.

Parenteral application:
Depending upon dosage, short-term fever reactions, nausea and vomiting can occur.

In individual cases, allergic reactions of the immediate type are possible.

Interactions with Other Drugs

None known.

Dosage

Unless otherwise prescribed:

Internal:
Daily dosage:
6 - 9 ml expressed juice;
equivalent preparations.

Parenteral:
Depends on individual kind and seriousness of condition as well as specific nature of the preparation. Parenteral application requires a gradation of dosage, especially for children; the manufacturer is required to show this information for the particular preparation.

External:
Semi-solid preparations containing at least 15 percent pressed juice.

Mode of Administration

Pressed juice and galenical preparations for internal and external use.

Duration of Administration

Preparations for parenteral use:
Not longer than 3 weeks.

Preparations for internal and external use:
Not longer than 8 weeks.

Actions

In human and/or animal experiments, *Echinacea* preparations given internally or parenterally have produced immune effects. Among others, the number of white blood cells and spleen cells is increased, the capacity for phagocytosis by human granulocytes is activated, and the body temperature is elevated.

Elder flower
Sambuci flos
Holunderblüten
Published March 13, 1986

Name of Drug
Sambuci flos, elder flower.

Composition of Drug
Elder flower consists of the dried, sifted inflorescence of *Sambucus nigra* L. [Fam. Caprifoliaceae], as well as its preparations in effective dosage.

Uses
Colds.

Contraindications
None known.

Side Effects
None known.

Interactions with Other Drugs
None known.

Dosage
Unless otherwise prescribed:
Average daily dosage:
   10 - 15 g drug;
   1.5 - 3 g fluidextract
     (according to *Erg. B. 6*);
   2.5 - 7.5 g tincture
     (according to *Erg. B. 6*);
equivalent preparations.

Mode of Administration
Whole herb and other galenical preparations for teas, 1 - 2 cups of tea sipped several times daily, as hot as possible.

Actions
Diaphoretic
Increased bronchial secretion

Eleuthero (Siberian Ginseng) root
Eleutherococci radix
Eleutherococcus-senticosus-Wurzel
Published January 17, 1991

Name of Drug
Eleutherococci radix, eleuthero, Siberian ginseng root.

Composition of Drug
Eleuthero consists of the dried roots and/or rhizome of *Eleutherococcus senticosus* Ruprecht et Maximowicz [syn. *Acanthopanax senticosus* (Rupr.et maxim ex maxim Harms)] [Fam. Araliaceae], as well as their preparations in effective dosage.

The root contains lignans and coumarin derivatives.

Uses
As tonic for invigoration and fortification in times of fatigue and debility or declining capacity for work and concentration, also during convalescence.

Contraindications
High blood pressure.*

Side Effects
None known.

Interactions with Other Drugs
None known.

Dosage
Unless otherwise prescribed:
Daily dosage:
    2 - 3 g of root;
    equivalent preparations.

Mode of Administration
Powdered or cut root for teas, as well as aqueous-alcoholic extracts for internal use.

Duration of Administration
Generally up to 3 months.
A repeated course is feasible.

Actions
In various stress models, e.g., immobilization test and coldness test, the endurance of rodents was enhanced.

With healthy volunteers, the lymphocyte count, especially that of T-lymphocytes, increased following intake of fluidextracts.

*[**Ed. note:** For a brief discussion on the potential hypertensive activity of Eleuthero, see the Introduction, pages 61-62.]

Ephedra
Ephedrae herba
Ephedrakraut
Published January 17, 1991

Name of Drug
Ephedrae herba, ephedra, ma huang.

Composition of Drug
Ephedra consists of the dried, young branchlets, harvested in the fall, of *Ephedra sinica* Stapf, *E. shennungiana* Tang [Fam. Ephedraceae], or other equivalent *Ephedra* species, as well as their equivalent preparations in effective dosage.

The herb contains alkaloids; main alkaloids are ephedrine and pseudoephedrine.

Uses
Diseases of the respiratory tract with mild bronchospasms in adults and children over the age of six.

Contraindications
Anxiety and restlessness, high blood pressure, glaucoma, impaired circulation of the cerebrum, adenoma of prostate with residual urine accumulation, pheochromocytoma, thyrotoxicosis.

Side Effects
Insomnia, motor restlessness, irritability, headaches, nausea, vomiting, disturbances of urination, tachycardia.
In higher dosage:
    drastic increase in blood pressure, cardiac arrhythmia, development of dependency.

Interactions with Other Drugs
In combination with:
- Cardiac glycosides or halothane: disturbance of heart rhythm.
- Guanethidine: enhancement of the sympathomimetic effect.

MAO-inhibitors:
- Greatly raising the sympathomimetic action of ephedrine.
- Secale alkaloid derivatives or oxytocin: development of hypertension.

Dosage
Unless otherwise prescribed:
Single dosage:
Adults:
Herb preparations corresponding to 15 - 30 mg total alkaloid, calculated as ephedrine.
Children:
Herb preparations corresponding to 0.5 mg total alkaloid per kg of body weight.

Maximum Daily Dosage
Adults:
Herb preparations corresponding to 300 mg total alkaloid, calculated as ephedrine.
Children:
2 mg total alkaloid per kg of body weight.

Mode of Administration
Comminuted herb, as well as other galenical preparations for internal use.

Duration of Administration
Ephedra preparations should only be used on a short-term duration because of tachyphylaxis and danger of addiction.

Note: Ephedrine-containing preparations are listed as addictive by the International Olympic Committee and the German Sports Association.

Actions
In animal experiments:
- antitussive
  Ephedrine acts by indirectly stimulating the sympathomimetic and central nervous system.
- Bacteriostatic

Eucalyptus leaf
Eucalypti folium
Eucalyptusblätter
Published September 24, 1986; Revised March 13, 1990

Name of Drug
Eucalypti folium, eucalyptus leaf.

Composition of Drug
Eucalyptus leaf consists of the dried, mature leaves from older trees of *Eucalyptus globulus* Labillardiere [Fam. Myrtaceae], as well as other preparations in effective dosage.

The leaves contain essential oil which consists mainly of 1,8-cineol and tannins.

Uses
Catarrhs of the respiratory tract.

Contraindications
Inflammation of the gastrointestinal tract and the bile ducts; serious liver diseases. Eucalyptus preparations should not be applied to the face, especially the nose, of babies and very young children.

Side Effects
In rare cases, after taking eucalyptus preparations nausea, vomiting, and diarrhea may occur.

Interactions with Other Drugs
None known.
Note: Eucalyptus oil induces the enzyme system of the liver involved in the detoxification process. Therefore, the effects of other drugs can be weakened and/or shortened.

Dosage
Unless otherwise prescribed:
Internal:
Average daily dosage:
 4 - 6 g of leaf;
 equivalent preparations.
Tincture (according to *Erg. B. 6*):
 Daily dosage 3 - 9 g.

Mode of Administration
Chopped leaf for infusions and other galenical preparations for internal and external application.

Actions
Secretomotory
Expectorant
Weakly antispasmodic

Eucalyptus oil
Eucalypti aetheroleum
Eucalyptusöl
Published September 24, 1986; Revised March 13, 1990

Name of Drug
Eucalypti aetheroleum, eucalyptus oil.

Composition of Drug
Eucalyptus oil consists of the volatile oil from various cineol-rich species of *Eucalyptus*, such as *Eucalyptus globulus* Labillardiere, *E. fructicetorum* F. Von Mueller (syn. *E. polybractea* R.T. Baker) and/or *E. smithii* R.T. Baker [Fam. Myrtaceae], as well as their preparations in effective dosage. The oil is obtained by steam distillation, followed by rectification of the fresh leaves and branch tops, and contains at least 70 percent (w/w) 1,8-cineol.

Uses
Internal and external:
 for catarrhs of the respiratory tract.
External:
 for rheumatic complaints.

Contraindications
Internal:
 Inflammatory diseases of the gastrointestinal tract and bile ducts, severe liver diseases.
External:
 For infants and young children, eucalyptus preparations should not be applied to areas of the face, especially the nose.

Side Effects
In rare cases, nausea, vomiting and diarrhea may occur after ingestion of eucalyptus preparations.

Interactions with Other Drugs
Eucalyptus oil induces the enzyme system of the liver involved in the detoxification process. Therefore, the effects of other drugs can be weakened and/or shortened.

Dosage

Unless otherwise prescribed:
Internal:
Average daily dosage:
    0.3 - 0.6 g eucalyptus oil;
    equivalent preparations.
External:
    5 - 20 percent in oil and semi-solid preparations;
    5 - 10 percent in aqueous-alcoholic preparations;
Essential oil:
    several drops rubbed into the skin.

Mode of Administration

Essential oil and other galenical preparations for internal and external application.

Actions

Secretomotory
Expectorant
Mildly antispasmodic
Mild local hyperemic

Fennel oil

Foeniculi aetheroleum
Fenchelöl
Published April 19, 1991

Name of Drug

Foeniculi aetheroleum, fennel oil

Composition of Drug

Fennel oil is the essential oil obtained from the dried, ripe fruits of the *Foeniculum vulgare* Miller var. *vulgare* (Miller) Thellung [Fam. Apiaceae], by water steam distillation, as well as its preparations in effective dosage.

    Fennel oil contains anethole, fenchone, and not more than 5 percent estragon.

Uses

Peptic discomforts, such as mild, spastic disorders of the gastrointestinal tract, feeling of fullness, flatulence.
Catarrhs of the upper respiratory tract.
Fennel honey:
    Catarrhs of the upper respiratory tract in children.

Contraindications

Fennel honey:
    None known.

Other preparations:
    Pregnancy. Not to be used for infants and toddlers.

Side Effects

In rare cases, allergic reactions affecting skin and respiratory system.

Interactions with Other Drugs

None known.

Dosage

Unless otherwise prescribed:
Daily dosage:
    0.1 - 0.6 ml, equivalent to 0.1 - 0.6 g of herb;
    equivalent preparations.
Fennel honey syrup with 0.5 g fennel oil/kg:
    10 - 20 g;
    equivalent preparations.

Mode of Administration

Essential oil and galenical preparations for internal use.

Duration of Administration
Unless otherwise advised by a physician or pharmacist, one should not consume fennel oil for an extended period (several weeks).
Note: Fennel syrup, fennel honey: Diabetics must consider sugar content of bread exchange units according to manufacturer's information.

Actions
Stimulation of gastrointestinal motility.
In higher concentrations, antispasmodic.
Experimentally, anethole and fenchone have shown a secretolytic action on the respiratory tract.
In vitro, antimicrobial.

Fennel seed
Foeniculi fructus
Fenchel
Published April 19, 1991

Name of Drug
Foeniculi fructus, fennel seed.

Composition of Drug
Fennel seed consists of the dried, ripe fruits of *Foeniculum vulgare* Miller var. *vulgare* (Miller) Thellung [Fam. Apiaceae], as well as their preparations in effective dosage.

The seeds contain at least 4 percent essential oil with not more than 5 percent estragon.

Uses
Dyspepsias such as mild, spastic gastrointestinal afflictions, fullness, flatulence.
Catarrh of the upper respiratory tract.
Fennel syrup, fennel honey: catarrh of the upper respiratory tract in children.

Contraindications
Herb for infusions and preparations containing an equivalent amount of the essential oil:
　None known.
Other preparations:
　Pregnancy.

Side Effects
In individual cases allergic reactions of skin and respiratory tract.

Interactions with Other Drugs
None known.

Dosage
Unless otherwise prescribed:
Daily dosage:
　5 - 7 g herb;
　10 - 20 g fennel syrup or honey (*Erg. B. 6*);
　5 - 7.5 g compound fennel tincture;
　equivalent preparations.

Mode of Administration
Crushed or ground seeds for teas, tea-like products, as well as other galenical preparations for internal use.

Duration of Administration
Fennel preparations should not be used on a prolonged basis (several weeks) without consulting a physician or pharmacist.
Note: Fennel syrup, fennel honey: Diabetics must consider sugar content of bread exchange units according to manufacturer's information.

Actions
Promotes gastrointestinal motility, in higher concentrations acts as an antispasmodic. Experimentally, anethole and fenchone have been shown to have a secretolytic action in the respiratory tract; in the frog, aqueous fennel extracts raise the mucociliary activity of the ciliary epithelium.

Fenugreek seed
Foenugraeci semen
Bockshornsamen
Published February 1, 1990

Name of Drug
Foenugraeci semen, fenugreek.

Composition of Drug
Fenugreek consists of the ripe, dried seed of *Trigonella foenum-graecum* L. [Fam. Fabaceae], as well as its preparations in effective dosage.

The drug contains mucilage and bitter principles.

Uses
Internal:
Loss of appetite.
External:
As poultice for local inflammation.

Contraindications
None known.

Side Effects
Repeated external applications can result in undesirable skin reactions.

Interactions with Other Drugs
None known.

Dosage
Unless otherwise prescribed:
Internal:
6 g drug; equivalent preparations.
External:
50 g powdered drug with ¼ liter water.

Mode of Administration
Liniments in the form of alcoholic solutions, ointments, gels, emulsions, oils. Also bath additive and as an inhalant.

Actions
Secretolytic
Hyperemic
Mild antiseptic

Fir Needle oil
Piceae aetheroleum
Fichtennadelöl
Published August 21, 1985; Revised March 13, 1990

Name of Drug
Piceae aetheroleum, fir needle oil, white spruce oil.

Composition of Drug
Fir needle oil is a volatile oil obtained from tips of branches or twigs of *Picea abies* (L.) Karsten (synonyms: *P. excelsa* (Lamarck) Link), *Abies alba* Miller, *A. sachalinensis* (Fr. Schmidt) Masters, or *A. sibirica* Ledebour [Fam. Pinaceae], as well as essential oil preparations thereof in effective dosage.

Uses

External and internal:
    For catarrhal illness of the upper and lower respiratory tract.
External:
    For rheumatic and neuralgic pains.

Contraindications

Bronchial asthma, whooping cough.

Side Effects

Increased irritation to the skin and mucous membranes can occur.
    Bronchospasms can be increased.

Interactions with Other Drugs

None known.

Dosage

Unless otherwise prescribed:
    Dosage is individualized according to the type and intensity of the illness, any special areas of use, as well as the mode of administration.

Mode of Administration

Liniments in the form of alcoholic solutions, ointments, gels, emulsions, oils. Also bath additive and as an inhalant.

Actions

Secretolytic
Hyperemic
Mild antiseptic

Fir Shoots, Fresh

Piceae turiones recentes
Frische Fichtenspitzen
Published October 15, 1987

Name of Drug

Piceae turiones recentes, fresh fir shoots.

Composition of Drug

Preparations from the fresh shoots, approximately 10-15 cm long, collected in spring, of *Picea abies* (L.) Karsten and/or *A. alba* Miller (syn. *A. pectinata* (Lamarck) de Candolle) [Fam. Pinaceae].
    It contains essential oil.

Uses

Internal use:
    Catarrh of the respiratory tract.
External use:
    Mild rheumatic or neuralgic pains.

Contraindications

None known.

Side Effects

None known.

Interactions with Other Drugs

None known.

Dosage

Unless otherwise prescribed:
Internal:
    Average daily dose is preparation equivalent to 5 - 6 g of drug.
External:
    In baths equivalent to 200 - 300 g drug for one full bath.

Mode of Administration

Galenical preparations for internal and external use.

Actions

Secretolytic
Mild antiseptic
Hyperemic

Flaxseed
Lini semen
Leinsamen
Published May 12, 1984

Name of Drug
Lini semen, flaxseed.

Composition of Drug
Flaxseed consists of the dried, ripe seed of the collective variations of *Linum usitatissimum* L. [Fam. Linaceae], as well as its preparations in effective dosage. The various cultivars of *L. usitatissimum* (L.) Vav. et Ell. are equally acceptable for the indications listed in this monograph. The seeds contain: fiber (hemicellulose, cellulose, and lignin), fatty oil with 52 - 76 percent linolenic acid esters, albumin, linustatin, and linamarin.

Uses
Internal:
 Chronic constipation, for colons damaged by abuse of laxatives, irritable colon, diverticulitis, as mucilage for gastritis and enteritis.
External:
 As cataplasm for local inflammation.

Contraindications
Ileus of any origin.

Side Effects
If directions are observed, i.e., especially if the concomitant administration of sufficient amounts of liquid (1:10) is observed, there are no known side effects.

Interactions with Other Drugs
As with any other mucilage, the absorption of other drugs may be negatively affected.

Dosage
Unless otherwise prescribed:
Internal:
 1 tablespoon of whole or "bruised" seed (not ground) with 150 ml of liquid 2 - 3 times daily.
 2 - 3 tablespoons of milled flaxseed for the preparation of flaxseed mucilage (gruel).
External:
 30 - 50 g flaxseed flour for a moist-heat cataplasm or compress.

Mode of Administration
Internal:
 As seed, as cracked or coarsely ground seed, in which only the cuticle and mucilage epidermis are damaged; as flaxseed mucilage (gruel) and other galenical preparations.
External:
 As flaxseed flour or flaxseed expellent.

Actions
Laxative effects due to increase in volume and consequent initiation of intestinal peristalsis due to stretching reflexes. Protective effect on the mucosa because of coating action.

Fumitory
Fumariae herba
Erdrauchkraut
Published September 18, 1986

Name of Drug
Fumariae herba, common fumitory.

Composition of Drug
Common fumitory herb consists of the dried, above-ground parts of *Fumaria officinalis* L. [Fam. Fumariaceae], gathered during the flowering season, as well as their preparations in effective dosage.

The herb contains isoquinolines as the main ingredient, and also contains flavonoid glycosides.

Uses
Spastic discomfort in the area of the gallbladder and bile ducts, as well as the gastrointestinal tract.

Contraindications
None known.

Side Effects
None known.

Interactions with Other Drugs
None known.

Dosage
Unless otherwise prescribed:
Average daily dosage:
    6 g of herb;
    equivalent preparations.

Mode of Administration
Cut herb and galenical preparations thereof for internal use.

Action
A light, antispasmodic effect on the upper digestive tract is sufficiently documented.

Galangal
Galangae rhizoma
Galangtwurzelstock
Published September 18, 1986; Revised March 13, 1990

Name of Drug
Galangae rhizoma, galangal rhizome, lesser galangal rhizome.

Composition of Drug
Galangal consists of the dried rhizome of *Alpinia officinarum* Hance [Fam. Zingiberaceae], as well as its preparations in effective dosage.

The rhizome contains essential oil, pungent principles, and flavonoids.

Uses
Dyspepsia, loss of appetite.

Contraindications
None known.

Side Effects
None known.

Interactions with Other Drugs
None known.

Dosage
Unless otherwise prescribed:
Daily dosage:
    Tincture (according to Erg. B. 6):
        2 - 4 g;
    Rhizome:
        2 - 4 g.

Mode of Administration
Comminuted drug, powder, as well as other galenical preparations for oral application.

Actions
Antispasmodic
Antiphlogistic (inhibition of prostaglandin synthesis)
Antibacterial

Garlic
Allii sativi bulbus
Knoblauchzwiebel
Published July 6, 1988

Name of Drug
Allii sativi bulbus, garlic clove.

Composition of Drug
Garlic bulbs, consisting of fresh or carefully dried bulbs that consist of the main bulb with several secondary bulbs (cloves) of *Allium sativum* L. [Fam. Alliaceae], as well as its preparations in effective dosage.
    Garlic contains alliin and its degradation products and sulfur-containing essential oil.

Uses
Supportive to dietary measures at elevated levels of lipids in blood.
    Preventative measures for age-dependent vascular changes.

Contraindications
None known.

Side Effects
In rare instances there may be gastrointestinal symptoms, changes to the flora of the intestine, or allergic reactions.
Note: The odor of garlic may pervade the breath and skin.

Interactions with Other Drugs
None known.

Dosage
Unless otherwise prescribed:
Average daily dosage:
    4 g fresh garlic;
    equivalent preparations.

Mode of Administration
The minced bulb and preparations thereof for internal use.

Actions
Antibacterial
Antimycotic
Lipid-lowering
Inhibition of platelet aggregation
Prolongation of bleeding and clotting time
Enhancement of fibrinolytic activity

Gentian root
Gentianae radix
Enzianwurzel
Published November 30, 1985; Revised March 13, 1990

Name of Drug
Gentianae radix, gentian root.

Composition of Drug
Gentian root consists of the dried, unfermented roots and rhizome of *Gentiana lutea* L. [Fam. Gentianaceae], containing a bitter value of not less than 10,000, as well as its preparations in effective dosage.

The drug contains bitter principles (amarogentin, gentiopicroside) and the bitter-tasting gentiobiose.

Uses
Digestive disorders, such as loss of appetite, fullness, flatulence.

Contraindications
Gastric and duodenal peptic ulcers.

Side Effects
Especially sensitive persons may occasionally experience headaches.

Interactions with Other Drugs
None known.

Dosage
Unless otherwise prescribed:
Daily dosage:
    Tincture (according to Erg. B. 6):
        1 - 3 g;
    Fluidextract (according to Erg. B. 6):
        2 - 4 g;
    Root:
        2 - 4 g.

Mode of Administration
Comminuted drug and dried extracts for infusions, bitter-tasting forms of medications for oral administration.

Actions
The essential active principles are the bitter substances contained in the herb. These bring about a reflex excitation of the taste receptors, leading to increased secretion of saliva and the digestive juices. Gentian root is therefore considered to be not simply a pure bitter, but also a roborant and tonic.

In animal experimentation there are indications that bronchial secretion is increased.

Ginger root
Zingiberis rhizoma
Ingwerwurzelstock
Published May 5, 1988; Revised March 13, 1990, and September 9, 1990

Name of Drug
Zingiberis rhizoma, ginger root.

Composition of Drug
Ginger root consists of the peeled, finger-long, fresh or dried rhizome of *Zingiber*

officinale Roscoe [Fam. Zingiberaceae], as well as its preparations in effective dosage

The rhizome contains essential oil and pungent principles.

Uses
Dyspepsia, prevention of motion sickness.

Contraindications
With gallstones, only to be used after consultation with a physician.
Note: No administration for morning sickness during pregnancy.
[**Ed. note:** A review of clinical literature could not justify this caution. There is no evidence that ginger causes harm to the mother or fetus. Please see Introduction, page 62]

Side Effects
None known.

Interactions with Other Drugs
None known.

Dosage
Daily dosage:
2 - 4 g rhizome;
equivalent preparations.

Mode of Administration
Chopped or comminuted rhizome and dry extracts for teas, other galenical preparations for internal use.

Actions
Antiemetic
Positively inotropic
Promoting secretion of saliva and gastric juices
Cholagogue
In animals:
antispasmodic
In humans:
increase in tonus and peristalsis in intestines.

Ginkgo Biloba Leaf Extract
Ginkgo folium
Ginkgo biloba blätter
Published July 19, 1994

Name of Drug
Dry extract (35 - 67:1) from *Ginkgo biloba* L. leaf [Fam. Ginkgoaceae], extracted with acetone/water. Active Ingredient Classification ASK No. 05939.

Composition of Drug
A dry extract from the dried leaf of *Ginkgo biloba* L. manufactured using acetone/water and subsequent purification steps without addition of concentrates or isolated ingredients.

The drug/extract ratio is 35 - 67:1, on average 50:1.

The extract is characterized by:
22 - 27 percent flavonone glycosides, determined as quercetin and kaempferol, including isorhamnetin (via HPLC) and calculated as flavones with a molar mass of $MM_r = 756.7$ (quercetin glycosides) and $M_r = 740.7$ (kaempferol glycosides); 5 - 7 percent terpene lactones, of which approximately 2.8 - 3.4 percent consists of ginkgolides A, B, and C, as well as approximately 2.6 - 3.2 percent bilobalide; below 5 ppm ginkgolic acids. The given ranges include manufacturing and analytical variances.

Pharmacological Properties, Pharmacokinetics, Toxicology

The following pharmacological effects have been established experimentally:

- Improvement of hypoxic tolerance, particularly in the cerebral tissue.
- Inhibition of the development of traumatically or toxically induced cerebral edema, and acceleration of its regression.
- Reduction of retinal edema and of cellular lesions in the retina.
- Inhibition in age-related reduction of muscarinergic cholinoceptors and 2-adrenoceptors as well as stimulation of choline uptake in the hippocampus.
- Increased memory performance and learning capacity.
- Improvement in the compensation of disturbed equilibrium.
- Improvement of blood flow, particularly in the region of microcirculation.
- Improvement of the rheological properties of the blood.
- Inactivation of toxic oxygen radicals (flavonoids).
- Antagonism of the platelet-activating factor/PAF (ginkgolides).
- Neuroprotective effect (ginkgolides A and B, bilobalide).

The pharmacokinetics have been investigated both in animal experiments and in trials involving humans. An absorption rate of 60 percent was found in rats for a radioactively labeled extract (as specified under **Composition of Drug**). In humans after application of an extract specified as above, absolute bioavailability was 98 - 100 percent for ginkgolide A, 79 - 93 percent for ginkgolide B and at least 70 percent for bilobalide.

Both the acute and the chronic toxicity of an extract as specified under **Composition of Drug** is very low; accordingly, the LD^{50} in the mouse was 7725 mg/kg body weight after oral application and 1100 mg/kg body weight after intravenous application.

Investigations with this extract as specified above showed no effects which were either mutagenic, carcinogenic, or toxic to reproduction.

No evaluation was performed on the transferability of the experimental results to extracts other than those investigated. [**Ed. note:** This statement refers to the fact that only a few proprietary ginkgo extracts were used in the studies upon which this monograph is based. Whether these results can be extrapolated to other ginkgo extracts is uncertain.]

Clinical Data

1. Uses

(a) For symptomatic treatment of disturbed performance in organic brain syndrome within the regimen of a therapeutic concept in cases of demential syndromes with the following principal symptoms:

- Memory deficits, disturbances in concentration, depressive emotional condition, dizziness, tinnitus, and headache.
- The primary target groups are dementia syndromes, including primary degenerative dementia, vascular dementia, and mixed forms of both.

Note: Prior to starting treatment with ginkgo extract, clarification should be obtained as to whether the pathological symptoms encountered are not based on an underlying disease requiring a specific treatment.

(b) Improvement of pain-free walking distance in peripheral arterial occlusive disease in Stage II of Fontaine (intermittent claudication) in a regimen of physical therapeutic measures, in particular walking exercise.

(c) Vertigo and tinnitus (ringing in the ear) of vascular and involutional origin.

2. Contraindications

Hypersensitivity to *Ginkgo biloba* preparations.

3. Side Effects
Very seldom stomach or intestinal upsets, headaches, or allergic skin reaction.

4. Special Cautions in Use
None known.

5. Use During Pregnancy and Lactation
No restrictions known.

6. Interactions with Other Drugs
None known.

7. Dosage and Administration
Unless otherwise prescribed:
Daily dosages:
Indication (a):
    120 - 240 mg native dry extract in 2 or 3 doses.
Indications (b) and (c):
    120 - 160 mg native dry extract in 2 or 3 doses.

Mode of Administration
In liquid or solid pharmaceutical forms, for oral intake.

Duration of Administration
Indication (a):
    Length of administration should be judged according to the severity of symptoms and should extend at least 8 weeks in the case of chronic illness. Administration for more than 3 months should be reviewed as to justification for continued administration.
Indication (b):
    Improvement of ambulatory range requires administration for not less than 6 weeks.
Indication (c):
    Administration for more than 6 - 8 weeks has no therapeutic benefit.

8. Overdosage
None known.

9. Special Warnings
None.

10. Effects on Operators of Vehicles and Machinery
None known.

Ginseng root
Ginseng radix
Ginsengwurzel
Published January 17, 1991

Name of Drug
Ginseng radix, ginseng root.

Composition of Drug
Ginseng root consists of the dried main and lateral root and root hairs of *Panax ginseng* C. A. Meyer [Fam. Araliaceae], as well as their preparations in effective dosage. The root contains at least 1.5 percent ginsenosides, calculated as ginsenoside Rg1.

Uses
As tonic for invigoration and fortification in times of fatigue and debility, for declining capacity for work and concentration, also during convalescence.

Contraindications
None known.

Side Effects
None known.

Interactions with Other Drugs
None known.

Dosage
Unless otherwise prescribed:
Daily dosage:
   1 - 2 g of root;
   equivalent preparations.

Mode of Administration
Cut root for teas, powder and galenical preparations for internal use.

Duration of Administration
Generally up to 3 months.
A repeated course is feasible.

Action
In various stress models, e.g., an immobilization test and the coldness test, the resistance of laboratory test animals (rodents) was increased.

Goldenrod
Solidago
Goldrute
Published October 15, 1987; Revised March 13, 1990

Name of Drug
Solidaginis virgaureae herba, European goldenrod herb.
Solidaginis herba, goldenrod herb.

Composition of Drug
European goldenrod herb consists of the above-ground parts of *Solidago virgaurea* L. [Fam. Asteraceae] gathered during the flowering season and dried carefully, as well as their preparations in effective dosage.

Goldenrod herb consists of the above-ground parts of *S. serotina* Aiton (synonym *S. gigantea* Willdenow), *S. canadensis* L. and hybrids thereof gathered during the flowering season and carefully dried, as well as their preparations in effective dosage.

The herb contains flavonoids, saponins, and phenol glycosides.

Uses
As irrigation therapy for inflammatory diseases of the lower urinary tract, urinary calculi and kidney gravel, as prophylaxis for urinary calculi and kidney gravel.

Contraindications
None known.
Note: No irrigation therapy in case of edema due to impaired heart and kidney function.

Side Effects
None known.

Interactions with Other Drugs
None known.

Dosage
Daily dosage:
   6 - 12 g herb;
   equivalent preparations.

Mode of Administration
Comminuted drug for teas and other galenical preparations for internal use.
Note: Observe copious intake of fluids.

Actions
Diuretic
Mildly antispasmodic
Antiphlogistic

Guaiac wood
Guajaci lignum
Guajakholz
Published April 23, 1987

Name of Drug
Guajaci lignum, guaiac wood.

Composition of Drug
Guaiac wood consists of the heartwood and sapwood of *Guaiacum officinale* L. and/or *G. sanctum* L. [Fam. Zygophyllaceae], as well as their preparations in effective dosage. The wood contains resin and saponins.

Uses
Supportive therapy for rheumatic complaints.

Contraindications
None known.

Side Effects
None known.

Interactions with Other Drugs
None known.

Dosage
Unless otherwise prescribed:
Average daily dosage:
    4.5 g of drug;
    equivalent preparations.

Mode of Administration
Comminuted wood for decoctions and other galenical preparations for internal use.
Note: The essential oil known as "guaiac wood oil" must be evaluated separately.

Gumweed herb
Grindeliae herba
Grindeliakraut
Published January 17, 1991

Name of Drug
Grindeliae herba, gumweed herb.

Composition of Drug
Gumweed herb consists of the dried tops and leaves of *Grindelia robusta* Nutt. and/or *G. squarrosa* (Pursh) Dunal [Fam. Asteraceae], gathered during flowering season, as well as their preparations in effective dosage.
    The drug contains essential oil.

Uses
Catarrhs of the upper respiratory tract.

Contraindications
None known.

Side Effects
In rare cases irritation of the gastric mucosa.

Interactions with Other Drugs
None known.

Dosage
Unless otherwise prescribed:
Daily dosage:
    4 - 6 g of drug or 3 - 6 g gumweed fluidextract (Erg. B. 6);
    tincture (1:10 or 1:5. ethanol 60 percent - 80 percent [v/v]), 1.5 - 3 ml; equivalent preparations.

Mode of Administration
Comminuted herb for teas and other galenical preparations for internal use.

Action
In vitro antibacterial

Haronga bark and leaf
Harunganae madagascariensis cortex et folium
Harongarinde und blätter
Published March 13, 1990

Name of Drug
Harunganae madagascariensis cortex et folium, haronga bark and leaf.

Composition of Drug
Haronga bark with dried leaves consists of the bark and leaves of *Harungana madagascariensis* Lamarck ex Poiret [Fam. Hypericaceae], as well as its preparations in effective dosage.

The bark contains 1,8-dihydroxyanthracene derivatives, such as harunganin and madagascin.

The leaf contains dimers of 1,8-dihydroxyanthracene derivatives, such as hypericin and pseudohypericin.

Uses
Dyspepsia, mild exocrine pancreatic insufficiency.

Contraindications
Acute pancreatitis and acute attacks of chronic recurring pancreatitis, severe liver function disorders, gallstones, obstruction of bile ducts, gallbladder empyema, ileus.

Side Effects
None known.
Warning: Photosensitivity is especially possible in fair-skinned individuals.

Interactions with Other Drugs
None known.

Dosage
Unless otherwise prescribed:
Average daily dosage:
    7.5 - 15 mg of an aqueous-alcoholic dry extract corresponding to 25 - 50 mg drug;
equivalent preparations.

Mode of Administration
Preparations of haronga bark with leaves for oral use.

Duration of Administration
Preparations of haronga bark with leaves must not be taken longer than 2 months.

Action
Stimulation of the excretory function of the pancreas
Stimulation of the gastric juice secretion
Choleretic
Cholecystokinetic

Hawthorn leaf with flower
Crataegi folium cum flore
Weißdornblätter mit Blüten
Published July 19, 1994

Name of Drug
Crataegi folium cum flore, hawthorn leaf with flowers.

Composition of Drug
Hawthorn leaf with flower, consisting of dried flowering twig tips of *Crataegus monogyna* Jaquin emend. Lindman or *C. laevigata* (Poiret) de Candolle [Fam. Rosaceae], or other members of the *Crataegus* genus cited in a valid pharmacopeia as well as preparations from them in an effective dosage.

The drug contains flavonoids (flavones, flavonols) including hyperoside, vitexin-rhamnose, rutin, and vitexin and oligomeric procyanidins (n=2 to n=8 catechins and/or epicatechins).

Pharmacological Properties, Pharmacokinetics, Toxicology
The following pharmacodynamic effects have been established in isolated organs or in animal experimentation with preparations from hawthorn leaf with flower (hydroalcoholic extract with defined content of oligomeric procyanidins and/or flavonoids: macerates, fresh plant extract) and with individual fractions (oligomeric procyanidins, biogenic amines): Positive inotropic effect, positive dromotropic effect, negative bathmotropic effect, increased coronary and myocardial circulatory perfusion, reduction in peripheral vascular resistance.

In cases of cardiac insufficiency according to Stage II New York Heart Association (NYHA), an improvement of subjective findings as well as an increase in cardiac work tolerance, a decrease in pressure/heart rate product, an increase in the ejection fraction and a rise in the anaerobic threshold have been established in human pharmacological studies following the administration of 160 to 900 mg aqueous-alcoholic extract per day (adjusted to oligomeric procyanidins and/or flavonoids) over periods lasting up to 56 days.

The pharmacokinetics of the drug have been investigated only in animal studies, and no scientific results are available in the context of human pharmacokinetics.

Investigations of acute toxicity using a hydroalcoholic dry extract (drug/extract ratio 5:1, standardized for oligomeric procyanidins) are available, according to which no fatal events occurred after oral or peritoneal administration in mice or rats in doses of up to 3 g per kg of body weight.

Symptoms of intoxication with an intraperitoneal administration of 3 g/kg body weight include sedation, piloerection, dyspnea, and tremor.

The oral administration of powdered herb at individual doses of 3 g per kg body weight in rats and 5 g per kg body weight in mice produce no fatal reactions.

No toxic effects were observed after oral administration of 30, 90, and 300 mg aqueous/ethanolic dry extract per kg body weight in rats and dogs over a period of 26 weeks. For this extract, the "no effect" dose was 300 mg per kg body weight in rats and dogs for 26 weeks. No fatal events and no toxic effects were observed after the oral administration of 300 and 600 mg drug powder per kg body weight over a period of four weeks.

No experimental data are available concerning embryonic and fetal toxicity, fertility, and post-natal development.

Although they have indeed produced different results, more recent studies are now available as regards testing the mutagenicity of *Crataegus* preparations. It is assumed that the mutagenic activity demonstrated on Salmonella is based on the quercetin content, and the induction of SCE particularly on the presence of flavone-C-glycosides as well as of flavone aglycones. By comparison with the quantity of quercetin ingested with the food, however, the content of quercetin in the drug is so low that a risk for humans may be practically excluded.

No experimental data are available regarding carcinogenicity. The findings regarding gene toxicity and mutagenicity give no indication of carcinogenic risk of the drug in human use.

Clinical Data

1. Uses
Decreasing cardiac output as described in functional Stage II of NYHA.*

2. Contraindications
None known.

3. Side Effects
None known.

4. Special Caution for Use
A physician must be consulted in cases where symptoms continue unchanged for longer than six weeks or in case of swelling of the legs. Medical diagnosis is absolutely necessary when pains occur in the region of the heart, spreading out to the arms, upper abdomen or the area around the neck, or in cases of respiratory distress (dyspnea).

5. Use During Pregnancy and Lactation
None known.

6. Interactions with Other Drugs
None known.

7. Dosage and Administration
Unless otherwise prescribed:
160 - 900 mg native, water-ethanol extract (ethanol 45 percent v/v or methanol 70 percent v/v, drug-extract ratio = 4 - 7:1, with defined flavonoid or procyanidin content), corresponding to 30 - 168.7 mg procyanidins, calculated as epicatechin, or 3.5 - 19.8 mg flavonoids, calculated as hyperoside in accordance with *DAB* 10, in two or three individual doses.

Hawthorn fluidextract *DAB* 10:
Equivalent individual or daily dosage must be confirmed by clinical-pharmacological experiment or clinical study.

Mode of Administration
Liquid or dry pharmaceutical forms, for oral intake.

Duration of Administration
6 weeks minimum.

8. Overdosage
Not known.

9. Special Warnings
None.

10. Effects on Operators of Vehicles and Machinery
None.
Note: The drug as well as aqueous, aqueous-ethanolic, and wine-based extracts and fresh juice from the plant are traditionally taken orally as a tonic and strengthener of the cardiac/circulatory functions. This information is based exclusively on tradition and long-term experience.

*[**Ed. note:** Stages I and II of NYHA refer to stages of heart disease in the New York Heart Association's 1994 *Revisions to Classification of Functional Capacity and Objective Assessment of Patients with Diseases of the Heart*: "Patients with cardiac disease but without resulting limitations of physical activity. They are comfortable at rest. Ordinary physical activity results in fatigue, palpitation, dyspnea, or anginal pain." Monopreparations of hawthorn flower, fruit, and leaf are discussed in the **Unapproved Herbs** section. A discussion of the reasons for approval of this hawthorn leaf with flower monograph and disapproval of other forms is found on pages 33, 39, and 63 of the Introduction.

Hay flower
Graminis flos
Heublumen
Published May 5, 1988

Name of Drug
Graminis flos, hay flower.

Composition of Drug
Hay flower consists of the inflorescence, fruits and above-ground parts of *Poaceae*.

Uses
Topical use:
  heat therapy for degenerative diseases, such as the various forms of arthritis.

Contraindications
Open injuries, acute arthritis attacks, acute inflammation.

Side Effects
Allergic skin reactions are possible in rare cases.

Interactions with Other Drugs
None known.

Dosage
Unless otherwise prescribed:
  Externally 1 - 2 times daily as moist heat in the form of compresses.
  The hay flower bag is heated to 42° C (ca. 108° F), directly applied to the part to be treated, covered over and left in place for 40 - 50 minutes.
  For reasons of hygiene, the contents of the bag should be used only once.

Actions
Topically hyperemic
Influence of the inner organs via cuti-visceral reflexes

Heart's Ease herb
Violae tricoloris herba
Stiefmütterchenkraut
Published March 13, 1986

Name of Drug
Viola tricoloris herba, heart's ease herb, viola, Johnny Jump-up.

Composition of Drug
Viola herb consists of the dried, above-ground parts of *Viola tricolor* L., mainly of the subspecies *V. vulgaris* (Koch) Oborny and subspecies *V. arvensis* (Murray) Gaudin [Fam. Violaceae], harvested at flowering season, as well as their preparations in effective dosage.

The herb contains flavonoids.

Uses
External:
Mild seborrheic skin diseases, milk scall in children.

Contraindications
None known.

Side Effects
None known.

Interactions with Other Drugs
None known.

Dosage
Unless otherwise prescribed:
1.5 g of drug per cup of water as tea, 3 times daily;
equivalent preparations.

Mode of Administration
Chopped herb for teas and decoctions and for other galenical preparations for external use.

Hempnettle herb
Galeopsidis herba
Hohlzahnkraut
Published April 23, 1987

Name of Drug
Galeopsidis herba, hempnettle.

Composition of Drug
Hempnettle consists of the above-ground parts of *Galeopsis segetum* Necker (synonym *G. ochroleuca* Lamarck) [Fam. Lamiaceae], gathered at flowering season, as well as their preparations in effective dosage.

The herb contains tannin and saponins.

Uses
Mild catarrhs of the respiratory tract.

Contraindications
None known.

Side Effects
None known.

Interactions with Other Drugs
None known.

Dosage

Unless otherwise prescribed:
Average daily dosage:
  6 g of herb;
  equivalent preparations.

Mode of Administration

Comminuted herb for teas and other galenical preparations for internal use.

Henbane leaf
Hyoscyami folium
Hyoscyamusblätter
Published May 5, 1988

Name of Drug
Hyoscyami folium, henbane leaf.

Composition of Drug
Henbane leaf consists of the dried leaves or the dried leaves and flowering tops of *Hyoscyamus niger* L. [Fam. Solanaceae], as well as their preparations in effective dosage.

The drug contains at least 0.05 percent total alkaloids, calculated as hyoscyamine. The alkaloids consist mainly of hyoscyamine and scopolamine.

Uses
Spasms of the gastrointestinal tract.

Contraindications
Tachycardiac arrhythmias, prostatic adenoma with urine retention, narrow-angle glaucoma, acute pulmonary edema, mechanical stenosis in any part of the gastrointestinal tract, megacolon.

Side Effects
Dryness of the mouth, disturbances of optic conditions, tachycardia, difficulty in urination.

Interactions with Other Drugs
Enhancement of anticholinergic action by tricyclic antidepressants, amantadine, antihistamines, phenothiazines, procainamide and quinidine.

Dosage
Unless otherwise prescribed:
Average single dosage:
  0.5 g of standardized henbane powder corresponding to 0.25 - 0.35 mg total alkaloid.
Maximum single dosage:
  1 g of standardized henbane powder corresponding to 0.5 - 0.7 mg total alkaloid.
Maximum daily dosage:
  3 g of standardized henbane powder corresponding to 1.5 - 2.1 mg total alkaloid, calculated as hyoscyamine.

Mode of Administration
Standardized henbane powder and galenical preparations for internal application.

Actions
Henbane preparations produce a parasympatholytic or anticholinergic effect by competitive inhibition of acetylcholine. This inhibition affects the muscarinic action of acetylcholine but not its nicotine-like effects on ganglia and motor end-plates.

Henbane preparations exert peripheral actions on the autonomic nervous system and on smooth muscle, as well as the central nervous system. Because of their parasympatholytic properties, they cause relaxation of organs containing smooth muscle, particularly in the region of the gastrointestinal tract. Furthermore, they relieve muscular tremors of central nervous origin.

The spectrum of actions of *Hyoscyamus niger* additionally includes a sedative effect.

Hops
Lupuli strobulus
Hopfenzapfen
Published December 5, 1984; Revised March 13, 1990

Name of Drug
Lupuli strobulus, hops strobile, hops.

Composition of Drug
Hops, consisting of the dried strobiles of *Humulus lupulus* L. [Fam. Moraceae], and their preparations in effective dosage.

The drug contains at least 0.35 percent (v/w) essential oil.

Other ingredients are α- and ß-bitter acids and 2-methyl-3-butanol.

Uses
Mood disturbances such as restlessness and anxiety, sleep disturbances.

Contraindications
None known.

Side Effects
None known.

Interactions with Other Drugs
None known.

Dosage
Unless otherwise prescribed:
Single dosage of drug:
   0.5 g.

Mode of Administration
Cut drug, powdered drug or dry extract powder for infusions or decoctions or other preparations. Liquid and solid preparations for internal use.

Note: Combinations with all other sedatives can be beneficial.

Actions
Calming
Sleep promoting

Horehound herb
Marrubii herba
Andornkraut
Published February 1, 1990

Name of Drug
Marrubii herba, horehound herb.

Composition of Drug
Horehound herb consists of the fresh or dried, above-ground parts of *Marrubium vulgare* L. [Fam. Lamiaceae], as well as their preparations in effective dosage.

The herb contains bitter principles and tannins.

Uses
Loss of appetite and dyspepsia, such as bloating and flatulence.

Contraindications
None known.

Side Effects
None known.

Interactions with Other Drugs
None known.

Dosage
Unless otherwise prescribed:
Daily dosage:
    4.5 g of drug;
    2 - 6 tbs. of pressed juice;
    equivalent preparations.

Mode of Administration
Comminuted herb, freshly expressed plant juice and other galenical preparations for internal use.

Action
Marrubinic acid works as a choleretic.

Horse Chestnut seed
Hippocastani semen
Roßkastaniensamen
Published December 5, 1984; Replaced April 15, 1994

Name of Drug
Hippocastani semen, horse chestnut seed.

Composition of Drug
A dry extract manufactured from horse chestnut seeds, *Aesculus hippocastanum* L. [Fam. Hippocastanaceae], adjusted to a content of 16 - 20 percent triterpene glycosides (calculated as anhydrous aescin).

Pharmacological Properties, Pharmacokinetics, Toxicology
As found in different animal experiments, the principal ingredient in horse chestnut seed extract is the triterpene glycoside mixture, aescin (escin), which has an anti-exudative and vascular-tightening effect.

There are indications that horse chestnut seed extract reduces the activity of lysosomal enzymes that is increased in chronic pathological conditions of the veins, so that the breakdown of glycoacalyx (mucopolysaccharides) in the region of the capillary walls is inhibited. The filtration of low-molecular proteins, electrolytes and water into the interstitium is inhibited through a reduction of vascular permeability.

Using placebo as reference, a significant reduction of transcapillary filtration has been demonstrated in pharmacological studies involving human subjects, and a significant improvement shown in the symptoms of chronic venous insufficiency (sensation of tiredness, heaviness and tension, pruritus, pain and swelling in the legs) in various randomized double-blind studies and/or cross-over studies.

Pilot studies are available on the toxicology of horse chestnut seed extract. The oral LD^{50} of the extract is 990 mg per kg body weight in the mouse, 2150 mg per kg body weight in the rat, 1530 mg per kg body weight in the rabbit, and 130 mg per kg body weight in the dog. In the rat, the "no effect" dose is between 9 and 30 mg per kg body weight after intravenous administration of horse chestnut seed extract over a period of 8 weeks. Chronic administration above 80 mg per kg body weight over a period of 34 weeks produced gastric irritation in dogs. In rats, no toxic changes were observed throughout the same period up to an oral dose of 400 mg per kg body weight.

Clinical Data

1. Indications
Treatment of complaints found in pathological conditions of the veins of the legs (chronic venous insufficiency), for example, pains and a sensation of heaviness in the legs, nocturnal systremma (cramps in the calves), pruritus and swelling of the legs.

Note: Other non-invasive treatment measures prescribed by a physician, such as leg compresses, wearing of supportive elastic stockings, or cold water applications, must be observed under all circumstances.

2. Contraindications
None known.

3. Side Effects
Pruritus, nausea, and gastric complaints may occur in isolated cases after oral intake.

4. Special Caution for Use
None.

5. Use During Pregnancy and Lactation
No restriction known.

6. Interaction with Other Drugs
None known.

7. Dosage and Mode of Administration
Daily dose:
100 mg aescin (escin) corresponding to 250 - 312.5 mg extract 2 times per day in delayed release form.

8. Overdosage
None known.

9. Special Warnings
None.

10. Effect on Operators of Vehicles and Machinery
None.

Horseradish
Armoraciae rusticanae radix
Meerrettich
Published May 5, 1988

Name of Drug
Armoraciae rusticanae radix, horseradish.

Composition of Drug
Horseradish consists of the fresh or dried roots of *Armoracia rusticana* Ph. Gaertner, B. Meyer et Scherbius (syn. *Cochlearia armoracia* L.) [Fam. Brassicaceae], as well as their preparations in effective dosage.

The drug contains mustard oil and mustard oil glycosides.

Uses
Internal:
Catarrhs of the respiratory tract; supportive therapy for infections of the urinary tract.
External:
Catarrhs of the respiratory tract; hyperemic treatment for minor muscle aches.

Contraindications
Internal:
Stomach and intestinal ulcers, kidney disorders. No administration to children under the age of 4.

Side Effects
Internal: Discomforts of the gastrointestinal tract.

Interactions with Other Drugs
None known.

Dosage
Unless otherwise prescribed:
Internal:
Average daily dosage:
20 g of fresh root;
equivalent preparations.
External:
Preparations with a maximum of 2 percent mustard oil.

Mode of Administration
Fresh or dried, cut or ground root, freshly pressed juice as well as other galenical preparations for internal or external applications.

Actions
Antimicrobial
Hyperemic

Horsetail herb
Equiseti herba
Schachtelhalmkraut
Published September 18, 1986

Name of Drug
Equiseti herba, horsetail herb.

Composition of Drug
Horsetail consists of the fresh or dried, green, sterile stems of *Equisetum arvense* L. [Fam. Equisetaceae], as well as its preparations in effective dosage.

The herb contains silicic acid and flavonoids.

Uses

Internal:
Post-traumatic and static edema.
Irrigation therapy for bacterial and inflammatory diseases of the lower urinary tract and renal gravel.

External:
Supportive treatment for poorly healing wounds.

Contraindications

None known.

Note: No irrigation therapy in case of edema due to impaired heart and kidney function.

Side Effects

None known.

Interactions with Other Drugs

None known.

Dosage

Unless otherwise prescribed:
Internal:
Average daily dosage:
6 g of herb;
equivalent preparations.
External use in compresses:
10 g of herb to 1 liter of water.

Mode of Administration

Internal:
Comminuted herb for infusions and other galenical preparations for oral administration.
For irrigation therapy, ensure an abundant fluid intake.

External:
Comminuted herb for decoctions and other galenical preparations.

Action

Mild diuretic

Iceland moss

Lichen islandicus
Isländisches Moos
Published March 2, 1989

Name of Drug

Lichen islandicus, Iceland moss.

Composition of Drug

Iceland moss consists of the dried thallus of *Cetraria islandica* (L.) Acharius s.l. [Fam. Parmeliaceae], as well as its preparations in effective dosage.

The herb contains mucilage and bitter principles.

Uses

(a) Irritation of the oral and pharyngeal mucous membranes and accompanying dry cough.
(b) Loss of appetite.

Contraindications

None known.

Side Effects

None known.

Interactions with Other Drugs

None known.

Dosage

Unless otherwise prescribed:
Average daily dosage:
4 - 6 g of herb;
equivalent preparations.

Mode of Administration

Use (a):
Comminuted herb for infusions and other galenical formulations for internal use.

Use (b):
Comminuted herb, preferably for cold macerates and other bitter-tasting preparations for internal use.

Actions
Soothing
Mildly antimicrobial

Indian Snakeroot
Rauwolfiae radix
Rauwolfiawurzel
Published September 18, 1986

Name of Drug
Rauwolfiae radix, Indian snakeroot

Composition of Drug
Indian snakeroot consists of the dried roots of *Rauvolfia serpentina* (L.) Bentham ex Kurz [Fam. Apocynaceae],* as well as their preparations in effective dosage.

The drug contains at least 1 percent alkaloids calculated as reserpine with reference to the dried drug.

Uses
Mild, essential hypertension (borderline hypertension), especially with elevated tension of the sympathetic nervous system, for example, sinus tachycardia, anxiety, tension and psychomotor irritation, when dietetic measures alone are not sufficient.

Contraindications
Depression, ulcer, pheochromocytoma, pregnancy and lactation.

Side Effects
Stuffy nose, depressive mood, fatigue, reduction in sexual potency.
Note: This preparation can change reaction time, even when used as directed, leading to decreased ability to drive in traffic or to operate machines. This effect is potentiated in connection with use of alcohol.

Interactions with Other Drugs
with:
Digitalis glycosides:
   bradycardia;
Neuroleptics:
   mutual potentiation;
Barbiturates:
   mutual potentiation;
Levodopa:
   reduced effectiveness, but undesired extrapyramidal motor symptoms can be increased;
Sympathomimetics (e.g., in cough/cold medications, and appetite suppressants):
   initial strong blood pressure increase.

Dosage
Unless otherwise prescribed:
Average daily dosage:
   600 mg drug corresponding to 6 mg total alkaloids.

Mode of Administration
Comminuted drug. Powdered drug as well as other galenical preparations for internal use.

Actions

Based on the strong sympathicolysis [alpha and beta receptor blocking action] (catecholamine reduction), blood pressure lowering and sedating. In addition there are direct central and peripheral receptor sites for specific alkaloids.

*[**Ed. note:** The original German monograph writes the genus name in the Latin binomial as *Rauwolfia*, a spelling commonly used. However, our taxonomic reviewers stipulate the spelling *Rauvolfia*.]

Ivy leaf
Hederae helicis folium
Efeublätter
Published July 6, 1988

Name of Drug
Hederae helicis folium, ivy leaf.

Composition of Drug
Ivy leaf consists of the dried leaf of *Hedera helix* L. [Fam. Araliaceae], as well as its preparations in effective dosage.

The drug contains saponins.

Uses
Catarrhs of the respiratory passages, symptomatic treatment of chronic inflammatory bronchial conditions.

Contraindications
None known.

Side Effects
None known.

Interactions with Other Drugs
None known.

Dosage
Unless otherwise prescribed:
 Average daily dosage:
 0.3 g of drug;
 equivalent preparations.

Mode of Administration
Comminuted drug and other galenical preparations for internal use.

Actions
Expectorant
Antispasmodic
Irritative to skin and mucosa

Jambolan bark
Syzygii cumini cortex
Syzygiumrinde
Published April 23, 1987

Name of Drug
Syzygii cumini cortex, jambolan bark.

Composition of Drug
Jambolan bark consists of the dried bark from the trunk of *Syzygium cumini* (L.) Skeels (synonym *S. jambolana* (Lam.) de Candolle) [Fam. Myrtaceae], as well as its preparations in effective dosage.

The bark contains tannins.

Uses
Internal:
Nonspecific acute diarrhea, topical therapy for mild inflammation of the oral-pharyngeal mucosa.
External:
Mild, superficial inflammation of the skin.

Contraindications
None known.

Side Effects
None known.

Interactions with Other Drugs
None known.

Dosage
Unless otherwise prescribed:
Average daily dosage:
3 - 6 g of drug;
equivalent preparations.

Mode of Administration
Comminuted herb for decoctions and other galenical preparations for internal use and local application.

Duration of Administration
If diarrhea persists for more than 3 - 4 days, consult a physician.

Action
Astringent

Java tea
Orthosiphonis folium
Orthosiphonblätter
Published March 13, 1986; Revised March 13, 1990

Name of Drug
Orthosiphonis folium, Java tea.

Composition of Drug
Java tea consists of the dried leaf and stem tips of *Orthosiphon spicatus* (Thunberg) Baker (syn. *O. stamineus* Bentham) [Fam. Lamiaceae], harvested shortly before flowering, as well as its preparations in effective dosage.

The herb contains lipophilic flavones (such as sinensetin, scutellarein-tetramethylether and eupatorin), essential oil, and large amounts of potassium salts.

Uses
Irrigation therapy for bacterial and inflammatory diseases of the lower urinary tract and renal gravel.

Contraindications
None known.
Warning: No irrigation therapy in case of edema due to limited heart and kidney function.

Side Effects
None known.

Interactions with Other Drugs
None known.

Dosage
Unless otherwise prescribed:
Daily dosage:
  6 - 12 g herb;
  equivalent preparations.

Mode of Administration
Cut herb for infusions and other galenical preparations for oral use.

Actions
Diuretic
Weakly antispasmodic

Juniper berry
Juniperi fructus
Wacholderbeeren
Published December 5, 1984

Name of Drug
Juniperi fructus, juniper berry.

Composition of Drug
Juniper berry is the ripe, fresh or dried spherical ovulate cone ("berry") of *Juniperus communis* L. [Fam. Cupressaceae], as well as its preparations in effective dosage. Juniper berry contains at least 1 percent (v/w) volatile oil in reference to the dried drug.

Main ingredients of the volatile oil are terpene hydrocarbons such as α-pinene, ß-pinene, myrcene, sabinene, thujone, and limonene. Also contained are sesquiterpene hydrocarbons such as caryophyllene, cadinene, and elemene and terpene alcohols such as 4-terpineol.

Furthermore, juniper berries contain flavonoid glycosides, tannins, sugar and resin- and wax-containing compounds.

Uses
Dyspepsia.

Contraindications
Pregnancy and inflammation of the kidneys.

Side Effects
Prolonged usage or overdosing may cause kidney damage.

Interactions with Other Drugs
None known.

Dosage
Unless otherwise prescribed:
Daily dose:
  2 to a maximum of 10 g of the
  dried juniper fruit, corresponding to
  20 - 100 mg of the essential oil.

Mode of Administration

Whole, crushed, or powdered drug for infusions and decoctions, alcohol extracts, and in wine. Essential oil. Liquid and solid medicinal forms only for oral application.
Warning: Combinations with other plant drugs in teas and similar preparations for treating bladder and kidney diseases may be helpful.

Action

Animal experiments have shown an increase in urine excretion as well as a direct effect on smooth muscle contraction.

Kava Kava

Piperis methystici rhizoma
Kava-kava-Wurzelstock
Published June 1, 1990

Name of Drug

Piperis methystici rhizoma, kava kava rhizome (root).

Composition of Drug

Kava kava rhizome consists of the dried rhizomes of *Piper methysticum* G. Forster [Fam. Piperaceae], as well as their preparations in effective dosage.

The drug contains kava-pyrones (kawain).

Uses

Conditions of nervous anxiety, stress, and restlessness.

Contraindications

Pregnancy, nursing, endogenous depression.

Side Effects

None known.
Note: Extended continuous intake can cause a temporary yellow discoloration of skin, hair and nails. In this case, further application of this drug must be discontinued. In rare cases, allergic skin reactions can occur. Also, accommodative disturbances, such as enlargement of the pupils and disturbances of the oculomotor equilibrium, have been described.

Interactions with Other Drugs

Potentiation of effectiveness is possible for substances acting on the central nervous system, such as alcohol, barbiturates and psychopharmacological agents.

Dosage

Unless otherwise prescribed:
Daily dosage:
   Herb and preparations equivalent to 60 - 120 mg kava pyrones.

Mode of Administration

Comminuted rhizome and other galenical preparations for oral use.

Duration of Administration

Not more than 3 months without medical advice.
Note: Even when administered within its prescribed dosages, this herb may adversely affect motor reflexes and judgment for driving and/or operating heavy machinery.

Actions
Anti-anxiety
In animal experiments a potentiation of narcosis (sedation), anticonvulsive, antispasmodic, and central muscular relaxant effects were described.

Kidney bean pods (without seeds)
Phaseoli fructus sine semine
Samenfreie Gartenbohnenhülsen
Published March 13, 1986; Revised March 13, 1990

Name of Drug
Phaseoli fructus sine semine, kidney bean pods (without seeds).

Composition of Drug
Seed-free pods of *Phaseolus vulgaris* L. [Fam. Fabaceae], as well as preparations in effective dosage.

The drug contains flavonoids, phaseolin and chemically related phytoalexins.

Uses
Supportive treatment for inability to urinate.

Contraindications
None known.

Interactions with Other Drugs
None known.

Dosage
Unless otherwise prescribed:
Daily dose:
  5 - 15 g of herb;
  equivalent preparations.

Mode of Administration
Comminuted herb for decoctions and other galenical preparations for internal use.

Action
Weakly diuretic

Knotweed herb
Polygoni avicularis herba
Vogelknöterichkraut
Published April 23, 1987; Revised March 13, 1990

Name of Drug
Polygoni avicularis herba, knotweed, knotgrass.

Composition of Drug
Knotweed herb consists of the dried herb, occasionally containing roots, of *Polygonum aviculare* L. [Fam. Polygonaceae], gathered during flowering season, as well as its preparations in effective dosage.

The drug contains tannin and silicic acid.

Uses
Mild catarrhs of the respiratory tract, inflammatory changes to the oral and pharyngeal mucosa.

Contraindications
None known.

Side Effects
None known.

Interactions with Other Drugs
None known.

Dosage
Daily dosage:
    4 - 6 g of drug;
    equivalent preparations.

Mode of Administration
Ground herb for teas and other galenical preparations for internal use and local application.

Actions
Astringent
Acetylcholinesterase inhibitor

Lady's Mantle
Alchemillae herba
Frauenmantelkraut
Published September 18, 1986

Name of Drug
Alchemillae herba, lady's mantle.

Composition of Drug
Lady's mantle herb consists of the fresh or dried, above-ground parts of *Alchemilla vulgaris* L. [Fam. Rosaceae], gathered at flowering time, as well as its preparations in effective dosage.

    The herb contains tannins and flavonoids.

Uses
Light and nonspecific diarrhea.

Contraindications
None known.

Side Effects
None known.

Interactions with Other Drugs
None known.

Dosage
Unless otherwise prescribed:
Average daily dosage:
    5 - 10 g of herb;
    equivalent preparations.

Mode of Administration
Cut herb for infusions and decoctions, as well as other galenical preparations for internal use.

Duration of Administration
If diarrhea persists longer than 3 - 4 days, consult with a physician.

Action
Astringent

Larch Turpentine
Terebinthina laricina
Lärchenterpentin
Published December 5, 1984; Revised March 13, 1990

Name of Drug
Terebinthina laricina, larch turpentine.
Terebinthina veneta, Venetian turpentine.

Composition of Drug
The balsam of *Larix decidua* Miller [Fam. Pinaceae], obtained by drilling into the trunks.

The balsam contains up to 20 percent essential oil.

Uses
Rheumatic and neuralgic discomforts, catarrhal diseases of the respiratory tract, furuncle.

Contraindications
Sensitivity to essential oils.
For inhalation:
acute inflammation of the respiratory tract.

Side Effects
Topical application can cause allergic skin reactions, as has been observed with all balsams.

Interactions with Other Drugs
None known.

Dosage
External:
Liquid and semi-solid preparations 10 - 20 percent.

Mode of Administration
Embrocations in the form of ointments, gels, emulsions and oils.

Actions
Hyperemic
Antiseptic

Lavender flower
Lavandulae flos
Lavendelblüten
Published December 5, 1984; Revised March 13, 1990

Name of Drug
Lavandulae flos, lavender flower.

Composition of Drug
Lavender flower consists of the dried flower of *Lavandula angustifolia* Miller [Fam. Lamiaceae], gathered shortly before fully unfolding, as well as its preparations in effective dosage.

The drug contains at least 1.5 percent (v/w) essential oil with linalyl acetate, linalool, camphor, ß-ocimene, and 1,8-cineol as its main components. Furthermore, the drug contains about 12 percent tannins unique to the family Lamiaceae.

Uses
Internal:
Mood disturbances such as restlessness or insomnia, functional abdominal complaints (nervous stomach irritations, Roehmheld syndrome,

meteorism, nervous intestinal discomfort).
For balneotherapy:
    Treatment of functional circulatory disorders.

Contraindications
None known.

Side Effects
None known.

Interactions with Other Drugs
None known.

Dosage
Unless otherwise prescribed:
Internal:
    As tea:
        1 - 2 teaspoons of drug per cup of water.
    Lavender oil:
        1 - 4 drops (ca. 20 - 80 mg), e.g., on a sugar cube.
    External use as bath additive:
        20 - 100 g of drug for a 20 liter bath.

Mode of Administration
As herb for preparations of tea, as extract and as bath additive.
Note: Combinations with other sedative and/or carminative herbs may be beneficial.

Actions
Internal:
    Sedative
    Antiflatulent

Lemon Balm
Melissae folium
Melissenblätter
Published December 5, 1984; Revised March 13, 1990

Name of Drug
Melissae folium, lemon balm, melissa.

Composition of Drug
Lemon balm contains the fresh or dried leaf of *Melissa officinalis* L. [Fam. Lamiaceae], as well as its preparations in effective dosage.

The leaf contains at least 0.05 percent (v/w) essential oil based on the dried herb. Main components are citronellal, citral a, and citral b, as well as other mono- and sesquiterpenes. Other ingredients are tannins unique to the Lamiaceae, such as triterpenylic acid, bitter principles, and flavonoids.

Uses
Nervous sleeping disorders. Functional gastrointestinal complaints.

Contraindications
None known.

Side Effects
None known.

Interactions with Other Drugs
None known.

Dosage
Unless otherwise prescribed:
    Several times daily, 1.5 - 4.5 g of herb per cup of tea, as needed.

Mode of Administration

Comminuted herb, herb powder, fluid-extracts or dry extracts for teas and other galenical preparations. Ground herb and its preparations for oral use.

Note: Combinations with other sedative and/or carminative herbs may be beneficial.

Actions

Sedative
Carminative

Licorice root

Liquiritiae radix

Süßholzwurzel

Published May 15, 1985; Revised March 13, 1990, April 19, 1991, and September 21, 1991

Name of Drug

Liquiritiae radix, licorice root.

Composition of Drug

Licorice root consists of unpeeled, dried roots and stolons of *Glycyrrhiza glabra* L. [Fam. Fabaceae], as well as their preparations in effective dosage. The unpeeled roots contain at least 4 percent glycyrrhizic acid and 25 percent water-soluble matter. Licorice root also consists of peeled, dried roots and stolons of *G. glabra* L. [Fam. Fabaceae], as well as their preparations in effective dosage. The peeled roots contain at least 20 percent water-soluble matter.

The root contains several flavonoids of flavanone and isoflavanone derivatives in addition to the potassium and calcium salts of the glycyrrhizic acid. It also contains phytosterols and coumarins.

Uses

For catarrhs of the upper respiratory tract and gastric/duodenal ulcers.

Contraindications

Cholestatic liver disorders, liver cirrhosis, hypertonia, hypokalemia, severe kidney insufficiency, pregnancy.

Side Effects

On prolonged use and with higher doses, mineralocorticoid effects may occur in the form of sodium and water retention and potassium loss, accompanied by hypertension, edema, and hypokalemia, and, in rare cases, myoglobinuria.

Interactions with Other Drugs

Potassium loss due to other drugs, e.g., thiazide diuretics, can be increased. With potassium loss, sensitivity to digitalis glycosides increases.

Dosage

Unless otherwise prescribed:
Average daily dosage:
    About 5 - 15 g of root, equivalent to 200 - 600 mg of glycyrrhizin;
As *Succus liquiritiae*:
    0.5 - 1 g for catarrhs of the upper respiratory tract, 1.5 - 3 g for gastric/duodenal ulcers;
equivalent preparations.

Mode of Administration

Powdered root, finely cut root or dry extracts for infusions, decoctions, liquid or solid dosage forms for internal use (*Succus liquiritiae*).

Duration of Administration
Not longer than 4 - 6 weeks without medical advice. There is no objection to using licorice root as a flavoring agent up to a maximum daily dosage equivalent to 100 mg glycyrrhizin.

Actions
According to controlled clinical studies, glycyrrhizic acid and the aglycone of glycyrrhizic acid accelerate the healing of gastric ulcers. Secretolytic and expectorant effects have been confirmed in tests on rabbits. In the isolated rabbit ileum, an antispasmodic action has been observed at concentrations of 1:2500 - 1:5000.

Lily-of-the-valley herb
Convallariae herba
Maiglöckchenkraut
Published April 23, 1987; Revised February 1, 1990

Name of Drug
Convallariae herba, lily-of-the-valley herb.

Composition of Drug
Lily-of-the-valley herb consists of the dried, above-ground parts of *Convallaria majalis* L. [Fam. Liliaceae], or closely related species, as well as their preparations in effective dosage. The herb is harvested during flowering season. The lily-of-the-valley contains cardioactive glycosides; the principal glycoside is convallotoxin.

Uses
Mild cardiac insufficiency, heart insufficiency due to old age, chronic cor pulmonale.

Contraindications
Therapy with digitalis glycosides, potassium deficiency.

Side Effects
Nausea, vomiting, cardiac arrhythmias.

Interactions with Other Drugs
Increased effectiveness and also side effects of simultaneously administered quinidine, calcium, saluretics, laxatives, and extended therapy with glucocorticoids.

Dosage
Unless otherwise prescribed:
Average daily dosage:
   0.6 g standardized lily-of-the-valley powder;
equivalent preparations.

Mode of Administration
Comminuted herb, as well as galenical preparations thereof for internal use.

Actions
Positive inotropic on the myocardium
Economizes heart performance
Lowers the elevated left-ventricular diastolic pressure, as well as pathologically elevated venous pressure
Tonic for the veins
Natriuretic
Kaliuretic

Linden flower
Tiliae flos
Lindenblüten
Published September 1, 1990

Name of Drug
Tiliae flos, linden flower.

Composition of Drug
Linden flower consists of the dried flower of *Tilia cordata* Miller and/or *Tilia platyphyllos* Scopoli [Fam. Tiliaceae], as well as its preparations in effective dosage. The drug contains flavonoids, tannins, and mucilage.

Uses
Colds and cold-related coughs.

Contraindications
None known.

Interactions with Other Drugs
None known.

Dosage
Unless otherwise prescribed:
Daily dosage:
   2 - 4 g of drug;
   equivalent preparations.

Mode of Administration
Comminuted herb for teas and other galenical preparations for internal use.

Action
Diaphoretic

Lovage root
Levistici radix
Liebstöckelwurzel
Published June 1, 1990

Name of Drug
Levistici radix, lovage root.

Composition of Drug
Lovage root consists of the dried rhizomes and roots of *Levisticum officinale* Koch [Fam. Apiaceae], as well as their preparations in effective dosage.
   The drug contains essential oil and coumarin derivatives.

Uses
Irrigation therapy for inflammation of the lower urinary tract and for prevention of kidney gravel.

Contraindications
Preparations of lovage should not be used if acute inflammation of the kidney parenchyma with impaired kidney function exists.
   No irrigation therapy in cases of edema due to limited heart and kidney function.

Side Effects
None known.

Interactions with Other Drugs
None known.

Dosage
Unless otherwise prescribed:
Daily dosage:
  4 - 8 g of drug;
  equivalent preparations.

Mode of Administration
Comminuted herb and other galenical preparations for internal use.

Note: Intense exposure to the sun and ultraviolet light should be avoided during extended use of lovage root.

Action
The ligustilide-containing essential oil is antispasmodic.

Mallow flower
Malvae flos
Malvenblüten
Published March 2, 1989

Name of Drug
Malvae flos, blue mallow flower.

Composition of Drug
Mallow flower consists of the dried flowers of *Malva sylvestris* L. and/or *Malva sylvestris* L. ssp. *mauritiana* (L.) Ascherson et Graebner [Fam. Malvaceae], as well as their preparations in effective dosage.
  The drug contains mucilage.

Uses
Irritations of the mucosa of the mouth and throat and associated dry, irritative cough.

Contraindications
None known.

Side Effects
None known.

Interactions with Other Drugs
None known.

Dosage
Unless otherwise prescribed:
Daily dosage:
  5 g of drug;
  equivalent preparations.

Mode of Administration
Comminuted herb for infusions and other preparations for internal use.

Action
Demulcent

Mallow leaf
Malvae folium
Malvenblätter
Published March 2, 1989

Name of Drug
Malvae folium, mallow leaf.

Composition of Drug
Mallow leaf consists of the dried leaves of *Malva sylvestris* L. and/or *M. neglecta* Wallroth [Fam. Malvaceae], or equivalent preparations in effective dosage.

The drug contains mucilage.

Uses
Irritations of mucosa of mouth and throat and associated dry, irritating cough.

Contraindications
None known.

Side Effects
None known.

Interactions with Other Drugs
None known.

Dosage
Unless otherwise prescribed:
Daily dose:
5 g of drug;
equivalent preparations.

Mode of Administration
Comminuted drug for infusions as well as other galenical preparations for internal use.

Action
Demulcent

Manna
Manna
Manna
Published February 1, 1990

Name of Drug
Manna, manna ash.

Composition of Drug
Manna consists of the dried sap generated from the slit bark of trunk and branches of *Fraxinus ornus* L. [Fam. Oleaceae], as well as its preparations in effective dosage.

The drug contains mannitol.

Uses
Constipation. Ailments where an easier elimination and a soft stool are desirable, such as anal fissures, hemorrhoids, and post-rectal/anal surgery.

Contraindications
Bowel obstruction.

Side Effects
Sensitive individuals can experience nausea and flatulence.

Interactions with Other Drugs
None known.

Dosage
Unless otherwise prescribed:
Daily dosage:
> For adults, 20 - 30 g of drug;
> For children, 2 - 16 g of drug;
> equivalent preparations.

Mode of Administration
Comminuted herb and other galenical preparations for internal use.

Duration of Administration
Laxatives should not be taken for an extended period of time without consulting a physician.

Action
Laxative

Marshmallow leaf
Althaeae folium
Eibischblätter
Published March 2, 1989

Name of Drug
Althaeae folium, marshmallow leaf.

Composition of Drug
Marshmallow leaf consists of the dried leaf of *Althaea officinalis* L. [Fam. Malvaceae], as well as its preparations in effective dosage.
   The drug contains mucilage.

Uses
Irritation of the oral and pharyngeal mucosa and associated dry cough.

Contraindications
None known.

Side Effects
None known.

Interactions with Other Drugs
None known.
Note: Absorption of other drugs taken simultaneously may be delayed.

Dosage
Unless otherwise prescribed:
Daily dosage:
> 5 g of leaf;
> equivalent preparations.

Mode of Administration
Cut leaves for aqueous extracts as well as other galenical preparations for internal use.

Action
Alleviates local irritation.

Marshmallow root
Althaeae radix
Eibischwurzel
Published March 2, 1989

Name of Drug
Althaeae radix, marshmallow root.

Composition of Drug
Marshmallow root consists of the dried root, unpeeled or peeled, of *Althaea officinalis* L. [Fam. Malvaceae], as well as its preparations in effective dosage.

Uses
(a) Irritation of the oral and pharyngeal mucosa and associated dry cough.
(b) Mild inflammation of the gastric mucosa.

Contraindications
None known.

Side Effects
None known.

Interactions with Other Drugs
None known.
Note: The absorption of other drugs taken simultaneously may be delayed.

Dosage
Unless otherwise prescribed:
Daily dosage:
    6 g of root;
    equivalent preparations.
Marshmallow syrup:
    Single dose:
        10 g.

Mode of Administration
Cut or ground root for aqueous extracts as well as other galenical preparations for internal use. Marshmallow syrup to be used only for use (a).
Note: Marshmallow syrup: diabetics need to allow for sugar concentration (according to declaration of manufacturer) ... percent (equivalent to...bread units).*

Actions
Alleviates local irritation
Inhibits mucociliary activity
Stimulates phagocytosis

*[**Ed. note:** This relates to the need for diabetics to consider and allow for the sugar content of the syrup as stated on the label and is written precisely as it appears in the original German.]

Maté
Mate folium
Mateblätter
Published May 5, 1988

Name of Drug
Mate folium, maté, yerba maté.

Composition of Drug
Maté consists of the dried leaf and leaf stem of *Ilex paraguariensis* de Saint-Hilaire

[Fam. Aquifoliaceae], as well as their preparations in effective dosage.

The herb contains caffeine.

Uses
Mental and physical fatigue.

Contraindications
None known.

Side Effects
None known.

Interactions with Other Drugs
None known.

Dosage
Unless otherwise prescribed:
Average daily dosage:
   3 g of drug;
   equivalent preparations.

Mode of Administration
Comminuted herb for teas, herb powder for other galenical preparations for internal use.

Actions
Analeptic
Diuretic
Positively inotropic
Positively chronotropic
Glycogenolytic
Lipolytic

Mayapple root and resin
Podophylli peltati rhizoma/resina
Podophyllumwurzelstock/Harz
Published March 13, 1986

Name of Drug
Podophylli peltati rhizoma, mayapple root, American mandrake.

Podophylli peltati resina, mayapple resin, American mandrake resin.

Composition of Drug
Mayapple root consists of the dried rhizome and connected roots of *Podophyllum peltatum* L. [Fam. Berberidaceae].

The root contains at least 4 percent resin with podophyllotoxin. Mayapple resin consists of the resin of the dried and stored (aged) rhizome of *P. peltatum* L., as well as its preparations in effective dosage.

Uses
External:
   Removal of pointed condyloma.

Contraindications
Pregnancy.

Side Effects
None known.

Interactions with Other Drugs
None known.

Dosage
Daily dosage:
   1.5 - 3 g root;
   1.5 - 3 g fluidextract (*Erg. B. 6*);
   2.5 - 7.5 g tincture (*Erg. B. 6*);
   equivalent preparations.

Mode of Administration
Dried rhizome for production of resin exclusively for external application.
Note: The treated skin surface must not be larger than 25 cm^2 [approx. 10 in. x 10 in.]. Be sure to protect skin adjacent to treated area.

Meadowsweet
Filipendula ulmaria
Mädesüß
Published March 2, 1989

Name of Drug
Spiraeae flos, meadowsweet flower.
Spiraeae herba, meadowsweet herb.

Composition of Drug
Meadowsweet flower consists of the dried flower of *Filipendula ulmaria* (L.) Maximowicz (syn. *Spiraea ulmaria* L.) [Fam. Rosaceae], as well as its preparations in effective dosage.

Meadowsweet herb consists of the dried, above-ground parts of *F. ulmaria* (L.) Maximowicz, harvested during flowering season, as well as its preparations in effective dosage.

The drug contains flavonoids and, mainly in the flowers, phenol glycosides, also essential oil.

Uses
As supportive therapy for colds.

Contraindications
None known.

Note: Meadowsweet flowers contain salicylate. They should not be used where a salicylate sensitivity exists.

Side Effects
None known.

Interactions with Other Drugs
None known.

Dosage
Unless otherwise prescribed:
Daily dosage:
  2.5 - 3.5 g meadowsweet flower or
  4 - 5 g meadowsweet herb;
equivalent preparations.

Mode of Administration
Comminuted herb and other galenical preparations for infusions; a cup of the infusion drunk as hot as possible several times a day.

Milk Thistle fruit
Cardui mariae fructus
Mariendistelfrüchte
Published March 13, 1986

Name of Drug
Cardui mariae fructus, milk thistle fruit.

Composition of Drug
Milk thistle fruit consists of ripe seed of *Silybum marianum* (L.) Gaertner [Fam. Asteraceae], freed from the pappus, and its preparations in effective dosage.

The drug contains silibinin, silydianin, and silychristin.

Uses
Crude drug:
  Dyspeptic complaints.

Formulations:*
Toxic liver damage; for supportive treatment in chronic inflammatory liver disease and hepatic cirrhosis.

Contraindications
None known.

Side Effects
Crude drug:
 None known.
Formulations:
 A mild laxative effect has been observed in occasional instances.

Interactions with Other Drugs
None known.

Dosage
Unless otherwise prescribed:
Average daily dose of drug:
 12 - 15 g;
 Formulations equivalent to 200 - 400 mg of silymarin, calculated as silibinin.

Mode of Administration
Powdered drug for making infusions and other galenical formulations to be taken by mouth.

Actions
Silymarin acts as an antagonist in many experimental liver-damage models: phalloidin and -amanitin (death-cap toxins), lanthanides, carbon tetrachloride, galactosamine, thioacetamide, and the hepatotoxic virus FV3 of cold-blooded vertebrates.

The therapeutic activity of silymarin is based on two sites or mechanisms of action:
(a) it alters the structure of the outer cell membrane of the hepatocytes in such a way as to prevent penetration of the liver toxin into the interior of the cell;
(b) it stimulates the action of nucleolar polymerase A, resulting in an increase in ribosomal protein synthesis, and thus stimulates the regenerative ability of the liver and the formation of new hepatocytes.

*[**Ed. note:** "Formulation" refers to an extract standardized to at least 70 percent silymarin, the collective name for the three compounds listed in the **Composition of Drug** section.]

Mint oil
Menthae arvensis aetheroleum
Minzöl
Published September 24, 1986; Revised March 13, 1990, September 1, 1990, and July 14, 1993

Name of Drug
Menthae arvensis aetheroleum, mint oil.

Composition of Drug
Mint oil consists of volatile oil obtained from *Mentha arvensis* L. var. *piperaescens* Holmes ex Christy [Fam. Lamiaceae], as well as its preparations in effective dosage. The oil is obtained by steam distillation of the fresh, flowering herb, followed by partial removal of menthol and rectification.

Mint oil contains at least 3 percent and at most 17 percent esters, calculated as menthyl acetate, at least 42 percent free alcohols, calculated as menthol, and at least 25 percent and at most 40 percent ketones, calculated as menthone.

Uses
Internal:
  flatulence, functional gastrointestinal and gallbladder disorders, catarrhs of the upper respiratory tract.
External:
  myalgia and neuralgic ailments.

Contraindications
Internal:
  obstruction of the bile ducts, inflammation of the gallbladder, severe liver damage. To be used only after consultation with a physician.
External:
  For infants and young children, mint oil-containing preparations should not be used on areas of the face and especially the nose.

Side Effects
Sensitive people may experience stomach disorders.

Interactions with Other Drugs
None known.

Dosage
Unless otherwise prescribed:
Internal:
  Average daily dosage: 3 - 6 drops;
Inhalation:
  3 - 4 drops in hot water;
External:
  Several drops rubbed into the skin; equivalent preparations.
  5 - 20 percent in oil and semi-solid preparations;
  5 - 10 percent in aqueous-alcoholic preparations;
  In nasal ointments, 1 - 5 percent essential oil.

Mode of Administration
Essential oil and other galenical preparations for internal and external application.

Actions
Carminative
Cholagogue
Antibacterial
Secretolytic
Cooling

Mistletoe herb
Visci albi herba
Mistelkraut
Published December 5, 1984

Name of Drug
Visci albi herba, mistletoe herb.

Composition of Drug
Mistletoe herb consists of fresh or dried younger branches with flowers and fruits of *Viscum album* L. [Fam. Viscaceae], as well as their preparations in effective dosage.

Uses
For treating degenerative inflammation of the joints by stimulating cuti-visceral reflexes following local inflammation brought about by intradermal injections.

As palliative therapy for malignant tumors through non-specific stimulation.

Contraindications
Protein hypersensitivity, chronic-progressive infections, e.g., tuberculosis.

Side Effects
Chills, high fever, headaches, angina, orthostatic circulatory disturbances and allergic reactions.

Interactions with Other Drugs
None known.

Dosage
Unless otherwise prescribed:
  According to directions of the manufacturer.

Mode of Administration
Fresh plant, cut and powdered herb for the preparation of solutions for injections.

Actions
Intracutaneous injections cause local inflammations which can progress to necrosis.

In animal experiments cytostatic, non-specific immune stimulation.

Note: The blood pressure-lowering effects and the therapeutic effectiveness for mild forms of hypertonia (borderline hypertonia) need further investigation.

Motherwort herb
Leonuri cardiacae herba
Herzgespannkraut
Published March 13, 1986

Name of Drug
Leonuri cardiacae herba, motherwort herb.

Composition of Drug
Motherwort herb consists of the above-ground parts of *Leonurus cardiaca* L. [Fam. Lamiaceae], gathered during flowering season, as well as their preparations in effective dosage.

The drug contains alkaloids (stachydrine), glycosides of bitter principles, and bufenolide.

Uses
Nervous cardiac disorders and as adjuvant for thyroid hyperfunction.

Contraindications
None known.

Side Effects
None known.

Interactions with Other Drugs
None known.

Dosage
Unless otherwise prescribed:
Average daily dosage:
  4.5 g herb;
  equivalent preparations.

Mode of Administration
Comminuted herb for infusions and other galenical preparations for internal use.

Mullein flower
Verbasci flos
Wollblumen
Published February 1, 1990

Name of Drug
Verbasci flos, mullein flower.

Composition of Drug
Mullein flower consists of the dried petals of *Verbascum densiflorum* Bertoloni and/or of *V. phlomoides* L. (syn. *V. thapsus* L.) [Fam. Scrophulariaceae], as well as their preparations in effective dosage.

The drug contains saponins and mucopolysaccharides.

Uses
Catarrhs of the respiratory tract.

Contraindications
None known.

Side Effects
None known.

Interactions with Other Drugs
None known.

Dosage
Unless otherwise prescribed:
Daily dosage:
   3 - 4 g of herb;
   equivalent preparations.

Mode of Administration
Comminuted herb for teas and other galenical preparations for internal use.

Actions
Alleviating irritation
Expectorant

Myrrh
Myrrha
Myrrhe
Published October 15, 1987

Name of Drug
Myrrha, myrrh [Somalian myrrh].

Composition of Drug
Myrrh consists of oleo-gum resin extruded from the stems of *Commiphora molmol* Engler [Fam. Burseraceae], then air-dried, as well as its preparations in effective dosage.

Myrrh can also originate from other *Commiphora* species, if the chemical composition is comparable to the official drug.

Uses
Topical treatment of mild inflammations of the oral and pharyngeal mucosa.

Contraindications
None known.

Side Effects
None known.

Interactions with Other Drugs
None known.

Dosage
Unless otherwise prescribed:
Myrrh tincture:
    Dab 2 - 3 times daily with undiluted tincture;

As a rinse or gargle:
    5 - 10 drops in a glass of water.
In dental powders:
    10 percent of powdered resin.

Mode of Administration
Powdered resin, myrrh tincture and other galenical preparations for topical use.

Action
Astringent

Niauli oil
Niauli aetheroleum
Niauliöl
Published August 29, 1992

Name of Drug
Niauli aetheroleum, niauli oil.

Composition of Drug
Niauli oil consists of the essential oil from the leaves of *Melaleuca viridiflora* Solander ex Gaertner [Fam. Myrtaceae], obtained by water distillation, as well as its preparations in effective dosage.

The drug contains 35 - 60 percent cineol.

Pharmacological Properties, Pharmacokinetics, Toxicology
In vitro antibacterial, stimulatory to circulation.

Clinical Data

1. Uses
Catarrhs of the upper respiratory tract.

2. Contraindications
Internal:
    Inflammatory diseases of the gastrointestinal tract and gall ducts, severe liver disease.
External:
    Preparations containing niauli oil should not be used in the facial areas, particularly the nose, of infants and toddlers.

3. Side Effects
In rare cases, nausea, vomiting, and diarrhea can occur with internal use.

4. Interactions with Other Drugs
Niauli oil contains 35 - 60 percent cineol. Cineol causes the induction of the enzymes involved in the detoxification of the liver. The effect of other drugs can, therefore, be reduced and/or shortened.

5. Dosage
Unless otherwise prescribed:
Internal:
    Single dose 0.2 g;
    Daily dosage 0.2 - 2 g;
Oily nose drops:
    2 - 5 percent in vegetable oil.

External:
    Preparations in oil 10 - 30 percent.

Mode of Administration
Drug and other galenical preparations for internal and external application.

Oak bark
Quercus cortex
Eichenrinde
Published February 1, 1990

Name of Drug
Quercus cortex, oak bark.

Composition of Drug
Oak bark consists of the dried bark of young branches and saplings of *Quercus robur* L. and/or *Q. petraea* (Mattuschka) Lieblein [Fam. Fagaceae], harvested in the spring, as well as their preparations in effective dosage.
    The drug contains tannins.

Uses
External:
    Inflammatory skin diseases.
Internal:
    Nonspecific, acute diarrhea, and local treatment of mild inflammation of the oral cavity and pharyngeal region, as well as genital and anal area.

Contraindications
Internal:
    None known.
External:
    Skin damage over a large area.
Baths:
    Full baths should not be taken, regardless of the active ingredients in the bath, under the following conditions: weeping eczema and skin damage covering a large area; febrile and infectious diseases; cardiac insufficiency stages III and IV (NYHA); hypertonia state IV (WHO).

Side Effects
None known.

Interactions with Other Drugs
External:
    None known.
Internal:
    The absorption of alkaloids and other alkaline drugs may be reduced or inhibited.

Dosage
Unless otherwise prescribed:
Internal:
    Daily dosage:
        3 g of drug;
        equivalent preparations.
For rinses, compresses and gargles:
    20 g drug per 1 liter of water;
    equivalent preparations.
For full and partial baths:
    5 g drug per 1 liter of water;
    equivalent preparations.

Mode of Administration
Comminuted herb for decoctions and other galenical preparations for internal and topical use.

Duration of Administration
If diarrhea persists longer than 3 - 4 days, a physician must be consulted.
Other areas of application:
    Not more than 2 - 3 weeks.

Actions
Astringent
Virustatic

Oat straw
Avenae stramentum
Haferstroh
Published October 15, 1987

Name of Drug
Avenae stramentum, oat straw.

Composition of Drug
Oat straw consists of the dried, threshed leaf and stem of *Avena sativa* L. [Fam. Poaceae], as well as its preparations in effective dosage.
    The drug contains silicic acid.

Uses
External application:
    Inflammatory and seborrheic skin disease, especially those with itching.

Contraindications
None known.

Side Effects
None known.

Interactions with Other Drugs
None known.

Dosage
Unless otherwise prescribed:
    100 g of herb for one full bath; equivalent preparations.

Mode of Administration
Comminuted herb for decoctions and other galenical preparations as bath additives.

Onion
Allii cepae bulbus
Zwiebel
Published March 13, 1986

Name of Drug
Allii cepae bulbus, onion.

Composition of Drug
Onion consists of the fresh or dried, thick and fleshy leaf sheaths and stipules of *Allium cepa* L. [Fam. Alliaceae], as well as their preparations in effective dosage.

It contains alliin and similar sulfur compounds, essential oil, peptides and flavonoids.

Uses
Loss of appetite, prevention of atherosclerosis.

Contraindications
None known.

Side Effects
None known.

Interactions with Other Drugs
None known.

Dosage
Unless otherwise prescribed:
   Average daily dosage:
      50 g of fresh onions or 20 g of dried drug;
      equivalent preparations.

Mode of Administration
Cut onions, pressed juice from fresh onions and other oral galenical preparations.

Duration of Administration
Note: If onion preparations are used over several months, the daily maximum amount for diphenylamine is 0.035 g.

Actions
Antibacterial
Lipid and blood pressure-lowering
Inhibition of thrombocyte aggregation

Orange peel
Citri sinensis pericarpium
Orangenschalen
Published February 1, 1990

Name of Drug
Citri sinensis pericarpium, orange peel.

Composition of Drug
Orange peel consists of the fresh or dried outer peel of ripe fruits of *Citrus sinensis* (L.) Osbeck [Fam. Rutaceae], separated from the white pulp layer, as well as its preparations in effective dosage.
   The drug contains essential oil and bitter principles.

Uses
Loss of appetite.

Contraindications
None known.

Side Effects
None known.

Interactions with Other Drugs
None known.

Dosage
Unless otherwise prescribed:
Daily dosage:
   10 - 15 g of herb;
   Preparations with equivalent
     bitter value.

Mode of Administration
Comminuted herb for teas and other bitter-tasting galenical preparations for oral application.

Paprika (Cayenne)
Capsici fructus, capsici fructus acer
Paprika
Published February 1, 1990

Name of Drug
Capsici fructus, paprika.
Capsici fructus acer, cayenne pepper.

Composition of Drug
Paprika consists of the dried fruits of various capsaicin-rich *Capsicum* species [Fam. Solanaceae], as well as its preparations in effective dosage.

Cayenne pepper consists of the dried, ripe, usually removed from the calyx, fruits of *Capsicum frutescens* L., as well as its preparations in effective dosage.

The drugs contain capsaicinoids.

Uses
Painful muscle spasms in areas of shoulder, arm and spine of adults and school-age children.

Contraindications
Application on injured skin, allergies to paprika preparations.

Side Effects
In rare cases hypersensitivity reaction can occur (urticaria).

Interactions with Other Drugs
None known.
Note: No additional heat application.

Dosage
Unless otherwise prescribed:
In semi-liquid preparations containing 0.02 - 0.05 percent capsaicinoids,
in liquid preparations containing 0.005 - 0.01 percent capsaicinoids,
in poultices containing 10 - 40 µg capsaicinoids per cm^2.

Mode of Administration
Preparations of paprika exclusively for external uses.

Duration of Administration
Not longer than 2 days; 14 days must pass before a new application can be used in the same location.

Longer use on the same area may cause damage to sensitive nerves.
Warning: Paprika preparations irritate the mucous membranes even in very low concentrations and cause a painful burning sensation. Contact of paprika preparations with mucous membranes, especially the eyes, must be avoided.

Actions
Local hyperemic
Local nerve-damaging

Parsley herb and root

Petroselini herba/radix
Petersilienkraut/wurzel
Published March 2, 1989

Name of Drug
Petroselini herba, parsley
Petroselini radix, parsley root

Composition of Drug
Parsley, consisting of the fresh or dried plant section of *Petroselinum crispum* (Miller) Nyman ex A. W. Hill [Fam. Apiaceae] and pharmaceutical preparations thereof.

Parsley root, consisting of the dried root of *P. crispum* (Miller) Nyman ex A. W. Hill and pharmaceutical preparations thereof.

Uses
Used in flushing out the efferent urinary tract in disorders of the same and in prevention and treatment of kidney gravel.

Contraindications
Pregnancy; inflammatory kidney conditions.

Precautions
Irrigation therapy (flushing out treatment) should not be carried out in the case of edema caused by impaired heart or kidney function.

Side Effects
Occasional allergic skin or mucous membrane reactions have been reported.

Interactions with Other Drugs
None known.

Dosage
Unless otherwise prescribed:
Daily dose:
    6 g of the prepared drug.

Mode of Administration
The crushed drug for infusions as well as other galenical preparations with a comparably small proportion of essential oil to be taken orally.
Warning: The essential oil should not be used in isolation because of its toxicity.

Irrigation Therapy
Large amounts of fluids must be taken.

Passionflower herb

Passiflorae herba
Passionsblumenkraut
Published November 30, 1985; Revised March 13, 1990

Name of Drug
Passiflorae herba, passionflower herb.

Composition of Drug
Passionflower herb consists of fresh or dried, above-ground parts of *Passiflora*

incarnata L. [Fam. Passifloraceae], as well as their preparations in effective dosage.

The drug contains flavonoids (vitexin), maltol, coumarin derivatives, and small amounts of essential oil.

The content of harman alkaloids varies; it must not exceed 0.01 percent.

Uses
Nervous restlessness.

Contraindications
None known.

Side Effects
None known.

Interactions with Other Drugs
None known.

Dosage
Daily dosage:
4 - 8 g of herb;
equivalent preparations.

Mode of Administration
Comminuted herb for tea and other preparations for internal use.

Action
A motility-inhibiting effect has been observed in animal experiments.

Peppermint leaf
Menthae piperitae folium
Pfefferminzblätter
Published November 30, 1985;
Revised March 13, 1990, and September 1, 1990

Name of Drug
Menthae piperitae folium, peppermint leaf.

Composition of Drug
Peppermint leaves consist of the fresh or dried leaf of *Mentha* x *piperita* L. [Fam. Lamiaceae], as well as its preparations in effective dosage.

The herb contains at least 1.2 percent (v/w) essential oil. Other ingredients are tannins characteristic of *Lamiaceae*.

Uses
Spastic complaints of the gastrointestinal tract as well as gallbladder and bile ducts.

Contraindications
In case of gallstones, use only after consultation with a physician.

Side Effects
None known.

Interactions with Other Drugs
None known.

Dosage
Internal:
3 - 6 g of leaf;
5 - 15 g of tincture
(according to *Erg. B. 6*);
equivalent preparations.

Mode of Administration
Cut herb for infusions, extracts of peppermint leaves for internal use.

Actions
Direct antispasmodic action on the

smooth muscle of the digestive tract
Choleretic
Carminative

Note: There is a separate monograph for peppermint oil.

Peppermint oil
Menthae piperitae aetheroleum
Pfefferminzöl
Published March 13, 1986; Revised March 13, 1990,
September 1, 1990, and July 14, 1993

Name of Drug
Menthae piperitae aetheroleum, peppermint oil.

Composition of Drug
Peppermint oil consists of the essential oil of *Mentha* x *piperita* L. [Fam. Lamiaceae], obtained by steam distillation from freshly harvested, flowering sprigs, and its preparations in effective dosage.

Peppermint oil contains a minimum of 4.5 percent and a maximum of 10 percent (w/w) esters, calculated as menthyl acetate, at least 44 percent (w/w) free alcohols, calculated as menthol and a minimum of 15 percent and maximum of 32 percent (w/w) ketones, calculated as menthone.

Uses
Internal:
   Spastic discomfort of the upper gastrointestinal tract and bile ducts, irritable colon, catarrhs of the respiratory tract, inflammation of the oral mucosa.
External:
   Myalgia and neuralgia.

Contraindications
Obstruction of bile ducts, gallbladder inflammation, severe liver damage. In case of gallstones, to be used only after consultation with a physician.

Preparations containing peppermint oil should not be used on the face, particularly the nose, of infants and small children.

Side Effects
None known.

Interactions with Other Drugs
None known.

Dosage
Unless otherwise prescribed:
Internal:
Average daily dosage:
   6 - 12 drops.
For inhalation:
   3 - 4 drops in hot water.
For irritable colon:
   Average single dose 0.2 ml;
   Average daily dose 0.6 ml in enterically coated form.
External:
   Some drops rubbed in the affected skin areas.
   In semi-solid and oily preparations 5 - 20 percent;
   In aqueous-ethanol preparations 5 - 10 percent;
   In nasal ointments 1 - 5 percent essential oil.

Mode of Administration
Essential oil and galenical preparations for internal and external application.

Actions
Antispasmodic
Carminative
Cholagogue
Antibacterial
Secretolytic
Cooling

Peruvian Balsam
Balsamum peruvianum
Perubalsam
Published September 18, 1986

Name of Drug
Balsamum peruvianum, Peruvian balsam, Balsam Peru.

Composition of Drug
Peruvian balsam consists of the balsam generated from scorched tree stems of *Myroxylon balsamum* (L.) Harms var. *pereira* (Royle) Harms [Fam. Fabaceae], as well as its preparations in effective dosage.

Peruvian balsam contains 50 - 70 percent of an ester mixture composed mainly of benzyl esters of benzoic and cinnamic acid.

Uses
External:
for infected and poorly healing wounds, for burns, decubitus ulcers, frost bite, ulcus cruris, bruises caused by prostheses, hemorrhoids.

Contraindications
Distinct allergic dispositions.

Side Effects
Allergic skin reactions.

Interactions with Other Drugs
None known.

Dosage
Unless otherwise prescribed:
Galenical preparations containing 5 - 20 percent Peruvian balsam, for extensive surface application not more than 10 percent Peruvian balsam.

Mode of Administration
Galenical preparations for external use.

Duration of Administration
Not longer than one week.

Actions
Antibacterial/antiseptic
Promotion of granulation process
Antiparasitic (especially for scabies)

Petasites root
Petasitidis rhizoma
Pestwurzelstock
Published July 27, 1990

Name of Drug
Petasitidis rhizoma, petasites root.

Composition of Drug
Petasites root consists of the dried underground parts of *Petasites hybridus* (L.) Ph. Gartn., B. Mey. et Scherb. [Fam. Asteraceae], as well as its preparations in effective dosage.

The drug contains sesquiterpenes such as petasin.

Petasites root also contains pyrrolizidine alkaloids with 1,2-unsaturated necine structure and their N-oxides.

Uses
Supportive therapy for acute spastic pain in the urinary tract, particularly if stones exist.

Contraindications
Pregnancy, nursing.

Side Effects
None known.

Interactions with Other Drugs
None known.

Dosage
Unless otherwise prescribed:
Daily dosage:
Preparations equivalent to 4.5 - 7 g drug.
The daily dose must not exceed 1 µg (mcg) of pyrrolizidine alkaloids with 1,2-necine structure, including their N-oxides.

Mode of Administration
Extracts obtained with ethanol or lipophilic solvents and other galenical preparations for internal use.

Duration of Administration
Not longer than 4 - 6 weeks per year.

Action
Antispasmodic

Pheasant's Eye herb
Adonidis herba
Adoniskraut
Published May 5, 1988; Revised February 1, 1990

Name of Drug
Adonidis herba, pheasant's eye herb, adonis.

Composition of Drug
Pheasant's eye herb consists of the dried above-ground parts of *Adonis vernalis* L. [Fam. Ranunculaceae], gathered during the flowering season, as well as its prepara-

tions in effective dosage. The herb contains cardioactive glycosides and flavonoids.

Uses
Mild impairment of heart function, especially when accompanied by nervous symptoms.

Contraindications
Therapy with digitalis glycosides, potassium deficiency.

Side Effects
None known.
Note: If overdosed: nausea, vomiting, rhythmic heart disorder.

Interactions with Other Drugs
Enhancement of effectiveness, and thus also of side effects, with simultaneous administration of quinidine, calcium, saluretics, laxatives, and extended therapy with glucocorticoids.

Dosage
Unless otherwise prescribed:
Average daily dosage:
   0.6 g of standardized adonis powder (DAB 9).
Maximum single dosage:
   1 g.
Maximum daily dosage:
   3 g.

Mode of Administration
Comminuted herb and preparations thereof for internal use.

Actions
Positively inotropic
Animal experiments showed a tonic effect on the veins.

Pimpinella root
Pimpinellae radix
Bibernellwurzel
Published June 1, 1990

Name of Drug
Pimpinellae radix, pimpinella root.

Composition of Drug
Pimpinella root consists of the dried rhizomes and roots of *Pimpinella saxifraga* L. s.l. and/or *P. major* (L.) Hudson s.l. [Fam. Apiaceae], as well as its preparations in effective dosage.
   The drug contains essential oil and saponins.

Uses
Catarrhs of the upper respiratory tract.

Contraindications
None known.

Side Effects
None known.

Interactions with Other Drugs
None known.

Dosage
Unless otherwise prescribed:
Daily dosage:
   6 - 12 g drug;
   6 - 12 g pimpinel tincture (1:5);
   equivalent preparations.

Mode of Administration
Comminuted herb for teas and other galenical preparations for internal use.

Pine Needle oil
Pini aetheroleum
Kiefernnadelöl
Published August 21, 1985; Revised March 13, 1990

Name of Drug
Pini aetheroleum, pine needle oil.

Composition of Drug
The essential oil obtained from fresh needles, tips of the boughs or fresh boughs with needles and tips of *Pinus sylvestris* L., *P. mugo* ssp. *pumilio* (Haenke) Franco, *P. nigra* Arnold or *P. pinaster* Soland [Fam. Pinaceae], as well as their preparations in effective dosage.

Uses
External and internal:
    For catarrhal diseases of the upper and lower respiratory tract.
External:
    for rheumatic and neuralgic ailments.

Contraindications
Bronchial asthma, whooping cough.

Side Effects
Intensified irritation may occur on skin and mucous membranes. Bronchospasms may be reinforced.

Interactions with Other Drugs
None known.

Dosage
For inhalation:
    Several drops into hot water, the vapors to be inhaled.
External application:
    Several drops to be rubbed onto the affected area, in liquid and semi-solid preparations in concentrations of 10 - 50 percent.

Mode of Administration
Ointment in the forms of alcoholic solutions, ointments, gels, emulsions, and oils. As inhalant.

Actions
Secretolytic
Hyperemic
Weakly antiseptic

Pine Sprouts
Pini turiones
Kiefernsprossen
Published September 18, 1986; Revised March 13, 1990

Name of Drug
Pini turiones, pine sprouts.

Composition of Drug
Pine sprouts consist of the fresh or dried, 3 - 5 cm long sprouts, collected in spring, of *Pinus sylvestris* L. [Fam. Pinaceae], as well as their preparations in effective dosage.
    Pine sprouts contain essential oil, resin.

Uses
Internal:
    catarrhal conditions of the upper and lower respiratory tract.
External:
    mild muscular pain and neuralgia.

Contraindications
None known.

Side Effects
None known.

Interactions with Other Drugs
None known.

Dosage
Unless otherwise prescribed:
Average daily dosage:
    2 - 3 g of drug;
    equivalent preparations.
Embrocation:
    Liquid or semi-solid preparations of extracts of pine sprouts corresponding to 20 - 50 percent.

Mode of Administration
Internal:
    comminuted herb for teas, syrup and tinctures.
External:
    alcoholic solutions, as oils or ointments.

Actions
Secretolytic
Mildly antiseptic
Stimulating peripheral circulation

Plantain
Plantaginis lanceolatae herba
Spitzwegerichkraut
Published November 30, 1985

Name of Drug
Plantaginis lanceolatae herba, plantain herb.

Composition of Drug
Plantain herb consists of the fresh or dried above-ground parts of *Plantago lanceolata* L. [Fam. Plantaginaceae], harvested at flowering season, as well as their preparations in effective dosage.
    Plantain contains mucilage, iridoid glycosides such as aucubin and catapol, and tannin.

Uses
Internal:
    Catarrhs of the respiratory tract, inflammatory alterations of the oral and pharyngeal mucosa.
External:
    Inflammatory reactions of the skin.

Contraindications
None known.

Side Effects
None known.

Interactions with Other Drugs
None known.

Dosage
Unless otherwise prescribed:
Average daily dosage:
    3 - 6 g of herb;
    equivalent preparations.

Mode of Administration
Comminuted herb and other galenical preparations for internal and external use.

Actions
Astringent
Antibacterial

Pollen
Pollen
Pollen
Published January 17, 1991

Name of Drug
Pollen, pollen.

Composition of Drug
Raw pollen of various flowering plants, as well as its preparations in effective dosage.

Uses
As a roborant for feebleness and loss of appetite.

Contraindications
Pollen allergy.

Side Effects
Rare: Discomforts of the gastrointestinal tract.

Interactions with Other Drugs
None known.

Dosage
Unless otherwise prescribed:
Daily dosage:
    30 - 40 g of drug;
    equivalent preparations.
Micronized pollen (<10 g):
    3 - 4 g;
    equivalent preparations.

Mode of Administration
Pollen and other forms of application for internal use.

Action
Appetite stimulating

Poplar bud
Populi gemma
Pappelknospen
Published February 1, 1990

Name of Drug
Populi gemma, poplar buds (balm of Gilead buds).

Composition of Drug
Poplar buds consist of the dried, unopened leaf buds of *Populus* species

[Fam. Salicaceae], as well as their preparations in effective dosage.

The herb contains essential oil, flavonoids, and phenol glycosides.

Uses
Superficial skin injuries, external hemorrhoids, frostbite and sunburn.

Contraindications
Sensitivity to poplar buds, propolis, Peruvian balsam or salicylate.

Side Effects
Occasional allergic skin reactions.

Interactions with Other Drugs
None known.

Dosage
Unless otherwise prescribed:
    Semi-solid preparations equivalent to 20 - 30 percent of drug.

Mode of Administration
Semi-solid preparations for application on the skin.

Actions
Antibacterial
Stimulates wound healing

Potentilla
Potentillae anserinae herba
Gänsefingerkraut
Published November 30, 1985; Revised March 13, 1990

Name of Drug
Potentillae anserinae herba, potentilla, silverweed.

Composition of Drug
Potentilla herb consists of the fresh or dried leaf and flowers of *Potentilla anserina* L. [Fam. Rosaceae], harvested shortly before or during flowering, as well as its preparations in effective dosage.

The herb contains at least 2 percent tannins when precipitated with casein, calculated as gallic acid ($C_7H_6O_5$, MW 170.1) and related to the dried herb. Other ingredients are tormentoside, phytosterols, flavonoids and anthocyanins.

Uses
Mild dysmenorrheal disorders, support for treatment of milder, nonspecific, acute diarrhea, light inflammation of the oral and pharyngeal mucosa.

Contraindications
None known.

Side Effects
Gastric irritations could be aggravated.

Interactions with Other Drugs
None known.

Dosage
Daily dosage:
    4 - 6 g of herb;
    equivalent preparations.

Mode of Administration
Cut herb for infusions and decoctions.
    Powdered herb and other galenical preparations for oral use.

Actions
Astringent, depending on tannin concentration.

Distinct increase in tonus and contraction frequency on the isolated uterus of various animals.

Primrose flower
Primulae flos
Schlüsselblumenblüten
Published July 6, 1988; Revised March 13, 1990

Name of Drug
Primulae flos, primrose flower. [This herb is not evening primrose, *Oenothera biennis*.]

Composition of Drug
Primrose flower consists of the dried, whole flowers with calyx of *Primula veris* L. and/or *P. elatior* (L.) Hill [Fam. Primulaceae], as well as its preparations in effective dosage.

The calyces contain saponins.

Uses
Catarrhs of the respiratory tract.

Contraindications
Known allergies to primrose.

Side Effects
Gastric discomforts and nausea can occasionally occur.

Interactions with Other Drugs
None known.

Dosage
Daily dosage:
   2 - 4 g of drug;
   2.5 - 7.5 g of tincture
     (according to *Erg. B. 6*);
   equivalent preparations.

Mode of Administration
Comminuted herb for teas and other galenical preparations for internal use.

Actions
Secretolytic
Expectorant

Primrose root
Primulae radix
Primelwurzel
Published July 6, 1988; Revised March 13, 1990

Name of Drug
Primulae radix, primrose root, cowslip root. [This herb is not evening primrose, *Oenothera biennis*.]

Composition of Drug
Primrose root consists of the dried rhizome with roots of *Primula veris* L. and/or *P. elatior* (L.) Hill [Fam. Primulaceae], as well as its preparations in effective dosage.

The drug contains saponins.

Uses
Catarrhs of the respiratory tract.

Contraindications
None known.

Side Effects
Stomach upsets and nausea can occasionally occur.

Interactions with Other Drugs
None known.

Dosage
Daily dosage:
 0.5 - 1.5 g of drug;
 1.5 - 3 g of tincture (according to the *Austrian Pharmacopoeia* 9);
 equivalent preparations.

Mode of Administration
Comminuted drug for teas and cold macerations, as well as other galenical preparations for internal use.

Actions
Secretolytic
Expectorant

Psyllium seed, Black
Psyllii semen
Flohsamen
Published November 30, 1985; Revised March 13, 1990

Name of Drug
Psyllii semen, black psyllium seed.

Composition of Drug
Black psyllium seed consists of the dried, ripe seed of *Plantago psyllium* L. (syn. *P. afra* L.) and of *P. indica* L. (syn. *P. arenaria* Waldstein et Kitaibel) [Fam. Plantaginaceae], with a swell index of at least 10, and its formulations in effective dosage.
 The drug contains mucilages.

Uses
Chronic constipation, irritable bowel.

Contraindications
Stenosis of the esophagus or the gastrointestinal tract.

Side Effects
In rare cases allergic reactions, especially with powdered drug and liquid preparations.

Interactions with Other Drugs
None known.

Dosage
Daily dosage:
 10 - 30 g drug;
 equivalent preparations.

Mode of Administration
Whole or ground seeds, other galenical preparations for oral application.
Note: Separate monographs have been issued for blonde psyllium seed and psyllium husk.

Action
Regulation of intestinal peristalsis

Psyllium seed, Blonde

Plantaginis ovatae semen
Indische Flohsamen
Published February 1, 1990; Revised April 19, 1991

Name of Drug
Plantaginis ovatae semen, psyllium seed, blonde psyllium seed.

Composition of Drug
Psyllium, consisting of the ripe seeds of *Plantago ovata* Forsskaol (syn. *P. isphagula* Roxburgh) [Fam. Plantaginaceae] and pharmaceutical preparations thereof.

The drug contains bulking agents.

Uses
Chronic constipation; disorders in which easy bowel movements with a loose stool are desirable, e.g., in patients with anal fissures, hemorrhoids, following anal/rectal surgery; during pregnancy; as a secondary medication in the treatment of various kinds of diarrhea and in the treatment of irritable bowel.

Contraindications
Stenosis of the gastrointestinal tract. Obstruction or threatening obstruction of the bowel (ileus). Difficulties in regulating diabetes mellitus.

Side Effects
In rare cases allergic reactions may occur.

Interactions with Other Drugs
The intestinal absorption of other medication taken simultaneously may be delayed.

Warning: There may need to be a reduction in the insulin dosage in diabetics who are insulin-dependent.

Dosage
Unless otherwise prescribed:
Daily dose:
  12 - 40 g of the drug;
  equivalent preparations.

Mode of Administration
The whole seeds as well as other galenical preparations to be taken orally.
Note: Sufficient fluids must be taken with the drug, e.g., 150 ml water to 5 g drug. The dose should be taken a half hour to one hour after taking other medication.

Duration of Administration
Warning: If diarrhea lasts for more than 3 - 4 days, a physician must be consulted.

Actions
Diarrhea:
  An increase of the passage time of the bowel content through bonding of water.
Constipation:
  A decrease of the passage time of the bowel content through increase in the volume of the stool.
  A lowering of the serum-cholesterol level.

Psyllium seed husk, Blonde
Plantaginis ovatae testa
Indische Flohsamenschalen
Published February 1, 1990; Revised April 19, 1991

Name of Drug
Plantaginis ovatae testa, psyllium seed husk, blonde psyllium seed husk.

Composition of Drug
Psyllium, consisting of the epidermis with bordering collapsed layers of *Plantago ovata* Forsskaol (syn. *P. isphagula* Roxburgh) [Fam. Plantaginaceae] and pharmaceutical preparations thereof.

The drug contains bulking agents.

Uses
Chronic constipation; disorders whereby easy bowel movements with a loose stool are desirable, e.g., in patients with anal fissures, hemorrhoids, following anal/rectal surgery; during pregnancy; as a secondary medication in the treatment of various kinds of diarrhea and in the treatment of irritable bowel.

Contraindications
Stenosis of the gastrointestinal tract. Obstruction or threatening obstruction of the bowel (ileus). Poorly controllable diabetes mellitus.

Side Effects
In rare cases allergic reactions may occur.

Interactions with Other Drugs
The intestinal absorption of other medication taken simultaneously may be delayed.

Warning: There may need to be a reduction in the insulin dosage in diabetics who are insulin-dependent.

Dosage
Unless otherwise prescribed:
Daily dose:
    4 - 20 g of the drug prepared accordingly.

Mode of Administration
The whole drug as well as other galenical preparations to be taken orally.
Note: Sufficient fluids must be taken with the drug, e.g., 150 ml water to 5 g drug. The dose should be taken a half hour to one hour after taking other medication.

Duration of Use
Warning: If diarrhea lasts for more than 3 - 4 days, a physician must be consulted.

Actions
Diarrhea:
    An increase of the passage time of the bowel content through bonding of water.
Constipation:
    A decrease of the passage time of the bowel content through increase of the volume of the stool.
A lowering of the serum-cholesterol level.
A reduction of the postprandial blood sugar increase.

Pumpkin seed
Cucurbitae peponis semen
Kürbissamen
Published November 30, 1985; Revised January 17, 1991

Name of Drug
Cucurbitae peponis semen, pumpkin seed.

Composition of Drug
Pumpkin seed consists of the ripe, dried seed of *Cucurbita pepo* L. and cultivated varieties of *C. pepo* L. [Fam. Cucurbitaceae], as well as its preparations in effective dosage.

The seed contain cucurbitin, phytosterol in free and bound forms, ß- and γ-tocopherol, and minerals, including selenium.

Uses
Irritated bladder condition, micturition problems of benign prostatic hyperplasia stages 1 and 2.

Contraindications
None known.

Side Effects
None known.

Interactions with Other Drugs
None known.

Dosage
Unless otherwise prescribed:
Average daily dosage:
   10 g of seed;
   equivalent preparations.

Mode of Administration
Whole and coarsely ground seed and other galenical preparations for internal uses.

Action
Due to the lack of suitable models, there are no pharmacological studies that substantiate the empirically found clinical activity.
Note: This medication relieves only the symptoms associated with an enlarged prostate without reducing the enlargement. Please consult a physician at regular intervals.

Radish
Raphani sativi radix
Rettich
Published September 24, 1986

Name of Drug
Raphani sativi radix, radish.

Composition of Drug
Radish consists of the fresh roots of *Raphanus sativus* L. var. *niger* (Miller) S. Kerner and/or of *R. sativus* L. ssp. *niger* (Miller) de Candolle var. *albus* de Candolle [Fam. Brassicaceae], as well as its preparations in effective dosage.

Radish contains mustard oil glycosides and essential oil.

Uses
Peptic disorders, especially those related to dyskinesia of the bile ducts, catarrhs of the upper respiratory tract.

Contraindications
Cholelithiasis.

Side Effects
None known.

Interactions with Other Drugs
None known.

Dosage
Unless otherwise prescribed:
Average daily dosage:
    50 - 100 ml pressed juice.

Mode of Administration
Pressed juice for oral use.

Actions
Secretagogue for the upper gastrointestinal tract
Motility promoting
Antimicrobial

Rhatany root
Ratanhiae radix
Ratanhiawurzel
Published March 2, 1989

Name of Drug
Ratanhiae radix, rhatany root.

Composition of Drug
Rhatany root consists of the dried root of *Krameria triandra* Ruíz et Pavón [Fam. Krameriaceae], as well as its preparations in effective dosage.
    The drug contains at least 10 percent tannins.

Uses
Topical treatment of mild inflammations of the oral and pharyngeal mucosa.

Contraindications
None known.

Side Effects
In very rare cases, allergic reactions of the mucous membranes may occur.

Interactions with Other Drugs
None known.

Dosage
Unless otherwise prescribed:
    About 1 g comminuted drug in 1 cup of water as a decoction or 5 - 10 drops of rhatany tincture in 1 glass of water, 2 - 3 times daily;
    Undiluted rhatany tincture painted on the affected surface 2 - 3 times daily; equivalent preparations.

Mode of Administration
Comminuted herb for decoctions and other galenical preparations for topical application.

Duration of Administration
Without medical advice, not longer than 2 weeks.

Action
Astringent

Rhubarb root

Rhei radix

Rhabarber

Published November 1, 1984; Revised December 5, 1984; Replaced July 21, 1993

Name of Drug
Rhei radix, rhubarb root.

Composition of Drug
Rhubarb consists of the dried underground parts of *Rheum palmatum* L., *R. officinale* Baillon or of both species [Fam. Polygonaceae], as well as their preparations in effective dosage. Stem parts, roots and most of the bark are removed from the rhizomes.

The bark contains anthranoids, mainly of the rhein and physcion type.

The drug must conform to currently valid pharmacopeia.

Pharmacological Properties, Pharmacokinetics, Toxicology
1,8-dihydroxy-anthracene derivatives have a laxative effect. This effect is primarily due to the influence of the herb on the motility of the colon, inhibiting stationary and stimulating propulsive contractions. This results in an accelerated intestinal passage and, because of the shortened contact time, a reduction in liquid absorption. In addition, stimulation of the active chloride secretion increases the water and electrolyte content of stool.

Systematic studies pertaining to the kinetics of rhubarb preparations are not available; however, it must be supposed that the aglycones contained in the drug are already absorbed in the upper small intestine. The ß-glycosides are prodrugs which are neither absorbed nor cleaved in the upper gastrointestinal tract. They are degraded in the colon by bacterial enzymes to anthrones. Anthrones are the laxative metabolites.

Active metabolites of other anthronoids, such as rhein, infiltrate in small amounts into the milk ducts. A laxative effect on nursing infants has not been observed. The placental permeability for rhein is very small.

Drug preparations [i.e., herbal stimulant laxative drugs] have a higher general toxicity than the pure glycosides, presumably due to the content of aglycones.

Experiments pertaining to the genotoxicity of rhubarb and its preparations are not available. Some positive data were obtained for aloe-emodin, emodin, physcion and chrysophanol. No data are available for carcinogenicity.

Clinical Data

1. Uses
Constipation.

2. Contraindications
Intestinal obstruction, acute intestinal inflammation, e.g., Crohn's disease, colitis ulcerosa, appendicitis, abdominal pain of unknown origin. Children under 12 years of age; pregnancy.

3. Side Effects
In single incidents, cramp-like discomforts of the gastrointestinal tract. These cases require a dosage reduction.
With chronic use or abuse:
Disturbances of electrolyte balance, especially potassium deficiency, albuminuria, and hematuria. Pigment implantation into the intestinal mucosa (pseudomelanosis coli) is harmless and usually reverses upon discontinuation of the drug. Potassium deficiency can lead to disorders of heart function and muscular weakness, especially with concurrent use of cardiac glycosides, diuretics, or corticoadrenal steroids.

4. Special Caution for Use
Stimulating laxatives must not be used over an extended period (1 - 2 weeks) without medical advice.

5. Use During Pregnancy and Lactation
Because of insufficient toxicological investigation, this drug should not be used during pregnancy and lactation.

6. Interactions with Other Drugs
With long-term use/abuse, due to loss in potassium, an increase in effectiveness of cardiac glycosides and an effect on antiarrhythmics is possible. Potassium deficiency can be increased by simultaneous application of thiazide diuretics, corticoadrenal steroids or licorice root.

7. Dosage and Administration
Cut bark, powder or dry extracts for teas, decoction, cold maceration or elixir.

Liquid or solid forms of medication exclusively for oral use.

Unless otherwise prescribed:
20 - 30 mg hydroxyanthracene derivatives/day, calculated as rhein.

The individually correct dosage is the smallest dosage necessary to maintain a soft stool.

Note: The form of administration should be smaller than the normal daily dosage. Rhubarb preparations rich in tannin and deficient in anthranoids can have a constipating effect.

8. Overdosage
Electrolyte and fluid imbalance.

9. Special Warnings
Use of a stimulating laxative for longer than the recommended short-term application can cause an increase in intestinal sluggishness.

The preparation should be used only if there are no results from a change of diet or usage of bulk-forming products.

10. Effects on Operators of Vehicles and Machinery
None known.

Rose flower
Rosae flos
Rosenblüten
Published September 1, 1990

Name of Drug
Rosae flos, rose flower.

Composition of Drug
Rose flower consists of the dried petal of *Rosa gallica* L., *R. centifolia* L. [Fam. Rosaceae], and their variations, collected prior to fully unfolding, as well as its preparations in effective dosage.

The herb contains tannins.

Uses
Mild inflammations of the oral and pharyngeal mucosa.

Contraindications
None known.

Side Effects
None known.

Interactions with Other Drugs
None known.

Dosage
Unless otherwise prescribed:
1 - 2 g of drug per cup (200 ml) of water for tea.

Mode of Administration
Comminuted herb for teas and other galenical preparations for mouth rinses.

Action
Astringent

Rosemary leaf
Rosmarini folium
Rosmarinblätter
Published November 30, 1985; Revised November 28, 1986, and March 13, 1990

Name of Drug
Rosmarini folium, rosemary leaf.

Composition of Drug
Rosemary leaf consists of the fresh or dried leaf, gathered while flowering, of *Rosmarinus officinalis* L. [Fam. Lamiaceae], as well as its preparations in effective dosage.

The drug contains at least 1.2 percent (v/w) essential oil, in reference to the dried leaves.

Uses
Internal:
Dyspeptic complaints.
External:
Supportive therapy for rheumatic diseases, circulatory problems.

Contraindications
None known.

Side Effects
None known.

Interactions with Other Drugs
None known.

Dosage
Internal:
Daily dosage:
4 - 6 g of herb;
10 - 20 drops of essential oil;*
equivalent preparations.
External:
50 g of herb for one full bath;
6 - 10 percent essential oil in semi-solid and liquid preparations;
equivalent preparations.

Mode of Administration
Cut drug for infusions, powder, dry extracts and other galenical preparations for internal and external use.

Actions
Experimental:
Antispasmodic on gall passages and small intestines;
Positive inotropic;
Increases flow through the coronary artery.
In humans:
Skin irritating;
Stimulates increased blood supply (external use).

*[**Ed. note:** The essential oil dosage appears excessive and possibly unsafe. A more reasonable dosage for internal use would be 2 drops (1 ml).]

Sage leaf
Salviae folium
Salbeiblätter
Published May 15, 1985; Revised March 13, 1990

Name of Drug
Salviae folium, sage leaf.

Composition of Drug
Sage leaf consists of the fresh or dried leaf of *Salvia officinalis* L. [Fam. Lamiaceae], and preparations thereof in effective dosage. The leaves contain at least 1.5 percent (v/w) thujone-rich essential oil, based on the dried herb.

Principal components of the essential oil, in addition to thujone, are cineol and camphor. In addition, the leaves contain tannins, diterpene bitter principles, triterpenes, steroids, flavones, and flavonoid glycosides.

Uses
External:
 Inflammations of the mucous membranes of nose and throat.
Internal:
 Dyspeptic symptoms, excessive perspiration.

Contraindications
The pure essential oil and alcoholic extracts should not be used internally during pregnancy.

Side Effects
After prolonged ingestion of alcohol extracts or of the pure essential oil, epileptiform convulsions can occur.

Interactions with Other Drugs
None known.

Dosage
Unless otherwise prescribed:
Internal:
Daily dosage:
 4 - 6 g of herb;
 0.1 - 0.3 g of essential oil;
 2.5 - 7.5 g of tincture (according to *Erg. B. 6*);
 1.5 - 3 g fluidextract (according to *Erg. B. 6*).
For gargles and rinses:
 2.5 g of herb or 2 - 3 drops of essential oil in 100 ml of water as infusion or 5 g of alcoholic extract in 1 glass water.
External:
 Undiluted alcohol extract.

Mode of Administration
Cut herb for infusions, alcoholic extracts and distillates for gargles, rinses and other topical applications, as well as for internal use. Also pressed juice of fresh plants.

Actions
Antibacterial
Fungistatic
Virustatic
Astringent
Secretion-promoting
Perspiration-inhibiting

Sandalwood, White
Santali lignum albi
Weisses Sandelholz
Published March 2, 1989

Name of Drug
Santali lignum albi, white sandalwood.

Composition of Drug
White sandalwood consists of the core wood of the trunk of the tree after removal of bark and of the branches of *Santalum album* L. [Fam. Santalaceae], as well as its preparations in effective dosages.

The drug contains essential oil.

Uses
For adjuvant therapy of infections of the lower urinary tract.

Contraindications
Diseases of the parenchyma of the kidney.

Side Effects
Nausea, sometimes itching of the skin.

Interaction with Other Drugs
None known.

Dosage
Daily dosage:
  1 - 1.5 g essential oil;
  10 - 20 g drug;
  equivalent preparations.

Mode of Administration
Comminuted drug for decoctions as well as other galenical preparations for oral intake.
Note: Isolated oil of sandalwood should be used in an enteric coated form.

Duration of Administration
Not more than 6 weeks without consultation of a physician.

Actions
Antibacterial
Spasmolytic

Sandy Everlasting
Helichrysi flos
Ruhrkrautblüten
Published July 6, 1988; Revised September 1, 1990

Name of Drug
Helichrysi flos, sandy everlasting, immortelle.

Composition of Drug
Immortelle consists of the dried flowers of *Helichrysum arenarium* (L.) Moench [Fam. Asteraceae], gathered shortly before fully unfolding, as well as their preparations in effective dosage.

The drug contains flavonoids.

Uses
Peptic discomforts.

Contraindications
Obstruction of bile ducts.
   In case of gallstones, to be used only after consultation with a physician.

Side Effects
None known.

Interactions with Other Drugs
None known.

Dosage
Unless otherwise prescribed:
Average daily dosage:
   3 g of drug;
   equivalent preparations.

Mode of Administration
Comminuted herb for teas and other galenical preparations for internal use.

Action
Mildly choleretic

Sanicle herb
Saniculae herba
Sanikelkraut
Published September 24, 1986; Revised March 13, 1990

Name of Drug
Saniculae herba, sanicle herb, wood sanicle.

Composition of Drug
Sanicle herb consists of the dried, above-ground parts of *Sanicula europaea* L. [Fam. Apiaceae], as well as their preparations in effective dosage.
   The herb contains saponins.

Uses
Mild catarrhs of the respiratory tract.

Contraindications
None known.

Side Effects
None known.

Interactions with Other Drugs
None known.

Dosage
Daily dosage:
   4 - 6 g of drug;
   equivalent preparations.

Mode of Administration
Comminuted drug for decoctions as well as other galenical preparations for internal use.

Saw Palmetto berry
Sabal fructus
Sabal früchte
Published March 2, 1989; Revised February 1, 1990, and January 17, 1991

Name of Drug
Sabal fructus, saw palmetto berry.

Composition of Drug
Saw palmetto berry consists of the ripe, dried fruit of *Serenoa repens* (Bartram) Small (syn. *Sabal serrulata* (Michaux) Nuttall ex Schultes) [Fam. Arecaceae], as well as its preparations in effective dosage.

The drug contains fatty oil with phytosterols and polysaccharides.

Uses
Urination problems in benign prostatic hyperplasia stages I and II.*

Contraindications
None known.

Side Effects
In rare cases, stomach problems.

Interactions with Other Drugs
None known.

Dosage
Daily dosage:
1 - 2 g saw palmetto berry or 320 mg lipophilic ingredients extracted with lipophilic solvents (hexane or ethanol 90 percent v/v);
equivalent preparations.

Mode of Administration
Comminuted herb and other galenical preparations for oral use.

Actions
Antiandrogenic
Anti-exudative
Note: This medication relieves only the symptoms associated with an enlarged prostate without reducing the enlargement. Please consult a physician at regular intervals.

*[**Ed. note:** Stage I is characterized by increase in frequency of urination, pollakiuria (abnormally frequent urination), nocturea (urination at night), delayed onset of urination, and weak urinary stream. Stage II is characterized by the beginning of the decompensation of the bladder function accompanied by formation of residual urine and urge to urinate.]

Scopolia root
Scopoliae rhizoma
Glockenbilsenkrautwurzelstock
Published September 24, 1986

Name of Drug
Scopoliae rhizoma, scopolia root.

Composition of Drug
Scopolia root consists of the dried rhizome of *Scopolia carniolica* Jacquin [Fam. Solanaceae], as well as its preparations in effective dosage.

The drug contains 0.3 - 0.8 percent alkaloids, less than 0.4 percent L-hyoscyamine and a trace of scopolamine.

Uses
Spasms of the gastrointestinal tract, bile ducts, and urinary tract for adults and for children over the age of 6.

Contraindications
Narrow-angle glaucoma, prostate adenoma with residual urine, tachycardia, stenosis of the gastrointestinal tract, megacolon.

Side Effects
Dryness of mouth, reduction in perspiration, reddening of skin, disturbance of ocular accommodation, hyperthermia, tachycardia, difficulties in urination. Attacks of glaucoma can occur.

Interactions with Other Drugs
Increased effectiveness of simultaneously administered tricyclic antidepressants, amantadine, and quinidine.

Dosage
Unless otherwise prescribed:
Average daily dosage:
    Equivalent to 0.25 mg total alkaloids, calculated as hyoscyamine.
Maximum single dosage:
    Equivalent to 1 mg total alkaloids, calculated as hyoscyamine.
Maximum daily dosage:
    Equivalent to 3 mg total alkaloids, calculated as hyoscyamine.

Mode of Administration
Comminuted root, powder, and other galenical preparations for oral application.

Action
Scopolia root acts as a parasympatholytic/anticholinergic via competitive antagonism of the neuromuscular transmitter acetylcholine. This antagonism affects more the muscarine-like effect of acetylcholine, less the nicotine-like effects at the ganglions and the neuromuscular end-plate. Scopolia root displays peripheral effects targeted on the vegetative nervous system and the smooth muscles, as well as central nervous effects. Because of its parasympatholytic properties, scopolia root causes relaxation of the smooth muscle organs and elimination of spastic conditions, especially of the gastrointestinal tract and the bile ducts. Conditions of muscular tremors and muscular rigidity, caused by central nervous impulses, disappear. The action on the heart is positively chronotropic and positively dromotropic.

Scotch Broom herb
Cytisi scoparii herba
Besenginsterkraut
Published January 17, 1991

Name of Drug
Cytisi scoparii herba, Scotch broom herb.

Composition of Drug
Scotch broom herb consists of the above-ground parts of *Cytisus scoparius* (L.) Link, as well as preparations thereof in effective dosage.

The drug contains alkaloids, primarily sparteine. Preparations contain not more than 1 mg/ml of sparteine.

Uses
Functional heart and circulatory disorders.

Contraindications
None known.

Side Effects
None known.

Interaction with Other Drugs
Due to the tyramine content, application of the drug can cause a blood pressure crisis by simultaneous administration of MAO-inhibitors.

Dosage
Unless otherwise prescribed:
Daily dosage:
    aqueous-ethanolic extracts equivalent to 1 - 1.5 g of drug.

Mode of Administration
Aqueous-ethanolic extracts for internal use.

Senega Snakeroot
Polygalae radix
Senegawurzel
Published March 13, 1986; Revised March 13, 1990

Name of Drug
Polygalae radix, senega snakeroot.

Composition of Drug
Senega snakeroot consists of the dried root with remains of aerial stems of *Polygala senega* L. and/or other closely related species or a mixture of *Polygala* species [Fam. Polygalaceae], as well as its preparations in effective dosage.

The roots contain saponins.

Uses
Catarrhs of the respiratory tract.

Contraindications
None known.

Side Effects
With prolonged use, gastrointestinal irritation.

Interactions with Other Drugs
None known.

Dosage
Daily dosage:
- 1.5 - 3 g root;
- 1.5 - 3 g fluidextract
  (following *Erg. B. 6*);
- 2.5 - 7.5 g tincture
  (following *Erg. B. 6*);
- equivalent preparations.

Mode of Administration
Comminuted root for decoctions and other galenical preparations for internal use.

Actions
Secretolytic
Expectorant

Senna leaf
Sennae folium
Sennesblätter
Published July 21, 1993

Name of Drug
Sennae folium, senna leaf.

Composition of Drug
Senna leaf consists of the dried leaflets (pinnulae) of *Cassia senna* L. (*C. acutifolia* Del.) [Fam. Fabaceae], known as Alexandrian or Khartoum senna, or of *C. angustifolia* Vahl [Fam. Fabaceae], known as Tinnevelly senna, as well as their preparations in effective dosage.
[**Ed. note:** Currently accepted nomenclature for all three cultivars is *Senna alexandrina* Miller.]

The leaves contain anthranoids, mainly of the bi-anthrone type. The content of anthranoids of the emodin and aloe-emodin type is usually higher in senna fruit.

The drug must conform to the currently valid pharmacopeia.

Pharmacological Properties, Pharmacokinetics, Toxicology
1,8-dihydroxy-anthracene derivatives have a laxative effect. This effect is due to the sennosides, specifically, their active metabolite in the colon, rheinanthrone. The effect is primarily caused by the influence on the motility of the colon by inhibiting stationary and stimulating propulsive contractions. This results in an accelerated intestinal passage and, because of the shortened contact time, a reduction in liquid absorbed through the lumen. In addition, stimulation of active chloride secretion increases water and electrolyte content of the contents of the intestine.

Systematic studies pertaining to the kinetics of senna leaf preparations are not available. However, it must be supposed that the aglycones contained in the drug are absorbed in the upper small intestine. The ß-glycosides are prodrugs that are neither absorbed nor cleaved in the upper gastrointestinal tract. They are degraded in the colon by bacterial enzymes to rheinanthrone. Rheinanthrone is the laxative metabolite. The systemic availability of rheinanthrone is very low. Animal experiments reveal that less than 5 percent is passed in the urine in the oxidized form and/or in conjugated form as rhein and sennodine. The major amount of rheinanthrone (more than 90 percent) is bound to the feces in the colon and excreted as a polymer.

Active metabolites, such as rhein, infiltrate in small amounts into the milk ducts. A laxative effect on nursing infants has not been observed. The placental permeability for rhein is very small, as was observed in animal experiments.

Drug preparations have a higher general toxicity than the pure glycosides, presumably due to the content of aglycones. Experiments with senna leaf preparations are not available. A senna extract showed mutagenic toxicity in vitro. The pure substance, sennoside A, B, showed no mutagenic toxicity in vitro. An in vivo study with a defined extract of senna fruit revealed no mutagenicity. Preparations with an anthranoid content of 1.4 - 3.5 percent (calculated as the sum of specific individual compounds) were used. These were potentially equivalent to 0.9 - 2.9 percent rhein, 0.05 - 0.15 percent aloe-emodin and 0.001 - 0.006 percent emodin. The results appear to be also applicable for specific senna leaf preparations. Some positive results have been observed for aloe-emodin and emodin. A study for carcinogenicity was performed with an enriched sennoside fraction containing about 40.8 percent anthranoids, of which 35 percent were sennosides (calculated as the sum of the individually determined compounds), equivalent to about 25.2 percent of the calculated potential rhein, 2.3 percent potential aloe-emodin and 0.007 percent potential emodin. The tested substance contained 142 ppm free aloe-emodin and 9 ppm free emodin. The study was conducted over 104 weeks, rats received up to 25 mg/kg body weight and showed no substance-dependent increase of tumors.

Clinical Data

1. Uses
Constipation.

2. Contraindications
Intestinal obstruction, acute intestinal inflammation, e.g., Crohn's disease, colitis ulcerosa, appendicitis, abdominal pain of unknown origin. Children under 12 years of age.

3. Side Effects
In single incidents, cramp-like discomforts of the gastrointestinal tract. These cases require a dosage reduction.
With chronic use or abuse:
> Disturbance of electrolyte balance, especially potassium deficiency, albuminuria and hematuria. Pigment implantation into the intestinal mucosa (*pseudomelanosis coli*) is harmless and usually reverses on discontinuation of the drug. Potassium deficiency can lead to disorders of heart function and muscular weakness, especially with concurrent use of cardiac glycosides, diuretics, or corticosteroids.

4. Special Caution for Use
Stimulating laxatives must not be used over a long period (more than 1 - 2 weeks) without medical advice.

5. Use During Pregnancy and Lactation
Due to insufficient toxicological investigation, this herb should not be used during pregnancy or lactation.

6. Interaction with Other Drugs
In cases of chronic use or abuse, loss of potassium may potentiate cardiac glycosides and have an effect on anti-arrhythmic medications.

Potassium deficiency may be exacerbated by simultaneous administration of thiazide diuretics, corticoadrenal steroids, or licorice root.

7. Dosage
Comminuted herb, powder or dried extracts for teas, decoctions, cold macerates, or elixirs. Liquid or solid forms of medication exclusively for oral use.
Unless otherwise prescribed:
> 20 - 30 mg hydroxyanthracene derivatives daily, calculated as sennoside B.

The individually correct dosage is the smallest dose necessary to maintain a soft stool.
Note: The form of administration should be smaller than the daily dose.

8. Overdosage
Electrolyte and fluid imbalance.

9. Special Warnings
Use of a stimulating laxative for longer than the recommended period can cause intestinal sluggishness.

This preparation should be used only if no effects can be obtained through changes in diet or the use of bulk-forming products.

10. Effects on Operators of Vehicles or Machinery
None known.

Senna pod
Sennae fructus
Sennesfrüchte
Published July 21, 1993

Name of Drug
Sennae fructus acutifoliae, Alexandrian senna pod.
Sennae fructus angustifoliae, Tinnevelly senna pod.

Composition of Drug
Alexandrian senna pod consists of the dried fruits of *Cassia senna* L. (*C. acutifolia* Del. [syn. *Senna alexandrina*]) [Fam. Fabaceae], as well as their preparations in effective dosage.

Tinnevelly senna pod consists of dried fruits of *C. angustifolia* Vahl [Fam. Fabaceae], as well as its preparations in effective dosage. [**Ed. note:** Currently accepted nomenclature for both cultivars is *Senna alexandrina* Miller.]

Sufficient pharmacological-toxicologic studies are available for preparations containing 1.4 - 3.5 percent anthranoids (calculated as sum of individually determined compounds), equivalent to 0.9 - 2.3 percent potential rhein, 0.05 - 0.15 percent potential aloe-emodin and 0.001 - 0.006 percent potential emodin.

The drug must conform to the currently valid pharmacopeia.

Pharmacological Properties, Pharmacokinetics, Toxicology
1,8-dihydroxy-anthracene derivatives have a laxative effect. This effect is due to the sennosides, i.e., their active metabolite in the colon, rheinanthrone. The effect is primarily caused by the influence on the motility of the colon by inhibiting stationary and stimulating propulsive contractions. This results in an accelerated intestinal passage and, because of the shortened contact time, a reduction in liquid absorbed through the lumen. In addition, stimulation of the active chloride secretion increases the water and electrolyte content of the stool.

Systematic studies pertaining to the kinetics of senna fruit preparations are not available. However, it must be supposed that the aglycones contained in the drug are already absorbed in the upper small intestine. The ß-glycosides are pro-drugs that are neither absorbed nor cleaved in the upper gastrointestinal tract. They are degraded in the colon by bacterial enzymes to rheinanthrone. Rheinanthrone is the laxative metabolite. The systemic availability of rheinanthrone is very low. Animal experiments revealed that less than 5 percent is passed in the urine in the oxidized form and/or in conjugated form as rhein and sennodine. The major amount of rheinanthrone (more than 90 percent) is bound to the feces in the colon and excreted as polymers.

Active metabolites, such as rhein, infiltrate in small amounts into the milk ducts. A laxative effect on nursing infants has not been observed. The placental permeability for rhein is very small, as was observed in animals.

Drug preparations have a higher general toxicity than the pure glycosides, presumably due to the content of aglycones. Experiments with senna leaf preparations are not available. A senna extract showed mutagenic toxicity in vitro; the pure substance, sennoside A, B, was negative. An in vivo study with a defined extract of senna fruit revealed no mutagenicity. Preparations with an anthranoid content of 1.4 - 3.5 percent were used (calculated as the sum of specific individual compounds) that were potentially equivalent to 0.9 - 2.9 percent rhein, 0.05 - 0.15 percent aloe-emodin and 0.001 - 0.006 percent emodin. The results appear to be also applicable for specific senna leaf preparations. Some positive results have been observed for aloe-emodin and emodin. A study for carcinogenicity was performed with an enriched sennoside fraction containing about 40.8 percent anthranoids, of which 35 percent were sennosides (calculated as sum of the individually determined compounds), equivalent to about 25.2 percent of the calculated potential rhein, 2.3 percent potential aloe-emodin and 0.007 percent potential emodin. The tested substance contained 142 ppm free aloe-emodin and 9 ppm free emodin. The study was conducted over 104 weeks. Rats received up to 25 mg/kg body weight and showed no substance-dependent increase of tumors.

Clinical Data

1. Uses
Constipation.

2. Contraindications
Intestinal obstruction, acute intestinal inflammation, e.g., Crohn's disease, colitis ulcerosa, appendicitis, abdominal pain of unknown origin. Children under 12 years of age.

3. Side Effects
In single incidents, cramp-like discomforts of the gastrointestinal tract. These cases require a dosage reduction.
With chronic use or abuse:
> Disturbance of electrolyte balance, especially potassium deficiency, albuminuria and hematuria. Pigment implantation into the intestinal mucosa (*pseudomelanosis coli*) is harmless and usually reverses on discontinuation of the drug. Potassium deficiency can lead to disorders of heart function and muscular weakness, especially with concurrent use of cardiac glycosides, diuretics, and corticosteroids.

4. Special Caution for Use
Stimulating laxatives must not be used over a long period (more than 1 - 2 weeks) without medical advice.

5. Use During Pregnancy and Lactation
During the first trimester of pregnancy, senna pod preparations should be used only if a therapeutic effect cannot be obtained with a change in diet or through

the use of swelling laxatives. Active metabolites, such as rhein, infiltrate into the milk ducts. A laxative effect on nursing infants has not been observed.

6. Interactions with Other Drugs
In cases of chronic use or abuse, loss of potassium may potentiate cardiac glycosides and have an effect on antiarrhythmic medications. Potassium deficiency may be exacerbated by simultaneous administration of thiazide diuretics, corticosteroids, or licorice root.

7. Dosage and Administration
Comminuted herb, powder or dried extracts for teas, decoctions, cold macerates, or elixirs. Liquid or solid forms of medication exclusively for oral use. Unless otherwise prescribed:
20 - 30 mg hydroxyanthracene derivatives daily, calculated as sennoside B.

The individually correct dosage is the smallest dose necessary to maintain a soft stool.
Note: The form of administration should be smaller than the daily dose.

8. Overdosage
Electrolyte and fluid imbalance.

9. Special Warnings
Use of a stimulating laxative for longer than the recommended period can cause intestinal sluggishness.

This preparation should be used only if no effects can be obtained through changes in diet or use of bulk-forming products.

10. Effects on Operators of Vehicles and Machinery
None known.

Shepherd's Purse
Bursae pastoris herba
Hirtentäschelkraut
Published September 18, 1986; Revised March 13, 1990

Name of Drug
Bursae pastoris herba, shepherd's purse herb.

Composition of Drug
Shepherd's purse herb consists of the fresh or dried, above-ground parts of *Capsella bursa pastoris* (L.) Medikus [Fam. Brassicaceae], as well as its preparations in effective dosage.

Uses
Internal:
Symptomatic treatment of mild menorrhagia and metrorrhagia, topical application for nose bleeds.

External:
Superficial, bleeding skin injuries.

Contraindications
None known.

Side Effects
None known.

Interactions with Other Drugs
None known.

Dosage
Unless otherwise prescribed:
Average daily dosage:
   10 - 15 g of drug;
   equivalent preparations.
Topical use:
   3 - 5 g of herb per ¾ cup of water as tea.
Fluidextract (according to *Erg. B. 6*):
   Daily dosage: 5 - 8 g.

Mode of Administration
Comminuted drug for tea and other galenical preparations for internal use and external application.

Actions
Parenteral application only:
Muscarine-like effects with dose-dependent lowering and elevation of blood pressure;
Positive inotropic and chronotropic cardiac effects;
Increased uterine contraction.

Soapwort root, Red
Saponariae rubrae radix
Rote Seifenwurzel
Published April 27, 1989

Name of Drug
Saponariae rubrae radix, red soapwort root.

Composition of Drug
Red soapwort root consists of the dried root, rhizome, and runner of *Saponaria officinalis* L. [Fam. Caryophyllaceae], as well as its preparations in effective dosage. The root contains saponins.

Uses
Catarrhs of the upper respiratory tract.

Contraindications
None known.

Side Effects
In rare cases, stomach irritation.

Interactions with Other Drugs
None known.

Dosage
Unless otherwise prescribed:
Daily dosage:
   1.5 g root or equivalent preparations.

Mode of Administration
Comminuted herb for teas and other galenical preparations for internal use.

Actions
Expectorant by irritation of the gastric mucosa
Cytotoxic, in high concentrations

Soapwort root, White
Gypsophilae radix
Weiße Seifenwurzel
Published June 1, 1990

Name of Drug
Gypsophilae radix, white soapwort root.

Composition of Drug
White soapwort root consists of the dried, underground parts of *Gypsophila* species, particularly *Gypsophila paniculata* L., [Fam. Caryophyllaceae], as well as preparations in effective dosage.

The drug contains saponins.

Uses
Catarrhs of the upper respiratory tract.

Contraindications
None known.

Side Effects
In rare cases irritation of the gastric mucosa.

Interactions with Other Drugs
None known.

Dosage
Unless otherwise prescribed:
Daily dosage:
   30 - 150 mg drug;
   3 - 15 mg gypsophila saponin;
   equivalent preparations.

Mode of Administration
Ground herb for teas, gypsophila saponin and other galenical preparations for internal use.

Actions
Irritates mucous membranes
In high dosage, cytotoxic

Soy Lecithin
Lecithinum ex soya
Sojalecithin
Published May 5, 1988

Name of Drug
Lecithinum ex soya, soy lecithin

Composition of Drug
Soy lecithin consists of the phospholipids extracted from the seeds of *Glycine max* (L.) Merrill [Fam. Fabaceae], as well as preparations thereof in effective dosage.

Soy lecithin contains (3-sn-phosphatidyl)choline, phosphatidyl ethanolamine and phosphatidyl-inositol.

Uses
Moderate disturbances of fat metabolism, especially hypercholesterolemia if dietary measures are not sufficient.

Contraindications
None known.

Interactions with Other Drugs
None known.

Dosage
Unless otherwise prescribed:
Average daily dosage:
Total phospholipids in their natural mixture composition corresponding to 3.5 g (3-sn-phosphatidyl)choline.

Mode of Administration
Preparations from soy beans for oral intake.

Action
Lipid-lowering.

Soy Phospholipid with 73 - 79% (3-sn phosphatidyl)-cholin

Phospholipide aus Sojabohnen mit 73 - 79% (3-sn Phosphatidyl)-cholin
Phosphalipide aus Sojahohnen
Published July 19, 1994

Composition of Drug
Lecithinum ex soja, lecithin from soybean, extracted from *Glycine max* (L.) Merrill [Fam. Fabaceae], enriched extract with 73 - 79 percent 3-sn-phosphatidylcholine. The extract also includes:
Phosphatidylethanolamine max. 7 percent,
Phosphatidylinositic acid <0.5 percent,
Oil 2 - 6 percent,
Vitamin E 0.2 - 0.5 percent.
The given range includes both production and analytical variances.

Pharmacological Properties, Pharmacokinetics, Toxicology
Lecithin extract from soybeans consists on the average of 76 percent phosphatidylcholine and almost entirely of phosphoglycerides, of which the fatty acid linoleic acid predominates. The quota of phospholipids, which are the chief constituents of cell membrane, are in major part obtained by eating (0.5 - 3 g/day from food) and in lesser degree from synthesis by the liver.

A deficiency in phospholipids is the inevitable result of chronic parenteric nutrition.

Under pharmacodynamic characteristics are "hepatoprotective" effects in numerous experimental models, e.g., protection against ethanol, alkyl alcohols, tetrachlorides, paracetamol and galactosamine. Furthermore, in chronic models (ethanol, thioacetamide, organic solvents), there appears a defense against steatosis and fibrosis of the liver. The compound works by speeding regeneration and stabilization of membranes, stopping lipid peroxidation and, it is assumed, by collagen synthesis.

The pharmacokinetics of orally administered lecithin have been examined in animal studies in which the phosphatidylcholine was radioactively marked, the marking on a fatty acid in position 1 or position 2, choline, or a phosphorous. The respective marker substitutions show the pharmacokinetics. Phospholipids are degraded to lyso-phosphatidylcholine in the intestine and absorbed primarily in this form. In the gut wall phospholipids are in part re-synthesized, then circulated through the lymphatic system. In part the resynthesized phosphatidylcholine is processed in the liver to form fatty acids, choline, and glycerine-3-phosphate. In plasma, phosphatidylcholine and other phosphoglycerides are tightly bound to lipoproteins and/or albumin.

Phosphatidylcholine and other phosphoglycerides are degraded chiefly through a series of so-called phospholipases to fatty acids, choline and "glycerin" metabolites to be in turn re-synthesized in the liver and other organs. The administered metabolites in large part may be integrated within a few hours into body phospholipids. Their removal corresponds to the excretion of phospholipids and their corresponding metabolites.

Toxicology

Doses of phosphatidylcholine of up to 10 g/kg body weight in mice and rats and 4.5 g/kg body weight in rabbits given intravenously, intraperitoneally, and orally in a single dose are not toxic. The "no-effect" dosage over 48 weeks administration to rats lies upward of 3750 mg/kg body weight per day. Repeated i.v. application over 12 weeks places the lowest systemic toxic dosage between 0.1 and 1 g/kg body weight and lowest local toxic dosage at over 1 g/kg body weight in rats, and application over 4 weeks to dogs places the lowest toxic dosage at more than 0.1 g/kg body weight in dogs.

Doses of up to 3750 mg/kg body weight in pregnant animals, animal embryos, and animal neonates showed no pathology of toxicity to reproduction. The lowest teratogenic or embryo-toxic dosage in rats in oral and intravenous administration was more than 1 g/kg body weight. In rabbits teratogenic dosages were greater than 1 g/kg body weight for oral administration and greater than 0.5 g/kg body weight in intravenous administration. Various in vitro tests cannot demonstrate any mutagenic potential. Carcinogenicity has not been tested.

Clinical Data

1. Uses

Less severe forms of hypercholesterolemia in which diet and other non-medical interventions (e.g., exercise program, weight control) have not shown results.

Improvement of subjective complaints, such as loss of appetite and feeling of pressure in region of liver in toxic/ nutritional liver disease and chronic hepatitis.

Prerequisite to the therapy of chronic liver disease is the recognition and avoidance of noxious agents — in the case of alcoholic liver disease, alcohol abstinence. In chronic hepatitis adjuvant therapy with phospholipids of soybeans is only indicated when improvement of symptoms is discernible from other therapy.

2. Contraindications
None known.

3. Side Effects
Occasional gastrointestinal effects, i.e., stomach pain, loose stool, and diarrhea.

4. Special Caution for Use
None.

5. Use During Pregnancy and Lactation
None.

6. Interactions with Other Drugs
None known.

7. Dosage and Mode of Administration
Unless otherwise prescribed:
Daily dosage:
    1.5 - 2.7 g phospholipids from soybean with 73 - 79 percent 3-sn-phosphatidylcholine in a single dose.

8. Overdosage
Not known.

9. Special Precautions
None.

10. Effects on Operators of Vehicles and Machinery
None.

Spiny Restharrow root
Ononidis radix
Hauhechelwurzel
Published April 23, 1987; Revised March 13, 1990

Name of Drug
Ononidis radix, spiny restharrow root

Composition of Drug
Spiny restharrow root consists of the dried roots and rhizomes of *Ononis spinosa* L. [Fam. Fabaceae], harvested in autumn, as well as their preparations in effective dosage.

The drug contains isoflavonoids, such as ononin, flavonoids and small amounts of essential oil.

Uses
Irrigation therapy for inflammatory diseases of the lower urinary tract. Also for prevention and treatment of kidney gravel.

Contraindications
None known.
Note: No irrigation therapy in case of edema due to impaired heart and kidney function.

Side Effects
None known.

Interactions with Other Drugs
None known.

Dosage
Unless otherwise prescribed:
Daily dosage:
6 - 12 g of drug;
equivalent preparations.

Mode of Administration
Comminuted herb for teas and other galenical preparations for internal use.
Warning: Observe ample fluid intake.

Action
Diuretic

Squill
Scillae bulbus
Meerzwiebel
Published August 21, 1985; Revised March 2, 1989

Name of Drug
Scillae bulbus, squill, sea onion.

Composition of Drug
Squill consists of the sliced, dried, fleshy middle scales of the onion of the white variety of *Urginea maritima* (L.) Baker [Fam. Liliaceae], harvested at flowering season, as well as their preparations in effective dosage.

Squill contains glycosides of the bufadienolide type. Main glycosides are scillaren A and proscillaridin A, flavonoids and anthocyanins.

Uses
Milder cases of heart insufficiency, also for diminished kidney capacity.

Contraindications
Therapy with digitalis glycosides, potassium deficiency.

Side Effects
Nausea, vomiting, stomach disorders, diarrhea, irregular pulse.

Interactions with Other Drugs
Increase of effectiveness and thus also of side effects by simultaneous administration of quinidine, calcium, saluretics, laxatives and extended therapy with glucocorticoids.

Dosage
Unless otherwise prescribed:
Average daily dosage:
 0.1 - 0.5 g of standardized sea onion; powder;
 equivalent preparations.

Mode of Administration
Comminuted drug and other galenical preparations for internal use.

Actions
Positively inotropic on myocardial work capacity
Negatively chronotropic
"Economizing" heart action
Lowering increased, left ventricular diastolic pressure and pathologically elevated venous pressure.

St. John's Wort
Hyperici herba
Johanniskraut
Published December 5, 1984; Revised March 13, 1990

Name of Drug
Hyperici herba, St. John's Wort.

Composition of Drug
St. John's Wort consists of the dried, above-ground parts of *Hypericum perforatum*

L. [Fam. Hypericaceae], gathered during flowering season, as well as their preparations in effective dosage.

Uses
Internal:
> Psychovegetative disturbances, depressive moods, anxiety and/or nervous unrest. Oily hypericum preparations for dyspeptic complaints.

External:
> Oily hypericum preparations for treatment and post-therapy of acute and contused injuries, myalgia and first-degree burns.

Contraindications
None known.

Side Effects
Photosensitization is possible, especially in fair-skinned individuals.

Interactions with Other Drugs
None known.

Dosage
Unless otherwise prescribed:
Average daily dosage for internal use:
> 2 - 4 g of drug or 0.2 - 1 mg of total hypericin in other forms of drug application.

Mode of Administration
Chopped herb, herb powder, liquid and solid preparations for internal use. Liquid and semi-solid preparations for external use. Preparations made with fatty oils for external and internal use.

Actions
A mild antidepressant action of the herb and its preparations has been observed and reported by numerous physicians. According to experimental observation, hypericin can be categorized among the MAO inhibitors. Oily hypericum preparations demonstrate an antiinflammatory action.
[**Ed. note:** The research suggesting MAO activity was experimental and not conducted in animal systems. Subsequent research has indicated either no or very slight MAO activity in St. John's Wort or its preparations.]

Star Anise seed
Anisi stellati fructus
Sternanis
Published July 6, 1988

Name of Drug
Anisi stellati fructus, star anise.

Composition of Drug
Star anise consists of the ripe syncarp of *Illicium verum* Hooker filius [Fam. Illiciaceae], as well as its preparations in effective dosage.
> The drug contains essential oil.

Uses
Catarrhs of the respiratory tract, peptic discomforts.

Contraindications
None known.

Side Effects
None known.

Interactions with Other Drugs
None known.

Dosage
Unless otherwise prescribed:
Average daily dosage:
    3 g of drug or 0.3 g essential oil;
    equivalent preparations.

Mode of Administration
Herb ground fresh just prior to use, and other galenical preparations for internal use.

Actions
Bronchial expectorant
Antispasmodic for gastrointestinal tract

Stinging Nettle herb and leaf
Urticae herba/-folium
Brennesselkraut/Brennesselblätter
Published April 23, 1987

Name of Drug
Urticae herba, stinging nettle herb.
Urticae folium, stinging nettle leaf.

Composition of Drug
Stinging nettle herb consists of fresh or dried above-ground parts of *Urtica dioica* L., *U. urens* L. [Fam. Urticaceae], and/or hybrids of these species, collected during flowering season, as well as their preparations in effective dosage.

Stinging nettle leaf consists of fresh or dried leaves of *U. dioica* L., *U. urens* L. and/or hybrids of these species, gathered during flowering season, as well as their preparations in effective dosage.

Stinging nettle leaf and herb contain mineral salts, mainly calcium and potassium salts, and silicic acid.

Uses
Internal and external application:
    As supportive therapy for rheumatic ailments.
Internal:
    As irrigation therapy for inflammatory diseases of the lower urinary tract and prevention and treatment of kidney gravel.

Contraindications
None known.
Note: No irrigation therapy if edema exists due to impaired heart or kidney function.

Side Effects
None known.

Interactions with Other Drugs
None known.

Dosage
Unless otherwise prescribed:
Average daily dosage:
    8 - 12 g of drug;
    equivalent preparations.

Mode of Administration
Comminuted herb for teas and other galenical preparations for internal use, as stinging nettle spirit for external application.
Note: In irrigation therapy, intake of copious amounts of fluids must be observed.

Stinging Nettle root
Urticae radix
Brennesselwurzel
Published September 18, 1986
Revised March 2, 1989, March 13, 1990, and January 17, 1991

Name of Drug
Urticae radix, nettle root, stinging nettle root.

Composition of Drug
Stinging nettle root consists of the underground parts of *Urtica dioica* L., *U. urens* L. and/or their hybrids [Fam. Urticaceae] as well as preparations from nettle root at an effective dose.

The drug contains ß-sitosterol in free forms and as glycosides, as well as scopoletin.

Uses
Difficulty in urination in benign prostatic hyperplasia stages 1 and 2.

Contraindications
None known.

Side Effects
Occasionally, mild gastrointestinal upsets.

Interactions with Other Drugs
None known.

Dosage
Unless otherwise prescribed:
Daily dose:
    4 - 6 g of drug;
    equivalent preparations.

Mode of Administration
Comminuted drug for infusions as well as other galenical preparations for oral use.

Actions
Increase of urinary volume
Increase of maximum urinary flow
Reduction of residual urine
Note: This drug only relieves the symptoms of an enlarged prostate without reducing the enlargement. Please consult a physician at regular intervals.

Sundew
Droserae herba
Sonnentaukraut
Published May 12, 1984

Name of Drug
Droserae herba, round-leafed sundew.

Composition of Drug
Sundew consist of the dried above- and below-ground parts of *Drosera rotundifolia* L., *D. ramentacea* Burch ex Harv. et Sound., *D. longifolia* L. p.p. and *D. interme-*

dia Hayne [Fam. Droseraceae], as well as their preparations in effective dosage.

The herb contains 0.14 - 0.22 percent naphthoquinone derivatives calculated as juglone in respect to the dry mass of the herb.

Uses
For coughing fits and dry cough.

Contraindications
None known.

Side Effects
None known.

Interactions with Other Drugs
None known.

Dosage
Unless otherwise prescribed:
Average daily dosage:
   3 g of herb.

Mode of Administration
Liquid and solid preparations for external and internal application.

Actions
Bronchoantispasmodic
Antitussive

Sweet Clover
Meliloti herba
Steinkleekraut
Published March 13, 1986; Revised March 13, 1990

Name of Drug
Meliloti herba, sweet clover, yellow melilot.

Composition of Drug
Sweet clover consists of the dried or fresh leaf and flowering branches of *Melilotus officinalis* (L.) Pallas and/or *M. altissimus* Thuillier [Fam. Fabaceae], as well as their preparations in effective dosage.

The herb contains 5,6-benzo-pyrone (coumarin).

Other ingredients are 3,4-dihydro-coumarin (melilotin), o-coumaric acid, the glycoside melilotoside and flavonoids.

Uses
Internal:
   Problems arising from chronic venous insufficiency, such as pain and heaviness in legs, night cramps in the legs, itching, and swelling. For the supportive treatment of thrombophlebitis, post-thrombotic syndromes, hemorrhoids, and lymphatic congestion.
External:
   Contusions and superficial effusions of blood.

Contraindications
None known.

Side Effects
In rare cases headaches.

Interactions with Other Drugs
None known.

Dosage
Unless otherwise prescribed:
Average daily dosage:
    Herb or preparation in amounts corresponding to 3 - 30 mg coumarin;
    Parenteral application corresponding to 1 - 7.5 mg coumarin.
The effective dosage for sweet clover preparations in fixed combinations must be documented for each specific preparation.

Mode of Administration
Comminuted herb for infusions and other galenical preparations for oral use.
    Liquid forms of medication for parenteral application.
    Ointments, liniments, cataplasms and herbal sachets for external use.
    Ointments and suppositories for rectal use.

Actions
Anti-edematous for inflammatory and congestive edema by increase of venous reflux and improvement of lymphatic kinetics.
    Animal experiments showed an increase in healing wounds.

Thyme
Thymi herba
Thymiankraut
Published December 5, 1984; Revised March 13, 1990, and December 2, 1992

Name of Drug
Thymi herba, thyme.

Composition of Drug
Thyme is constituted of the stripped and dried leaves and flowers of *Thymus vulgaris* L., *T. zygis* L. [Fam. Lamiaceae], or both species as well as their preparations in effective dosage.
    The herb contains at least 0.5 percent phenols, calculated as thymol ($C_{10}H_{14}O$, MW=150.2) based on the dried herb.

Uses
Symptoms of bronchitis and whooping cough.
    Catarrhs of the upper respiratory tracts.

Contraindications
None known.

Side Effects
None known.

Interactions with Other Drugs
None known.

Dosage
Unless otherwise prescribed:
    1 - 2 g of herb for 1 cup of tea, several times a day as needed;
    1 - 2 g fluidextract 1 - 3 times daily;
    5 percent infusion for compresses.

Mode of Administration
Cut herb, powder, liquid extract or dry extract for infusions and other galenical preparations. Liquid and solid medicinal forms for internal and external application.
Note: Combinations with other herbs that have expectorant action could be appropriate.

Actions
Bronchoantispasmodic
Expectorant
Antibacterial

Thyme, Wild
Serpylli herba
Quendelkraut
Published October 15, 1987; Revised March 13, 1990

Name of Drug
Serpylli herba, wild thyme.

Composition of Drug
Wild thyme consists of the dried, flowering, above-ground parts of *Thymus serpyllum* L. [Fam. Lamiaceae], as well as its preparations in effective dosage.

The drug contains essential oil, principally carvacrol and/or thymol.

Uses
Catarrhs of the upper respiratory tract.

Contraindications
None known.

Side Effects
None known.

Interactions with Other Drugs
None known.

Dosage
Unless otherwise prescribed:
Average daily dose:
  6 g of herb;
  equivalent preparations.

Mode of Administration
Cut herb for infusions and other preparations for internal use.

Action
Antimicrobial

[**Ed. note:** Commercially, *Thymus pulegioides* L. and *T. praecox* Opiz subsp. *arcticus* (Dur.) Jalas are also offered as and mixed with *T. serpyllum* L.]

Tolu Balsam
Balsamum tolutanum
Tolubalsam
Published September 18, 1986

Name of Drug
Balsamum tolutanum, tolu balsam, balsam tolu.

Composition of Drug
Tolu balsam consists of the balsam generated from the slit tree trunks of *Myroxylon*

balsamum (L.) var. *balsamum* Harms (syn. *M. balsamum* var. *genuinum*) (Baill.) (Harms) [Fam. Fabaceae] as well as its preparations in effective dosage. This balsam is purified by melting, straining, and solidifying.

Tolu balsam contains benzoic and cinnamic acids, as well as their esters and essential oils.

Uses
Catarrhs of the respiratory tract.

Contraindications
None known.

Side Effects
None known.

Interaction with Other Drugs
None known.

Dosage
Unless otherwise prescribed:
Average daily dosage:
   0.6 g of herb;
   equivalent preparations.

Mode of Administration
Preparations of tolu balsam for internal use.

Tormentil root
Tormentillae rhizoma
Tormentillwurzelstock
Published May 5, 1988; Revised March 13, 1990

Name of Drug
Tormentillae rhizoma, tormentil root

Composition of Drug
Tormentil root consists of the dried rhizome taken from the root of *Potentilla erecta* (L.) Raüschel (synonym: *P. tormentilla* Necker) [Fam. Rosaceae] and preparations thereof.

Uses
Unspecified diarrhea disorders; mild mucous membrane inflammations of the mouth and pharynx.

Contraindications
None known.

Side Effects
Stomach complaints in sensitive subjects.

Interaction with Other Drugs
None known.

Dosage
When not otherwise prescribed:
average daily dose:
   4 - 6 g of the drug;
   equivalent preparations.
Tormentil tincture:
   10 - 20 drops to one glass of water daily to rinse out the mouth and throat.

Mode of Administration
Crushed drug for boiling and infusing, as well as in other galenical preparations to be taken orally and applied locally.

Duration of Administration
Should the diarrhea last more than 3 - 4 days, a physician should be consulted.

Turmeric root
Curcumae longae rhizoma
Curcumawurzelstock
Published November 30, 1985; Revised September 1, 1990

Name of Drug
Curcumae longae rhizoma, turmeric root.

Composition of Drug
Turmeric root consists of the finger-like, often tuber-like, scalded and dried rhizomes of *Curcuma longa* L. (syn. *C. domestica* Valeton and *C. aromatica* Salisbury) [Fam. Zingiberaceae], and their preparations in effective dosage.

The drug contains not less than 3 percent dicinnamoylmethane derivatives, calculated as curcumin, and not less than 3 percent volatile oil, both calculated on a dry-weight basis of the drug.

Uses
Dyspeptic conditions.

Contraindications
Obstruction of bile passages. In case of gallstones, use only after consulting with a physician.

Side Effects
None known.

Interactions with Other Drugs
None known.

Dosage
Unless otherwise prescribed:
Average daily dosage:
   1.5 - 3 g of drug;
   equivalent preparations.

Mode of Administration
Comminuted drug, as well as other galenical preparations for internal use.

Actions
The choleretic action of curcumin is experimentally well documented. Further indications exist for a cholecystokinetic and a clear antiinflammatory action.

Turmeric root, Javanese
Curcumae xanthorrhizae rhizoma
Javanische Gelbwurz
Published July 6, 1988; Revised September 1, 1990

Name of Drug
Curcumae xanthorrhizae rhizoma, Javanese turmeric.

Composition of Drug
Javanese turmeric consists of the sliced, dried, tuberous rhizomes of *Curcuma xanth-*

orrhiza Roxburgh (syn. *Curcuma xanthorrhiza* D. Dietrich) [Fam. Zingiberaceae], as well as its preparations in effective dosage.

The rhizome contains essential oil and dicinnamoylmethane derivatives.

Uses
Peptic disorders.

Contraindications
Obstruction of bile ducts, gallstones. In case of gallstone, use only after consultation with a physician.

Side Effects
After prolonged use, stomach problems.

Interactions with Other Drugs
None known.

Dosage
Unless otherwise prescribed:
Average daily dosage:
2 g of rhizome;
equivalent preparations.

Mode of Administration
The crushed drug for infusions and other galenical forms for internal use.

Action
Choleretic

Turpentine oil, Purified
Terebinthinae aetheroleum rectificatum
Gereinigtes Terpentinöl
Published May 15, 1985; Revised March 13, 1990

Name of Drug
Terebinthinae aetheroleum rectificatum, purified turpentine oil.

Composition of Drug
Purified turpentine oil is the essential oil obtained from the turpentine of *Pinus* species, especially *P. palustris* Miller (syn. *P. australis* Michaux filius), and *P. pinaster* Aiton [Fam. Pinaceae].

Uses
External and internal:
  Chronic disease of the bronchii with heavy secretion.
External:
  Rheumatic and neuralgic ailments.

Contraindications
Sensitivity to essential oils.
Inhalation:
  Acute inflammation of the respiratory tract.

Side Effects
Topical application to extensive surface areas can cause symptoms of poisoning, e.g., damage to kidneys and the central nervous system.

Interactions with Other Drugs
None known.

Dosage
Unless otherwise prescribed:
For inhalation:
  several drops in hot water with the vapors to be inhaled.
For external application:
  several drops to be rubbed onto the affected area, in liquid and semi-solid preparations 10 - 50 percent.

Mode of Administration
Semi-solid preparations in the form of ointments, gels, emulsion, and oils, and as plaster and inhalant.

Actions
Hyperemic
Antiseptic
Reduces bronchial secretion

Usnea
Usnea species
Bartflechten
Published April 27, 1989

Name of Drug
Usnea species, usnea.

Composition of Drug
Usnea consists of the dried thallus of *Usnea* species, primarily of *U. barbata* (L.) Wiggers emend. Mot., *U. florida* (L.) Fries, *U. hirta* (L.) Hoffmann and *U. plicata* (L.) Fries [Fam. Usneaceae], as well as preparations of *Usnea* in effective dosage.

The herb contains lichenic acid.

Uses
Mild inflammations of the oral and pharyngeal mucosa.

Contraindications
None known.

Side Effects
None known.

Interactions with Other Drugs
None known.

Dosage
Unless otherwise prescribed:
Lozenges with preparations equivalent to 100 mg herb, 3 - 6 times daily, 1 lozenge.

Mode of Administration
Preparations of herb for lozenges and equivalent solid forms of medication.

Action
Antimicrobial

Uva Ursi leaf
Uvae ursi folium
Bärentraubenblätter
Published June 15, 1994

Name of Drug
Uvae ursi folium, uva ursi leaf, bearberry.

Composition of Drug
Uva ursi (bearberry) leaves, consisting of the dried leaves of *Arctostaphylos uva ursi* (L.) Sprengel [Fam. Ericaceae] and pharmaceutical preparations thereof.

Pharmacological Characteristics, Pharmacokinetics, Toxicology

Preparations made from bearberries act antibacterially in vitro against *Proteus vulgaris, E. coli, Ureaplasma urealyticum, Mycoplasma hominis, Staphylococcus aureus, Pseudomonas aerginosa,* Friedländer's pneumonia, *Enterococcus faecalis,* and *Streptococcus* strains, as well as against *Candida albicans.* The antimicrobial effect is associated with the aglycone hydroquinone released from arbutin (transport form) or arbutin waste products in the alkaline urine. A methanol extract of the drug (50 percent) is said to have an inhibiting effect on tyrosinase activity. The forming of melanin from DOPA using tyrosinase as well as from DOPA-CHROM through auto-oxidation is also said to be inhibited by the drug.

There are indications that after uva ursi tea (3 g/150 ml) has been taken, hydroquinone glucuronides occur predominately alongside low levels of hydroquinone.

Clinical Data

1. Uses
Inflammatory disorders of the efferent urinary tract.

2. Contraindications
Pregnancy, lactation, children under 12.

3. Side Effects
Nausea and vomiting may occur in persons with sensitive stomachs.

4. Special Caution for Use
None known.

5. Use During Pregnancy and Lactation
Should not be administered during pregnancy.

The occurrence of arbutin/hydroquinone in the breast milk has not been researched. The drug, therefore, should not be administered during lactation.

6. Interaction with Other Drugs
Uva ursi preparations should not be administered with any substances which cause acidic urine since this reduces the antibacterial effect.

7. Dosage and Mode of Administration
Unless otherwise prescribed:
Single dose:
    3 g drug to 150 ml water as an infusion or cold maceration or 100 - 210 mg hydroquinone derivatives, calculated as water-free arbutin.
Daily dose:
    3 g drug to 150 ml water as an infusion or cold maceration up to 4 times a day or 400 - 840 mg hydroquinone derivatives calculated as water-free arbutin.

Mode of Administration
Crushed drug.
    Drug powder for infusions or cold macerations; extracts and solid forms for oral administration.

Duration of Treatment
Medication containing arbutin should not be taken for longer than a week or more than five times a year without consulting a physician.

8. Overdosage
None known.

9. Special Precautions
None known.

10. Effects on Operators of Vehicles and Machinery
None known.

Uzara root
Uzarae radix
Uzarawurzel
Published September 1, 1990

Name of Drug
Uzarae radix, uzara root.

Composition of Drug
Uzara root consists of the dried, underground parts of 2 - 3 year-old plants of *Xysmalobium undulatum* (L.) R. Brown [Fam. Asclepiadaceae], as well as their preparations in effective dosage.

The drug contains glycosides with cardenolide structure.

Uses
Nonspecific, acute diarrhea.

Contraindications
Therapy with cardiac glycosides.

Side Effects
None known.

Interactions with Other Drugs
None known.

Dosage
Unless otherwise prescribed:
Adults:
    Initial single dosage:
      preparations equivalent to 1 g herb or 75 mg total glycosides.
    Daily dosage:
      equivalent to 45 - 90 mg of total glycosides, calculated as uzarin.

Mode of Administration
Ethanol-water extracts in liquid form, or as dry extracts obtained from methanol-water extractions for internal use.

Duration of Administration
If diarrhea persists for more than 3 - 4 days, consult a physician.

Actions
Inhibits intestinal motility
In high dosage, digitalis-like effects on the heart.

Valerian root
Valerianae radix
Baldrianwurzel
Published May 15, 1985; Revised March 13, 1990

Name of Drug
Valerianae radix, valerian root.

Composition of Drug
Valerian root, consisting of fresh underground plant parts, or parts carefully dried below 40°C, of the species *Valeriana officinalis* L. [Fam. Valerianaceae], and its preparations in effective dosage.

The roots contain essential oil with monoterpenes and sesquiterpenes (valerenic acids). Preparations of valerian used therapeutically (infusion, extract, fluidextract, tincture) no longer contain the thermolabile and chemically unstable valepotriates.

Uses
Restlessness, sleeping disorders based on nervous conditions.

Contraindications
None known.

Side Effects
None known.

Interactions with Other Drugs
None known.

Dosage
Unless otherwise prescribed:
Infusions:
   2 - 3 g of drug per cup,
   once to several times per day.
Tincture:
   ½ - 1 teaspoon (1 - 3 ml),
   once to several times per day.
Extracts:
   Amount equivalent to 2 - 3 g of drug,
   once to several times per day.
External Use:
   100 g for one full bath;
   equivalent preparations.

Mode of Administration
Internal:
   As expressed juice from fresh plants, tincture, extracts, and other galenical preparations.
External:
   As a bath additive.

Actions
Sedative
Sleep-promoting

Walnut leaf
Juglandis folium
Walnußblätter
Published June 1, 1990

Name of Drug
Juglandis folium, walnut leaf.

Composition of Drug
Walnut leaf consists of the dried leaf of *Juglans regia* L. [Fam. Juglandaceae], as well as its preparations in effective dosage.
   The drug contains tannins.

Uses
External:
   Mild, superficial inflammations of the skin; excessive perspiration, e.g., of the hands and feet.

Contraindications
None known.

Side Effects
None known.

Interactions with Other Drugs
None known.

Dosage
Unless otherwise prescribed:
For compresses and partial baths:
    2 - 3 g herb per 100 ml water;
    equivalent preparations.

Mode of Administration
Comminuted drug for decoctions and other galenical preparations for external use.

Action
Astringent

Watercress
Nasturtii herba
Brunnenkressekraut
Published February 1, 1990

Name of Drug
Nasturtii herba, watercress.

Composition of Drug
Watercress consists of the fresh or dried, above-ground parts of *Nasturtium officinale* R. Brown [Fam. Brassicaceae], as well as their preparations in effective dosage.

The herb contains mustard glycosides and mustard oil.

Uses
Catarrh of respiratory tract.

Contraindications
Gastric and intestinal ulcers, inflammatory kidney diseases.

No application for children under the age of four.

Side Effects
In rare cases, gastrointestinal complaints.

Interactions with Other Drugs
None known.

Dosage
Unless otherwise prescribed:
Daily dosage:
    4 - 6 g dried herb;
    20 - 30 g fresh herb;
    60 - 150 g freshly pressed juice;
    equivalent preparations.

Mode of Administration
Cut herb, freshly pressed juice, as well as other galenical preparations for internal use.

White Dead Nettle flower
Lamii albi flos
Weiße Taubnesselblüten
Published April 23, 1987

Name of Drug
Lamii albi flos, white dead nettle flower.

Composition of Drug
White dead nettle flower consists of the dried petal with attached stamens of

Lamium album L. [Fam. Lamiaceae], as well as its preparations in effective dosage.

The flowers contain tannin, mucilage and saponins.

Uses
Internally, for catarrh of the upper respiratory passages, topical treatment of mild inflammation of the mucous membranes of the mouth and throat, and for non-specific fluor albus (leukorrhea).

Externally, for mild, superficial inflammation of the skin.

Contraindications
None known.

Side Effects
None known.

Interactions with Other Drugs
None known.

Dosage
Unless otherwise prescribed:
Internal:
Average daily dosage:
   3 g of drug.
External:
   5 g of flowers for one sitz bath; equivalent preparations.

Mode of Administration
Flowers for teas and other galenical preparations for internal applications, rinses, baths and moist compresses.

White Mustard seed
Sinapis albae semen
Weiße Senfsamen
Published February 1, 1990

Name of Drug
Sinapis albae semen, white mustard seed.

Composition of Drug
White mustard seed consists of the ripe, dried seed of *Sinapis alba* L. [Fam. Brassicaceae], as well as its preparations in effective dosage.

White mustard seeds contain mustard oil glycosides and mustard oils.

Uses
External:
   Poultices for catarrhs of the respiratory tract, as well as for segment therapy of chronic degenerative diseases affecting the joints and soft tissues.

Contraindications
No applications for children under the age of six.

Note: Since mustard oils are absorbed by the skin, these preparations should not be used when kidney disorders exist.

Side Effects
Prolonged application may result in skin and nerve damage.

Interactions with Other Drugs
None known.

Dosage
Unless otherwise prescribed:
External:
   Just prior to application, mix 4 table-

spoons of powdered seeds with warm water for a poultice.

Mode of Administration
External: Ground or powdered seeds for poultices. The poultices are applied for 5 - 10 minutes to children, 10 - 15 minutes to adults.

For sensitive skin, the application time must be decreased on an individual basis.

Duration of Administration
Up to 2 weeks.

Actions
Irritating to the skin
Bacteriostatic

White Willow bark
Salicis cortex
Weidenrinde
Published May 12, 1984

Name of Drug
Salicis cortex, white willow bark.

Composition of Drug
White willow bark consists of the bark of the young, 2 - 3-year-old branches harvested during early spring of *Salix alba* L., *S. purpurea* L., *S. fragilis* L. and other comparable *Salix* species [Salicaceae], as well as their preparations in effective dosage. The bark contains at least 1 percent total salicin derivatives, calculated as salicin ($C_{13}H_{18}O_7$, MW 286.3) and related to the dried herb.

Uses
Diseases accompanied by fever, rheumatic ailments, headaches.

Contraindications
See **Interactions with Other Drugs**

Side Effects
See **Interactions with Other Drugs**

Interactions with Other Drugs
Because of white willow bark's active constituents, interactions like those encountered with salicylates may arise. However, in reviewing the scientific literature available so far, there are no definite indications for this.

Dosage
Unless otherwise prescribed:
Average daily dosage corresponding to 60 - 120 mg total salicin.

Mode of Administration
Liquid and solid preparations for internal use.
Note: Combinations with diaphoretic drugs could be considered.

Actions
Antipyretic
Antiphlogistic
Analgesic

Witch Hazel leaf and bark
Hamamelidis folium et cortex
Hamamelisblätter und-rinde
Published August 21, 1985; Revised March 13, 1990

Name of Drug
Hamamelidis folium, witch hazel leaf.
Hamamelidis cortex, witch hazel bark.

Composition of Drug
Witch hazel leaf consists of the dried leaf of *Hamamelis virginiana* L. [Fam. Hamamelidaceae], as well as its preparations in effective dosage.

The drug contains 3 - 8 percent tannin, mainly gallotannins. Other ingredients are flavonoids and essential oil.

Witch hazel bark consists of the dried bark of the trunk and branches of *H. virginiana* L., as well as its preparations in effective dosage.

The drug contains at least 4 percent tannins. Characteristic ingredients of witch hazel bark are ß-hamamelitannin and γ-hamamelitannin, the depside ellagitannin, catechin derivatives, and free gallic acid.

Fresh leaf and twigs of *H. virginiana* L., consists of leaves and twigs collected in spring and early summer for the production of water distillates.

Uses
Minor injuries of skin, local inflammation of skin and mucous membranes. Hemorrhoids. Varicose veins.

Contraindications
None known.

Side Effects
None known.

Interactions with Other Drugs
None known.

Dosage
Unless otherwise prescribed:
External:
  Water steam distillate (witch hazel water) undiluted or diluted 1:3 with water;
  For poultices, 20 - 30 percent in semi-solid preparations.
Extract preparations:
  Semi-solid and liquid preparations, corresponding to 5 - 10 percent drug.
Drug:
  Decoctions of 5 - 10 g of herb per cup (250 ml) of water for compresses and irrigations.
Internal use (mucous membranes):
Suppositories:
  1 - 3 times daily, the amount of a preparation corresponding to 0.1 - 1 g drug to be applied 1 - 3 times a day.
Other preparations:
  Several times daily, corresponding to 0.1 - 1 g drug in preparations, or witch hazel water undiluted or diluted with water.

Mode of Administration
Witch hazel leaves and bark:
  Cut drug or extracts for internal and external use.
Fresh leaves and bark of *Hamamelis*:
  Steam distillate for internal and external use.

Actions
Astringent
Antiinflammatory
Locally hemostatic

Woody Nightshade stem
Dulcamarae stipites
Bittersüßstengel
Published June 1, 1990

Name of Drug
Dulcamarae stipites, woody nightshade.

Composition of Drug
Woody nightshade consists of the dried, 2 - 3-year-old stems of *Solanum dulcamara* L. [Fam. Solanaceae], harvested in spring prior to leafing or late autumn after leaves have dropped, as well as its preparations in effective dosage.

The drug contains tannins, steroid alkaloids and steroid saponins.

Uses
As supportive therapy for chronic eczema.

Contraindications
None known.

Side Effects
None known.

Interactions with Other Drugs
None known.

Dosage
Unless otherwise prescribed:
Internal:
Daily dosage:
    1 - 3 g of drug;
    equivalent preparations.
External:
    Infusions or decoctions equivalent to 1 - 2 g of drug per 250 ml (1 cup) of water.

Mode of Administration
Comminuted herb for teas and other galenical preparations for internal use, and for compresses and rinses.

Actions
Astringent
Antimicrobial
Irritative to mucous membranes
Steroid alkaloid: Anticholinergic
Solasodin: Antiphlogistic

Wormwood
Absinthii herba
Wermutkraut
Published December 5, 1984

Name of Drug
Absinthii herba, wormwood.

Composition of Drug
Wormwood consists of the fresh or dried upper shoots and leaves, or the fresh or dried basal leaves, or a mixture of the above plant parts from *Artemisia absinthium* L. [Fam. Asteraceae], harvested during flowering season, as well as its preparations in effective dosage. The herb contains at least 0.3 percent (v/w) volatile oil and has

a bitter value of not less than 15,000. The volatile oil contains thujone. Additionally, the herb contains bitter principles of the sesquiterpene lactone type such as absinthin, anabsinthin, artabsin, anabsin, also flavones, ascorbic acid, and tannins.

Uses
Loss of appetite, dyspepsia, biliary dyskinesia.

Contraindications
None known.

Side Effects
None known.

Interactions with Other Drugs
None known.

Dosage
Unless otherwise prescribed:
Daily dosage:
 2 - 3 g of herb as water infusion.

Mode of Administration
Cut herb for infusions and decoctions, herb powder, also extracts and tinctures as liquid or solid forms of medication for oral administration.

Warning: Combinations with other bitters or aromatics may be advantageous. In toxic doses, thujone, the active component of the oil, acts as a convulsant poison. Therefore, the essential oil must not be used except in combinations.

Action
The effectiveness as an aromatic bitter is based on the bitter principles and volatile oil. Useful experimental pharmacological data of recent years are not available.

Yarrow
Millefolii herba/flos
Schafgarbe
Published February 1, 1990

Name of Drug
Millefolii herba, yarrow herb.
Millefolii flos, yarrow flower.

Composition of Drug
Yarrow herb consists of the fresh or dried, above-ground parts of *Achillea millefolium* L. [Fam. Asteraceae], harvested at flowering season, as well as its preparations in effective dosage.

Yarrow flower consists of the dried inflorescence of *A. millefolium* L. s.l. [Fam. Asteraceae], as well as its preparations in effective dosage.

The drug contains essential oil and proazulene.

Uses
Internal:
 Loss of appetite, dyspeptic ailments, such as mild, spastic discomforts of the gastrointestinal tract.
As sitz bath:
 Painful, cramp-like conditions of psychosomatic origin (in the lower part of the female pelvis).

Contraindications
Allergy to yarrow and other composites.

Side Effects
None known.

Interactions with Other Drugs
None known.

Dosage
Unless otherwise prescribed:
Daily dosage:
    4.5 g yarrow herb;
    3 tsp. pressed juice from fresh plants;
    3 g yarrow flowers;
      equivalent preparations.
For sitz baths:
    100 g yarrow per 20 l (5 gal.) of water.

Mode of Administration
Comminuted drug for teas and other galenical preparations for internal use and for sitz baths, pressed juice of fresh plants for internal use.

Actions
Choleretic
Antibacterial
Astringent
Antispasmodic

Yeast, Brewer's
Faex medicinalis
Medizinische Hefe
Published May 5, 1988

Name of Drug
Faex medicinalis, medicinal yeast.

Composition of Drug
Medicinal yeast consists of fresh or dried cells of *Saccharomyces cerevisiae* Meyer [Fam. Saccharomycetaceae] and/or of *Candida utilis* (Hennenberg) Rodden et Kreyer Van Rey [Fam. Cryptococcaceae], as well as their preparations in effective dosage.

    Medicinal yeast contains vitamins, particularly B complex, glucans and mannans.

Uses
Loss of appetite and as a supplement for chronic forms of acne and furunculosis.

Contraindications
None known.

Side Effects
Migraine-like headaches can occur in sensitive individuals. The intake of fermentable yeast may cause flatulence.

Interactions with Other Drugs
None known.

Note: Simultaneous intake of monoamine oxidase inhibitors can cause an increase in blood pressure.

Dosage
Unless other prescribed:
Average daily dosage:
    6 g;
    equivalent preparations.

Mode of Administration
Medicinal yeast and galenical preparations for internal use.

Actions
Antibacterial
Stimulation of phagocytosis

Yeast, Brewer's/Hansen CBS 5926

Saccharomyces cerevisiae Hansen CBS 5926
Trokenhefe aus Saccharomyces cerevisiae Hansen CBS 5926
Published April 15, 1994

Constituents of Drug

Brewer's yeast from *Saccharomyces cerevisiae* Hansen CBS 5926 (syn. *S. boulardii*) [Fam. Saccharomycetaceae] and genetically identical strains in lyophilized form. One gram of the lyophilisate contains 885 mg *S. cerevisiae* Hansen CBS 5926 corresponding to 1 times 10^{10} viable organisms.

Pharmacological Properties, Pharmacokinetetics, Toxicology

The effectiveness of brewer's yeast depends on the viability of the organism.

Brewer's yeast can bind fimbriated, pathogenic bacteria. In vitro, growth inhibition was demonstrated by co-culturing brewer's yeast with the following organisms: *Proteus mirabilis* and *vulgaris*, *Salmonella typhi* and *typhimurium*, *Pseudomonas aeruginosa*, *Staphyloccus aureus*, *Escherichia coli*, certain *Shigella* and *Candida albicans*. Concentration dependencies for growth inhibitions were not given. Brewer's yeast can also inhibit the growth of *Clostridium difficile*, as well as the diarrhea-causing effect of enterotoxic strains of *E. coli*. On the isolated intestinal loop model, sodium and water influx into the intestinal lumen was induced by incubation with the toxin from the cholera vibrio; this reaction was reduced by 40 percent in the presence of brewer's yeast. Intestinal preparations were also employed to show the reversal of the increased chloride transport induced by prostaglandins E2 and I2 in the presence of brewer's yeast as compared to untreated controls.

An increase in the activity of the disaccharidases saccharidase, lactase, and maltase, which are located in the intestinal membrane, was observed in animal experiments, as well as in humans. In animal experiments, the secretory immunoglobulin (sIgA) was increased in the gastrointestinal tract after oral intake of brewer's yeast.

With a single oral dosage of 3 g/kg body weight of brewer's yeast, no toxic reactions were observed in mice and rats. No substance-dependent changes were observed with a dosage of 330 mg/kg body weight over 6 weeks (6 days/week) given to dogs, and about 100 mg/kg body weight given daily over 6 months to rats and rabbits. The Ames test with *Salmonella typhimurium* TA 90, TA 100, TA 1335, TA 1337, and TA 1338 revealed no mutagenic effects, with or without activation of SY-mix. Experiments for embryocytic and carcinogenic effects are not available.

Clinical Data

1. Indications

For symptomatic treatment of acute diarrhea.

For prophylactic and symptomatic treatment of diarrhea during travel and diarrhea occurring while tube feeding. As an adjuvant for chronic forms of acne.

2. Contraindications

Not to be used in case of yeast allergies.
Warning: infants and small children are excluded from self-medication in any case.

3. Side Effects

Oral intake may cause flatulence.

In individual cases, intolerance (incompatibilities) may occur in the form of itching, urticaria, local or general exanthemas, and Quincke's edema.

4. Special Precaution for Usage

In case of diarrhea, replacement of fluids and electrolytes is an important therapeutic measure, especially for children. Diarrhea of infants and small children requires consultation with a physician.

Diarrheas lasting longer than 2 days, containing blood, or accompanied by fever, require medical attention.

If during therapy with brewer's yeast microbiological tests are performed on stool samples, the intake of yeast must be reported to the laboratory, since false positive results may be reported.

5. Usage During Pregnancy and Lactation

No data available.

6. Interaction with Other Drugs

The simultaneous intake of brewer's yeast and antimycotics can influence the activity of brewer's yeast.

Warning: Simultaneous intake of MAO-inhibitors may cause increased blood pressure.

7. Dosage and Mode of Administration

Unless otherwise prescribed:
Daily dosage (children older than 2 years/adults):
   For prevention of travel diarrhea, beginning 5 days prior to journey:
      250 - 500 mg daily.
   For therapy of diarrhea:
      250 - 500 mg daily.
   For diarrhea due to tube feeding:
      add 500 mg brewer's yeast/liter of nutrient solution.
   Suggestion: The treatment should be continued for several days after diarrhea has ceased.
   For acne:
      750 mg daily.

Mode of Administration

Lyophylisate in capsules for internal use as well as addition to tubal feed mixtures.

8. Overdosage

None known.

9. Special Warnings

None known.

10. Effects on Operators of Vehicles and Machinery

None known.

Chapter 3

Approved Component Characteristics

Cajeput oil
Cajeputi aetheroleum
Cajeputöl
Published July 14, 1993

Name of Drug
Cajeputi aetheroleum, cajeput oil.

Composition of Drug
Cajeput oil consists of the essential oil from the fresh leaf and branch tops of various species of *Melaleuca leucodendra* L. [Fam. Myrtaceae], obtained by water distillation, as well as preparations thereof in effective dosage.

Pharmacological Properties, Pharmacokinetics, Toxicology
In vitro antimicrobial, hyperemic.

Clinical Data

1. Combination Partner in the Following Herb Combinations
1. Cajeput oil, peppermint oil, clove oil, menthol, camphor.
2. Cajeput oil, peppermint oil, clove oil, eucalyptus oil.
3. Cajeput oil, sage oil, clove oil, eucalyptus oil.
4. Cajeput oil, clove oil, eucalyptus oil.
5. Cajeput oil, peppermint oil, eucalyptus oil.
6. Cajeput oil, rosemary oil, arnica tincture.
7. Cajeput oil, niauli oil (from *Melaleuca viridiflora*), peppermint oil, eucalyptus oil.
8. Cajeput oil, peppermint oil, eucalyptus oil.
9. Cajeput oil, eucalyptus oil.
10. Cajeput oil, dwarf pine oil, clove oil, juniper oil, peppermint oil, eucalyptus oil, wintergreen oil, menthol.
11. Cajeput oil, peppermint oil, eucalyptus oil, juniper oil, wintergreen oil.
12. Cajeput oil, peppermint oil, spearmint oil, eucalyptus oil, juniper oil, wintergreen oil, bergamot oil, star anise oil, cinnamon oil, pine needle oil.
13. Cajeput oil, peppermint oil, spearmint oil, eucalyptus oil, juniper oil, wintergreen oil, bergamot oil, star anise oil, cinnamon oil, pine needle oil.
14. Cajeput oil, St. John's Wort flower, dwarf pine oil, rosemary oil.
15. Cajeput oil, castor fiber, bitter tincture, cinchona bark, peppermint oil, caraway oil, valerian tincture, ethyl ether.
16. Cajeput oil, eucalyptus oil, menthol, clove oil, peppermint oil, juniper berry oil, cinnamon oil, lemon balm oil, wintergreen oil, star anise oil.
17. Cajeput oil, dwarf pine oil, rosemary oil, niauli oil, juniper berry oil, peppermint oil, eucalyptus oil.

18. Cajeput oil, camphor, menthol, rosemary oil, cayenne, methyl salicylate, benzyl nicotinate.
19. Cajeput oil, arnica herb, witch hazel leaf, niauli oil, peppermint oil, Peruvian balsam, eucalyptus oil, 2 homeopathic preparations.
20. Cajeput oil, spruce needle oil, rosemary oil, eucalyptus oil, purified turpentine.
21. Cajeput oil, thyme oil, dwarf pine oil, rosemary oil, Siberian fir oil, juniper berry oil, menthol, camphor, eucalyptus oil.
22. Cajeput oil, purified turpentine, camphor, 10 percent ammonia solution.
23. Cajeput oil, eucalyptus oil, Peruvian balsam, blackthorn fruits, 2 homeopathic preparations.
24. Cajeput oil, arbor vitae leaf oil, sassafras root oil, cognac oil, 1 homeopathic preparation.
25. Cajeput oil, arbor vitae leaf oil, sassafras root oil, concentrated Virginian juniper wood oil, sulfurated turpentine.
26. Cajeput oil, fennel oil, caraway oil, juniper berry oil, turpentine, laurel berry oil.
27. Cajeput oil, camphor, rosemary oil, spruce needle oil, turpentine, sage oil, methyl salicylate.
28. Cajeput oil, anise oil, lemon oil, eucalyptus oil, fennel oil, caraway oil, menthol, clove oil, peppermint oil, juniper berry oil, cinnamon oil, citronella oil, rosemary oil, dwarf pine oil, pine needle oil, thyme oil, wintergreen oil, garlic oil, bitter orange peel oil, sassafras root oil, dill oil, spearmint oil, convolvulus root oil.
29. Cajeput oil, juniper berry oil, rosemary oil, essential nutmeg oil, rosin, marjoram oil, fatty nutmeg oil, turpentine, rue oil, spruce resin, juniper wood oil, purified turpentine, laurel fruit oil, star anise oil.
30. Cajeput oil, anise oil, eucalyptus oil, clove oil, peppermint oil, juniper berry oil, cinnamon oil, citronella oil, rosemary oil, dwarf pine oil, sage oil, wintergreen oil.
31. Cajeput oil, anise oil, lemon oil, eucalyptus oil, fennel oil, glycerol, caraway oil, menthol, myrrh tincture, clove oil, peppermint oil, vanillin, cinnamon oil, thyme oil, sage oil, lemon balm oil.
32. Cajeput oil, camphor, 10 percent ammonia solution, sodium hydroxide, turpentine, cayenne, ceresin, potassium hydroxide.
33. Cajeput oil, camphor, eucalyptus oil, purified turpentine, rosemary oil, spruce needle oil, allantoin, sage oil, methyl salicylate, sodium pentadecyl sulfonate, chlorophyll nonoxinol, dodecylpoly (oxyethylene)-x-hydrogen sulfate.
34. Cajeput oil, aloe, myrrh gum, calendula flower, rosemary leaf, arnica leaf, Peruvian balsam, 1 homeopathic preparation.
35. Cajeput oil, camphor, aloe, myrrh gum, calendula flower, rosemary leaf, arnica flower, Peruvian balsam, 1 homeopathic preparation.
36. Cajeput oil, St. John's Wort, aloe, myrrh gum, calendula flower, rosemary leaf, arnica flower, Peruvian balsam, 1 homeopathic preparation.
37. Cajeput oil, purified turpentine, bitter orange flower oil, Chinese cinnamon oil, camphor, herb Robert (*Geranium robertianum*), St. John's Wort, galbanum gum, figwort herb, calendula herb, oak bark, mugwort herb, blue malva flower, goldenrod herb, pine sprouts.
38. Cajeput oil, pine needle oil, herb Robert, St. John's Wort, figwort herb, calendula herb, oak bark, mugwort, mallow flower, goldenrod herb, pine sprouts.
39. Cajeput oil, camphor, eucalyptus oil, menthol, purified turpentine, juniper berry oil, Siberian fir oil, rosemary oil, pine needle oil, thyme oil, pine sprouts.

40. Cajeput oil, camphor, eucalyptus oil, menthol, purified turpentine, juniper berry oil, Siberian fir oil, rosemary oil, pine needle oil, chlorophyll, pine sprouts, 1 homeopathic preparation.
41. Cajeput oil, niauli oil, sage oil, seven chemically defined components.
42. Cajeput oil, eucalyptus oil, camphor, menthol, thyme oil, niauli oil, rosemary oil, dwarf pine oil, spruce needle oil, fir oil, sage oil, arborvitae leaf oil, fir cone oil, spearmint oil, -cetyl stearyl-t-hydroxypoly-(oxyethylene)-12.
43. Cajeput oil, menthol, peppermint oil, spearmint oil, eucalyptus oil, juniper berry oil, wintergreen oil, bergamot oil, cinnamon oil, pine needle oil.

2. Claimed Uses for the Above-Named Combinations (by corresponding number)

1. Muscle and joint pain associated with rheumatic disease; also arthrosis, neuralgia, sciatica, lumbago, intervertebral disc and lower back problems, muscle strain, such as stiff neck, pain connected with sport injuries, such as sprains, contusions, strains, symptoms of cold, such as nasal catarrh, cough, sore throat, bronchial discomforts, itching due to insect bites, for sports massage.
2. For increased chance of infections, for catarrhal diseases, antiinflammatory, disinfectant, refreshing for sports massage.
3. For poorly healing and infected wounds, leg ulcers.
4. Hemorrhoids.
5. Internally for cough, hoarseness, congestion, gastric discomfort, flatulence. Externally for arthritis, lumbago, headaches.
6. Rheumatism of all origins, neuralgia, lumbago, sciatica, tendovaginitis, periostitis, epicondylitis.
7. Externally for catarrhal diseases, arthritis, neuralgia. Internally for spasms of the gastrointestinal tract and for helminthiasis.
8. Colds, nasal catarrhs, pain of nerves and limbs, lumbago, arthritis, first aid for toothache.
9. Protection for sore throat, nose and pharynx, improved blood supply for the respiratory system, soothing, calming.
10. Nervous headache, colds, nerve pain, neuralgia, nervous stomach, overexertion, exhaustion, flatulence, hematoma, intestinal catarrh, insect bites, calf cramps, toothache.
11. Cooling, calming, pain-relieving, promoting increased blood circulation, disinfectant for sprains, strains, contusions, dislocations, calf cramps, protection for insect bites.
12. Disinfectant for oral and pharyngeal cavity, for hoarseness, sore throat, cough, congestion.
13. Colds, cough, hoarseness, nasal catarrh, catarrh, headaches, exhaustion, abdominal and stomach pain of nervous origin, intestinal catarrh, nerve pain and neuralgia, rheumatic conditions, sprains, calf cramps, minor wounds, toothache.
14. Neuralgia, rheumatism, lumbago, sciatica, disorders of the vertebra, arthritis, arthrosis.
15. As a stomachic.
16. Internally for shortness of breath, for bronchial asthma (calming cough irritation, expectorant), cardiac asthma, for catarrhal diseases, disturbances of the digestive system, gastric spasms, flatulence. Externally for rheumatic discomforts, lumbago, migraine, and insect bites.
17. Headaches, nerve pain, influenza symptoms, fever, rheumatic pain, sciatica, lumbago, colds, cough, nasal catarrh, hoarseness.
18. Neuralgia, rheumatism, sciatica, lumbago.
19. Percutaneous liniment for catarrhal diseases of the respiratory tract, for arthritis, rheumatism, and insect bites.
20. Supportive treatment of circulatory disorders, for increased blood supply,

frostbite, for all forms of rheumatism.
21. Muscle rheumatism, joint rheumatism, pain in the limbs, sciatica, lumbago, insufficient blood supply, lower back pain, for all rheumatic diseases, muscle pain, back pain, shoulder pain, pain in the arms, tendonitis, stiffness of the joints, bruises, sprains.
22. Rheumatism, lumbago, sciatica, muscle and nerve pain, trigeminal neuralgia, inflammation of the joints, sprains, dislocations, contusions, hematoma.
23. Catarrh of the nasal mucosa, hypertrophy of the mucous membrane, hay fever (also prophylactic), as an adjuvant for ailments of the paranasal sinuses.
24. Any kind of skin disorder, eczema, fistulae, furuncles.
25. Dyscratic symptoms, "humoral disorders," rashes, psoriasis, eczema.
26. Flatulence and abdominal spasms.
27. Adjuvant to circulatory and metabolic disorders.
28. For prophylaxis of muscle soreness, before and after exertion in sport and work, during the season of increased danger of infections as a preventative for colds, for oral hygiene, for foot care before and after strenuous walking and extended standing, for promotion of blood circulation, for inhalation, mucolytic, prophylactic of the respiratory organs.
29. Rheumatic muscle and joint pain, tendovaginitis, sciatica, prophylaxis of phlebitis, sport injuries, massages for nerve pain.
30. Oral remedy: colds, cough, hoarseness, nasal catarrh, flu-like infections, nervous gastric discomfort, nausea, as a gargle for infections of the throat, as an inhalant for cough, hoarseness, nasal catarrh.
31. As a tonic for the nerves, for sensitivity to changes in the weather, fatigue, drowsiness and restlessness, after physical and mental exertion, for daily oral hygiene, for discomfort due to dentures, as prophylaxis for colds, for danger of infection, for hoarseness and voice care, for insect bites, for prevention of skin blemishes and athlete's foot, for promotion of physical resistance and daily fitness to variations in temperature, as a deodorant, for care of the muscles and sports massage, as support for the digestive process, as prophylaxis for gastrointestinal discomforts, such as feeling of fullness and bloating.
32. As hyperemic, segment therapy, pain of various origins, acute and chronic rheumatoid disorders, lumbago, arthritis, bronchitis, symptomatic for flu-like infections.
33. Supportive treatment for circulatory disorders, for increased blood supply, frostbite, for all types of rheumatism.
34. As a nourishing ointment for wounds, skin and healing, restoration of the skin and promotion to granulation.
35. Disc damage, brachialgia, osteochondritis, radiculitis, spondylitis, arthrosis deformans.
36. Arthritis, arthrosis, sciatica, neuralgia, rheumatism, strains, dislocations, bruises, contusions, muscle cramps after overexertion, periodontitis, gingivitis, furunculosis, sore throat, frostbite.
37. Metabolic hypofunction of the intestinal tract and tissues, intestinal sluggishness, wounds, gout, rheumatism, ulcerations, skin problems, frost impacts, myocardial insufficiency, muscular atrophy, dystrophic nervous disturbances.
38. Metabolic hypofunction of the intestinal tract and tissues, intestinal sluggishness, wounds, gout, rheumatism, ulcerations, skin problems, frostbite, myocardial insufficiency, muscular atrophy, dystrophic nervous disturbances.
39. As a liniment for rheumatic discomforts, pain in the limbs, painful strains, for migraine-like headaches, as an ointment and inhalant for cough and bronchitis.

40. Rheumatic pain of muscles and joints, sciatica, lumbago, strains, neuralgia, fatigue after sports exertion.
41. Infectious, allergic and atrophic diseases of the mucous membrane of the oral-pharyngeal cavity, nasal catarrh, hay fever, congestion and dry irritations of the nose, acute and chronic catarrhs.
42. Catarrhs of the upper respiratory tract, influenza-like infections, cough, acute and chronic catarrh, acute, chronic and spastic bronchitis, circulatory disturbances of the skin, frostbite, heavy and painful legs, discomforts of rheumatic origin, pain of the limbs and muscles, lumbago, nervous disorders, conditions of fatigue, psychogenic heart problems, headaches.
43. Cooling and ice-treatment for sports injuries without wounds, pain-relieving for contusions, muscle spasms, strains, cryotherapy for swellings, muscular pain, sprains, tendonitis (tennis elbow). Disorders of tendons, prevention of hematomas and secondary symptoms.

3. Contraindications
For infants and small children, cajeput preparations should not be applied in the facial areas, especially the nose.

Dosage and Mode of Administration
No data are available indicating the dosage for the drug in combination preparations. According to information in the literature, cajeput oil as a mono-preparation is used externally as a 5 percent alcohol solution. The dosage depends in each case on the contribution of the individual drugs in the respective combinations and must be documented specifically for each preparation.

Evaluation
Because of the cineol content and the documented experience for the use of the drug as a rubefacient, a qualitatively positive contribution to the effectiveness of the combinations for external use for rheumatic and neuralgic discomforts can be assumed. No information is available for internal use.

Nasturtium
Tropaeolum majus
Kapuzinerkresse
Published August 29, 1992

Composition of Drug
Nasturtium consists of the above-ground parts, seeds or leaf of *Tropaeolum majus* L. [Fam. Tropaeolaceae], as well as preparations thereof in effective dosage.

Pharmacological Properties, Pharmacokinetics, Toxicology
Benzyl mustard oil (benzyl isothiocyanate) obtained from *Tropaeolum majus* has, in vitro, a bacteriostatic, virustatic and antimycotic effect. Mustard oil is accumulated and excreted mainly in the respiratory and urinary tract.
External:
    hyperemic.

Clinical Data
Recent medical and/or clinical reports are not available. Old clinical data show efficacy for urinary tract infection and catarrh of the upper respiratory tract.

1. Components of the Following Drug Combinations

a) Nasturtium herb, peppermint leaf, lady's mantle, couch grass, horsetail herb, dead nettle herb, meadowsweet, white dead nettle flower, alpine lady's mantle, white clover flower.
b) Nasturtium herb, peppermint leaf, lady's mantle, couch grass, silver weed, calendula flower, agrimony leaf, common avens root, alpine plantain herb, alpine lady's mantle, bearswort.
c) Nasturtium herb, meadowsweet herb, silver weed, knotweed, *Ilex aquifolium* leaf, dead nettle herb, meadowsweet flower, white dead nettle flower, oat straw, cleavers herb.
d) Nasturtium herb, arnica flower, valerian root, chamomile, salvia leaf, thyme, mullein, yarrow, common avens root.
e) Nasturtium seed, dandelion herb and root, kava kava root, bryony root, rusty-leafed rhododendron leaf.
f) Nasturtium herb, dried yeast (*Saccharomyces bryonia*), echinacea herb and root, witch hazel leaf, night-blooming cereus, white cedar tips (arbor vitae), monk's hood herb, propolis.
g) Nasturtium herb, thyme, plantain herb, echinacea root, garden cress herb.
h) Nasturtium herb, *Brassica oleracea*, rosemary, St. John's Wort, watercress, dandelion, menthol, camphor, citronella oil.
i) Nasturtium seed, dandelion herb and root, kava kava root, bryonia root, mountain laurel leaf, marsh tea, bittersweet stems, rusty-leafed rhododendron leaf.
j) Nasturtium herb, horseradish root, horseradish root oil, myrrh gum, 1 homeopathic component.
k) Nasturtium herb, horsetail herb, birch leaf, squill, cocoa, Scotch broom herb, madder root, restharrow root, goldenrod herb, lovage root, saw palmetto fruit, guaiazulene.
l) Nasturtium, echinacea, 3 homeopathic components.

2. Claimed Uses of the Above Combinations

a) Strengthening female organs, improvement of weak conditions.
b) Increase in defense capacity for catarrhs, halting invading infections.
c) Care of sensitive urinary tract and bladder conditions.
d) As tea for mouthwashes for periodontal inflammation, canker, dental fistula, ulceration of the gums, toothache, trigeminal pain.
e) Attrition and degenerative manifestations of the joints, rheumatic arthritis and muscular inflammations, lumbago, muscular myogelosis and abnormal conditions of muscular tone.
f) Bacterial and thrush infections of the respiratory tract, infections of the lower urinary tract, cystitis, pyelonephritis, prostatitis, irritable bladder.
g) Bacterial and thrush infections of the respiratory tract, infections of the lower urinary tract, cystitis, pyelonephritis, prostatitis, irritable bladder, urethral catarrh.
h) Rheumatism, neuralgic diseases.
i) Chronic degenerative arthritis.
j) Influenza-like infections, inflammatory diseases of the tonsils, nose, paranasal sinus, tracheobronchitis, infections of the urinary tract.
k) Biological protection for influenza by increase of the individual immune reaction against infectious agents.

3. Contraindications

Not to be used for infants and small children.
Oral use:
    gastric and intestinal ulcers,
        kidney diseases.

4. Side Effects
Nasturtium contains benzyl mustard oil (benzyl isothiocyanate). Benzyl mustard oil can cause skin and mucosal irritations. Used internally, gastrointestinal disorders may occur. One case of the occurrence of a transient, urticarial exanthem was reported after ingestion of mustard oil from nasturtium. Benzyl mustard oil acts as a contact allergen if applied to the skin.

5. Special Cautions for Use
None known.

6. Use During Pregnancy and Lactation
None known.

7. Interactions with Other Drugs
None known.

8. Dosage and Mode of Administration
In older studies, mono-preparations of extracts were applied in daily dosages equivalent to 3 times 14.4 mg benzyl mustard oil. The dosage for combinations depends on the contribution of the herb in the specific combination, which in each case must be documented.

9. Overdosage
Overdosing can cause albuminuria, which apparently is due to damage to the glomerulus and tubulus system.

10. Special Cautions
None known.

11. Effects on Operators of Vehicles and Machinery
None known.

Assessment
Based on the pharmacological properties, a qualitatively positive contribution to the effectiveness of combinations for supportive treatment of infections of the lower urinary tract, catarrhs of the respiratory system, as well as topical application for mild muscular pain can be assumed.

Chapter 4

Approved Fixed Combinations

Fixed Combinations of Angelica root, Gentian root, and Caraway seed
Published March 11, 1992

Name of Drug
Fixed combinations of angelica root, gentian root, and caraway seed.

Composition of Drug
Fixed combinations consisting of:
- Angelica root with herb corresponding to the monograph published March 16, 1990;
- Gentian root corresponding to the monograph published November 11, 1985;
- Caraway seed corresponding to the monograph published December 14, 1989;
- as well as their preparations in effective dosage.

Uses
Loss of appetite, peptic discomfort, such as sensation of fullness and flatulence, mild, spastic discomfort in the gastrointestinal area.

Contraindications
Gastric and duodenal ulcers.

Side Effects
Particularly predisposed individuals may occasionally experience headaches.

Furanocoumarin, contained in angelica root, renders the skin photosensitive and in combination with ultraviolet light can cause inflammation of the skin. Prolonged sun bathing and exposure to UV light, therefore, should be avoided during the course of therapy with angelica root.

Interactions with Other Drugs
None known.

Dosage
Unless otherwise prescribed:
- Caraway must be present in the dosage given in its monograph.
- Angelica root and gentian root must be at the concentration of 50 - 75 percent of the daily dosage given in the individual monographs.

Deviating dosages must be justified specifically for the preparation (e.g., comparison of bitter values).

Mode of Administration
Comminuted drug for tea and other bitter-tasting galenical preparations for oral use.

Action
A carminative action is documented for angelica root, gentian root, and caraway seed. Pharmacological experiments for the fixed combinations are not available.

Fixed Combinations of Angelica root, Gentian root, and Fennel

Published December 18, 1991

Name of Drug
Fixed combinations of angelica root, gentian root, and fennel.

Composition of Drug
Fixed combinations consisting of:
Angelica root corresponding to B. Anz. 101, June 1, 1990;
Gentian root corresponding to B. Anz. 223, November 30, 1985;
Fennel corresponding to B. Anz. 74, April 19, 1991;
and their preparations in effective dosage.

Uses
Loss of appetite; dyspeptic disorders, such as sensation of fullness and flatulence; mild, spastic disturbances of the gastrointestinal tract.

Contraindications
Gastric and duodenal ulcers.
Pregnancy:
Preparations other than teas and preparations with essential oil contents comparable to those of teas.

Side Effects
In individual cases, allergic reactions of the skin and respiratory tract. Occasionally, headaches.
Warning: Furanocoumarin contained in this preparation causes light-sensitivity of the skin and may lead to inflammation of the skin in combination with UV exposure. During use of this preparation, extended sun bathing and intensive UV radiation should be avoided.

Interactions with Other Drugs
None known.

Dosage
Unless otherwise prescribed:
Fennel must be present in the dosage recommended in the monograph. Angelica root and gentian root must be present at a concentration of 50 - 75 percent of the daily dosage recommended in the monographs for the individual herbs. Deviating dosages must be documented for the specific preparation (e.g., through comparison of bitter values).

Mode of Administration
Bitter-tasting galenical preparations for oral intake.

Duration of Use
Fennel preparations should not be used over extended periods of time (several weeks) without medical advice.

Actions
An appetite-stimulating action with increased gastric secretion has been documented for preparations of angelica root and gentian root. Fennel has a spasmolytic action. Pharmacological tests for the effectiveness of fixed combinations are not available.

Fixed Combinations of Angelica root, Gentian root, and Bitter Orange peel

Published December 18, 1991

Name of Drug
Fixed combinations of angelica root, gentian root and bitter orange peel.

Composition of Drug
Fixed combinations consisting of:
Angelica root corresponding to
B. Anz. 101, June 1, 1990;
Gentian root corresponding to
B. Anz. 223, November 30, 1985;
Bitter Orange peel corresponding to
B. Anz. 193, October 15, 1987;
and their preparations in
effective dosage.

Uses
Loss of appetite; dyspeptic disorders, such as sensation of fullness and flatulence.

Contraindications
Gastric and duodenal ulcers.

Side Effects
Furanocoumarin contained in this preparation causes light-sensitivity of the skin and may lead to inflammation of the skin in combination with UV exposure. During use of angelica root, gentian root and bitter orange peel, or preparations thereof, extended sun bathing, and intensive UV radiation should be avoided.

Interactions with Other Drugs
None known.

Dosage
Unless otherwise prescribed:
The individual components of the combination must be present in amounts corresponding to 30 - 50 percent of the daily dosage indicated in the monographs for the individual herbs. Deviating dosages must be documented for the specific preparation (e.g., through comparison of bitter values).

Mode of Administration
Comminuted herbs and other bitter tasting preparations for oral use.

Actions
An appetite-stimulating action with increased gastric secretion has been documented for preparations of angelica root, gentian root and bitter orange peel. Pharmacological tests for the effectiveness of fixed combinations are not available.

Fixed Combinations of Angelica root, Gentian root, and Wormwood

Published March 11, 1992

Name of Drug
Fixed combinations of angelica root, gentian root, and wormwood.

Composition of Drug
Fixed combinations consisting of:
Angelica root with herb corresponding to the monograph published March 16, 1990;
Gentian root corresponding to the monograph published November 11, 1985;
Wormwood corresponding to the monograph published November 1, 1984;
as well as their preparations in effective dosage.

Uses
Loss of appetite, peptic discomfort, such as sensation of fullness and flatulence.

Contraindications
Gastric and duodenal ulcers.

Side Effects
Furanocoumarin, contained in angelica root, renders the skin photosensitive and in combination with ultraviolet light can cause inflammation of the skin. Prolonged sun bathing and exposure to UV light, therefore, should be avoided during the course of therapy with angelica root.

Interactions with Other Drugs
None known.

Dosage
Unless otherwise prescribed:
The single combination components must be at the concentration of 30 - 50 percent of the daily dosage given in the individual monographs. Deviating dosages must be justified specifically for the preparation (e.g., comparison of bitter values).

Mode of Administration
Comminuted drug for tea and other bitter-tasting galenical preparations for oral use.

Actions
Appetite-stimulating and gastric juice-secreting actions are documented for preparations of angelica root, gentian root, and wormwood herb. Pharmacological experiments for fixed combinations are not available.

Fixed Combinations of Angelica root, Gentian root, Wormwood, and Peppermint oil

Published December 18, 1991

Name of Drug
Fixed combinations of angelica root, gentian root, wormwood, and peppermint oil.

Constituents
Fixed combinations consisting of:
Angelica root corresponding to
B. Anz. 101, June 1, 1990;
Gentian root corresponding to
B. Anz. 223, November 30, 1985;
Wormwood corresponding to
B. Anz. 228, December 5,1984;
Peppermint oil corresponding to
B. Anz. 50, March 13, 1986;
and their preparations in
effective dosage.

Uses
Loss of appetite; dyspeptic disorders, such as sensation of fullness and flatulence; mild, spastic discomfort of the gastrointestinal tract.

Contraindications
Gastric and duodenal ulcers. Obstruction of the biliary tract, gallbladder inflammation, severe liver damage. If suffering from gallstones, use only after consultation with a physician or pharmacist.

Side Effects
Sensitive patients may suffer from gastric discomfort. Furanocoumarin contained in this preparation causes light-sensitivity of the skin and may lead to inflammation of the skin in combination with UV exposure. During use of angelica root or preparations thereof, extended sun bathing and intensive UV radiation should be avoided.

Interactions with Other Drugs
None known.

Dosage
Unless otherwise prescribed:
Peppermint oil must be present at the amount given in the monograph. The other individual components of the combination must be present in amounts corresponding to 30 - 50 percent of the daily dosage indicated in the monographs for the individual herbs.
Deviating dosages must be documented for the specific preparation (e.g., through comparison of bitter values).

Mode of Administration
Comminuted drug, as well as essential oil and other bitter-tasting galenical preparations for oral intake.

Actions
An appetite-stimulating action with increased gastric secretion has been documented for preparations of angelica root, gentian root and wormwood. For peppermint leaves and Angelica root, a spasmolytic and carminative effect is known. Pharmacological tests for the effectiveness of fixed combinations are not available.

Fixed Combinations of Anise oil, Fennel oil, and Caraway oil

Published August 13, 1991

Composition of Drug
Fixed combinations consisting of:
Anise oil corresponding to April 11, 1988 (B. Anz. p. 2943);
Fennel oil corresponding to March 11, 1991 (B. Anz. p. 2742);
Caraway oil corresponding to December 14, 1989 (B. Anz. 22a, February 1, 1990);
and their preparations in effective dosage.

Uses
Dyspeptic discomfort, especially with mild spasms of the gastrointestinal region, flatulence, and a sensation of fullness.

Contraindications
Oversensitivity to anise, fennel, or anethole. Pregnancy. Not to be used for infants and small children.

Side Effects
In individual cases, allergic reactions of the skin, respiratory tract, and gastrointestinal tract.

Interactions with Other Drugs
None known.

Dosage
Unless otherwise prescribed:
The individual components of the combination must be present at 30 - 50 percent of the recommended daily dosage in the monographs for the individual herbs.

Mode of Administration
Essential oils and other galenical preparations for oral intake.

Duration of Use
Fennel preparations should not be taken over extended time periods (several weeks) without consultation with a physician or pharmacist.

Actions
A spasmolytic and antibacterial effect is documented for preparations of caraway oil, fennel oil, and anise oil. Pharmacological tests for the effectiveness of fixed combinations are not available.

Fixed Combinations of Anise oil, Fennel oil, Licorice root, and Thyme

Published April 4, 1992; Revised September 9, 1992

Composition of Drug
Fixed combinations consisting of:
 Anise oil corresponding to
  B. Anz 122, July 6, 1988;
 Fennel oil corresponding to
  B. Anz 74, April 19, 1991;
 Licorice root corresponding to
  B. Anz 90, May 15, 1985;
 Thyme according to
  B. Anz 228, December 5, 1984;
 and their preparations in
  effective dosage.

Uses
Colds and diseases of the upper respiratory tract with viscous phlegm.

Contraindications
For a daily dosage up to 100 mg glycyrrhizin:
 Oversensitivity to anise and anethole. Pregnancy. Not to be used for infants and small children.
For a daily dosage of more than 100 mg glycyrrhizin:
 Cholestatic liver diseases, liver cirrhosis, hypertonia, hypokalemia, severe kidney insufficiency, pregnancy. Allergies to anise and anethole. Not to be used for infants and small children.

Side Effects
For a daily dosage up to 100 mg glycyrrhizin:
 Occasionally, allergic reactions of the skin, respiratory tract, and gastrointestinal tract.
For a daily dosage of more than 100 mg glycyrrhizin:
 Extended use and higher dosages may cause mineralocorticoid effects in the form of sodium and water retention, potassium loss with hypertonia, edema and hypokalemia with muscular asthenia, and, in rare cases, myoglobinuria. Occasionally, allergic reactions of skin, respiratory tract, and gastrointestinal tract may occur.

Interactions with Other Drugs
For a daily dosage up to 100 mg glycyrrhizin:
 None known.
For a dosage above 100 mg glycyrrhizin:
 Loss of potassium can be increased through other drugs, e.g., thiazide and loop diuretics. Sensitivity to digitalis glycosides increased through loss of potassium.

Dosage
Unless otherwise prescribed:
 The individual four components of the combination must be present at 25 - 40 percent of the recommended daily dosage in the monographs for the individual herbs.

Mode of Administration
Comminuted drug and essential oils, as well as galenical preparations for oral intake.

Duration of Use
Not longer than 4 - 6 weeks without medical advice.

Actions
The following actions are documented: a secretolytic effect for licorice root and fennel oil; an expectorant effect for licorice root, thyme, and anise oil; a bronchospasmolytic and antibacterial effect for thyme and anise oil. Pharmacological tests for the effectiveness of fixed combinations are not available.

Fixed Combinations of Anise oil and Iceland moss
Published April 4, 1992

Composition of Drug
Fixed combinations consisting of:
Anise oil corresponding to
B. Anz. 122, July 6, 1988;
Iceland moss corresponding to
B. Anz. 43, March 2, 1989;
and their preparations in
effective dosage.

Uses
Catarrhs of the upper respiratory tract with dry cough.

Contraindications
Allergy to anise and anethole.

Side Effects
Occasionally, allergic reactions of the skin, respiratory tract, and gastrointestinal tract.

Interactions with Other Drugs
None known.

Dosage
Unless otherwise prescribed:
The individual components of the combination must be present at the recommended daily dosage in the monographs for the individual herbs.

Mode of Administration
Comminuted drug and essential oil, as well as galenical preparations for oral intake.

Actions
For preparations of anise oil, an expectorant action is documented; also, mild spasmolytic and antibacterial actions are documented. Iceland moss has a soothing effect and a mild antibacterial action. Pharmacological tests for the effectiveness of fixed combinations are not available.

Fixed Combinations of Anise oil, Primrose root, and Thyme
Published April 4, 1992

Composition of Drug
Fixed combinations consisting of:
Anise oil corresponding to
B. Anz. 122, July 6, 1988;
Primrose root corresponding to
B. Anz. 122, July 6, 1988;
Thyme herb corresponding to
B. Anz. 228, December 5, 1984;
and their preparations in
effective dosage.

Uses
Colds and diseases of the upper respiratory tract with viscous phlegm.

Contraindications
Oversensitivity to anise and anethole.

Side Effects
Occasionally, allergic reactions of the skin, respiratory tract, and gastrointestinal tract. Individual cases of gastric discomfort and nausea may occur.

Interactions with Other Drugs
None known.

Dosage
Unless otherwise prescribed:
> The individual components of the combination must correspond to 30 - 50 percent of the daily dosage given in the monographs for the individual herbs.

Mode of Application
Comminuted drug and galenical preparations for oral intake.

Actions
An expectorant effect is documented for anise oil, primrose root, and thyme. In addition, anise oil and thyme have an antibacterial and bronchospasmolytic action. Primrose has a secretolytic action. Pharmacological tests for the effectiveness of fixed combinations are not available.

Fixed Combinations of Anise seed, Ivy leaf, Fennel seed, and Licorice root
Published April 4, 1992; Revised September 9, 1992

Composition of Drug
Fixed combinations consisting of:
> Anise seed corresponding to
> B. Anz. 122, July 6, 1988;
> Ivy leaf corresponding to
> B. Anz. 122, July 6, 1988;
> Fennel seed corresponding to
> B. Anz. 74, April 19, 1991;
> Licorice root corresponding to
> B. Anz. 90, May 15, 1985;
> and their preparations in
> effective dosage.

Uses
Colds and diseases of the upper respiratory tract with viscous phlegm.

Contraindications
For a daily dosage up to 100 mg glycyrrhizin:
> Oversensitivity to anise and anethole. Pregnancy: Preparations other than teas and preparations with essential oil contents comparable to those of teas.

For a daily dosage of more than 100 mg glycyrrhizin:
> Cholestatic liver diseases, liver cirrhosis, hypertonia, hypokalemia, severe kidney insufficiency, pregnancy. Allergies to anise and anethole.

Side Effects
For a daily dosage up to 100 mg glycyrrhizin:
> Occasionally allergic reactions of the skin, respiratory tract, or gastrointestinal tract.

For a daily dosage of more than 100 mg glycyrrhizin:
> Extended use and higher dosages may cause mineralocorticoid effects in the form of sodium and water retention, potassium loss with hypertonia, edema, and hypokalemia with muscular asthenia, and in rare cases myoglobinuria. Occasionally, allergic reactions of the skin, respiratory tract, or gastrointestinal tract may occur.

Interactions with Other Drugs
For a daily dosage up to 100 mg glycyrrhizin: None known.

For a dosage above 100 mg glycyrrhizin: Loss of potassium can be increased through other drugs, e.g., thiazide and loop diuretics. Sensitivity to digitalis glycosides increased through loss of potassium.

Dosage
Unless otherwise prescribed:
The individual components of the combination must be present at 25 - 40 percent of the amounts recommended as daily dosage in the monographs for the individual herbs.

Mode of Administration
Preparations for oral intake.

Duration of Use
Not longer than 4 - 6 weeks without medical advice.

Actions
Licorice root has a secretolytic and expectorant effect, fennel is secretolytic, anise and ivy leaves are expectorant and spasmolytic; anise also has an antibacterial action. Pharmacological tests for the effectiveness of fixed combinations are not available.

Fixed Combinations of Anise seed, Marshmallow root, Eucalyptus oil, and Licorice root
Published April 4, 1992

Composition of Drug
Fixed combinations consisting of:
Anise seed corresponding to
B. Anz. 122, July 6, 1988;
Marshmallow root corresponding to
B. Anz. 43, March 2, 1989;
Eucalyptus oil corresponding to
B. Anz. 177a, September 24, 1986;
Licorice root corresponding to
B. Anz. 90, May 15, 1985;
and their preparations in effective dosage.

Uses
Colds and diseases of the upper respiratory tract with dry cough.

Contraindications
For a daily dosage up to 100 mg glycyrrhizin:
Oversensitivity to anise and anethole. Inflammatory diseases of the gastrointestinal tract and biliary tract; severe liver diseases.

For a daily dosage of more than 100 mg glycyrrhizin:
Cholestatic liver diseases, liver cirrhosis and other severe liver diseases, hypertonia, hypokalemia, severe kidney insufficiency, pregnancy. Allergies to anise and anethole. Inflammatory diseases of the gastrointestinal tract and biliary tract.

Side Effects

For a daily dosage up to 100 mg glycyrrhizin:
Occasionally, allergic reactions of the skin, respiratory tract, and gastrointestinal tract. In rare cases, gastric disturbances, nausea, and diarrhea may occur.

For a daily dosage of more than 100 mg glycyrrhizin:
Extended use and higher dosages may cause mineralocorticoid effects in the form of sodium and water retention, potassium loss with hypertonia, edema and hypokalemia with muscular asthenia, and in rare cases myoglobinuria. Occasionally, allergic reactions of the skin, respiratory tract, and gastrointestinal tract may occur. In rare cases, gastric disturbances, nausea, and diarrhea may occur.

Interactions with Other Drugs

For a daily dosage up to 100 mg glycyrrhizin:
Eucalyptus oil causes the induction of the enzyme system in the liver responsible for the breakdown of foreign materials. The effect of other medications may, therefore, be reduced and/or shortened.

For a dosage above 100 mg glycyrrhizin:
Loss of potassium can be increased through other drugs, e.g., thiazide and loop diuretics. Sensitivity to digitalis glycosides is increased through loss of potassium. Eucalyptus oil causes the induction of the enzyme system in the liver responsible for the breakdown of foreign materials. The effect of other medications may, therefore, be reduced and/or shortened.

Warning: The absorption of other, simultaneously taken medications can be delayed.

Dosage

Unless otherwise prescribed:
Marshmallow must be at the concentration given in the monograph. Licorice root, eucalyptus oil, and anise must be present at 30 - 50 percent of the amounts recommended as daily dosage in the monographs for the individual herbs.

Mode of Administration

Comminuted drug and galenical preparations for oral intake.

Duration of Use

Not longer than 4 - 6 weeks without medical advice.

Actions

An expectorant action is documented for preparations of licorice root, eucalyptus oil, and anise. A secretolytic effect has been shown for licorice root, and a secretomotory action for eucalyptus oil. Anise has also an antibacterial action. Marshmallow has a soothing effect and inhibits in-vitro the mucociliary activity. In addition, anise and eucalyptus oil have a mild spasmolytic action. Pharmacological tests for the effectiveness of fixed combinations are not available.

Fixed Combinations of Anise seed, Marshmallow root, Iceland moss, and Licorice root

Published April 4, 1992

Composition of Drug
Fixed combinations consisting of:
Anise seed corresponding to
B. Anz. 122, July 6, 1988;
Marshmallow root corresponding to
B. Anz. 43, March 2, 1989;
Iceland moss corresponding to
B. Anz. 43, March 2, 1989;
Licorice root corresponding to
B. Anz. 90, May 15, 1985;
and their preparations in
effective dosage.

Uses
Catarrhs of the upper respiratory tract with dry cough.

Contraindications
For a daily dosage up to 100 mg glycyrrhizin:
Oversensitivity to anise and anethole.
For a daily dosage of more than 100 mg glycyrrhizin:
Cholestatic liver diseases, liver cirrhosis, hypertonia, hypokalemia, severe kidney insufficiency, pregnancy. Allergies to anise and anethole.

Side Effects
For a daily dosage up to 100 mg glycyrrhizin:
Occasionally, allergic reactions of the skin, respiratory tract, and gastrointestinal tract.
For a daily dosage of more than 100 mg glycyrrhizin:
Extended use and higher dosages may cause mineralocorticoid effects in the form of sodium and water retention, potassium loss with hypertonia, edema, and hypokalemia with muscular asthenia, and, in rare cases, myoglobinuria. Occasionally, allergic reactions of the skin, respiratory tract, and gastrointestinal tract may occur.

Interactions with Other Drugs
For a daily dosage up to 100 mg glycyrrhizin:
None known.
Warning: The absorption of other, simultaneously taken medications may be delayed.
For a dosage above 100 mg glycyrrhizin:
Loss of potassium can be increased through other drugs, e.g., thiazide and loop diuretics. Sensitivity to digitalis glycosides is increased through loss of potassium.
Warning: The absorption of other, simultaneously taken medications may be delayed.

Dosage
Unless otherwise prescribed:
Marshmallow and Iceland moss must each be at the concentration equivalent to 50 - 75 percent of the daily dosage given in the monographs for individual herbs. Also, licorice root and anise must be present at concentrations corresponding to 50 - 75 percent of the daily dosage recommended in the monographs for the individual herbs.

Mode of Administration
Comminuted drug and galenical preparations for oral intake.

Duration of Use
Not longer than 4 - 6 weeks without medical advice.

Actions
An expectorant action is documented for preparations of licorice root and anise. A secretolytic effect has been shown for licorice root. Anise also has an antibacterial and mildly spasmolytic action. Marshmallow and Iceland moss have a soothing effect; Iceland moss has, in addition, a mild antibacterial action. Pharmacological tests for the effectiveness of fixed combinations are not available.

Fixed Combinations of Anise seed, Marshmallow root, Primrose root, and Sundew
Published April 4, 1992

Composition of Drug
Fixed combinations consisting of:
Anise seed corresponding to
B. Anz. 122, July 6, 1988;
Marshmallow root corresponding to
B. Anz. 43, March 2, 1989;
Primrose root corresponding to
B. Anz. 122, July 6, 1988;
Sundew corresponding to
B. Anz. 228, December 5, 1984;
and their preparations in effective dosage.

Uses
Catarrhs of the upper respiratory tract with spastic, dry cough.

Contraindications
Allergy to anise and anethole.

Side Effects
Occasionally allergic reactions of the skin, respiratory tract, and gastrointestinal tract. Individual cases of gastric disorders and nausea may occur.

Interactions with Other Drugs
None known.

Warning: The absorption of other, simultaneously taken medications may be delayed.

Dosage
Unless otherwise prescribed:
Marshmallow and sundew herb must be at the concentration given in the monographs. The other components of the combination must be each equivalent to 50 - 75 percent of the daily dosage given in the monographs for the individual herbs.

Mode of Administration
Comminuted drug and galenical preparations for oral intake.

Actions
For preparations of primrose root and anise an expectorant action is documented. Anise and sundew have, in addition, a spasmolytic effect. Primrose root is secretolytic, anise is antibacterial and sundew is antitussive. Marshmallow has a soothing effect and inhibits in-vitro mucociliary activity. Pharmacological tests for the effectiveness of fixed combinations are not available.

Fixed Combinations of Anise seed, Fennel seed and Caraway seed
Published August 13, 1991

Composition of Drug
Fixed combinations consisting of:
Anise seed corresponding to
April 11, 1988 (*B. Anz.* p. 2943);
Fennel seed corresponding to
March 11, 1991 (*B. Anz.* p. 2742);
Caraway seed corresponding
to December 14, 1989
(*B. Anz.* 22a, February 1, 1990);
and their preparations in
effective dosage.

Uses
Dyspeptic discomfort, especially with mild spasms of the gastrointestinal region, flatulence, and a sensation of fullness.

Contraindications
Oversensitivity to anise, fennel, or anethole.
Pregnancy:
Preparations other than teas and preparations with essential oil contents comparable to those of teas.

Side Effects
In individual cases, allergic reactions of the skin, respiratory tract, and gastrointestinal tract.

Interactions with Other Drugs
None known.

Dosage
Unless otherwise prescribed:
The individual components of the combination must each be present at 30 - 55 percent of the amounts recommended as daily dosage in the monographs for the individual herbs.

Mode of Administration
Comminuted drug for teas and other galenical preparations for oral intake.

Duration of Use
Fennel preparations should not be taken over extended time periods (several weeks) without consultation with a physician or pharmacist.

Actions
A spasmolytic and antibacterial effect is documented for preparations of anise, fennel, and caraway. Pharmacological tests for the effectiveness of fixed combinations are not available.

Fixed Combinations of Anise seed, Linden flower, and Thyme
Published April 4, 1992

Composition of Drug
Fixed combinations consisting of:
Anise seed corresponding to
B. Anz. 122, July 6, 1988;
Linden flower corresponding to
B. Anz 164, September 1, 1990;
Thyme corresponding to
B. Anz 228, December 5, 1984;
and their preparations in
effective dosage.

Uses
Catarrhs of the upper respiratory tract with dry cough.

Contraindications
Oversensitivity to anise and anethole.

Side Effects
Occasionally, allergic reactions of skin, respiratory tract, and gastrointestinal tract.

Interactions with Other Drugs
None known.

Dosage
Unless otherwise prescribed:
    Linden flower must be present at the dosage given in the monograph. The other components of the combination must be present at 50 - 75 percent of the daily dosage given in the monographs for the individual herbs.

Mode of Administration
Comminuted drug for teas and other galenical preparations for oral intake.

Actions
An expectorant, antibacterial, and mild spasmolytic effect is documented for preparations of anise seed and thyme. A diaphoretic action is documented for linden flower. Pharmacological tests for the effectiveness of the fixed combinations are not available.

Fixed Combinations of Birch leaf, Goldenrod, and Java tea
Published August 29, 1992

Name of Drug
Fixed combinations of birch leaf, goldenrod, and Java tea.

Composition of Drug
Fixed combinations consisting of:
    Birch leaf corresponding to the monograph published March 13, 1986;
    Goldenrod herb corresponding to the monograph published October 15, 1987;
    Java tea corresponding to the monograph published March 13, 1986;
    as well as their preparations in effective dosage.

Uses
For irrigation therapy of inflammatory diseases of the lower urinary tract, and for prophylaxis of kidney stones.

Contraindications
None known.
Note: No irrigation therapy in case of edema due to insufficient heart and kidney function.

Side Effects
None known.

Interactions with Other Drugs
None known.

Dosage
Unless otherwise prescribed:
    The individual combination components must correspond to a concentration of 30 - 50 percent given as daily dosage in the monographs of the single drug.

Mode of Administration
For oral application, comminuted drug or extracts for tea.
Note: Copious intake of fluids must be observed.

Actions
A diuretic action is documented for birch leaf, goldenrod, and Java tea. Goldenrod and Java tea have also a mild antispasmodic action. In addition, goldenrod has an antiphlogistic effect. Pharmacological experiments for the fixed combinations are not available.

Fixed Combinations of Camphor, Eucalyptus oil, and Purified Turpentine oil
Published July 14, 1993

Name of Drug
Fixed combinations of camphor, eucalyptus oil, and purified turpentine oil.

Composition of Drug
Fixed combinations consisting of:
- Camphor corresponding to publication of November 1, 1984 (B. Anz. p. 13326);
- Eucalyptus oil corresponding to publication of July 21, 1986 (B. Anz. 177a of September 24, 1986, supplement);
- Purified Turpentine oil corresponding to publication of May 6, 1985 (B. Anz. p. 4953);
- as well as their preparations in effective dosage.

Pharmacological Properties, Pharmacokinetics, Toxicology
For preparations of camphor, eucalyptus oil and purified turpentine, hyperemization and secretolytic action is documented. In addition, eucalyptus oil acts as an expectorant and mild antispasmodic, purified turpentine as an antiseptic. Upon oral application, camphor acts also as an analeptic for the respiratory and circulatory systems, and as a bronchoantispasmodic. Pharmacological studies on the effectiveness of the fixed combinations are not available.

Clinical Data

1. Uses
For inhalation and external:
- Catarrhs of the respiratory tract.

External:
- Pain in the muscles and joints of non-inflammatory, rheumatic diseases.

2. Contraindications
Hypersensitivity to essential oils.
Inhalation:
- Acute pneumonia.

External:
- Injured skin (burns). For infants and small children, camphor and eucalyptus preparations should not be used in the facial area, especially around the nose.

3. Side Effects
Contact eczema is possible. External use on large surfaces could cause symptoms of poisoning (damage to kidneys and central nervous system).
Note: If used other than officially recommended (oral intake), nausea, vomiting and diarrhea may result.

4. Interactions with Other Drugs
None known.

5. Dosage
Unless otherwise prescribed:
The individual combination partners must be present at a concentration of 30 - 50 percent of the daily dosage specified in the respective monographs.
Sufficient data are not available concerning the dosage of this combination for infants and small children.

6. Mode of Administration
Internal:
For inhalation, use several drops in hot water and inhale the steam.
External:
For colds, rub semi-solid and liquid preparations onto chest and back.
For muscle and joint pains, apply semi-solid and liquid preparations to the affected areas.

Fixed Combinations of Caraway oil and Fennel oil
Published August 13, 1991

Composition of Drug
Fixed combinations consisting of:
Caraway oil corresponding to December 14, 1989 (B. Anz. 22a, February 1, 1990);
Fennel oil corresponding to March 11, 1991 (B. Anz. p. 2742);
and their preparations in effective dosage.

Uses
Dyspeptic discomfort, especially with mild spasms in the gastrointestinal region, flatulence, and a sensation of fullness.

Contraindications
Pregnancy. Not to be used for infants and small children.

Side Effects
In individual cases, allergic reaction of the skin and respiratory tract.

Interactions with Other Drugs
None known.

Dosage
Unless otherwise prescribed:
The individual components must be present in amounts equivalent to 50 - 75 percent of the daily dosage indicated in the monographs for the individual oils.

Mode of Administration
Essential oil and galenical preparations thereof for oral intake.

Duration of Application
Fennel preparations should not be taken over extended time periods (several weeks) without consultation of a physician or pharmacist.

Actions
A spasmolytic, carminative and antibacterial effect is documented for caraway oil and fennel oil. Pharmacological tests for the effectiveness of fixed combinations are not available.

Fixed Combinations of Caraway oil, Fennel oil, and Chamomile flower

Published August 13, 1991; Revised September 3, 1992

Composition of Drug
Fixed combinations consisting of:
Caraway oil corresponding to December 14, 1989 (*B. Anz.* 22a, February 1, 1990);
Fennel oil corresponding to March 11, 1991 (*B. Anz.* p. 2742);
Chamomile flower corresponding to November 1, 1984 (*B. Anz.* p.13327);
and their preparations in effective dosage.

Uses
Dyspeptic discomfort, especially with mild spasms in the gastrointestinal region, flatulence, and a sensation of fullness.

Contraindications
Pregnancy. Not to be used for infants and small children.

Side Effects
In individual cases, allergic reaction of skin and respiratory tract.

Interactions with Other Drugs
None known.

Dosage
Unless otherwise prescribed:
The individual components of the combination must be present in amounts equivalent to 30 - 50 percent of the daily dosage indicated in the monographs for the individual herbs.

Mode of Administration
Essential oil, comminuted drug and galenical preparations thereof for oral intake.

Duration of Application
Fennel preparations should not be taken over extended time periods (several weeks) without consultation of a physician or pharmacist.

Actions
A spasmolytic and antibacterial effect is documented for caraway oil, fennel oil, and chamomile flower. Pharmacological tests for the effectiveness of fixed combinations are not available.

Fixed Combinations of Caraway seed and Fennel seed

Published August 13, 1991

Composition of Drug
Fixed combinations consisting of:
Caraway seed corresponding to December 14, 1989 (*B. Anz.* 22a, February 1, 1990);
Fennel seed corresponding to March 11, 1991 (*B. Anz.* p. 2742);
and their preparations in effective dosage.

Uses
Dyspeptic discomfort, especially with mild spasms in the gastrointestinal region, flatulence, and a sensation of fullness.

Contraindications
In pregnancy, preparations other than teas and preparations with essential oil contents comparable to those of teas.

Side Effects
In individual cases, allergic reaction of the skin and respiratory tract.

Interaction with Other Drugs
None known.

Dosage
Unless otherwise prescribed:
The individual components must be present equivalent to 50 - 75 percent of the daily dosage indicated in the monographs for the individual herbs.

Mode of Administration
Comminuted drug for teas and other galenical preparations thereof for oral intake.

Duration of Application
Fennel seed preparations should not be taken over extended time periods (several weeks) without consultation of a physician or pharmacist.

Actions
A spasmolytic and carminative effect is documented for caraway seed and fennel seed. Pharmacological tests for the effectiveness of fixed combinations are not available.

Fixed Combinations of Caraway seed, Fennel seed and Chamomile flower

Published August 13, 1991

Composition of Drug
Fixed combinations consisting of:
Caraway seed corresponding to December 14, 1989 (*B. Anz.* 22a, February 1, 1990);
Fennel seed corresponding to March 11, 1991 (*B. Anz.* p. 2742);
Chamomile flower corresponding to November 1, 1984 (*B. Anz.* p.13327);
and their preparations in effective dosage.

Uses
Dyspeptic discomfort, especially with mild spasms in the gastrointestinal region, flatulence, and a sensation of fullness.

Contraindications
In pregnancy, preparations other than teas and preparations with essential oil contents comparable to those of teas.

Side Effects
In individual cases, allergic reaction of the skin and respiratory tract.

Interaction with Other Drugs
None known.

Dosage
Unless otherwise prescribed:
The individual components of the combination must be present in amounts equivalent to 30 - 50 percent of the daily dosage indicated in the monographs for the individual herbs.

Mode of Administration
Comminuted drug for teas and other galenical preparations thereof for oral intake.

Duration of Application
Fennel preparations should not be taken over extended time periods (several weeks) without consultation of a physician or pharmacist.

Action
A spasmolytic effect is documented for caraway seed, fennel seed, and chamomile flower. Pharmacological tests for the effectiveness of fixed combinations are not available.

Fixed Combinations of Dandelion root with herb, Celandine herb, and Artichoke leaf

Published December 18, 1991

Name of Drug
Fixed combinations of dandelion root with herb, celandine herb, and artichoke leaf.

Composition of Drug
Fixed combinations consisting of:
Dandelion root with herb corresponding to B. Anz. 228, December 5, 1984;
Celandine herb corresponding to B. Anz. 90, May 15, 1985;
Artichoke leaf corresponding to B. Anz. 122, July 6, 1988;
and their preparations in effective dosage.

Uses
Spastic epigastric discomfort due to functional disorders of the biliary system.

Contraindications
Obstruction of the biliary tract, empyema of gallbladder, ileus. Allergies to artichoke and other composites. In case of gallbladder diseases, to be used only after consultation with a physician or pharmacist.

Side Effects
None known.

Interactions with Other Drugs
None known.

Dosage
Unless otherwise prescribed:
Celandine herb must be present in the amount given in the monograph. The other two components of the combination must each be equivalent to 50 - 75 percent of the daily dosage indicated in the monographs for the individual herbs.

Mode of Administration
Comminuted drug and galenical preparations for oral intake.

Actions
A cholagogic effect has been documented for dandelion root with herb and artichoke leaf. Celandine herb has a papaverine-like, mildly spasmolytic effect on the upper gastrointestinal tract. Pharmacological tests for the effectiveness of combinations are not available.

Fixed Combinations of Dandelion root with herb, Celandine herb, and Wormwood
Published March 11, 1992

Name of Drug
Fixed combinations of dandelion root with herb, celandine herb, and wormwood.

Composition of Drug
Fixed combinations consisting of:
Dandelion root with herb corresponding to the monograph published November 1, 1984 (B. Anz. p. 13327);
Celandine herb corresponding to the monograph published May 6, 1985 (B. Anz. p. 4952);
Wormwood herb corresponding to the monograph published November 1, 1984 (B. Anz. p. 13327);
as well as their preparations in effective dosage.

Uses
Dyspeptic complaints, particularly for functional disorders of the gallbladder drainage system.

Contraindications
Obstruction of the bile ducts, empyema of the gallbladder, ileus. In case of gallstones, to be used only after consultation with a physician.

Side Effects
None known.

Interactions with Other Drugs
None known.

Dosage
Unless otherwise prescribed:
Celandine must be present at the concentration given in the monograph. Dandelion root with herb and wormwood must be at 50 - 75 percent of the daily dosage given in the monographs for the individual herb.
Deviating dosages must be justified for the specific preparation (e.g., comparison of bitter values).

Mode of Administration
Liquid and solid preparations for oral application.

Actions
Stimulation of gall secretion and appetite has been established for dandelion root with herb and wormwood herb. Celandine herb shows a papaverine-like, mild antispasmodic action on the upper intestinal tract. Pharmacological tests for the effectiveness of fixed combinations are not available.

Fixed Combinations of Dandelion root with herb, Peppermint leaf, and Artichoke leaf
Published December 18, 1991

Name of Drug
Fixed combinations of dandelion root with herb, peppermint leaf, and artichoke leaf.

Composition of Drug
Fixed combinations consisting of:
Dandelion root with leaf corresponding to B. Anz. 228, December 5, 1984;
Peppermint leaf corresponding to B. Anz. 223, November 30, 1985;
Artichoke leaf corresponding to B. Anz. 122, July 6, 1988;
and their preparations in effective dosage.

Uses
Spastic epigastric discomfort due to functional disorders of the biliary system.

Contraindications
Obstruction of the biliary tract, empyema of gallbladder, ileus. Known allergies to artichoke and other composites. In case of gallbladder disease, to be used only after consultation with a physician or pharmacist.

Side Effects
None known.

Interactions with Other Drugs
None known.

Dosage
Unless otherwise prescribed:
Peppermint leaves must be present in the amount given in the monograph. The other two components of the combination must be each equivalent to 50 - 75 percent of the daily dosage indicated in the monographs for the individual herbs.
Deviating dosages must be justified for the specific preparation (e.g., comparison of bitter values).

Mode of Administration
Comminuted drug and galenical preparations for oral intake.

Actions
A cholagogic effect has been documented for dandelion root with herb and artichoke leaf. Peppermint leaf has a direct spasmolytic effect on the smooth muscles of the gastrointestinal tract. Pharmacological tests for the effectiveness of fixed combinations are not available.

Fixed Combinations of Eucalyptus oil and Pine Needle oil

Published July 14, 1993

Name of Drug
Fixed combinations of eucalyptus oil and pine needle oil.

Composition of Drug
Fixed combinations consisting of:
Eucalyptus oil according to the notice of 21 July 1986 (*B. Anz.* p. 177a of September 24, 1986, Supplement); Pine needle oil according to the notice of August 13, 1986 (*B. Anz.* 9943);
as well as preparations in effective dosage.

Pharmacological Properties, Pharmacokinetics, Toxicology
For preparations from eucalyptus oil and pine needle oil a hyperemic and secretolytic effect is proven. In addition, eucalyptus oil is an expectorant and is weakly spasmolytic. Pine needle oil is weakly antiseptic. Pharmacological studies about the effects of the fixed combination are unknown.

Clinical Data

1. Uses
For inhalation and external application in case of illnesses of the respiratory tract caused by a cold.

2. Contraindications
Bronchial asthma. Whooping cough.
External:
In the case of babies and small children, eucalyptus-containing preparations should not be applied in the area of the face, especially the nose.

3. Side Effects
On the skin and mucous membranes irritation phenomena can appear. Bronchial spasms can increase.
Note: If not used according to directions (e.g., swallowing), nausea, vomiting and diarrhea can occur.

4. Interactions with Other Drugs
None known.

5. Dosage
Unless otherwise prescribed:
Eucalyptus oil and pine needle oil each time, 3 - 10 percent in semisolid preparations.
Mixture of the essential oils 50 percent of the dose.

6. Mode of Administration
Semisolid preparations are rubbed on the chest and back.
For inhalation:
Hot water is poured over 1 - 5 g of ointment and the vapors are inhaled.
Hot water is poured over 1 - 5 drops of the essential oil mixture and the vapors are inhaled, or in the case of babies and small children 1 - 5 drops are given on a cloth.

Fixed Combinations of Eucalyptus oil, Primrose root, and Thyme

Published April 4, 1992

Composition of Drug
Fixed combinations consisting of:
Eucalyptus oil corresponding to B. Anz. 177a, September 24, 1986;
Primrose root corresponding to B. Anz. 122, July 6, 1988;
Thyme corresponding to B. Anz. 228, December 5, 1984;
and their preparations in effective dosage.

Uses
Colds and diseases of the upper respiratory tract with viscous phlegm.

Contraindications
Inflammatory diseases of the gastrointestinal and biliary regions; severe liver diseases.

Side Effects
Occasionally, gastric discomfort, nausea, vomiting and diarrhea may occur.

Interactions with Other Drugs
Eucalyptus oil induces the enzyme system responsible for the breakdown of foreign substances in the liver. The effectiveness of other medications may, therefore, be diminished and/or shortened.

Dosage
Unless otherwise prescribed:
The individual components of the combination must each be present at 30 - 50 percent of the daily dosage given in the monographs for the individual herbs.

Mode of Administration
Comminuted drug and galenical preparations for oral intake.

Actions
An expectorant effect is documented for preparations of primrose root, thyme, and eucalyptus oil. In addition, eucalyptus oil and primrose root have secretolytic action. Eucalyptus oil and thyme have a mild spasmolytic action, and thyme, an antibacterial action. Pharmacological tests for the effectiveness of fixed combinations are not available.

Fixed Combinations of Ginger root, Gentian root, and Wormwood

Published December 18, 1991

Name of Drug
Fixed combinations of ginger root, gentian root, and wormwood.

Composition of Drug
Fixed combinations consisting of:
 Ginger root corresponding to
  B. Anz. 85, May 5, 1988;
 Gentian root corresponding to
  B. Anz. 223, November 30, 1985;
 Wormwood corresponding to
  B. Anz. 228, December 5, 1984;
 and their preparations in effective
  dosage.

Uses
Loss of appetite, dyspeptic discomfort such as a sensation of fullness and flatulence.

Contraindications
Gastric and duodenal ulcers.

Side Effects
None known.

Interactions with Other Drugs
None known.

Dosage
Unless otherwise prescribed:
 The individual components must each be present at 30 - 50 percent of the daily dosage given in the monographs for the individual herbs.
 Deviating dosages must be justified for the specific preparations (e.g., comparative bitter values).

Mode of Administration
Comminuted drug and bitter-tasting galenical preparations for oral intake.

Actions
For preparations of ginger root, gentian root, and wormwood, an appetite-stimulating effect with promotion of gastric secretion is documented. Pharmacological tests for the effectiveness of fixed combinations are not available.

Fixed Combinations of Gumweed herb, Primrose root, and Thyme

Published April 4, 1992

Composition of Drug
Fixed combinations consisting of:
 Gumweed herb corresponding to
  B. Anz. 11, January 17, 1991;
 Primrose root corresponding to
  B. Anz. 122, July 6, 1988;
 Thyme corresponding to B. Anz. 228,
  December 5, 1984;
 and their preparations in effective
  dosage.

Uses
Colds and diseases of the upper respiratory tract with viscous phlegm.

Contraindications
None known.

Side Effects
Occasionally gastric discomfort and nausea.

Interactions with Other Drugs
None known.

Dosage
Unless otherwise prescribed:
The individual components of the combination must each be present at 30 - 50 percent of the daily dosage given in the monographs for the individual herbs.

Mode of Administration
Comminuted drug and galenical preparations for oral intake.

Actions
An expectorant effect is documented for preparations of primrose root and thyme. Gumweed herb and thyme also have antibacterial action. Primrose root has secretolytic action and thyme, bronchospasmolytic action. Pharmacological tests for the effectiveness of fixed combinations are not available.

Fixed Combinations of Ivy leaf, Licorice root, and Thyme
Published April 4, 1992; Revised September 3, 1992

Composition of Drug
Fixed combinations of:
Ivy leaf corresponding to
B. Anz. 122, July 6, 1988;
Licorice root corresponding to
B. Anz. 90, May 15, 1985;
Thyme corresponding to
B. Anz. 228, December 5, 1984;
and their preparations in effective dosage.

Uses
Colds and diseases of the upper respiratory tract with viscous phlegm.

Contraindications
For a daily dosage up to 100 mg glycyrrhizin:
None known.
For a daily dosage of more than 100 mg glycyrrhizin:
Cholestatic liver diseases, liver cirrhosis, hypertonia, hypokalemia, severe kidney insufficiency, pregnancy.

Side Effects
For a daily dosage up to 100 mg glycyrrhizin:
None known.
For a daily dosage of more than 100 mg glycyrrhizin:
Extended administration and higher dosages may cause mineralocorticoid effects in the form of sodium and water retention, loss of potassium with hypertonia, edema, and hypokalemia with muscular asthenia, and, in rare cases, myoglobinuria.

Interactions with Other Drugs
For a daily dosage up to 100 mg glycyrrhizin:
  None known.
For a daily dosage of more than 100 mg glycyrrhizin:
  Loss of potassium through other medications can be increased, e.g., thiazide and loop diuretics. The sensitivity toward digitalis glycosides increases with loss of potassium.

Dosage
Unless otherwise prescribed:
  The individual components of the combination must each be present at 30 - 50 percent of the daily dosage given in the monographs for the individual herbs.

Mode of Administration
Drug extracts for oral intake.

Actions
An expectorant and spasmolytic effect is documented for thyme, ivy leaf, and licorice root. In addition, thyme has antibacterial action. Pharmacological tests for the effectiveness of fixed combinations are not available.

Fixed Combinations of Javanese Turmeric root, Celandine herb, and Wormwood
Published December 18, 1991; Revised September 3, 1992

Name of Drug
Fixed combinations of Javanese turmeric root, celandine herb, and wormwood.

Composition of Drug
Fixed combinations consisting of:
  Javanese turmeric root corresponding to B. Anz. 122, July 6, 1988;
  Celandine herb corresponding to B. Anz. 90, May 15, 1985;
  Wormwood corresponding to B. Anz. 228, December 5, 1984;
  and their preparations in effective dosage.

Uses
Spastic epigastric discomfort due to functional disorders of the biliary tract.

Contraindications
Obstruction of the biliary tract. If suffering from gallstones, to be used only after consultation with a physician or pharmacist.

Side Effects
Gastric discomfort may occur with extended use.

Interactions with Other Drugs
None known.

Dosage
Unless otherwise prescribed:
  Celandine herb must be present at the dosage given in the monograph. The other components of the combination must each be present at 30 - 50 percent of the daily dosage given in the monographs for the individual herbs.
  Deviating dosages must be justified for the specific preparations (e.g., comparative bitter values).

Mode of Administration
Comminuted drug and galenical preparations thereof for oral intake.

Actions

For preparations of wormwood and Javanese turmeric root, a choleretic effect is documented; for celandine herb a papaverine-like, mildly spasmolytic effect on the gastrointestinal tract is known. Pharmacological tests for the effectiveness of fixed combinations are not available.

Fixed Combinations of Javanese Turmeric root, Peppermint leaf, and Wormwood

Published December 18, 1991

Name of Drug

Fixed combinations of Javanese turmeric root, peppermint leaf and wormwood.

Composition of Drug

Fixed combinations consisting of:
Javanese turmeric root corresponding to B. Anz. 122, July 6, 1988;
Peppermint leaf corresponding to B. Anz. 223, November 30, 1985;
Wormwood corresponding to B. Anz. 228, December 5, 1984;
and their preparations in effective dosage.

Uses

Dyspeptic discomfort, especially due to functional disorders of the biliary tract.

Contraindications

Obstruction of the biliary tract. If suffering from gallstones, to be used only after consultation with a physician or pharmacist.

Side Effects

Gastric discomfort may occur with extended use.

Interactions with Other Drugs

None known.

Dosage

Unless otherwise prescribed:
The individual components must each be present at 30 - 50 percent of the daily dosage given in the monographs for the individual herbs.

Deviating dosages must be justified for the specific preparations (e.g., comparative bitter values).

Mode of Administration

Comminuted drug and galenical preparations thereof for oral intake.

Actions

For preparations of Javanese turmeric root, peppermint leaf, and wormwood, a choleretic and carminative effect is documented; for peppermint leaf also a spasmolytic action. Pharmacological tests for the effectiveness of fixed combinations are not available.

Fixed Combinations of Licorice root and German Chamomile flower

Published July 14, 1993

Name of Drug
Fixed combinations of licorice root and chamomile flower.

Composition of Drug
Fixed combinations consisting of:
Licorice root with herb corresponding to the monograph published May 6, 1985 (*B. Anz.* p. 4953);
Chamomile flower corresponding to the monograph published November 1, 1984 (*B. Anz.* p. 13326);
as well as their preparations in effective dosage.

Pharmacological Properties, Pharmacokinetics, Toxicology
For preparations of licorice and chamomile, an antispasmodic action is documented. Chamomile has an antiphlogistic and wound healing effect.

Glycyrrhizic acid and the aglycone of glycyrrhizic acid enhance the healing of gastric ulcers, according to controlled, clinical studies. Pharmacological studies pertaining to the fixed combination are not available.

Clinical Data

1. Uses
For symptomatic treatment of irritated (nervous) stomach and simple gastric ulcers.

2. Contraindications
For a daily dosage up to 100 mg glycyrrhizin:
None known.
For a daily dosage of more than 100 mg of glycyrrhizin:
Cholestatic liver disorders, liver cirrhosis, hypertonia, hypokalemia, severe kidney insufficiency, pregnancy.

3. Side Effects
For a daily dosage up to 100 mg glycyrrhizin:
None known.
For a daily dosage of more than 100 mg of glycyrrhizin:
Extended use and higher dosages can cause mineralocorticoid effects, such as sodium and water retention, loss of potassium with high blood pressure, edema and hypokalemia with muscle weakness, and, in rare cases, myoglobinuria.

4. Interactions with Other Drugs
For a daily dosage up to 100 mg glycyrrhizin:
None known.
For a daily dosage of more than 100 mg of glycyrrhizin:
Loss of potassium due to other medications, e.g., thiazide and loop diuretics, can be intensified. Loss of potassium increases the sensitivity to digitalis glycosides.

5. Dosage
Unless otherwise prescribed:
The individual combination partners must be present at the concentration of 50 - 75 percent of the daily dosage given in the individual monographs.

6. Mode of Administration
Comminuted herb and preparations for oral use.

7. Duration of Administration
Without medical advice, not longer than 4 - 6 weeks.

Fixed Combinations of Licorice root, Peppermint leaf, and German Chamomile flower

Published March 11, 1992

Name of Drug
Fixed combinations of licorice root, peppermint leaf and chamomile flower.

Composition of Drug
Fixed combinations consisting of:
Licorice root corresponding to the monograph published May 15, 1985;
Peppermint leaf corresponding to the monograph published November 11, 1985;
Chamomile flower corresponding to the monograph published November 1, 1984;
as well as their preparations in effective dosage.

Uses
Acute and chronic inflammation of the gastric mucosa with spastic discomforts in the gastrointestinal area.

Contraindications
Cholestatic liver disorders, cirrhosis of the liver, hypertonia, hypokalemia, severe kidney insufficiency, pregnancy.

In case of gallstones, to be used only after consultation with a physician.

Side Effects
For a daily dosage up to 100 mg glycyrrhizin:
None known.
For a daily dosage of more than 100 mg of glycyrrhizin:
Extended use and higher dosages can cause mineralocorticoid effects, such as sodium and water retention, potassium loss with high blood pressure, edema and hypokalemia with muscle weakness, and, in rare cases, myoglobinuria.

Interactions with Other Drugs
Loss of potassium due to other medication, e.g., thiazide and loop diuretics, can be intensified. Loss of potassium increases the sensitivity to digitalis glycosides.

Dosage
Unless otherwise prescribed:
Licorice root, peppermint leaf and chamomile flower must be at the concentration of 50 - 75 percent of the daily dosage given in the individual monographs.
Deviating dosages must be justified specifically for the preparation.

Mode of Administration
Liquid and solid preparations for oral application.

Duration of Administration
Without medical advice, not longer than 4 - 6 weeks.

Actions
An antispasmodic effect is documented for licorice root, peppermint leaf, and chamomile flower. Chamomile flower has in addition an antiphlogistic and wound-healing action, glycyrrhizic acid and the aglycone of glycyrrhizic acid enhance the healing of gastric ulcers, according to controlled clinical studies. Pharmacological experiments for fixed combinations are not available.

Fixed Combinations of Licorice root, Primrose root, Marshmallow root, and Anise seed
Published March 11, 1992

Name of Drug
Fixed combinations of licorice root, primrose root [*Primula*, not *Oenothera* (evening primrose)], marshmallow root and anise seed.

Composition of Drug
Fixed combinations consisting of:
Licorice root corresponding to the monograph published May 6, 1985;
Primrose root corresponding to the monograph published April 11, 1988;
Marshmallow root corresponding to the monograph published January 5, 1989;
Anise seed corresponding to the monograph published April 11, 1988;
as well as their preparations in effective dosage.

Uses
Catarrh of the upper respiratory tract and resulting dry cough.

Contraindications
For daily dosages of less than 100 mg glycyrrhizin:
Hypersensitivity to anise and anethole.
For daily dosages of more than 100 mg glycyrrhizin:
Cholestatic liver disorders, cirrhosis of the liver, hypertonia, hypokalemia, severe kidney insufficiency, pregnancy. Hypersensitivity to anise and anethole.

Side Effects
For daily dosages below 100 mg glycyrrhizin:
Occasionally allergic reactions involving skin, respiratory tract and gastrointestinal tract. Isolated stomach discomforts and nausea can occur.
For daily dosages above 100 mg glycyrrhizin:
Extended use and higher dosages can cause mineralocorticoid effects, such as sodium and water retention, loss of potassium coupled with high blood pressure, edema and hypokalemia with weakness of the muscles, and, in rare cases, myoglobinuria. Occasionally allergic reactions involving skin, respiratory tract and gastrointestinal tract. Isolated stomach discomforts and nausea can occur.

Interactions with Other Drugs
For daily dosages below 100 mg glycyrrhizin:
None known.
For daily dosages above 100 mg glycyrrhizin:
Loss of potassium due to other medications, e.g., thiazide and loop diuretics, can be increased. Loss of potassium can increase the sensitivity to digitalis glycosides.

Note: The absorption of other, simultaneously administered drugs can be delayed.

Dosage
Unless otherwise prescribed:
Marshmallow root must be present in the dosage given in its monograph.
Licorice root, primrose root, and anise must be at the concentration of 30 - 50 percent of the daily dosage given in the individual monographs.
Deviating dosages must be justified specifically for the preparation.

Mode of Administration
Liquid and solid forms of preparations for oral use.

Duration of Administration
Without medical advice, not longer than 4 - 6 weeks.

Actions
An expectorant effect is documented for Licorice root, primrose root and anise seed. In addition, a secretolytic action is shown for licorice root and primrose root. Anise has an antibacterial and mild antispasmodic action; marshmallow root has a soothing action and inhibits ciliary activity in vitro. Pharmacological experiments for the fixed combinations are not available.

Fixed Combinations of Marshmallow root, Fennel seed, Iceland moss, and Thyme
Published April 4, 1992

Composition of Drug
Fixed combinations consisting of:
Marshmallow root corresponding to
  B. Anz. 43, March 2, 1989;
Fennel seed corresponding to
  B. Anz. 74, April 19, 1991;
Iceland moss corresponding to
  B. Anz. 43, March 2, 1989;
Thyme corresponding to
  B. Anz. 228, December 5, 1984;
and their preparations in
  effective dosage.

Uses
Colds and diseases of the upper respiratory tract with dry cough.

Contraindications
Pregnancy:
  Other preparations of fennel, except for teas and preparations with essential oil contents comparative to teas.

Side Effects
In individual cases, allergic reactions of the skin and respiratory tract.

Interactions with Other Drugs
None known.
Warning: The absorption of other, simultaneously taken drugs can be delayed.

Dosage
Unless otherwise prescribed:
  Marshmallow root and Iceland moss must each be present at 50 - 75 percent of the daily dosage given in the monographs for the individual herbs. Also, fennel and thyme must each be present at 50 - 75 percent of the daily dosage given in the monographs for the individual herbs.

Mode of Administration
Comminuted drug and galenical preparations for oral intake.

Duration of Use
Preparations of fennel should not be taken over an extended period of time (several weeks) without consultation with a physician or pharmacist.

Actions

A bronchospasmolytic action is demonstrated for preparations of thyme and fennel seed. Marshmallow root and Iceland moss have a soothing effect. Thyme and Iceland moss have antibacterial action, and thyme, in addition, has an expectorant action. Pharmacological tests for the effectiveness of fixed combinations are not available.

Fixed Combinations of Marshmallow root, Primrose root, Licorice root, and Thyme oil
Published April 4, 1992

Composition of Drug
Fixed combinations of:
  Marshmallow root corresponding to
    B. Anz. 43, March 2, 1989;
  Primrose root corresponding to
    B. Anz. 122, July 6, 1989;
  Licorice root corresponding to
    B. Anz. 90, May 15, 1985;
  Thyme oil corresponding to
    B. Anz. 228, December 5, 1984;
  and their preparations in effective
    dosage.

Uses
Catarrhs of the upper respiratory tract with dry cough.

Contraindications
For a daily dosage up to 100 mg glycyrrhizin:
  None known.
For a daily dosage of more than 100 mg glycyrrhizin:
  Cholestatic liver diseases, liver cirrhosis, hypertonia, hypokalemia, severe kidney insufficiency, pregnancy.

Side Effects
For a daily dosage up to 100 mg glycyrrhizin:
  Isolated cases of gastric discomfort and nausea.
For a daily dosage of more than 100 mg glycyrrhizin:
  Extended administration and higher dosages may cause mineralocorticoid effects in the form of sodium and water retention, loss of potassium with hypertonia, edema, and hypokalemia with muscular asthenia, and in rare cases, myoglobinuria. Isolated cases of gastric discomfort and nausea.

Interactions with Other Drugs
For a daily dosage up to 100 mg glycyrrhizin:
  None known.
Warning: The absorption of other, simultaneously taken drugs can be delayed.
For a daily dosage of more than 100 mg glycyrrhizin:
  Loss of potassium through other medications can be increased, e.g., thiazide and loop diuretics. The sensitivity toward digitalis glycosides increases with loss of potassium.
Warning: The absorption of other, simultaneously taken medications can be delayed.

Dosage
Unless otherwise prescribed:
  Marshmallow root must be present at the concentration given in the monograph. Licorice root, primrose root, and

thyme oil must each be present at 30 - 50 percent of the daily dosage given in the monographs for the individual herbs.

Mode of Administration
Liquid and solid forms of administration for oral intake.

Duration of Use
Not longer than 4 - 6 weeks without the advice of a physician.

Actions
An expectorant effect is documented for licorice root, primrose root, and thyme oil; for licorice root and primrose root, also a secretolytic action. In addition, thyme oil has a soothing effect and inhibits mucociliary activity in-vitro. Pharmacological tests for the effectiveness of fixed combinations are not available.

Fixed Combinations of Milk Thistle fruit, Peppermint leaf, and Wormwood
Published December 18, 1991

Name of Drug
Fixed combinations of milk thistle fruit, peppermint leaf, and wormwood.

Composition of Drug
Fixed combinations consisting of:
Milk Thistle fruit corresponding to
B. Anz. 50, March 13, 1986;
Peppermint leaf corresponding to
B. Anz. 223, November 30, 1985;
Wormwood corresponding to
B. Anz. 228, December 5, 1984;
and their preparations in effective dosage.

Uses
Dyspeptic discomfort, especially functional disorders of the biliary tract.

Contraindications
In case of gallstones, to be taken only after consultation with a physician or pharmacist.

Side Effects
None known.

Interaction with Other Drugs
None known.

Dosage
Unless otherwise prescribed:
The components of the combination must each be present at 30 - 50 percent of the daily dosage given in the monographs for the individual herbs.

Deviating dosages must be justified for the specific preparation (e.g., comparative bitter values).

Mode of Administration
Comminuted drug and galenical preparations thereof for oral use.

Actions
A choleretic and carminative effect is documented for preparations of milk thistle fruit, peppermint leaf, and wormwood. Peppermint leaf also has a spasmolytic action. Pharmacological tests for the effectiveness of fixed combinations are not available.

Fixed Combinations of Passionflower herb, Valerian root, and Lemon Balm

Published May 25, 1991

Name of Drug
Fixed combinations of passionflower herb, valerian root, and lemon balm

Composition of Drug
Fixed combinations consisting of:
Passionflower herb corresponding to November 11, 1985 (B. Anz. p. 14335);
Valerian root corresponding to May 6, 1985 (B. Anz. p. 4953);
Lemon balm corresponding to November 1, 1984 (B. Anz. p. 13327);
and their preparations in effective dosage.

Uses
Conditions of unrest, difficulty in falling asleep due to nervousness.

Contraindications
None known.

Side Effects
None known.

Interactions with Other Drugs
None known.

Dosage
Unless otherwise prescribed:
The individual components must each be present at 30 - 50 percent of the daily dosage given in the monographs for the individual herbs.

Mode of Administration
Comminuted drug for teas and other galenical preparations for oral intake.

Actions
A sedative, sleep-promoting effectiveness is documented for preparations of lemon balm, passionflower herb, and valerian root. Pharmacological tests for the effectiveness of the fixed combination are not available.

Effects on Operators of Vehicles or Machinery
Medications with sleep-promoting actions can change the ability to react, so that participation in traffic or operation of machinery is impaired, even when taken under strict direction.

This action is enhanced in combination with alcohol.

Fixed Combinations of Peppermint leaf and Caraway seed

Published August 13, 1991

Composition of Drug
Fixed combinations consisting of:
Peppermint leaf corresponding to November 11, 1985 (B. Anz. p. 14335);
Caraway seed corresponding to December 14, 1989 (B. Anz. 22a, February 1, 1990);
and their preparations in effective dosage.

Uses
Dyspeptic discomfort, especially with mild spasms in the gastrointestinal region, flatulence, and a sensation of fullness.

Contraindications
In case of gallbladder disease, only to be used after consultation with a physician or pharmacist.

Side Effects
None known.

Interactions with Other Drugs
None known.

Dosage
Unless otherwise prescribed:
The individual components of the combination must be equivalent to 50 - 75 percent of the daily dosage given in the monographs for the individual herbs.

Mode of Administration
Comminuted drug for teas and other galenical preparations for oral use.

Actions
A spasmolytic and carminative effect is documented for peppermint leaf and caraway seed. Pharmacological tests for the effectiveness of fixed combinations are not available.

Fixed Combinations of Peppermint leaf, Caraway seed, and Fennel seed

Published August 13, 1991

Composition of Drug
Fixed combinations consisting of:
Peppermint leaf corresponding to November 11, 1985 (B. Anz. p. 14335);
Caraway seed corresponding to December 14, 1989 (B. Anz. 22a, February 1, 1990);
Fennel seed corresponding to March 11, 1991 (B. Anz. p. 2742);
and their preparations in effective dosage.

Uses
Dyspeptic discomfort, especially with mild spasms in the gastrointestinal region, flatulence, and a sensation of fullness.

Contraindications
In case of gallbladder disease, only to be used after consultation with a physician or pharmacist.
Pregnancy:
Preparations other than teas and preparations with essential oil contents comparable to those of teas.

Side Effects
In individual cases, allergic reactions to the skin and respiratory tract.

Interactions with Other Drugs
None known.

Dosage
Unless otherwise prescribed:
The individual components of the combination must be equivalent to 30 - 50 percent of the daily dosage given in the monographs for the individual herbs.

Mode of Administration
Comminuted drug for teas and other galenical preparations for oral use.

Duration of Application
Fennel seed preparations should not be used over extended time periods (several weeks) without consultation with a physician or pharmacist.

Actions
A spasmolytic and carminative effect is documented for peppermint leaf, caraway seed, and fennel seed. Pharmacological tests for the effectiveness of fixed combinations are not available.

Fixed Combinations of Peppermint leaf, Caraway seed, and Chamomile flower
Published August 13, 1991

Composition of Drug
Fixed combinations consisting of:
Peppermint leaf corresponding to November 11, 1985 (B. Anz. p. 14335);
Caraway seed corresponding to publication of December 14, 1989 (B. Anz. 22a, February 1, 1990);
Chamomile flower corresponding to publication of November 1, 1984 (B. Anz. p. 13327);
and their preparations in effective dosage.

Uses
Dyspeptic discomfort, especially with mild spasms in the gastrointestinal region, flatulence, and a sensation of fullness.

Contraindications
In case of gallbladder disease, only to be used after consultation with a physician or pharmacist.

Side Effects
None known.

Interactions with Other Drugs
None known.

Dosage
Unless otherwise prescribed:
The individual components of the combination must be equivalent to 30 - 50 percent of the daily dosage given in the monographs for the individual herbs.

Mode of Administration
Comminuted drug for teas and other galenical preparations for oral use.

Actions
A spasmolytic and carminative effect is documented for peppermint leaf, caraway seed, and chamomile flower. Pharmacological tests for the effectiveness of fixed combinations are not available.

Fixed Combinations of Peppermint leaf, Caraway seed, Chamomile flower, and Bitter Orange peel
Published December 18, 1991

Name of Drug
Fixed combinations of peppermint leaf, caraway seed, chamomile flower, and bitter orange peel.

Composition of Drug
Fixed combinations consisting of:
Peppermint leaf corresponding to November 11, 1985 (B. Anz. p. 14335);
Caraway seed corresponding to December 14, 1989 (B. Anz. 22a, February 1, 1990);
Chamomile flower corresponding to November 1, 1984 (B. Anz. p. 13327);
Bitter orange peel corresponding to October 15, 1987 (B. Anz. 193);
and their preparations in effective dosage.

Uses
Loss of appetite; dyspeptic discomfort, such as sensation of fullness and flatulence.

Contraindications
In case of gallbladder disease, only to be used after consultation with a physician or pharmacist.

Side Effects
Furanocoumarins contained in this preparation render the skin light sensitive, which, in connection with exposure to UV light may cause inflammation of the skin. For the duration of administration of bitter orange peel or preparations thereof, extended exposure to sun and UV light should be avoided.

Interactions with Other Drugs
None known.

Dosage
Unless otherwise prescribed:
The individual components of the combination must be equivalent to 25 - 40 percent of the daily dosage given in the monographs for the individual herbs.

Mode of Administration
Comminuted drug for teas and other galenical preparations for oral use.

Actions
A spasmolytic effect is documented for preparations of peppermint leaf, caraway seed, and chamomile flower; a carminative effect for peppermint leaf and bitter orange peel. Pharmacological tests for the effectiveness of fixed combinations are not available.

Fixed Combinations of Peppermint leaf, Caraway seed, Fennel seed, and Chamomile flower
Published August 13, 1991

Composition of Drug
Fixed combinations consisting of:
Peppermint leaf corresponding to November 11, 1985 (B. Anz. p. 14335);
Caraway seed corresponding to December 14, 1989 (B. Anz. 22a, February 1, 1990);
Fennel seed corresponding to March 11, 1991 (B. Anz. p. 2742);
Chamomile flower corresponding to November 1, 1984 (B. Anz. p. 13327);
and their preparations in effective dosage.

Uses
Dyspeptic discomfort, especially with mild spasms in the gastrointestinal region, flatulence, and a sensation of fullness.

Contraindications
In case of gallbladder disease, only to be used after consultation with a physician or pharmacist.
Pregnancy:
Preparations other than teas and preparations with essential oil contents comparable to those of teas.

Side Effects
In individual cases, allergic reactions of the skin and respiratory tract.

Interactions with Other Drugs
None known.

Dosage
Unless otherwise prescribed:
The individual components of the combination must be equivalent to 20 - 40 percent of the daily dosage given in the monographs for the individual herbs.

Mode of Administration
Comminuted drug for teas and other galenical preparations for oral use.

Duration of Application
Fennel preparations should not be used over extended time periods (several weeks) without consultation with a physician or pharmacist.

Actions
A spasmolytic and carminative effect is documented for peppermint leaf, caraway seed, fennel seed, and chamomile flower. Pharmacological tests for the effectiveness of fixed combinations are not available.

Fixed Combinations of Peppermint leaf and Fennel seed

Published August 13, 1991

Composition of Drug
Fixed combinations consisting of:
  Peppermint leaf corresponding to November 11, 1985 (B. Anz. p. 14335);
  Fennel seed corresponding to March 11, 1991 (B. Anz. p. 2742);
  and their preparations in effective dosage.

Indications
Dyspeptic discomfort, especially with mild spasms in the gastrointestinal region, flatulence, and a sensation of fullness.

Contraindications
In case of gallbladder disease, only to be used after consultation with a physician or pharmacist.
Pregnancy:
  Preparations other than teas and preparations with essential oil contents comparable to those of teas.

Side Effects
In individual cases, allergic reactions to the skin and respiratory tract.

Interactions with Other Drugs
None known.

Dosage
Unless otherwise prescribed:
  The individual components of the combination must be equivalent to 50 - 75 percent of the daily dosage given in the monographs for the individual herbs.

Mode of Administration
Comminuted drug for teas and other galenical preparations for oral use.

Duration of Application
Fennel preparations should not be used over extended time periods (several weeks) without consultation with a physician or pharmacist.

Actions
A spasmolytic and carminative effect is documented for peppermint leaf and fennel seed. Pharmacological tests for the effectiveness of fixed combinations are not available.

Fixed Combinations of Peppermint leaf, Fennel seed, and Chamomile flower

Published August 13, 1991

Composition of Drug
Fixed combinations consisting of:
  Peppermint leaf corresponding to November 11, 1985 (B. Anz. p. 14335);
  Fennel seed corresponding to March 11, 1991 (B. Anz. p. 2742);
  Chamomile flower corresponding to publication of November 1, 1984 (B. Anz. p. 13327);
  and their preparations in effective dosage.

Uses
Dyspeptic discomfort, especially with mild spasms in the gastrointestinal region, flatulence, and a sensation of fullness.

Contraindications
In case of gallbladder disease, only to be used after consultation with a physician or pharmacist.
Pregnancy:
> Preparations other than teas and essential oil contents comparable to those of teas.

Side Effects
In individual cases, allergic reactions to the skin and respiratory tract.

Interactions with Other Drugs
None known.

Dosage
Unless otherwise prescribed:
> The individual components of the combination must be equivalent to 30 - 50 percent of the daily dosage given in the monographs for the individual herbs.

Mode of Administration
Comminuted drug for teas and other galenical preparations for oral use.

Duration of Application
Fennel preparations should not be used over extended time periods (several weeks) without consultation with a physician or pharmacist.

Actions
A spasmolytic and carminative effect is documented for peppermint leaf and fennel seed. Pharmacological tests for the effectiveness of fixed combinations are not available.

Fixed Combinations of Peppermint leaf, German Chamomile flower, and Caraway seed
Published February 27, 1991

Name of Drug
Fixed combinations of peppermint leaf, chamomile flower and caraway seed.

Composition of Drug
Fixed combinations consisting of:
> Peppermint leaf corresponding to the monograph published November 30, 1985;
> Chamomile flower corresponding to the monograph published December 5, 1984;
> Caraway seed corresponding to the monograph published February 1, 1990;
> as well as their preparations in effective dosage.

Uses
Dyspeptic discomforts, particularly with mild spasms in the area of the gastrointestinal tract, flatulence, feeling of fullness.

Contraindications
None known.

Side Effects
None known.

Interactions with Other Drugs
None known.

Dosage
Unless otherwise prescribed:
> The individual combination components must be at a concentration of 30 - 50 percent of the daily or single dosage given in the monograph for the single drug.
> Deviating dosages must be specifically justified for each preparation.

Mode of Administration
Comminuted drug for tea and other galenical preparations for oral applications.

Action
An antispasmodic action is documented for preparations of peppermint leaf, chamomile, and caraway. Pharmacological experiments concerning the action of the fixed combinations are not available.

Fixed Combinations of Peppermint oil and Caraway oil
Published August 13, 1991

Composition of Drug
Fixed combinations consisting of:
> Peppermint oil corresponding to February 18, 1986 (B. Anz. p. 3077);
> Caraway oil corresponding to December 14, 1989 (B. Anz. 22a, February 1, 1990);
> and their preparations in effective dosage.

Uses
Dyspeptic discomfort, especially with mild spasms in the gastrointestinal region, flatulence, sensation of fullness.

Contraindications
Obstruction of biliary tract, cholecystitis, severe liver diseases. In case of gallbladder disease, only to be used after consultation with a physician or pharmacist.

Side Effects
Sensitive individuals may experience gastric discomfort.

Interactions with Other Drugs
None known.

Dosage
Unless otherwise prescribed:
> The individual components of the combination must be equivalent to 50 - 75 percent of the daily dosage given in the monographs for individual herbs.

Mode of Administration
Essential oils and other galenical preparations thereof for oral use.

Actions
A spasmolytic, carminative and antibacterial effect is documented for peppermint oil and caraway oil. Pharmacological tests for the effectiveness of fixed combinations are not available.

Fixed Combinations of Peppermint oil, Caraway oil, and Chamomile flower

Published August 13, 1991

Composition of Drug

Fixed combinations consisting of:
Peppermint oil corresponding to February 18, 1986 (*B. Anz.* p. 3077);
Caraway oil corresponding to December 14, 1989 (*B. Anz.* 22a, February 1, 1990);
Chamomile flower corresponding to November 1, 1984 (*B. Anz.* p. 13327);
and their preparations in effective dosage.

Uses

Dyspeptic discomfort, especially with mild spasms in the gastrointestinal region, flatulence, and a sensation of fullness.

Contraindications

Obstruction of biliary tract, cholecystitis, severe liver diseases. If suffering from gallstones, to be used only after consultation with a physician or pharmacist.

Side Effects

Sensitive individuals may experience gastric discomfort.

Interactions with Other Drugs

None known.

Dosage

Unless otherwise prescribed:
The individual components of the combination must be equivalent to 30 - 50 percent of the daily dosage given in the monographs for the individual herbs.

Mode of Administration

Essential oil, comminuted drug, and galenical preparations thereof for oral use.

Actions

A spasmolytic, carminative, and antibacterial effect is documented for peppermint oil, caraway oil, and chamomile flower. Pharmacological tests for the effectiveness of fixed combinations are not available.

Fixed Combinations of Peppermint oil, Caraway oil, and Fennel oil

Published August 13, 1991

Composition of Drug

Fixed combinations consisting of:
Peppermint oil corresponding to February 18, 1986 (*B. Anz.* p. 3077);
Caraway oil corresponding to December 14, 1989 (*B. Anz.* 22a, February 1, 1990);
Fennel oil corresponding to publication of March 11, 1991 (*B. Anz.* p. 2742);
and their preparations in effective dosage.

Uses
Dyspeptic discomfort, especially with mild spasms in the gastrointestinal region, flatulence, sensation of fullness.

Contraindications
In case of gallbladder disease, only to be used after consultation with a physician or pharmacist.

Not to be used in case of obstruction of biliary tract, cholecystitis, severe liver diseases, pregnancy, for infants and small children.

Side Effects
In individual cases, allergic reactions of the skin and respiratory tract. Sensitive individuals may experience gastric discomfort.

Interactions with Other Drugs
None known.

Dosage
Unless otherwise prescribed:
The individual components of the combination must be equivalent to 30 - 50 percent of the daily dosage given in the monographs for the individual herbs.

Mode of Administration
Essential oil and galenical preparations thereof for oral use.

Duration of Application
Fennel preparations should not be used over extended time periods (several weeks) without consultation with a physician or pharmacist.

Actions
Spasmolytic, carminative and antibacterial effects are documented for peppermint oil, caraway oil, and fennel oil. Pharmacological tests for the effectiveness of fixed combinations are not available.

Fixed Combinations of Peppermint oil, Caraway oil, Fennel oil, and Chamomile flower
Published August 13, 1991

Composition of Drug
Fixed combinations consisting of:
Peppermint oil corresponding to February 18, 1986 (*B. Anz.* p. 3077);
Caraway oil corresponding to December 14, 1989 (*B. Anz.* 22a, February 1, 1990);
Fennel oil corresponding to March 11, 1991 (*B. Anz.* p. 2742);
Chamomile flower corresponding to November 1, 1984 (*B. Anz.* p. 13327);
and their preparations in effective dosage.

Uses
Dyspeptic discomfort, especially with mild spasms in the gastrointestinal region, flatulence, sensation of fullness.

Contraindications
In case of gallbladder disease, only to be used after consultation with a physician or pharmacist.

Not to be used in case of biliary tract obstruction, cholecystitis, severe liver diseases, pregnancy, or for infants and small children.

Side Effects
In individual cases, allergic reactions of the skin and respiratory tract. Sensitive individuals may experience gastric discomfort.

Interactions with Other Drugs
None known.

Dosage
Unless otherwise prescribed:
The individual components of the combination must be equivalent to 25 - 40 percent of the daily dosage given in the monographs for the individual herbs.

Mode of Administration
Essential oil, comminuted drug, and galenical preparations thereof for oral use.

Duration of Application
Fennel preparations should not be used over extended time periods (several weeks) without consultation with a physician or pharmacist.

Actions
Spasmolytic, carminative, and antibacterial effects are documented for peppermint oil, caraway oil, fennel oil, and chamomile flower. Pharmacological tests for the effectiveness of fixed combinations are not available.

Fixed Combinations of Peppermint oil and Fennel oil
Published August 13, 1991

Composition of Drug
Fixed combinations consisting of:
Peppermint oil corresponding to February 18, 1986 (B. Anz. p. 3077);
Fennel oil corresponding to March 11, 1991 (B. Anz. p. 2742);
and their preparations in effective dosage.

Uses
Dyspeptic discomfort, especially with mild spasms in the gastrointestinal region, flatulence, sensation of fullness.

Contraindications
In case of gallbladder disease, only to be used after consultation with a physician or pharmacist.
Not to be used by those suffering from obstruction of the biliary tract, cholecystitis, severe liver damage, pregnancy, or for infants and small children.

Side Effects
In individual cases, allergic reactions of the skin and respiratory tract. Sensitive individuals may experience gastric discomfort.

Interactions with Other Drugs
None known.

Dosage
Unless otherwise prescribed:
The individual components of the combination must be equivalent to 50 - 75 percent of the daily dosage given in the monographs for individual herbs.

Mode of Administration
Essential oil and other galenical preparations thereof for oral use.

Duration of Application
Fennel oil should not be used over extended time periods (several weeks) without consultation with a physician or pharmacist.

Actions
Spasmolytic, carminative and antibacterial effects are documented for preparations of peppermint oil and fennel oil. Pharmacological tests for the effectiveness of fixed combinations are not available.

Fixed Combinations of Peppermint oil, Fennel oil, and Chamomile flower
Published August 13, 1991

Composition of Drug
Fixed combinations consisting of:
Peppermint oil corresponding to February 18, 1986 (B. Anz. p. 3077);
Fennel oil corresponding to March 11, 1991 (B. Anz. p. 2742);
Chamomile flower corresponding to November 1, 1984 (B. Anz. p. 13327);
and their preparations in effective dosage.

Uses
Dyspeptic discomfort, especially with mild spasms in the gastrointestinal region, flatulence, and a sensation of fullness.

Contraindications
In case of gallbladder disease, only to be used after consultation with a physician or pharmacist.
Not be used by those with obstruction of the biliary tract, cholecystitis, severe liver damage, pregnancy, or for infants and small children.

Side Effects
In individual cases allergic reactions of skin and respiratory tract. Sensitive individuals may experience gastric discomfort.

Interactions with Other Drugs
None known.

Dosage
Unless otherwise prescribed:
The individual components of the combination must be equivalent to 30 - 50 percent of the daily dosage given in the monographs for the individual herbs.

Mode of Administration
Essential oil, comminuted drug, and other galenical preparations for oral use.

Duration of Application
Fennel oil should not be used over extended time periods (several weeks) without consultation with a physician or pharmacist.

Actions
Spasmolytic, carminative and antibacterial effects are documented for preparations of peppermint oil, fennel oil, and chamomile flower. Pharmacological tests for the effectiveness of fixed combinations are not available.

Fixed Combinations of Pheasant's Eye fluidextract, Lily-of-the-valley powdered extract, Squill powdered extract, and Oleander leaf powdered extract

Published September 24, 1993

Name of Drug

Fixed combinations of Pheasant's Eye fluidextract, Lily-of-the-valley powdered extract, Squill powdered extract, and Oleander leaf powdered extract.

Composition of Drug

Fixed combinations consisting of:

Pheasant's Eye fluidextract obtained by extracting the herb with 80 percent ethanol after preconditioning with 80 percent ethanol and calcium hydroxide (herb: native extract = 3.2:1). The extract contains at least 0.1 percent total glycosides calculated as cymarin, determined as the sum of all glycosides obtained by HPLC. Total glycosides comprise 3 - 20 percent adonitoxin and 1 - 10 percent cymarin. The fluidextract has a potency on guinea pigs of 1.2 - 9.6 mg/g (related to cymarin).

Lily-of-the-valley dry extract obtained by extracting the herb after preconditioning with 92 - 96 percent ethanol and calcium hydroxide (herb: native extract=14.5 - 17.5:1). The dry extract contains at least 0.4 percent total glycosides calculated as convallatoxin, determined as the sum of all glycosides obtained by HPLC. The total glycosides comprise 4 - 35 percent convallatoxin, 1.5 - 20 percent sarhamnolosid, 10 - 20 percent desglucocheirotoxol and 1 - 25 percent desglucocheirotoxin. The dry extract has a potency on guinea pigs of 6.2 - 37.2 mg/g (related to convallatoxin).

Squill bulb fermented with water and then extracted with ethyl acetate (herb: native extract=1000:1). The extract is concentrated and again extracted with ethanol; the residue of the ethanol extract is used. The extract contains at least 25 percent total glycosides calculated as proscillaridin A, determined as the sum of all glycosides obtained by HPLC. The total glycosides comprise 35 - 60 percent proscillaridin A, 8 - 25 percent 19-oxo-proscillaridin and a maximum of 8 percent of other glycosides. The dry extract has a potency on guinea pigs of 346-968 mg/g (related to proscillaridin A).

Oleander dry extract obtained by extracting the leaves after fermentation with water and calcium hydroxide (herb: native extract=10 - 12:1). The dry extract contains at least 1 percent total glycosides calculated as oleandrin, determined as the sum of all glycosides obtained by HPLC. The total glycosides comprise 10-45 percent oleandrin and a maximum of 5 percent gentiobiosyloleandrin. The dry extract has a potency on the guinea pig of 3.45 - 20.7 mg/g (related to oleandrin).

The extracts were mixed corresponding to the guinea pig units (GPU) of 25:15:25:25. The dosage determination of the various forms of administration was based on the experimentally defined therapeutic value of the extract mixture. The formulation of the combinations is as follows:

Solid, single dosed preparations:
  25 GPU Pheasant's Eye fluidextract equivalent to 0.03 mg total glycosides, calculated as cymarin;
  5 GPU Lily-of-the-valley dry extract equivalent to 0.005 mg total glycosides, calculated as convallatoxin;
  25 GPU Squill dry extract equivalent to 0.009 mg total lycosides, calculated as proscillaridin A;
  25 GPU Oleander dry extract equivalent to 0.004 mg total glycosides, calculated as leandrin;
Liquid, not individualized dosage forms/100 ml:
  5000 GPU Pheasant's Eye fluidextract equivalent to 5.99 mg total glycosides, calculated as cymarin;
  3125 GPU Lily-of-the-valley dry extract equivalent to 0.97 mg total glycosides, calculated as convallatoxin;
  5000 GPU Squill dry extract equivalent to 1.73 mg total glycosides, calculated as proscillaridin A;
  5000 GPU Oleander dry extract equivalent to 0.86 mg total glycosides, calculated as leandrin.

Pharmacological Properties, Pharmacokinetics, Toxicology

The principal glycoside of Pheasant's Eye herb is cymarin, of Lily-of-the-valley leaf is convallatoxin, of Squill is proscillaridin A, and of Oleander leaf is oleandrin. The actions of cardiac glycosides on the heart are:
  positive inotropic (increasing contractile strength and velocity while delaying relaxation), negative chronotropic (decreasing the time or rate of contraction), negative dromotropic (decreasing stimulus conduction), positive bathmotropic (increasing stimulation of the ventricular muscle).

Pharmacokinetics

Cymarin:
  The indication for the absorption of cymarin lies between 15 and 47 percent. The half-life of elimination is given as 13-23 hours. Elimination of cymarin occurs mainly by renal discharge. The subsidence rate is 50 percent.
  Recent investigations, particularly of the substance reacting in combinations, are not available.

Convallatoxin:
  For convallatoxin an absorption rate of 10 percent and a subsidence rate of 40 - 50 percent are given. The absorption rate is supposedly increased by saponins contained in the herb. No information is available concerning its metabolism in humans. A renal/biliary excretion is assumed. The binding to plasma proteins lies between 16 and 23 percent.
  Recent investigations, particularly of the substance reacting in combinations, are not available.

Proscillaridin A:
  Proscillaridin A is absorbed at a rate of 20 - 30 percent. The half-life value is 45 - 50 hours. The plasma protein binding is about 85 percent. Proscillaridin A is removed by biliary excretion after conjugation with glucuronic and sulfuric acid. There is an indication for an enterohepatic circulation.
  Recent investigations, particularly of the substance reacting in combinations, are not available.

Oleandrin:
  For oleandrin, an absorption rate of 86 percent is given.
  Recent investigations, particularly of the substance reacting in combinations, are not available.

Clinical Data

Uses

Mild, limited heart action and circulatory instability.

Contraindications
Heart insufficiency NYHA functional levels III and IV, therapy with digitalis glycosides, digitalis intoxication, hypercalcemia, potassium deficiency, bradycardia, ventricular tachycardia.

Side Effects
Nausea, vomiting, gastric disorders, diarrhea, irregular pulse, and cardiac dysrhythmia may occur.

Special Caution for Use
Caution in case of stimulus conduction disorders and i.v. calcium therapy.

Use During Pregnancy and Lactation
None known.

Interactions with Other Drugs
Increased effectiveness and thus also increased side effects with concurrently administered quinidine, calcium, saluretics, laxatives, and long-term therapy with glucocorticoids.

Dosage
Unless otherwise prescribed:
Daily dosage of adults:
Solid, individually dosed preparations:
  equivalent to 270 - 540 GPU;
Liquid, not individually dosed preparations:
  equivalent to 310 GPU.

Mode of Administration
Aqueous-alcoholic solutions and solid preparations for oral use.

Overdosage
Corresponding overdosage will result in basically the same symptoms as obtained with digitalis intoxication.

Main symptoms are disturbances of the heart rhythm, gastrointestinal and central nervous symptoms.

The sequence of therapeutic action depends on the severity of intoxication. For slight overdosing, discontinuation of the glycoside and careful monitoring of the patient would be sufficient.

Influences which lead to changes in digitalis tolerance are to be avoided or corrected (disturbances of the electrolyte, acid and base balance)

Patients with dangerous cardiac irregularity should be admitted to intensive care units and placed on monitors.

Depending on clinical situations, the following drugs may be administered:

For hypokalemia, the serum potassium level must be raised to the high normal range (KI:AV-block).

In the case of severe intoxication, often dangerous hyperkalemia occurs initially. For the treatment of this hyperkalemia, intravenous infusions of high concentrations of glucose with insulin are indicated.

For complex ventricular arrhythmias, diphenylhydantoin (phenytoin sodium) or lidocaine should be administered.

For bradycardiac rhythmic disturbances, parasympatholytics are applied, e.g., atropine, ipatropium bromide. If necessary, a transvenous pacemaker is temporarily implanted.

Life-threatening intoxications:
  Ingestion of extreme dosages, accidentally or with suicidal intent, basic poison elimination is indicated: irrigation of the stomach after initial application of atropine, followed by active charcoal, cholestyramin or cholestipol.

Forced diuresis, peritoneal- and hemodialysis have proven to be unsuccessful for digoxin elimination.

Special Warnings
None known.

Fixed Combinations of Primrose root, Marshmallow root, and Anise seed

Published March 11, 1992

Name of Drug
Fixed combinations of primrose root [*Primula*, not *Oenothera* (evening primrose)], marshmallow root, and anise seed.

Composition of Drug
Fixed combinations consisting of:
Primrose root corresponding to the monograph published April 11, 1988;
Marshmallow root corresponding to the monograph published January 5, 1989;
Anise seed corresponding to the monograph published April 11, 1988;
as well as their preparations in effective dosage.

Uses
Catarrh of the upper respiratory tract and resulting dry cough.

Contraindications
Hypersensitivity to anise and anethole.

Side Effects
Occasionally allergic reactions involving skin, respiratory tract and gastrointestinal tract. Isolated stomach discomforts and nausea can occur.

Interactions with Other Drugs
Note: The absorption of other, simultaneously administered medicines can be delayed.

Dosage
Unless otherwise prescribed:
Marshmallow root must be present in the dosage given in its monograph.
Primrose root and anise must be at the concentration of 50 - 75 percent of the daily dosage given in the individual monographs.
Deviating dosages must be justified specifically for the preparation.

Mode of Administration
Liquid and solid forms of preparations for oral use.

Actions
An expectorant effect is documented for primrose root and anise seed; in addition, a secretolytic action is shown for primrose root. Anise has an antibacterial and mild antispasmodic action, marshmallow root has a soothing action and inhibits ciliary activity in vitro. Pharmacological experiments for the fixed combinations are not available.

Fixed Combinations of Primrose root, Sundew, and Thyme

Published April 4, 1992

Composition of Drug
Fixed combinations consisting of:
Primrose root corresponding to
B. Anz. 122, July 6, 1988;
Sundew corresponding to
B. Anz. 228, December 5, 1984;
Thyme corresponding to
B. Anz. 228, December 5, 1984;
and their preparations in
effective dosage.

Uses
Catarrhs of the respiratory tract with spastic cough.

Contraindications
None known.

Side Effects
Occasionally, gastric discomforts and nausea may occur.

Interactions with Other Drugs
None known.

Dosage
Unless otherwise prescribed:
The individual components of the combination must each be present at 50 - 75 percent of the daily dosage given in the monographs for the individual herbs.

Mode of Administration
Comminuted drug and galenical preparations for oral intake.

Actions
An expectorant effect is documented for preparations of primrose root and thyme. Thyme and sundew have bronchospasmolytic action, primrose root has secretolytic action, and sundew has antitussive action. Pharmacological tests for the effectiveness of fixed combinations are not available.

Fixed Combinations of Primrose root and Thyme

Published April 4, 1992

Composition of Drug
Fixed combinations consisting of:
Primrose root corresponding to
B. Anz. 122, July 6, 1988;
Thyme corresponding to
B. Anz. 228, December 5, 1984;
and their preparations in
effective dosage.

Uses
Colds and disease of the upper respiratory tract with viscous phlegm.

Contraindications
None known.

Side Effects
Occasionally, gastric discomforts and nausea may occur.

Interactions with Other Drugs
None known.

Dosage
Unless otherwise prescribed:
> The individual components of the combination must each be present at 50 - 75 percent of the daily dosage given in the monographs for the individual herbs.

Mode of Administration
Comminuted drug and galenical preparations for oral intake.

Actions
An expectorant effect is documented for preparations of primrose root and thyme. In addition, thyme has antibacterial and bronchospasmolytic action. Primrose root has secretolytic action. Pharmacological tests for the effectiveness of fixed combinations are not available.

Fixed Combinations of Senna leaf and Blonde Psyllium seed husk
Published November 25, 1993

Name of Drug
Fixed combinations of senna leaf and blonde psyllium seed husk.

Composition of Drug
Fixed combinations consisting of:
> Senna leaf corresponding to monograph B. Anz. 133 of July 21, 1993;
> Blonde Psyllium seed husk corresponding to monograph B. Anz. 22a of February 1, 1990;
> as well as their preparations in effective dosage.

Pharmacological Properties, Pharmacokinetics, Toxicology
A laxative effect is documented for preparations of senna leaf and blonde psyllium seed husk; 1,8-dihydroxy-anthracene derivatives have a laxative effect. This effect is based on the sennosides, i.e., on their active metabolite in the colon, rheinanthrone. The effect is primarily caused by the influence on the motility of the colon as an inhibition of stationary and stimulation of propulsive contractions. This results in an accelerated intestinal passage and, because of the shortened contact time, a reduction in liquid absorption. In addition, stimulation of the active chloride secretion increases water and electrolyte content.

Blonde psyllium seed husk has a laxative effect because of bulk formation due to water absorption resulting in an increased filling pressure.

The effectiveness of the combination is additive, resulting from the effects of the combination partners.

Pharmacological studies concerning the effectiveness of the fixed combination are not available.

Clinical Data

1. Uses
Constipation.

2. Contraindications

Pathological narrowings in the gastrointestinal tract, intestinal obstructions, difficult-to-control diabetes mellitus, acutely inflamed intestinal diseases, e.g., Crohn's disease, ulcerative colitis, appendicitis, abdominal pain of unknown origin. Children under 12 years of age.

3. Side Effects

In single incidents, allergic reactions may occur.

Chronic use/abuse:
 loss of electrolytes, especially loss of potassium, albuminuria and hematuria, pigment implantation into the intestinal mucosa (*pseudo melanosis coli*), which is harmless and usually is reversed upon discontinuation of the drug.

Potassium deficiency can lead to disorders of heart function and muscular weakness, especially with concomitant use of heart glycosides, diuretics and corticoadrenal steroids.

4. Special Caution for Use

Stimulating laxatives must not be used over an extended period of time (1 - 2 weeks) without medical advice.

5. Use During Pregnancy and Lactation

Because of insufficient toxicological investigations, this drug should not be used during pregnancy and lactation.

6. Interactions with Other Drugs

With chronic use/abuse:
 due to loss in potassium, an increase in effectiveness of cardiac glycosides and an effect on antiarrhythmic drugs is possible. Potassium deficiency can be increased by simultaneous application of thiazide diuretics, corticoadrenal steroids and licorice root.

Note: A reduction of the dosage of insulin may be necessary for insulin-dependent diabetics.

7. Dosage

Unless otherwise prescribed:
 The individual combination partners must be contained at concentrations of 50 - 75 percent of the daily dosage specified in the respective monographs. The individually correct dosage is the smallest dosage necessary to maintain a soft stool.

Mode of Administration

Solid preparations for oral use.

Note: Intake of copious amounts of fluid must be observed. Also, the fixed combination should not be administered until one-half to one hour after intake of other medications.

Any single dose should be less than the common daily dosage.

8. Overdosage

Actions influencing electrolyte and water balance.

9. Special Warnings

Usage of a stimulating laxative for longer than the recommended short-term application can cause an increase in intestinal sluggishness.

The preparation should only be used if no effects can be obtained through change of diet or usage of bulk-forming products.

10. Effects on Operators of Vehicles and Machinery

None known.

Fixed Combinations of Senna leaf, Peppermint oil, and Caraway oil

Published January 27, 1991; Replaced November 25, 1993

Name of Drug
Fixed combinations of senna leaf, peppermint oil and caraway oil.

Composition of Drug
Fixed combinations consisting of:
Senna leaf, corresponding to monograph B. Anz. 133 of July 21, 1993;
Peppermint oil corresponding to monograph B. Anz. 50 of March 13, 1986;
Caraway oil corresponding to monograph in the B. Anz. 22a of February 1, 1990;
as well as their preparations in effective dosage.

Pharmacological Properties, Pharmacokinetics, Toxicology
1,8-dihydroxy-anthracene derivatives have a laxative effect. This laxative effect is based on the sennosides, i.e., on their active metabolite in the colon, rheinanthrone. The effect is primarily caused by the influence on the motility of the colon as an inhibition of stationary and stimulation of propulsive contractions. This results in an accelerated intestinal passage and, because of the contact time, a reduction in liquid absorption. In addition, stimulation of the active chloride secretion increases the water and electrolyte content.

An antispasmodic action is documented for preparations of peppermint oil and caraway oil.

The effect of the combination is additive-synergistic.

Pharmacological studies concerning the effectiveness of the fixed combination are not available.

Clinical Data

1. Uses
Constipation, especially with spastic-like discomforts.

2. Contraindications
Intestinal obstructions, acutely inflamed intestinal diseases, e.g., Crohn's disease, ulcerative colitis, appendicitis, abdominal pain of unknown origin. Children under 12 years of age. In case of gallstones, to be used only after consultation with a physician.

3. Side Effects
In single incidents, spastic gastrointestinal discomforts. In these cases, a dosage reduction is required.

Chronic use/abuse:
loss of electrolytes, especially loss of potassium, albuminuria and hematuria, pigment implantation into the intestinal mucosa (*pseudomelanosis coli*), which is harmless and usually reverses upon discontinuation of the drug. Potassium deficiency can lead to disorders of heart function and muscular weakness, especially with concurrent use of cardiac glycosides, diuretics and corticoadrenal steroids.

4. Special Caution for Use
Stimulating laxatives must not be used over an extended period of time (1 - 2 weeks) without medical advice.

5. Use During Pregnancy and Lactation
Because of insufficient toxicological investigations, this drug should not be used during pregnancy and lactation.

6. Interactions with Other Drugs
By chronic use/abuse, due to loss in potassium, an increase in effectiveness of cardiac glycosides and an effect on antiarrhythmic drugs is possible. Potassium deficiency can be aggravated by simultaneous administration of the fixed combination and thiazide diuretics, corticoadrenal steroids, or licorice root.

7. Dosage
Unless otherwise prescribed:
   Senna leaf must be contained in the amount specified in the monograph. The essential oils must be present at concentrations of 50 - 70 percent of the daily dosage specified in the respective individual monographs.
   A deviating dosage of the essential oils must be specifically determined for each preparation.
   The individually correct dosage is the smallest dosage necessary to maintain a soft stool.

Mode of Administration
Liquid and solid preparations for oral use.
Note: A single administration should be less than the common daily dosage.

8. Overdosage
Actions influencing electrolyte and water balance.

9. Special Warnings
Usage of a stimulating laxative for longer than the recommended short-term application can cause an increase in intestinal sluggishness. The preparation should be used only if no effects can be obtained through change of diet or usage of bulk-forming products.

10. Effects on Operators of Vehicles and Machinery
None known.

Fixed Combinations of Star Anise seed and Thyme
Published April 4, 1992

Composition of Drug
Fixed combinations consisting of:
   Star anise seed corresponding to B. Anz. 122, July 6, 1988;
   Thyme corresponding to B. Anz. 228, December 5, 1984;
   and their preparations in effective dosage.

Uses
Colds and diseases of the upper respiratory tract.

Contraindications
None known.

Side Effects
None known.

Interactions with Other Drugs
None known.

Dosage
Unless otherwise prescribed:
> The individual components of the combination must each be present at 50 - 75 percent of the daily dosage given in the monographs for the individual herbs.

Mode of Administration
Comminuted drug for teas and other galenical preparations for oral intake.

Actions
A bronchospasmolytic and expectorant effect is documented for preparations of thyme; a bronchosecretolytic effect is documented for star anise seed. Pharmacological tests for the effectiveness of fixed combinations are not available.

Fixed Combinations of Sundew and Thyme
Published April 4, 1992

Composition of Drug
Fixed combinations consisting of:
> Sundew corresponding to
>   B. Anz. 228, December 5, 1984;
> Thyme corresponding to
>   B. Anz. 228, December 5, 1984;
> and their preparations in effective dosage.

Uses
Catarrhs of the respiratory tract with spastic cough.

Contraindications
None known.

Side Effects
None known.

Interactions with Other Drugs
None known.

Dosage
Unless otherwise prescribed:
> The individual components of the combination must each be present at 50 - 75 percent of the daily dosage given in the monographs for the individual herbs.

Mode of Administration
Comminuted drug and galenical preparations for oral intake.

Actions
A bronchospasmolytic effect is documented for preparations of thyme and sundew. Thyme has, in addition, an expectorant and antibacterial action; sundew, an antitussive action. Pharmacological tests for the effectiveness of fixed combinations are not available.

Fixed Combinations of Thyme and White Soapwort root
Published April 4, 1992

Composition of Drug
Fixed combinations consisting of:
  Thyme corresponding to B. Anz. 228, December 5, 1984
  White Soapwort root corresponding to B. Anz. 101, June 1, 1990;
  and their preparations in effective dosage.

Uses
Colds and disease of the upper respiratory tract with viscous phlegm.

Contraindications
None known.

Side Effects
In rare cases, irritation of the gastric mucosa.

Interactions with Other Drugs
None known.

Dosage
Unless otherwise prescribed:
  The individual components of the combination must each be present at 50 - 75 percent of the daily dosage given in the monographs for the individual herbs.

Mode of Administration
Comminuted drug and galenical preparations for oral intake.

Actions
Bronchospasmolytic, expectorant, and antibacterial effects are documented for preparations of thyme; an irritating effect on the mucosal membranes is documented for white soapwort root. Pharmacological tests for the effectiveness of fixed combinations are not available.

Fixed Combinations of Turmeric root and Celandine herb
Published December 12, 1991

Name of Drug
Fixed combinations of turmeric root and celandine herb.

Composition of Drug
Fixed combinations consisting of:
  Turmeric root corresponding to B. Anz. 223, November 30, 1985;
  Celandine herb corresponding to B. Anz. 90, May 15, 1985;
  and their preparations in effective dosage.

Uses
Spastic discomfort in the epigastric region, due to functional disorders of the biliary tract.

Contraindications
Obstruction of the biliary tract. If suffering from gallstones, only to be used after consultation with a physician or pharmacist.

Side Effects
None known.

Interactions with Other Drugs
None known.

Dosage
Unless otherwise prescribed:
The individual components of the combination must be equivalent to the daily dosage given in the monographs for the individual herbs.

Mode of Administration
Fluid and dry extracts for liquid and solid forms of administration for oral intake.

Actions
A choleretic effectiveness is documented for preparations of turmeric root. Indications for a cholecystokinetic action are known. Celandine herb has a confirmed papaverine-like, mildly spasmolytic effect on the upper gastrointestinal tract. Pharmacological tests for the effectiveness of fixed combinations are not available.

Fixed Combinations of Uva Ursi leaf, Goldenrod, and Java tea
Published August 29, 1992

Name of Drug
Fixed combinations of uva ursi leaf, goldenrod herb, and java tea.

Composition of Drug
Fixed combinations consisting of:
Uva ursi leaf corresponding to the monograph published December 5, 1984;
Goldenrod herb corresponding to the monograph published October 15, 1987;
Java tea corresponding to the monograph published March 13, 1986;
as well as their preparations in effective dosage.

Uses
Supportive therapy of inflammatory diseases of the lower urinary tract.

Contraindications
None known.
Note: No irrigation therapy in case of edema due to insufficient heart and kidney function.

Side Effects
Children and patients with a sensitive stomach may experience nausea and vomiting.

Interactions with Other Drugs
Uva ursi preparations should not be given simultaneously with medications designed to acidify the urine.

Dosage
Unless otherwise prescribed:
Uva ursi leaf must be present at a concentration given in the monograph for the single herb. The other combination components must each correspond to a

concentration of 30 - 50 percent of the daily dosage given in the monographs of the single drug.

Mode of Administration
For oral application, comminuted drug or extracts for tea.
Note: Copious intake of fluids must be observed.

Duration of Administration
Not longer than 14 days without the consent of a physician.

Actions
A diuretic and mildly antispasmodic action is documented for goldenrod and Java tea. In addition, goldenrod has an antiphlogistic effect. Uva ursi leaf has a bacteriostatic effect in an alkaline (pH 8) urine, due to the formation of hydroquinone glucuronides and hydroquinone sulfuric acid esters from arbutin by metabolic reactions in the organism. Pharmacological experiments for the fixed combination are not available.

Fixed Combinations of Valerian root and Hops
Published February 27, 1991

Name of Drug
Fixed combinations of valerian root and hops.

Composition of Drug
Fixed combinations consisting of:
Valerian root corresponding to the monograph published May 15, 1985;
Hops corresponding to the monograph published December 5, 1984;
as well as preparations in effective dosage.

Uses
Nervous sleeping disorders, conditions of unrest.

Side Effects
None known.

Interactions with Other Drugs
None known.

Dosage
Unless otherwise prescribed:
The individual combination components must be at a concentration of 50 - 75 percent of the daily or single dosage given in the monograph for the single herb. Deviating dosages must be specifically justified for each preparation.

Mode of Administration
Comminuted drug for tea and other galenical preparations for oral applications.

Actions
A sedative and sleep-promoting action is documented for preparations of valerian and hops. Pharmacological experiments with this combination gave indication of a sedative and sleep-promoting action.

Fixed Combinations of Valerian root, Hops, and Lemon Balm

Published May 8, 1991

Name of Drug
Fixed combinations of valerian root, hops, and lemon balm.

Composition of Drug
Fixed combinations consisting of:
Valerian root corresponding to
B. Anz. 90, May 15, 1985;
Hops corresponding to B. Anz. 228, December 5, 1984;
Lemon Balm corresponding to
B. Anz. 228, December 5, 1984;
and their preparations in effective dosage.

Uses
Difficulty in falling asleep due to nervousness, unrest.

Contraindications
None known.

Side Effects
None known.

Interactions with Other Drugs
None known.

Dosage
Unless otherwise prescribed:
In a combination of two components of the above given three possibilities, the individual combination components must be present at 50 - 75 percent of the daily dosage recommended in the monographs for the individual herbs. In combinations of all three components, each component must be at 30 - 50 percent of the daily dosage recommended in the monographs for the individual herbs.

Mode of Administration
Comminuted drug for teas and other galenical preparations for oral intake.

Action
A sedative, sleep-promoting effectiveness is documented for valerian root, hops, and lemon balm. Pharmacological tests for the effectiveness of the combination indicated a sedative, sleep-promoting effectiveness.

Effects on Operators of Vehicles and Machinery
Medications with sleep-promoting actions can change the ability to react, so that participation in traffic or operation of machinery is impaired, even when taken under strict directions.

This action is enhanced in combination with alcohol.

Fixed Combinations of Valerian root, Hops, and Passionflower herb

Published May 8, 1991

Name of Drug
Fixed combinations of valerian root, hops, and passionflower herb.

Composition of Drug
Fixed combinations consisting of:
   Valerian root corresponding to
      B. Anz. 90, May 15, 1985;
   Hops corresponding to B. Anz. 228,
      December 5, 1984;
   Passionflower herb corresponding
      to B. Anz. 223, November 30, 1985;
   and their preparations in effective
      dosage.

Uses
Difficulty in falling asleep due to nervousness, unrest.

Contraindications
None known.

Side Effects
None known.

Interactions with Other Drugs
None known.

Dosage
Unless otherwise prescribed:
   In combinations of two components of the above given three possibilities, the individual combination components must each be present at 50 - 75 percent of the daily dosage recommended in the monographs for the individual herbs. In combinations of all three components, each component must be at 30 - 50 percent of the daily dosage recommended in the monographs for the individual herbs.

Mode of Administration
Comminuted drug for teas and other galenical preparations for oral intake.

Actions
A sedative, sleep-promoting effectiveness is documented for valerian root, hops, and passionflower herb. Pharmacological tests for the effectiveness of the combination indicated a sedative, sleep-promoting effectiveness.

Effects on Operators of Vehicles and Machinery
Medications with sleep-promoting actions can change the ability to react, so that participation in traffic or operation of machinery is impaired, even when taken under strict directions.
   This action is enhanced in combination with alcohol.

Chapter 5

Unapproved Herbs

The herbs in this section received negative evaluations by Commission E. These evaluations are based on lack of adequate scientific evidence to document current or historical usage and/or the potential or documented risks associated with the herb. Unapproved herb monographs contain a section called "Uses" in which the uses listed refer to observations of historical and/or current use in Germany which were not documented by the available scientific literature. The "Uses" section does not connote approved use by Commission E. See Chapter 11 for an index of Side Effects of Unapproved Herbs and Chapter 13 for an index of Pharmacological Actions of Unapproved Herbs. An index of Contraindications of Unapproved Herbs is located in the Addendum.

Alpine Lady's Mantle herb
Alchemillae alpinae herba
Frauenmantelkraut
Published August 29, 1992

Name of Drug
Alchemillae alpinae herba, alpine lady's mantle herb.

Composition of Drug
Alpine lady's mantle herb consists of the fresh or dried, above-ground parts of *Alchemilla alpina* L. [Fam. Rosaceae], as well as preparations thereof.

Pharmacological Properties, Pharmacokinetics, Toxicology
Not known.

Clinical Data

1. Uses
Preparations of alpine lady's mantle are used as a diuretic, antispasmodic and cardioactive agent, as well as for female complaints.

The effectiveness for the claimed applications is not documented.

2. Risks
None known.

Evaluation
Since the effectiveness for the claimed uses is not documented, a therapeutic application cannot be recommended.

Angelica seed and herb

Angelicae fructus, Angelicae herba
Angelikafrüchte/-kraut
Published June 1, 1990

Name of Drug
Angelicae fructus, angelica seed.
Angelicae herba, angelica herb.

Composition of Drug
Angelica seed consists of the fruit of *Angelica archangelica* L. [Fam. Apiaceae], as well as preparations thereof.
  Angelica herb consists of the above-ground parts of *A. archangelica* L., as well as preparations thereof.

Uses
Preparations of angelica seed and herb are used as a diuretic and diaphoretic. The effectiveness for these applications is not documented.

Risks
The herb contains furanocoumarin, which renders the skin photosensitive.

Evaluation
Since the effectiveness for the claimed uses has not been documented, and considering the risks, a therapeutic application cannot be justified.
[**Ed. note:** Angelica root is an approved herb.]

Ash bark and leaf

Fraxinus excelsior
Esche
Published February 1, 1990

Name of Drug
Fraxini cortex, ash bark.
Fraxini folium, ash leaf.

Composition of Drug
Ash bark consists of the bark of young branches of *Fraxinus excelsior* L. [Fam. Oleaceae], as well as preparations thereof.
  Ash leaf consists of the leaf of *F. excelsior* L., as well as preparations thereof.

Uses
Preparations of ash bark are used for fever and as a tonic. Their effectiveness is not verified. Preparations of ash leaf are used for arthritis, gout, and bladder complaints, as a laxative and as a diuretic.
  The effectiveness for the claimed applications has not been documented.

Risks
None known.

Evaluation
Since the effectiveness for the claimed applications has not been documented, a therapeutic application cannot be recommended.
  The effectiveness of ash in fixed combinations must be verified specifically by each preparation to receive a positive evaluation.

Actions

Preparations of fresh ash bark showed an analgesic, anti-exudative, and antiphlogistic action.

Asparagus herb
Asparagi herba
Spargelkraut
Published July 12, 1991

Name of Drug
Asparagi herba, asparagus herb.

Composition of Drug
Asparagus herb consists of the above-ground parts of *Asparagus officinalis* L. [Fam. Liliaceae], as well as preparations thereof.

Uses
Preparations of asparagus herb are used as a diuretic. The effectiveness for the claimed applications has not been sufficiently documented.

Risks
In rare cases, allergic skin reactions may occur.

Evaluation
Since the efficacy has not been sufficiently documented, a therapeutic application cannot be recommended.

Action
Animal experiments are available that indicate a slight diuretic action.

Barberry
Berberis vulgaris
Berberitze
Published March 2, 1989

Name of Drug
Berberidis fructus, barberry.
Berberidis cortex, barberry bark.
Berberidis radicis cortex, barberry root bark.
Berberidis radix, barberry root.

Composition of Drug
Barberry consists of the fruits of *Berberis vulgaris* L. [Fam. Berberidaceae], as well as preparations thereof.

Barberry bark consists of the bark of the above-ground parts of *B. vulgaris* L., as well as preparations thereof.

Barberry root bark consists of the bark of the underground parts of *B. vulgaris* L., as well as preparations thereof.

Barberry root consists of the underground parts of *B. vulgaris* L., as well as preparations thereof.

Uses

Barberry is used for ailments and discomforts of the kidneys and urinary tract, the gastrointestinal tract, for liver diseases, bronchial discomforts, spleen ailments, spasms, and as a stimulant for the circulatory system.

The effectiveness for the claimed applications is not documented.

Barberry root, bark, and/or root bark are used for ailments and complaints of the gastrointestinal tract, liver, gallbladder, kidney and urinary tract, respiratory tract, and heart and circulatory system, also as a febrifuge and "blood purifier."

The effectiveness for the claimed applications is not documented.

Risks

Barberry fruit:
  None known.
Other parts of *Berberis vulgaris*:
  Other parts of *B. vulgaris* contain alkaloids. The main alkaloid is berberine. Berberine is well tolerated up to 0.5 g. With accidental intake of more than 0.5 g of berberine, the following symptoms have been described:
  Lethargy, nose bleed, dyspnea, skin and eye irritation. Also kidney irritation and nephritis have been reported. Even lethal poisonings have been observed from overdoses of berberine. Disturbances of the gastrointestinal tract with nausea, vomiting and diarrhea have been noted.

The LD_{50} for berberine sulfate in mice is 24.3 mg/kg in intraperitoneal application.

Berberine in small dosages stimulates the respiratory system, while high dosages lead to severe dyspnea and spasms ending in lethal primary paralysis of the respiratory system. Lethal dosages also cause hemorrhagic nephritis.

Death due to respiratory paralysis occurred in anesthetized cats and dogs at 25 mg/kg. In addition, a noticeable inhibition of the heart action was observed.

No reports of poisonings with this herb (i.e., the herb barberry) are known.

Evaluation

Since the effectiveness for the claimed applications is not documented, a therapeutic use of this herb cannot be recommended.

[**Ed. note:** The risks listed above have been observed with the purified alkaloid berberine, not the parts of the herb barberry.]

Basil herb
Basilici herba
Basilikumkraut
Published March 18, 1992

Name of Drug
Basilici herba, basil herb.

Composition of Drug
Basil herb consists of the dried, aboveground parts of *Ocimum basilicum* L. [Fam. Lamiaceae], as well as preparations thereof.

Pharmacological Properties, Pharmacokinetics, Toxicology
In vitro antimicrobial.

Uses

Preparations of basil are used for supportive therapy for feelings of fullness and flatulence, for the stimulation of appetite and digestion, and as a diuretic.

The effectiveness for the claimed applications is not documented.

Risks

The herb contains about 0.5 percent essential oil with up to 85 percent estragole. Estragole, after metabolic activation, has a mutagenic effect. Animal experiments indicated a carcinogenic effect, which demands further investigation. Because of the high estragole content in the essential oil, the herb should not be taken during pregnancy, nursing, by infants or toddlers, or over extended periods of time.

Evaluation

Since the effectiveness for the claimed use is not documented, and because of the risks involved, a therapeutic application cannot be justified.

There is no objection to its use as an aroma or flavor corrigent in preparations containing up to 5 percent.

Bilberry leaf
Myrtilli folium
Heidelbeerblätter
Published April 23, 1987

Name of Drug

Myrtilli folium, bilberry leaf, blueberry leaf.

Composition of Drug

Bilberry leaf consists of the leaf of *Vaccinium myrtillus* L. [Fam. Ericaceae], as well as preparations thereof.

Uses

Bilberry leaf is used for diabetes mellitus, for the prevention and treatment of diseases and complaints of the gastrointestinal tract, kidney and urinary tract, for arthritis, gout, dermatitis, hemorrhoids, poor circulation, functional heart problems, as well as for "metabolic stimulation and blood purification."

The efficacy of the claimed uses has not been documented.

Risks

With higher dosages or on prolonged use, chronic intoxication may arise. The symptoms of chronic intoxication in animal experiments were initially cachexia, anemia, icterus, acute excitation, and disturbances of tonus, which, after chronic administration of 1.5 g/kg/day, could finally end in death.

Evaluation

Since the efficacy has not been documented, a therapeutic use of bilberry leaf preparation is not justifiable in view of the risks involved.

Bishop's Weed fruit
Ammeos visnagae fructus
Ammi-visnaga-Früchte
Published March 13, 1986; Replaced April 15, 1994

Name of Drug
Ammeos visnagae fructus; ammi visnaga berries, bishop's weed.

Composition of Drug
Bishop's weed berries, consisting of the dried ripened berries of *Ammi visnaga* (L.) Lamarck [syn. *A. daucoides* Gaertn.] [Fam. Apiaceae], as well as pharmaceutical preparations of same.

Pharmacological Properties, Pharmacokinetics, Toxicology
The results of pharmacological, pharmacokinetic and toxicological research on one have focused on a dry extract of bishop's weed berries corresponding to 10.5 percent gamma pyrones calculated as khellin (extraction medium: methanol/water 70 - 30, 70 - 99 percent natural extract, drug-extract ratio = 6.2:10.1).

In the modified Langendorff heart preparation for the guinea pig, a slight (8.8 percent) and brief increase of the coronary perfusion (starting with a concentration of 20 µ/ml) was observed to occur within the first 10 minutes.

In rats an increase of the heart minute volume occurs after an infusion of the extract of 1 mg/kg of body weight x min; the effect lasts for about an hour after the infusion has been discontinued.

The heartbeat of rats increases significantly after a 30-minute infusion of 1 mg/kg body weight x min.

KCl - or noradrenalin-induced spasms in the aorta of guinea pigs are relaxed by the extract as well as by the substances khellin, visnadin and visnagin in micromolar concentration in the extract. The extract at its highest concentration (316 µg/ml) causes a 46.3 percent reduction in the K+ spasms and a 64.9 percent reduction in the noradrenalin induced spasms.

After oral administration of 140 mg extract, khellin and visnadin were found in the plasma of six of the test subjects. No traces of visnagin were found; the maximum concentration of khellin was reached between 20 and 60 minutes at 29.4 and 276.5 ng/ml. Elimination occurred quickly; after 10 hours khellin was no longer detectable. For khellin the mean value was C_{max} value of 98.3 ng/ml. The LD_{50} of the extract administered orally is greater than 2000 mg/kg body weight for rats and mice.

After dosing rats with 10, 150 and 6000 mg extract/kg body weight over a period of four weeks, a minimal toxic level was reached at between 10 and 150 mg. After a 600 mg dose had been administered a mild to medium grade centrolobular hypertrophy of the liver parenchym with hepatocellular degeneration occurred.

There are no studies available on chronic toxicity, carcinogenicity, mutagenicity or teratogenicity.

Clinical Data

1. Uses
a) Indications established through research.
b) Claimed areas of use and explanation of rejection.
   Preparations of Bishop's Weed berries are used in the treatment of angina pectoris, coronary insufficiency, paroxsysmal tachycardia, extra systoles, presbycardia with hypertonia, asthma, whooping cough and cramp-like complaints of the abdomen. In

combination preparations Bishop's Weed berries are used as secondary treatments of early ageing in the area of the heart and the circulatory and vascular systems, after cardiac arrest, in nervous complaints of the heart, hypertonia; in bronchitis, bronchial asthma and coughs; spasms of the gastrointestinal tract, gallbladder and urinary tract; in disorders of the hepatobiliary system, kidney stones, tendency to form stones after surgery, kidney insufficiency, in the reduction of hormone-based ureter dilation in the second and third trimesters of pregnancy and on taking contraceptives; as a secondary antibacterial treatment of acute and chronic pyelonephritis in therapy-resistant cases; in climacteric complaints, depressions and in the prevention of hardening of the arteries and accompanying symptoms. The efficacy of the drug in the above-named areas has not been sufficiently proven. (Only one therapeutic observation has been reported.)

2. Risks

In rare cases pseudoallergic reactions, reversible cholostatic icterus/jaundice.

The khellin contained in the drug sensitizes the skin to light. For the duration of the treatment, therefore, long periods of exposure to the sun and concentrated ultraviolet radiation should be avoided.

After higher doses of khellin (100 mg daily administered orally), increased activity of the liver transaminases and of the gamma-glutamyltransferase have been observed.

Evaluation

Due to the insufficiently proven efficacy of the drug and its pharmaceutical preparations, as well as the associated risks, therapeutic use cannot be recommended.

How effective any spasmolytic action of the drug is when used in fixed preparations must be tested and proven for each individual preparation.

[**Ed. note:** This monograph was originally published on March 13, 1986, as approved. Due to new information on potential risks, its status changed to unapproved on April 15, 1994. See page 33.]

Bitter Orange flower
Aurantii flos
Pomeranzenblüten
Published July 14, 1993

Name of Drug

Aurantii flos, bitter orange flower.
Aurantii flos aetheroleum, bitter orange flower oil.

Composition of Drug

Bitter orange flower consists of the dried flowers of *Citrus aurantium* L. subspecies *aurantium* (syn. *C. aurantium* L. ssp. *amara* Engler) [Fam. Rutaceae], as well as preparations thereof in effective dosage.
Bitter orange flower oil consists of the volatile oil of *C. aurantium* L. subspecies *aurantium* (syn. *C. aurantium* L. ssp. *amara* Engler), as well as preparations thereof in effective dosage. The oil is obtained by steam distillation of the fresh, fully opened flowers.

Pharmacological Properties, Pharmacokinetics, Toxicology
Not documented.

Clinical Data

1. Uses
Preparations of orange flower and orange flower oil are used as a preventive measure for gastric and nervous complaints, gout, sore throat, as a sedative, for nervous tension and sleeplessness.

In combinations, orange flower and orange flower oil are mainly used for gastrointestinal disturbances, ulcus duodeni et ventriculi, for constipation, regulation of the lipid level in the blood, lowering the blood sugar in diabetics, blood purification, functional disorders of liver and gallbladder, stimulation of the heart and circulation, diseases of the respiratory tract, colds, frost bite, as a sedative for sleep disorders, kidney and bladder diseases, general feebleness, anemia, imbalances of mineral metabolism, impurities of the skin, loss of hair, and externally for inflammations of the eye (lid, conjunctiva, and cornea), retinal hemorrhage, exhaustion accompanying colds, headaches, neuralgia and muscular pain, rheumatic discomforts, bruises, phlebitis, and decubitus.

The effectiveness for the claimed applications has not been validated.

2. Risks
None known.

Evaluation
Since the effectiveness for the claimed uses has not been demonstrated, a therapeutic application cannot be recommended.

There are no concerns about the use of the herb as a taste or flavor additive.

Blackberry root
Rubi fruticosi radix
Brombeerwurzel
Published February 1, 1990

Name of Drug
Rubi fruticosi radix, blackberry root.

Composition of Drug
Blackberry root consists of the underground parts of *Rubus fruticosus* L. [Fam. Rosaceae], as well as preparations thereof.

Uses
Blackberry root is used as a preventative for dropsy.

The claimed efficacy has not been documented.

Risks
None known.

Evaluation
Since the efficacy has not been documented, a therapeutic application cannot be justified.

Blackthorn flower
Pruni spinosae flos
Schlehdornblüten
Published June 1, 1990

Name of Drug
Pruni spinosae flos, blackthorn flower.

Composition of Drug
Blackthorn flower consists of the dried flowers of *Prunus spinosa* L. [Fam. Rosaceae], as well as preparations thereof.

Uses
Preparations of blackthorn flower are used for common colds, diseases and ailments of the respiratory tract, as a laxative, for diarrhea, for prophylaxis and therapy of gastric spasms, bloating, intestinal diseases and dyspepsia, also for dropsy, ailments of the kidneys and bladder, bladder spasms, as a diuretic, diaphoretic, and for general exhaustion, convalescence, and, externally, for rashes, skin impurities and for "blood purification."

Risks
None known.

Evaluation
Since the effectiveness is not sufficiently documented, a therapeutic application cannot be recommended.

There is no concern for the use of the herb as a coloring agent for tea mixtures.

Bladderwrack
Fucus
Tang
Published June 1, 1990

Name of Drug
Fucus, bladderwrack.

Composition of Drug
Bladderwrack consists of the dried thallus of *Fucus vesiculosus* L. [Fam. Fucaceae], of *Ascophyllum nodosum* Le Jolis [Fam. Fucaceae], or of both species, as well as preparations thereof.

Uses
Preparations of bladderwrack are used for diseases of the thyroid, obesity, overweight, arteriosclerosis and digestive disorders, as well as for "cleansing the blood."

The effectiveness for the claimed applications is not verified.

Risks
Preparations containing a maximum daily dosage of 150 µg of iodine:
None known.

Above the dosage of 150 µg of iodine per day, there is danger that hyperthyroidism may be induced or existing hyperthyroidism may be made worse. In rare cases allergic reactions involving serious overall reactions may occur.

Evaluation

Since the efficacy of a dosage below 150 µg iodine/day has not been substantiated for the conditions listed, therapeutic use of the herb cannot be advocated. In view of the risks, the therapeutic use of doses above 150 µg iodine/day cannot be justified on the grounds of lack of activity.

Borage
Borago
Boretsch
Published July 12, 1991

Name of Drug
Boraginis flos, borage flower.
Boraginis herba, borage herb.

Composition of Drug
Borage flower consists of the flowers of *Borago officinalis* L. [Fam. Boraginaceae], as well as preparations thereof.

Borage herb consists of the fresh or dried, above-ground parts of *B. officinalis* L., as well as preparations thereof.

Uses
Preparations of borage flower and herb are used for blood purification and diuresis, as a preventative for inflammation of the lungs and peritoneum, for arthritis of the joints, as an expectorant, antiinflammatory agent, for pain relief, cardiac tonic, sedative, diaphoretic, for increase of circulatory capacity and for phlebitis, and for menopausal disorders.

The effectiveness for the claimed applications is not documented.

Risks
Borage contains variable amounts of toxic pyrrolizidine alkaloids (PA). Organotoxic, particularly hepatotoxic, effects are known for these alkaloids. Animal experiments showed carcinogenic effects for PA, with a mechanism of action genotoxicity.

Evaluation
Considering the risks and the undocumented effectiveness for the claimed uses, a therapeutic application of borage flower and herb cannot be justified.

Bryonia root
Bryoniae radix
Zaunrübenwurzel
Published July 6, 1988

Name of Drug
Bryoniae radix, bryonia root.

Composition of Drug
Bryonia root consists of the dried taproot of *Bryonia cretica* L. ssp. *dioica* (Jacquin) Tutin and/or *B. alba* L. [Fam. Cucurbitaceae], as well as preparations thereof.

Uses
Bryonia root is used as a laxative, emetic,

and diuretic, also in combinations for various diseases of the gastrointestinal tract, the respiratory tract, for all forms of arthritis, for metabolic disorders, for liver diseases, and as prophylaxis and therapy of acute and chronic infections.

The emetic and laxative effectiveness is undisputed.

The effectiveness of the other applications is not verified.

Risks

The following effects have been observed following ingestion of bryonia root preparations: dizziness, vomiting, severe colic, severe watery and sometimes bloody diarrhea, kidney damage, abortion, nervous excitement, and convulsions.

Bryonia contains cucurbitacins, some of which have strong cytotoxic properties.

Evaluation

Since the effectiveness of bryonia preparations for the claimed applications is not documented, and since the use of it as a drastic laxative and emetic is obsolete, a therapeutic administration cannot be justified because of the risks involved.

Buchu leaf
Barosmae folium
Buccoblätter
Published February 1, 1990

Name of Drug
Barosmae folium, buchu leaf.

Composition of Drug
Buchu leaf consists of the dried leaves of *Barosma betulina* Bartl. (syn. *Agathosma betulina* (Berg) Pill.) [Fam. Rutaceae], as well as preparations thereof.

Uses
Buchu leaf is used for inflammation and infection of the kidneys and urinary tract, for bladder irritations, as a disinfectant of the urinary tract, and as a diuretic.

The effectiveness for the claimed applications is not documented.

Risks
Buchu has essential oil that contains diosmin and pulegone, which can cause irritation. There are no reports of cases of poisoning.

Evaluation
Since the claimed effectiveness has not been documented, the application of buchu leaf cannot be recommended.

The use of buchu leaf as an aroma or flavor corrigent in tea mixture is acceptable.

Burdock root
Bardanae radix
Klettenwurzel
Published February 1, 1990

Name of Drug
Bardanae radix, burdock root.

Composition of Drug
Burdock root contains the fresh or dried, underground parts of *Arctium lappa* L., *A. minus* (Hill) Bernhardi and/or *A. tomentosum* Miller [Fam. Asteraceae], as well as preparations thereof.

Uses
Preparations of burdock root are used for ailments and complaints of the gastrointestinal tract, gout, arthritis, as a diaphoretic and diuretic, as well as for "blood purifying," and externally for ichthyosis, psoriasis, impure skin, and skin diseases.

The claimed efficacies have not been documented.

Risks
None known.

Evaluation
Since the claimed efficacies have not been documented, a therapeutic application cannot be recommended.

Calendula herb
Calendulae herba
Ringelblumenkraut
Published July 14, 1993

Name of Drug
Calendulae herba, calendula herb.

Composition of Drug
Calendula herb consists of the fresh or dried above-ground parts of *Calendula officinalis* L. [Fam. Asteraceae], harvested during flowering season, as well as preparations thereof in effective dosage.

Pharmacological Properties, Pharmacokinetics, Toxicology
Not known.

Clinical Data

1. Uses
Preparations of calendula herb are used as a stimulant for circulation, promotion of healing, as a releasing, lancing and purging agent, as well as for gastric hemorrhage, ulcers, spasms, swelling of the glands, jaundice, anemia, spleen disorders. Topically they are used for putrid or cancerous abscesses, wounds, bleeding and eczema.

In combinations, preparations of calendula herb are used for nausea, loss of appetite, disorders of the gastrointestinal tract and the liver-gallbladder system, as a laxative for metabolic disorders, for stimulation of the liver-gallbladder function, for constitutional abnormalities, blood purification, mobilization of endogenous defense mechanism, for disturbances of the cardiac and circulatory system, arteriosclerosis, heart problems, weakness of the heart muscle, headache, dizziness, tinnitus, conditions of anxiety, abnormal sensation of cold in hands and feet, tiredness, sleeplessness, as support for the bronchial system, preventative for mucous formation and cough, for influenza, stones, hemorrhoids, weak veins, stimulating urination and excretion of uric acid, for dropsy, for prevention of prostatitis, bladder irritation, prostate hypertrophy, ischuria (retention or suppression of urine), epididymitis, gout, rheumatism, abscesses, skin diseases, frostbite, muscular atrophy, dystrophic nervous disturbances, and topically for ulcers of the leg, putrid or slow-to-heal wounds, and for abnormalities of the connective tissue.

The effectiveness for the claimed applications has not been demonstrated.

2. Risks
None known.

Evaluation
Since the effectiveness for the claimed uses has not been demonstrated, a therapeutic application cannot be recommended.

Cat's Foot flower
Antennariae dioicae flos
Katzenpfötchenblüten
Published August 29, 1992

Name of Drug
Antennariae dioicae flos, cat's foot flower (cat's ear flower).

Composition of Drug
Cat's foot flower consists of the fresh or dried flowers of *Antennaria dioica* (L.) Gaertner [Fam. Asteraceae], as well as preparations thereof.

Pharmacological Properties, Pharmacokinetics, Toxicology
None known.

Clinical Data

1. Uses
Preparations of cat's foot flower are used for intestinal diseases. Its effectiveness for the claimed application is not documented.

2. Risks
None known.

Evaluation
Since the effectiveness for the claimed uses is not documented, a therapeutic application cannot be recommended. There is no objection to its use as a brightening agent in teas.

Celery
Apium graveolens
Sellerie
Published July 12, 1991

Name of Drug
Apium graveolens, celery.
Apii radix, celery root.
Apii herba, celery herb.
Apii fructus, celery seed.

Composition of Drug
Celery consists of the fresh, whole plant of *Apium graveolens* L. [Fam. Apiaceae], for the preparation of pressed juice.

Celery root consists of the fresh or dried, underground parts of *A. graveolens* L., as well as preparations thereof.

Celery herb consists of the fresh or dried, above-ground parts of *A. graveolens* L., as well as preparations thereof.

Celery seed consists of the fruits of *A. graveolens* L., as well as preparations thereof.

Uses
Preparations of celery are used as a diuretic, for "blood purification," for regulating elimination of the bowels, for glandular stimulation, rheumatic complaints, gout, stone diseases, for weight loss due to malnutrition, prophylactic for nervous unrest, for loss of appetite and exhaustion.

The effectiveness for the claimed applications is not documented.

Risks
Celery can cause allergic reactions, even ending in anaphylactic shock (celery-carrot-mugwort-syndrome).
Warning: Celery can contain large amounts of phototoxic furanocoumarin.

Evaluation
Since the effectiveness for the claimed uses is not documented, and since an allergic risk exists, a therapeutic application cannot be recommended.

Action
Animal experiments showed indications of a diuretic action.

Chamomile flower, Roman
Chamomillae romanae flos
Römische Kamillenblüten
Published November 25, 1993

Name of Drug
Chamomillae romanae flos, Roman chamomile.

Composition of Drug
Roman chamomile consists of the dried flowers of the cultivated double flowered variety of *Chamaemelum nobile* (L.) Allioni

(syn. *Anthemis nobilis* L.) [Fam. Asteraceae], as well as preparations thereof.

Pharmacological Properties, Pharmacokinetics, Toxicology
Not known.

Clinical Data

1. Uses
a) Uses as a result of evaluation: None.
b) Claimed uses which have been negatively evaluated:
Preparations of Roman chamomile are used for feeling of fullness, bloating and mild spasmodic gastrointestinal disturbances, inflammation of the oral and pharyngeal cavities, gastritis, nasal catarrh, and sinusitis, as well as externally for eczemas, wounds and inflammations.

In combinations, preparations of Roman chamomile are used for liver and gallbladder diseases, cholelithiasis, fatty liver, chronic heartburn, loss of appetite, feeling of fullness, bloating, upset stomach, digestive disturbances, Roemheld's syndrome, fermentative dyspepsia, dyspepsia of infants, spastic constipation, as a "blood purification remedy," as a general tonic during puberty and menopause, as a preventative for menstrual discomforts, for missed periods, painful, insufficient or irregular periods, as well as steam baths for catarrh of the frontal sinus, hay fever, swellings of the nasal and pharyngeal mucosa, inflammation of the ears, and externally for wounds, burns, frostbite, diaper rash on infants and toddlers, decubitus and hemorrhoids.

The effectiveness of the claimed indications is not documented.

2. Risks
Not to be used if allergies to Roman chamomile and other composites exist.

The sensitization potency is moderate, the frequency rare. There are case reports on allergic reactions. Cross reactions with yarrow, German chamomile, lettuce and chrysanthemum have been experimentally observed. Occasionally, a positive reaction to Roman chamomile has been seen in individuals allergic to composites.

One case of anaphylactic shock after ingestion of Roman chamomile tea has been observed. The occurrence of rhinitis is possible in individuals with atopic allergy to mugwort.

Evaluation
Since the effectiveness for the claimed uses is not documented, a therapeutic application cannot be recommended. There is no concern for the use of the herb as a brightening agent (1 percent) in tea mixtures, if the allergic risk is declared.

Chestnut leaf
Castaneae folium
Kastanienblätter
Published April 23, 1987

Name of Drug
Castaneae folium, chestnut leaf.

Composition of Drug
Chestnut leaf consists of the leaf of *Castanea sativa* Miller (syn. *C. vesca*

Gaertner, *C. vulgaris* Lamarck) [Fam. Fagaceae], as well as preparations thereof.

Uses
Chestnut leaf is used for complaints affecting the respiratory tract, such as bronchitis and whooping cough, and for disorders affecting the legs and the circulation.

Effectiveness for the claimed indications has not been documented.

Risks
None known.

Evaluation
Since the effectiveness for the claimed applications has not been documented, a therapeutic administration cannot be recommended.

Cinnamon flower
Cinnamomi flos
Zimtblüten
Published March 11, 1992

Name of Drug
Cinnamomi flos, cinnamon flower.

Composition of Drug
Cinnamon flower consists of the dried flowers of *Cinnamomum aromaticum* Nees (syn. *C. cassia* Blume) [Fam. Lauraceae], collected after withering, as well as preparations thereof.

Uses
Preparations of cinnamon flower are used for "blood purification." The effectiveness for the claimed application is not documented.

Risks
Frequently allergic reactions in skin and mucosa.

Not to be used in case of sensitivity to cinnamon or Peruvian balsam and during pregnancy.

Evaluation
Since the effectiveness for the claimed use is not documented, and because of the risks involved, a therapeutic application cannot be recommended. There is no objection to its use as a flavor corrigent.

Cocoa
Cacao testes
Kakaoschalen
Published February 27, 1991

Name of Drug
Cacao testes, cocoa.

Composition of Drug
Cocoa consists of the testae of *Theobroma cacao* L. [Fam. Sterculiaceae], as well as preparations thereof.

Uses
Preparations of cocoa are used for liver, bladder, and kidney ailments, diabetes, as a tonic and general remedy, and as an astringent for diarrhea.

The effectiveness for the claimed application is not documented.

Risks
Cocoa and cocoa products can cause allergic skin reactions and migraine headaches.

Evaluation
Since the efficacy has not been documented, a therapeutic application cannot be recommended.

Actions
Cocoa can result in constipation.
Cocoa contains methylxanthine, which acts as a diuretic.

Colocynth
Colocynthidis fructus
Koloquinthen
Published September 1, 1990

Name of Drug
Colocynthidis fructus, colocynth.

Composition of Drug
Colocynth consists of the ripe fruit of *Citrullus colocynthis* L. Schrader [Fam. Cucurbitaceae], freed from the outer shell of the pericarp, as well as preparations thereof.

The drug contains cucurbitacin.

Uses
Preparations of colocynth are used exclusively in fixed combinations for acute and chronic constipation of various origins, also during pregnancy and in case of liver and gallbladder ailments.

Colocynth preparations have a drastic laxative effect.

The effectiveness for the other claimed applications is not documented.

Risks
Colocynth contains up to 3 percent cucurbitacin. For the drug and its preparations, drastic irritations of the gastrointestinal mucosa to the extent of hemorrhagic diarrhea are documented. Partial absorption can lead to kidney damage and hemorrhagic cystitis. An abortive action is not known.

Evaluation
The use of colocynth as a drastic laxative can no longer be justified because of the high risks involved.

For the other claimed uses, the application cannot be justified because of risks and undocumented effectiveness.

Coltsfoot
Farfarae flos/-herba/-radix
Huflattichblüten/-kraut/-wurzel
Published July 27, 1990

Name of Drug
Farfarae flos, coltsfoot flower.
Farfarae herba, coltsfoot herb.
Farfarae radix, coltsfoot root.

Composition of Drug
Coltsfoot flower consists of the fresh or dried flowers of *Tussilago farfara* L. [Fam. Asteraceae], as well as preparations thereof.

Coltsfoot herb consists of the fresh or dried above-ground parts of *T. farfara* L., as well as preparations thereof.

Coltsfoot root consists of the fresh or dried underground parts of *T. farfara* L., as well as preparations thereof.

Uses
Preparations of coltsfoot are used for treatment and prevention of diseases and ailments of the respiratory tract, such as cough, hoarseness, bronchial catarrh, acute and chronic bronchitis, asthma, colds, influenza, inflammation and irritation of the oral and pharyngeal mucosa, sore throat, tonsillitis, rickets, swelling of the glands and tuberculosis of the lymph nodes, catarrhs of the gastrointestinal tract, diarrhea, for the stimulation of the metabolism, for "blood purification," as a diuretic and diaphoretic, and externally for wound treatment.

Coltsfoot is contained in tonics with claims of diverse indications.

The effectiveness for the claimed uses is not documented.

Risks
All plant parts of coltsfoot contain pyrrolizidine alkaloids (PA) in greatly varying amounts. Organotoxic, especially hepatotoxic, effects are known for these compounds. Animal experiments proved PA to be carcinogenic with a genotoxic mechanism of action.

Evaluation
In consideration of the risks and lack of documentation for the effectiveness of this herb for the claimed uses, a therapeutic application of coltsfoot flower, herb and root cannot be justified.

Corn Poppy flower
Rhoeados flos
Klatschmohnblüten
Published May 5, 1988

Name of Drug
Rhoeados flos, corn poppy flower.

Composition of Drug
Corn poppy flower consists of the dried petals of *Papaver rhoeas* L. [Fam. Papaveraceae], as well as preparations thereof.

Uses
Corn poppy flower is used for diseases and discomforts of the respiratory tract, for disturbed sleep and as a sedative, and for the relief of pain.

Effectiveness in the conditions indicated has not been established.

Risks
None known.

Evaluation
Since the efficacy of corn poppy flower for its claimed applications is not documented, therapeutic administration cannot be recommended.

There are no concerns regarding the use of this herb as a brightening agent in tea mixtures.

Cornflower
Centaurea cyanus
Kornblume
Published March 2, 1989

Name of Drug
Centaurea cyanus, cyani flos, cornflower, cyani flower.

Composition of Drug
Cornflower flower consists of the dried flowers of *Centaurea cyanus* L. [Fam. Asteraceae], freed from the receptacles and calyces, as well as preparations thereof.

The whole inflorescence and its preparations are also used.

Uses
Cornflower flowers and their preparations are used for fever, menstrual disorders, vaginal candidiasis, as a laxative, tonic, bitter, also as a diuretic and an expectorant, as well as a stimulant for liver and gallbladder function.

The effectiveness for the claimed applications is not documented.

Risks
None known.

Evaluation
Since the effectiveness for the claimed applications is not documented, a therapeutic use of this herb cannot be recommended.

There is no concern regarding the use as a coloring agent in herbal teas.

Damiana leaf and herb
Turnera diffusa
Damianablätter/-kraut
Published March 2, 1989

Name of Drug
Turnerae diffusae folium, damiana leaf. Turnerae diffusae herba, damiana herb.

Composition of Drug
Damiana leaf consists of the leaf of *Turnera diffusa* Willdenow [Fam. Turneraceae],

and its variations, as well as preparations of damiana leaves.

Damiana herb consists of the leaf and branch of *T. diffusa* Willdenow [Fam. Turneraceae], and its variations, as well as preparations of damiana herb.

Uses
Damiana preparations are used as an aphrodisiac, for prophylaxis and treatment of sexual disturbances, for strengthening and stimulation during exertion (overwork), also for boosting and maintaining mental and physical capacity.

The effectiveness for the claimed applications is not verified.

Risks
None known.

Evaluation
Since the effectiveness of Damiana preparations for the claimed applications is not documented, a therapeutic administration cannot be recommended.

Delphinium flower
Delphinii flos
Ritterspornblüten
Published April 27, 1989

Name of Drug
Delphinii flos, delphinium flower.

Composition of Drug
Delphinium flower consists of the flowers of *Delphinium consolida* L. [Fam. Ranunculaceae], as well as preparations thereof.

Uses
Preparations of Delphinium flower are used as a diuretic and vermifuge, as a sedative and an appetite-stimulating remedy. The effectiveness for the claimed applications is not documented.

Risks
Warning: The alkaloids of *Delphinium* lead to bradycardia, lowering of blood pressure, and cardiac arrest. Also, they have a central paralyzing and curare-like effect on the respiratory system.

Dependable information on the alkaloid content in the flowers is not available.

Evaluation
Since the effectiveness of Delphinium and its preparations is not documented, a therapeutic administration cannot be recommended.

There are no objections for its use as a brightening agent (under 1 percent) in tea mixtures.

Dill weed
Anethi herba
Dillkraut
Published October 15, 1987

Name of Drug
Anethi herba, dill herb, dill weed.

Composition of Drug
Dill herb consists of the fresh or dried leaf and upper stem of *Anethum graveolens* L. s.l. [Fam. Apiaceae], as well as preparations thereof.

Uses
Dill herb is used for prevention and treatment of diseases and disorders of the gastrointestinal tract, kidney and urinary tract, for sleep disorders, and for spasms.

The effectiveness of the claimed indications is not documented.

Risks
None known.

Evaluation
Since the effectiveness for the claimed applications is not documented, the therapeutic administration of this herb cannot be recommended.

Echinacea Angustifolia herb and root/Pallida herb
Echinaceae angustifoliae/pallidae herba
Echinaceae angustifoliae radix
schmalblättriges Sonnenhutkraut/blaßfarbenes Kegelblumenkraut
schmalblättriges Sonnenhutwurzel
Published August 29, 1992

Name of Drug
Echinacea angustifolia/pallidae herba, echinacea angustifoliae/pallidae herb; echinacea angustifolia radix, echinacea augustifolia root.

Composition of Drug
The fresh or dried roots, or the fresh or dried above-ground parts collected at the time of flowering, of *Echinacea angustifolia* D. C. [Fam. Asteraceae], as well as their preparations.

The fresh or dried above-ground parts, collected at the time of flowering, of *E. pallida* (Nutt.) Nutt., as well as their preparations.

On the market, preparations of *E. pallida* are to some extent incorrectly labeled as "*Echinacea angustifolia.*"

Pharmacological Properties, Pharmacokinetics, Toxicology
Animal experiment: In the carbon-clearance test, alcoholic root extracts as well as extracts of the above-ground herb show a rate increase in elimination of carbon particles.

In vitro: Alcoholic root extracts show an increase in phagocytic elements of 23 percent when tested in granulocyte smears.

Experiments reported in older publications cannot be definitely assigned to either of these species.

Uses

Preparations of "*Echinacea angustifolia*" are used to support and promote the natural powers of resistance of the body, especially in infectious conditions (influenza and colds, etc.) in the nose and throat, as an alterative in influenza, inflammatory and purulent wounds, abscesses, furuncles, ulcus cruris (indolent leg ulcers), herpes simplex, inflammation of connective tissue, wounds, headaches, metabolic disturbances, diaphoretic, and antiseptic. Activity for the uses listed has not been authenticated.

Risks

Internal use:

Not to be used in systemic diseases such as tuberculosis, leukosis, collagenosis, multiple sclerosis, AIDS, HIV infection, and other autoimmune diseases.

Parenteral use:

Depending upon dosage, chills, short-term fever reactions, nausea and vomiting may occur. In rare cases allergic reactions of the immediate type are possible.

If there is a tendency for allergy, especially against Asteraceae, and during pregnancies, do not apply parenterally.

Warning: The metabolic condition in diabetics can decline upon parenteral application.

Evaluation

Since the activity of the herb for the conditions listed above has not been substantiated, its therapeutic use cannot be recommended. Because of the risks, the use of parenteral preparations is not justified. [**Ed. note:** *Echinacea pallida* root is an approved herb, as is *E. purpurea* herb. The *E. purpurea* root monograph is in the **Unapproved Component Characteristics** section. See Introduction (page 61) for a discussion of positive and negative evaluations of *Echinacea* preparations.]

Elecampane root
Helenii radix
Alantwurzel
Published May 5, 1988

Name of Drug
Helenii radix, elecampane root.

Composition of Drug
Elecampane consists of the dried, cut root and rhizome of *Inula helenium* L. [Fam. Asteraceae], harvested in autumn from 2 - 3-year-old plants, as well as preparations thereof in effective dosage.

The herb contains essential oil and bitter principles.

Uses
Elecampane preparations are used for diseases of the respiratory tract, gastrointestinal tract, and kidney and lower urinary tract.

The effectiveness for the claimed applications has not been adequately documented.

Risks
The sesquiterpene lactones present in ele-

campane, principally alantolactone, irritate the mucous membranes. These lactones are sensitizing and cause allergic contact dermatitis. Alantolactone is bound as a hapten to the proteins of the skin. The adduct induces hypersensitivity to alantolactone and other compounds with a 2-methylene–γ-lactone (cross-reaction). Large amounts of the herb lead to vomiting, diarrhea, cramps, and symptoms of paralysis.

Evaluation
Since the activity of the herb and its preparations in the areas indicated has not been adequately substantiated, in view of the risks of an allergy its therapeutic use cannot be justified.

Ergot
Secale cornutum
Mutterkorn
Published September 18, 1986

Name of Drug
Secale cornutum, ergot.

Composition of Drug
Ergot consists of the sclerotium of *Claviceps purpurea* (Fries) Tulasne [Fam. Clavicipitaceae], grown on rye, as well as preparations thereof.

Uses
Ergot and ergot preparations are used in gynecology and obstetrics, e.g., hemorrhages, climacteric hemorrhages, menorrhagia and metrorrhagia, before and after abortions, for removal of the placenta. These preparations are also used for secondary bleeding and shortening of the afterbirth period, and for atonia of the uterus.

Risks
The alkaloids contained in the drug and its preparations exhibit an extremely differing action spectrum. The application of the alkaloids as, e.g., total extract is not reasonable. Partially synthetically modified ergot alkaloids show far less toxicity at the same or higher specific effectiveness.

Evaluation
Based on the risks, the therapeutic application of ergot and ergot preparations is not justified.

Eyebright
Euphrasia officinalis
Augentrost
Published August 29, 1992

Name of Drug
Euphrasia officinalis, eyebright. Euphrasiae herba, eyebright herb.

Composition of Drug
Eyebright consists of the whole plant of *Euphrasia officinalis* L. p. p. [Fam.

Scrophulariaceae] gathered during flowering season, as well as preparations thereof.

Eyebright herb consists of the fresh or dried, above-ground parts of E. officinalis L. p. p., as well as preparations thereof.

Pharmacological Properties, Pharmacokinetics, Toxicology
Not known.

Clinical Data

1. Uses
Eyebright preparations are used externally as lotions, poultices, and eye-baths, for eye complaints associated with disorders and inflammation of the blood vessels, inflammation of the eyelids and conjunctiva, as a preventive measure against mucus and catarrh of the eyes, "glued" and inflamed eyes, for coughs, colds, catarrh, and as a stomachic and against skin conditions. Activity for the indications listed has not been substantiated.

The effectiveness of the herb for its claimed uses is not documented.

2. Risks
None known.

Evaluation
Since the effectiveness of the herb for its claimed uses is not documented, a therapeutic application cannot be recommended because of hygienic reasons.

Figs
Caricae fructus
Feigen
Published June 1, 1990

Name of Drug
Caricae fructus, figs.

Composition of Drug
Figs consists of the dried fruits of *Ficus carica* L. [Fam. Moraceae], as well as preparations thereof.

Uses
Fig preparations are used as a laxative.
The claimed efficacy has not been sufficiently documented.

Risks
None known.

Evaluation
Since the claimed efficacy has not been sufficiently documented, a therapeutic application cannot be justified. There are no objections to the use of figs as an additive or flavor corrigent.

Ginkgo Biloba leaf
Ginkgo folium
Ginkgoblätter
Published July 19, 1994

Composition of Drug
Ginkgo leaf, ASK No. 05152 and preparations thereof.

Ginkgo leaf, dry extract without further detail, ASK No. 16640.

Ginkgo leaf, dry extract with ethanol/ethanol-water, ASK No. 19769.

Ginkgo leaf, dry extract with methanol/methanol-water, ASK No. 11837.

Ginkgo leaf, fluidextract with ethanol/ethanol-water, ASK No. 09119.

Ginkgo leaf, fluidextract with ethanol/wine, ASK No 12220.

Pharmacological Properties, Pharmacokinetics, Toxicology
There is no adequate scientific data for the pharmacology and toxicology of these preparations.

Clinical Data

1. Uses
Ginkgo leaf and preparations as specified above in monopreparations are applied in arterial circulatory disturbances, cerebral circulatory disturbances, and for deficiencies of cerebral circulation. They are also applied in:

Vertigo, improved circulation and strengthening of circulatory system, especially veins, as a strengthening and stress-relieving agent for the circulation, as a psychopharmaceutical and neurotropic agent.

In compound preparations these additional following syndromes are addressed:

Strengthening of reduced sexual activity, reduced libido, premature ejaculation, sexual neurasthenia, for increased potency, against premature aging, against psychogenic and body-produced mood disturbances, regulation of the pH value of the stomach and intestine, for liver and gallbladder function, for redox potential, cell poisoning, breakdown of fermentation products, for regulation of bacterial flora, restoration of balance to lymph and collateral circulation, increasing blood pressure in hypotonia, heart and circulatory disorders from low blood pressure, hypertension, heart trouble, circulatory problems, complex symptoms related to senile hypertension, arteriosclerosis, treatment of insufficient circulation in the elderly, strengthening of mental and physical performance deficiencies, amelioration of stress and over-strain, return of performance after illness, stimulation against age-related performance deficiencies and lack of concentration.

The efficacy of the preparations described has not been confirmed for the indications claimed.

2. Risks
Due to the content of ginkgolic acids, which are potent contact allergens, an allergic risk is not ruled out.
[**Ed. note:** This applies to various preparations made from the whole leaf. The approved standardized extract has had the ginkgolic acids reduced. For more on this subject, see Gingko section in the Introduction (pages 62 and 63.)]

Evaluation
Since the efficacy of the above preparations for their listed indications has not

been confirmed, no therapeutic application is approved.

[**Ed. note:** An approved ginkgo leaf extract preparation is listed in the **Approved Herbs** section.]

Goat's Rue herb
Galegae officinalis herba
Geißrautenkraut
Published September 24, 1993

Name of Drug
Galegae officinalis herba, goat's rue herb.

Composition of Drug
Goat's rue herb consists of the dried, above-ground parts of *Galega officinalis* L. [Fam. Fabaceae], harvested during the flowering season, as well as preparations thereof.

Pharmacological Properties, Pharmacokinetics, Toxicology
The herb contains galegin, which affects blood sugar. The blood sugar-lowering effect of goat's rue herb has not been documented.

Clinical Data

1. Uses
a) Uses as result of evaluation:
   None.
b) Claimed uses which have been negatively evaluated:
   Preparations of goat's rue herb are used as a diuretic, as well as supportive therapy for diabetes.

In combinations, preparations containing goat's rue herb are also used as a stimulant for the adrenal glands and the pancreas, for "glandular disturbances," for "blood purification," as a purifying remedy for the mesenchyma, for disturbances pertaining to the secretion of digestive fluids in the gastrointestinal tract, fermentative dyspepsia, Roemheld syndrome, diarrhea, abnormal bacterial flora in the colon, as a galactogogue, as an alterative, as a liver-protective remedy, for "status lymphaticus," as well as for exudative diathesis.

The effectiveness for the claimed applications is not documented.

2. Risks
The herb contains galegin, which, like the synthetic guanidine derivatives, has a hypoglycemic action. A therapeutic application for diabetes mellitus, however, cannot be justified because of the uncertain effectiveness of the herb, the severity of the disease, and the therapeutic alternatives available.

Poisoning by goat's rue herb has been observed in grazing animals.

Evaluation
Since the effectiveness for the claimed uses is not documented, a therapeutic application cannot be recommended. It cannot be justified for diabetes mellitus because of the severity of the disease and the availability of effective therapeutic alternatives.

Hawthorn berry
Crataegi fructus
Weißdornfrüchte
Published July 19, 1994

Name of Drug
Crataegi fructus, hawthorn berry.

Composition of Drug
Hawthorn berry consists of the dried fruit of *Crataegus monogyna* Jaquin emend. Lindman or *C. laevigata* (Poiret) de Candolle or others in a valid pharmacopeia citing *Crataegus* [Fam. Rosaceae], as well as preparations thereof.

Pharmacological Properties, Pharmacokinetics, Toxicology
There are no scientific data on which to base the pharmacology and toxicology of the herb. Spectrographic analysis of the chemical constituents of the herb distinguishes only quantitative differences between preparations from the fruit and preparations combining leaf and flower. One may assume pharmacodynamics similar to those shown for the preparation containing both leaf and flower.

Clinical Data

1. Claimed Areas of Application
Preparations of hawthorn berry may be applied to the treatment of coronary circulation, coronary complications and weak heart, heart and circulatory disturbances, hypotension, and arteriosclerosis.

2. Risks
None known.

Evaluation
Since the effectiveness of hawthorn berry for its claimed applications has not been documented, therapeutic use cannot be recommended.

The herb as a water extract, water-alcohol extract, wine infusion and fresh juice has been utilized traditionally to strengthen and invigorate heart and circulatory function.

These statements are based exclusively on historical record and long experience. [**Ed. note:** A preparation from Hawthorn leaf with flower is listed in the **Approved Herbs** section.]

Hawthorn flower
Crataegi flos
Weißdornblüten
Published July 19, 1994

Name of Drug
Crataegi flos, hawthorn flower.

Composition of Drug
Hawthorn flower consists of the dried flower of *Crataegus monogyna* Jaquin emend. Lindman or *C. laevigata* (Poiret)

de Candolle or others in a valid pharmacopeia citing *Cratageus* [Fam. Rosaceae], as well as preparations thereof.

Pharmacological Properties, Pharmacokinetics, Toxicology
There are no scientific data on which to base the pharmacology and toxicology of the herb. Spectrographic analysis of the chemical constituents of the herb distinguishes only quantitative differences between leaf and flower preparations. One may assume pharmacodynamics similar to those shown for preparations from leaf.

Clinical Data

1. Claimed Areas of Application
Preparations of hawthorn flowers may be applied to the treatment of coronary circulation, support of the heart muscle and attendant improvement in provision for the coronary artery, autonomic heart trouble, autonomic circulatory disturbances, geriatric heart disease, enhancing activity of myocardium, preventing stress-related heart disease, cardiac boost for the elderly, strengthening the heart and circulatory system, strengthening nerves, for coronary insufficiency, angina pectoris, cardiac neurasthenia, cardiac asthma, and arrhythmia.

2. Risks
None known.

Evaluation
Since the effectiveness of hawthorn flower for its claimed applications has not been documented, therapeutic use cannot be recommended.

The herb as a water extract, water-alcohol extract, wine infusion and fresh juice has been utilized traditionally to strengthen and invigorate heart and circulatory function.

These statements are based exclusively on historical record and experience.
[**Ed. note:** A preparation from Hawthorn leaf with flower is listed in the **Approved Herbs** section.]

Hawthorn leaf
Crataegi folium
Weißdornblätter
Published July 19, 1994

Name of Drug
Crataegi folium, hawthorn leaf.

Composition of Drug
Hawthorn leaf consists of the dried leaf of *Crataegus monogyna* Jaquin emend. Lindman or *C. laevigata* in a valid pharmacopeia citing *Cratageus* [Fam. Rosaceae], as well as preparations thereof.

Pharmacological Properties, Pharmacokinetics, Toxicology
There are no scientific data on which to base the pharmacology and toxicology of the herb. Spectrographic analysis of the chemical constituents of the herb distinguishes only quantitative differences between leaf and flower preparations. One may assume pharmacodynamics similar to those shown for preparations from flower.

Clinical Data

1. Claimed Areas of Application
Hawthorn leaf preparations may be applied prophylactically to impeded circulation in the coronary artery, for psychogenic disturbances of the heart and circulatory system, to improve the perfusion and nutrition of the myocardium, for simple circulatory disorders of the coronary artery not needing treatment with digitalis, beginnings of diminished cardiac output due to hypertension and pulmonary disease during and after infection, chronic disturbance of heart rhythm, to enhance treatment with cardiac glycosides, for hypotension, for heart trouble in menopause and advanced age as well as unregulated cardiac output in children.

2. Risks
None known.

Evaluation
Since the effectiveness of hawthorn leaf for its claimed applications has not been documented, therapeutic use cannot be recommended.

The herb as a water extract, water-alcohol extract, wine infusion and fresh juice has been utilized traditionally to strengthen and invigorate heart and circulatory function.

These statements are based exclusively on historical record and experience. [**Ed. note:** A preparation from Hawthorn leaf with flower is listed in the **Approved Herbs** section.]

Heather herb and flower
Callunae vulgaris herba/-flos
Heidekraut /Heidekrautblüten
Published June 1, 1990

Name of Drug
Callunae vulgaris herba, heather herb. Callunae vulgaris flos, heather flower.

Composition of Drug
Heather herb consists of the fresh or dried leaf, flower, and plant top of *Calluna vulgaris* (L.) Hull [Fam. Ericaceae], as well as preparations thereof.

Heather flower consists mainly of the flowers of *C. vulgaris* L., as well as preparations thereof.

Uses
Preparations of heather and/or heather flowers are used for diseases and ailments of the kidneys and the lower urinary tract, enlargement of the prostate, as a diuretic, for prophylaxis of stone ailments, vaginal discharge, diseases and ailments of the gastrointestinal tract, diarrhea, spasms of the stomach and intestines, colic, diseases of the liver and gallbladder, for gout, arthritis, diseases and disorders of the respiratory tract, cough, colds, sleep disorders, restlessness, as eye baths for inflamed eyes, treatment of wounds, for fever, spleen, and as a diaphoretic.

Combinations with heather and/or heather flower are additionally used as an adjuvant for diabetes, menstrual discomforts, menopause, for nervous exhaustion, for stimulation of digestion, and for the regulation of the circulatory system.

The effectiveness for the claimed uses is not documented.

Risks
None known.

Evaluation
Since the effectiveness for the claimed uses is not documented, a therapeutic application cannot be recommended.

There are no objections to the use of this herb as a brightening agent or flavor corrigent.

Hibiscus
Hibisci flos
Hibiscusblüten
Published February 1, 1990

Name of Drug
Hibisci flos, hibiscus flowers.

Composition of Drug
Hibiscus flowers consist of the calyces of *Hibiscus sabdariffa* L. var. *sabdariffa ruber* [Fam. Malvaceae], as well as preparations thereof.

Uses
Hibiscus flowers are used for loss of appetite, for colds, catarrhs of the upper respiratory tract and stomach, to dissolve phlegm, as a gentle laxative, diuretic, and for disorders of circulation.

The claimed efficacies are not substantiated.

Risks
None known.

Evaluation
Since the claimed efficacies of hibiscus flowers have not been documented, a therapeutic use cannot be justified. There are no concerns for the use of this herb for decorative purposes or as a flavor corrigent.

Hollyhock flower
Malvae arboreae flos
Stockrosenblüten
Published March 2, 1989

Name of Drug
Malvae arboreae flos, hollyhock flower.

Composition of Drug
Hollyhock flower consists of the flowers of *Alcea rosea* L. (syn. *Althaea rosea* (L.) Cavanilles) [Fam. Malvaceae], as well as preparations thereof.

Uses
Hollyhock flower is used as mucilage for prophylaxis and therapy of diseases and discomforts of the respiratory tract and the gastrointestinal tract, for urinary complaints and externally for ulcers and inflammations.

The effectiveness for the claimed applications is not verified.

Risks
None known.

Evaluation
Since the effectiveness for the claimed applications is not documented, a therapeutic administration cannot be recommended.

There is no concern for the use as a brightening agent in herbal tea mixtures.

Horse Chestnut leaf
Hippocastani folium
Roßkastanienblätter
Published July 14, 1993

Name of Drug
Hippocastani folium, horse chestnut leaf.

Composition of Drug
Horse chestnut leaf consists of the fresh or dried leaf of *Aesculus hippocastanum* L. [Fam. Hippocastanaceae], as well as preparations thereof.

Pharmacological Properties, Pharmacokinetics, Toxicology
2 ml and 8 ml/kg of an insufficiently defined extract of horse chestnut leaves, if injected intraperitoneally, caused edema inhibition in a model of dextran-induced edema in rat paws.

No data are available for pharmacokinetics.

The LD_{50} of an insufficiently defined horse chestnut extract is 137.6 ml/kg body weight for the Wistar rat and 220 ml/kg body weight for the DD mouse, intraperitoneal administration.

Clinical Data

1. Uses
Preparations of horse chestnut leaf are used for eczema, discomfort due to varicose veins, i.e., pain and feeling of heaviness in the legs, swellings of the legs when static, supportive for medical treatment of varicose ulcers, phlebitis and thrombophlebitis, hemorrhoids, spastic pains before and during menstruation, soft tissue swellings due to bone fractures and sprains, and complaints after concussion.

In combinations, preparations of horse chestnut leaf are used for discomfort due to hemorrhoids, anal fissures and rhagades, follow-up treatment for hemorrhoid surgery, stasis in the colon, prevention of weaknesses of the veins, strengthening of the venous walls, maintenance of normal blood supply in tissue, strengthening of venous blood circulation, prevention of fatigue of legs and feet, for severe disorders of the varicose system, such as varices, phlebitis, phlebectasia, endangiitis obliterans, angioneurosis, postphlebitic syndrome, ulcus cruris, edema, for prevention of thrombo-embolism, arteriosclerosis, arthrosis deformans, arthritis, sciatica, rheumatism, lumbago, neuralgia, accidental injuries, hematoma, bruises, brachialgia, and as a diuretic and purifying remedy.

The effectiveness for the claimed uses has not been demonstrated.

2. Risks
One case is cited in the literature in which an intramuscular injection of an extract of horse chestnut leaf induced cholestatic liver damage. Due to insufficient information, this case cannot be clearly credited to the herb.

Evaluation
Since the effectiveness for the claimed uses is not documented, a therapeutic application cannot be recommended.

[**Ed. note:** A monograph for Horse Chestnut seed extract is listed in the **Approved Herbs** section.]

Hound's Tongue
Cynoglossi herba
Hundszungenkraut
Published March 2, 1989

Name of Drug
Cynoglossi herba, hound's tongue.

Composition of Drug
Hound's Tongue herb consists of the above-ground parts of *Cynoglossum officinale* L. (syn. *C. clandestinum* Desfontaines) [Fam. Boraginaceae], as well as preparations thereof.

Uses
Preparations of Hound's Tongue are used as an antidiarrheal and an expectorant.

Fixed combinations containing Hound's Tongue are used for ailments and complaints of the gastrointestinal tract, infections, skin diseases, and bronchitis; and externally for diseases and painful discomfort of extremities, myalgia, neuralgia, trauma, nervous diseases, and care of scar tissue.

The effectiveness of the herb for the claimed applications is not documented.

Risks
Hound's Tongue contains large amounts of the hepatotoxic pyrrolizidine alkaloids.

Evaluation
Since the effectiveness for the claimed applications is not documented, a therapeutic administration cannot be justified due to the risks.

Hyssop
Hyssopus officinalis
Ysop
Published August 29, 1992

Name of Drug
Hyssopi herba, hyssop herb.
Hyssopi aetheroleum, hyssop oil.

Composition of Drug
Hyssop herb consists of the fresh or dried, above-ground parts of *Hyssopus officinalis* L. [Fam. Lamiaceae], as well as preparations thereof.

Hyssop oil consists of the essential oil of *H. officinalis* L., obtained by water steam distillation, as well as preparations thereof.

Pharmacological Properties, Pharmacokinetics, Toxicology

Hyssop herb:
    None known.
    Hyssop oil causes, in rats, clonic spasms and toniclonic spasms, using a dosage of 0.13 g/kg intraperitoneally.

Clinical Data

1. Uses
Preparations of hyssop herb are used for the gentle stimulation of circulation, for intestinal catarrhs, for diseases of the respiratory tract, colds, chest and lung ailments, for the prevention of frostbite damage, digestive disorders, intestinal ailments, menstrual complaints, heart problems and eye pain.
    The effectiveness for the claimed applications is not documented.

2. Risks
Hyssop herb:
    None known.
Hyssop oil:
    Three cases of poisoning have been registered resulting in clonic and/or clonic-tonic spasms. In adults a dosage of 10 and 30 drops was used, and, in a 6-year-old child, the dosage was 2 - 3 drops over several days.

Evaluation
Since the effectiveness for the claimed uses is not documented, a therapeutic application cannot be justified.
    There is no objection to the use of hyssop herb below 5 percent as a flavor corrigent in tea mixtures.

Jambolan seed
Syzygii cumini semen
Syzygiumsamen
Published April 23, 1987

Name of Drug
Syzygii cumini semen, jambolan seed.

Composition of Drug
Jambolan seed consists of the dried seed of *Syzygium cumini* (L.) Skeels (syn. *S. jambolana* (Lam.) de Candolle) [Fam. Myrtaceae], as well as preparations thereof.

Uses
Jambolan seed is used for diabetes and also in combination preparations for atonic and spastic constipation, diseases of the pancreas, gastric and pancreatic complaints, nervous disorders, depression and exhaustion. It is also used as a carminative, antispasmodic, stomachic, roborant, and aphrodisiac.
    The effectiveness for the claimed applications has not been documented.

Risks
The therapeutic use of jambolan seed for the various forms of diabetes cannot be justified because of other established therapeutic possibilities.

Action
The blood sugar-lowering effect of jambolan seed is uncertain and could not be established by several researchers.

Jimsonweed leaf and seed
Stramonii folium/-semen
Stramoniumblätter/-samen
Published February 1, 1990

Name of Drug
Stramonii folium, jimsonweed leaf, thorn apple.
Stramonii semen, jimsonweed seed.

Composition of Drug
Jimsonweed leaf consists of the dried leaf, or the dried leaves and flowering tops of *Datura stramonium* L. [Fam. Solanaceae], as well as preparations thereof.

Jimsonweed seed consists of the ripe seed of *D. stramonium* L., as well as preparations thereof.

Uses
Jimsonweed preparations are used for asthma, spastic or convulsive cough, pertussis during bronchitis and influenza, and as basic therapy for diseases of the autonomic nervous system.

The effectiveness for the claimed applications is not sufficiently documented.

Risks
Jimsonweed leaf and seed contain 0.1 - 0.6 percent alkaloids. Main alkaloids are L-hyoscyamine and L-scopolamine.

Poisonings with fatal consequences are described. The amount of available alkaloids in inhalant therapies, such as fumigations and "asthma cigarettes" cannot be calculated.

Because of the euphoric action of this herb, abuse and dependency occurs.

Evaluation
Since the effectiveness is not sufficiently documented, the application of jimsonweed leaf and seed and their preparations cannot be justified because of their risks.

Kelp
Laminariae stipites
Laminariastiele
Published July 14, 1993

Name of Drug
Laminariae stipites, kelp.

Composition of Drug
Kelp consists of the dried, stem-like parts of the thallus of *Laminaria hyperborea* (Gunn.) Foslie (syn. *L. cloustonii* (Edmondston) Lejolis) [Fam. Laminariaceae], as well as preparations thereof.

Pharmacological Properties, Pharmacokinetics, Toxicology
Not known.

Clinical Data

1. Uses
Preparations of kelp are used for the regulation of thyroid function, as well as in combination for goiter.

The effectiveness for the claimed applications is not verified.

2. Risks

Preparations containing a maximum daily dosage of 150 µg of iodine:
None known.

Above the dosage of 150 µg of iodine per day, there is danger that hyperthyroidism is induced or made worse. In rare cases allergic reactions involving serious overall reactions may occur.

Evaluation

Since the effectiveness for the claimed applications using a dosage below 150 µg iodine per day is not documented, a therapeutic administration cannot be recommended.

Above a dosage of 150 µg iodine per day, a therapeutic application cannot be recommended, because the effectiveness is not verified and the risks cannot be justified.

Lemongrass, Citronella

Cymbopogon species
Cymbopogon-Arten
Published February 1, 1990

Name of Drug

Cymbopoginis nardi herba, Ceylon citronella grass.
Cymbopoginis citrati herba, West Indian lemongrass.
Cymbopoginis citrati aetheroleum, West Indian lemongrass oil.
Cymbopoginis winteriani aetheroleum, Java citronella oil.

Composition of Drug

Ceylon citronella grass consists of the above-ground parts of *Cymbopogon nardus* Rendle [Fam. Poaceae], as well as preparations thereof.

West Indian lemongrass consists of the above-ground parts of *C. citratus* (DC) Stapf, as well as preparations thereof.

West Indian lemongrass oil consists of the essential oil from *C. citratus* (DC) Stapf, as well as preparations thereof.

Java citronella oil consists of the essential oil from *C. winterianus* Jowitt, as well as preparations thereof.

Uses

Lemongrass is used as a mild astringent and a tonic for the stomach.

Lemongrass, lemongrass oil and citronella oil preparations are used almost exclusively in combinations for disorders and discomforts of the gastrointestinal tract, muscle pain and neuralgia, colds, various nervous disturbances, and for conditions of exhaustion. Citronella is also used as an insect repellent. It is ingested orally or applied topically.

The effectiveness for the claimed applications is not documented.

Risks

Allergic reactions are rare, if preparations of the herb are topically applied to the skin. Two cases of toxic alveolitis have been reported after inhalation of an unknown amount of lemongrass oil. After an accidental ingestion of an insect repellent which contained citronella oil, a child was fatally poisoned.

Evaluation

Since the effectiveness of the claimed uses is not documented, a therapeutic application cannot be recommended.

There is no reservation about using citral-pool herbs and essential oils as an aroma or taste corrigent.

Linden Charcoal
Tiliae carbo
Lindenholzkohle
Published September 1, 1990

Name of Drug
Tiliae carbo, linden charcoal.

Composition of Drug
Linden charcoal consists of the charcoal obtained from the wood of *Tilia cordata* Miller and/or *T. platyphyllos* Scopoli [Fam. Tiliaceae], as well as preparations thereof.

Uses
Preparations of linden charcoal are used for intestinal disorders and, externally, for abscesses of the lower leg.

Risks
None known.

Evaluation
Since the effectiveness for the claimed applications is not documented, a therapeutic administration cannot be recommended.

Linden flower, Silver
Tiliae tomentosae flos
Silberlindenblüten
Published September 1, 1990

Name of Drug
Tiliae tomentosae flos, silver linden flower.

Composition of Drug
Silver linden flower consists of the dried flowers of *Tilia tomentosa* Moench (synonym *T. argentea* Desfontaines) [Fam. Tiliaceae], as well as preparations thereof.

Uses
Preparations of silver linden flower are used for catarrhs of the respiratory tract, as an antispasmodic, expectorant, diaphoretic, and a diuretic.

The effectiveness for the claimed applications is not documented.

Risks
None known.

Evaluation
Since the effectiveness for the claimed uses is not documented, a therapeutic application cannot be recommended.

There are no objections to its use as a corrigent for aroma and flavor.

Linden leaf
Tiliae folium
Lindenblätter
Published September 1, 1990

Name of Drug
Tiliae folium, linden leaf.

Composition of Drug
Linden leaf consists of the dried leaf of *Tilia cordata* Miller and/or *T. platyphyllos* Scopoli [Fam. Tiliaceae], as well as preparations thereof.

Uses
Preparations of linden leaf are used as a diaphoretic. The effectiveness for the claimed application is not documented.

Risks
None known.

Evaluation
Since the effectiveness for the claimed use is not documented, a therapeutic application cannot be recommended. There is no concern for the use of this herb as a filler in tea mixtures.

Linden wood
Tiliae lignum
Lindenholz
Published September 1, 1990

Name of Drug
Tiliae lignum, linden wood, lime tree wood.

Composition of Drug
Linden wood consists of the dried sap wood of *Tilia cordata* Miller and/or *T. platyphyllos* Scopoli [Fam. Tiliaceae], as well as preparations thereof.

Uses
Preparations of linden wood are used for diseases and ailments of the liver-gallbladder system, as well as for cellulitis. The effectiveness for the claimed applications is not documented.

Risks
None known.

Evaluation
Since the effectiveness for the claimed uses is not documented, a therapeutic application cannot be recommended.

Liverwort herb
Hepatici nobilis herba
Leberblümchenkraut
Published July 14, 1993

Name of Drug
Hepatici nobilis herba, liverwort herb.

Composition of Drug
Liverwort consists of the fresh or dried above-ground parts of *Hepatica nobilis* Gars. [Fam. Ranunculaceae], as well as preparations thereof.

Pharmacological Properties, Pharmacokinetics, Toxicology
None known.

Clinical Data

1. Uses
Preparations of liverwort herb are used for liver ailments, liver diseases of all origins, jaundice, gallstones and gravel, enlargement and congestion of the liver, icterus, portal vein problems, as an auxiliary agent for hepatitis and liver cirrhosis, for gastric and digestive discomforts, for stimulation of appetite, as a general tonic, for sensation of fullness, for the regulation of bowel function, stimulation of pancreatic function, regulation of the blood lipid level, for varicose veins, hemorrhoids, stimulation of circulation, cardiocirculatory stimulation, increase in the blood supply in the myocardium, as a sedative, for strengthening of the nerves, for blood purification and stimulation of the metabolism, and for the relief of menopausal symptoms.

The claimed efficacy has not been documented.

2. Risks
The plant contains protoanemonin. It is known that severe irritations with itching and pustule formation (ranunculus dermatitis) occur on skin and mucous membranes when preparations of fresh protoanemonin-containing plants or protoanemonin are applied. Upon internal use, higher dosages may lead to irritations of the kidneys and urinary tract.

Application is contraindicated during pregnancy.

Protoanemonin is destroyed upon drying.

Evaluation
Since the effectiveness for the claimed uses has not been documented, and considering the risks, a therapeutic application of protoanemonin-containing preparations cannot be justified.

Loofa
Luffa aegyptiaca
Luffaschwamm
Published September 24, 1993

Name of Drug
Luffa aegyptiaca, loofa, sponge cucumber.

Composition of Drug
Loofa sponge consists of the dried fiber structure of the ripe cucumber-like fruits of *Luffa aegyptiaca* Miller [Fam. Cucurbitaceae], as well as preparations thereof.

Pharmacological Properties, Pharmacokinetics, Toxicology
None known.

Uses
a) Uses as result of evaluation:
   None.
b) Claimed uses which have been negatively evaluated:
   Preparations of loofah sponge are used as a preventive for infections or colds, as a remedy for colds, nasal catarrhs, as well as sinusitis and suppuration of the sinus.
   The effectiveness for the claimed applications is not documented.

Risks
None known.

Evaluation
Since the effectiveness for the claimed uses is not documented, a therapeutic application cannot be recommended.

Lungwort
Pulmonariae herba
Lungenkraut
Published October 15, 1987

Name of Drug
Pulmonariae herba, lungwort

Composition of Drug
Lungwort, consisting of the dried plant section of *Pulmonaria officinalis* L. [Fam. Boraginaceae] and effective pharmaceutical preparations of same.

Uses
Lungwort preparations are used in the treatment of illnesses and conditions of the respiratory tract, the gastrointestinal tract, the kidney and urinary tract, and also are used as an astringent and in the treatment of wounds.
Efficacy in the areas of use has not been sufficiently proven.

Risks
None known.

Recommendation
Since the efficacy of the lungwort preparations has not been sufficiently documented in the above-named areas, its therapeutic use cannot be recommended.

Madder root
Rubiae tinctorum radix
Krappwurzel
Published September 18, 1986; Replaced August 29, 1992

Name of Drug
Rubiae tinctorum radix, madder root.

Composition of Drug
Madder root consists of the dried root of *Rubia tinctorum* L. [Fam. Rubiaceae], as

well as preparations thereof in effective dosage. The herb contains lucidin.

Pharmacological Properties, Pharmacokinetics, Toxicology

In rats, oral intake of fresh madder root (10 percent of the food) decreased stone formation in bladder and kidney induced by 3 percent $CaCO_3$. In rabbits, oral intake of madder root extract (150 - 200 mg/kg) caused decreased calcium oxalate crystallization in the kidney.

An increase in death rate was observed with feeding experiments of rats. Furthermore, feeding experiments with rabbits showed hepatotoxic effects. Genotoxic effects were observed in bacterial as well as in mammalian cell test systems.

Clinical Data

1. Uses

a) Application as a result of evaluation: None.
b) Claimed uses with negative evaluation: kidney stones and disintegration of kidney stones.

Because of the risks and the insufficiently documented effectiveness, the risk/benefit evaluation is negative.

2. Risks

Madder root contains lucidin. Lucidin is positive in various bacterial strains using the Ames test. The substance induces concentration-dependent gene mutations and DNA strand cleavage in V79 cells, causes transformation in the C3H/M2 cell transformation test, and is positive in the DNA-repair-test on rat hepatocytes. In vivo, a clear covalent bonding of lucidin to rat liver DNA has been observed. Therefore, there exists a strong indication that lucidin is mutagenic and carcinogenic.

3. Evaluation

Based on the genotoxic risk, combined with the fact that the claimed applications may involve an extended therapy and the insufficiently documented effectiveness, a therapy with madder root is not justified.
Note: After intake of madder root, occasional cases of red coloration of the urine, saliva, perspiration, and milk have been observed.

Male Fern
Filicis maris folium, herba, rhizoma
Wurmfarn
Published September 24, 1993

Name of Drug
Filicis maris folium, male fern leaf.
Filicis maris herba, male fern herb.
Filicis maris rhizoma, male fern rhizome.

Composition of Drug
Male fern leaf consists of the fresh or dried leaf of *Dryopteris filix-mas* (L.) Schott [Fam. Aspleniaceae], as well as preparations thereof.

Male fern herb consists of the fresh or dried above-ground parts of *D. filix-mas* (L.) Schott, as well as preparations thereof. Male fern rhizome consists of the fresh or dried rhizomes with leaf scars freed from attached roots, harvested in autumn, of *D. filix-mas* (L.) Schott, as well as preparations thereof.

Pharmacological Properties, Pharmacokinetics, Toxicology

Male fern rhizome has an anthelmintic effect and is strongly cytotoxic.

Clinical Data

1. Uses

a) Uses as a result of evaluation:
   None.
b) Claimed uses which have been negatively evaluated:
   Preparations of male fern herb are used externally for rheumatism, sciatica, muscle pain, neuralgia, earache and toothache, for teething in infants and sleep disorders, as well as internally for tapeworms and flukes.

In combinations, preparations of male fern are used externally for inflamed hallux valgus, painful bunion, pains in the feet and legs, cracks (fissures) of the soles of the feet, paresthesia, frostbite, circulatory disturbances, venectasia, minor ulcers, discogenic consecutive symptoms, lumbar syndrome, cervical syndrome, spondylarthritis, acute and chronic inflammations of the joints, ischialgia, lumbago, rheumatic diseases, arthritis deformans, arthritis, cicatricial keloid, scar tissue contraction, and neuralgia.

For treatment of worm diseases, safer and more effective therapeutic alternatives are available.

The effectiveness for the claimed applications is not documented.

2. Risks

Numerous poisonings, some with fatal consequences, have been reported regarding ingestion of preparations of male fern rhizome in therapeutic dosage. Observed symptoms of poisoning include visual disturbances including blindness, headache, dizziness, nausea, confusion, diarrhea, severe abdominal spasms, dyspnea, respiratory and cardiac insufficiency, arrhythmia, tremor, convulsions, stimulation of the uterus muscle, albuminuria and bilirubinuria. Side effects are supposedly increased by simultaneous intake of fats and oils, as well as of alcohol. A case of poisoning of a child with a decoction of male fern herb has been reported.

Internal use of male fern is obsolete.

Evaluation

Oral administration cannot be justified because of the high risks involved. External application cannot be recommended, since the effectiveness for the claimed uses is not documented.

Marjoram

Majoranae herb, aetheroleum
Majoran
Published December 2, 1992

Name of Drug

Majoranae herba, marjoram herb. Majoranae aetheroleum, marjoram oil.

Composition of Drug

Marjoram herb consists of the dried leaf and flower of *Origanum majorana* L (synonym *Majorana hortensis* Moench) [Fam. Lamiaceae], gathered during the flowering season and stripped off the stems, as well as preparations thereof.

Marjoram oil consists of the essential oil of *O. majorana* L. (syn. *M. hortensis* Moench), obtained by water steam distillation of the leaves and flowers freed from the stems and harvested during flowering season, as well as preparations thereof.

Pharmacological Properties, Pharmacokinetics, Toxicology

Marjoram herb and marjoram oil have an antibacterial action.

Clinical Data

1. Uses

Application as a result of evaluation:
   None.
Claimed uses with negative evaluation:
   Rhinitis and cold in infants; rhinitis in toddlers.

In combinations, marjoram and marjoram oil are used for the stimulation of appetite, to promote digestion, strengthening of the stomach, for acute and chronic gastritis, ulcus ventriculi, as an antispasmodic, for flatulence, for colic-like nervous gastrointestinal disorders, for a diathermic effect in the case of circulatory deficiencies in the abdominal region, for the support of intestinal activity, for purification of the system, supportive for acute inflammatory liver diseases, for functional regulation of diseases involving gallstones, for dry irritative coughs, for swellings of the nasal and pharyngeal mucosa, inflammation of the ears, headaches, for lowering the blood sugar in diabetics, promotion of milk secretion, as a tonic for nerves, heart and circulation system, for the promotion of healthy sleep, for mood swings, as a tonic (especially during convalescence), as a blood builder, for anorexia, sprains, bruises, lumbago, as an astringent, for dysmenorrhea, for climacteric complaints, for strengthening the female organs, as adjuvant for discharge, for beginning adnexitis, menstrual disturbances, for urogenital bleeding and a diuretic.

The effectiveness for the claimed uses is not sufficiently documented. A positive contribution in combinations for "dyspeptic disorders," "liver and gall preparations," for "colds" and for diseases of the urogenital tract, for diabetes, as a tonic, as a tea for the stimulation of milk secretion and for bruises and similar conditions, cannot be determined.

2. Risks

Marjoram herb contains arbutin and hydroxyquinone in low concentrations. Therefore, the herb is not suited for extended use. Hydroxyquinone is carcinogenic as tested in animals. Topical application of hydroxyquinone leads to depigmentation of the skin. There are no reports of similar side effects with marjoram ointment.

Evaluation

Since the effectiveness for the claimed applications is not sufficiently documented, a therapeutic administration of marjoram herb cannot be recommended.

Considering that the risks are not sufficiently clarified, a topical use of ointments containing marjoram extracts should not be used for the claimed indications in infants and small children.

Marsh Tea
Ledi palustris herba
Sumpfporstkraut
Published September 24, 1986

Name of Drug
Ledi palustris herba, marsh tea.

Composition of Drug
Marsh tea consists of the dried herb of *Ledum palustre* L. [Fam. Lamiaceae], as well as preparations thereof.

The herb contains essential oil.

Uses
Marsh tea is used for rheumatic discomforts and whooping cough, also as an emetic, diaphoretic, and diuretic.

The effectiveness for the claimed applications has not been documented.

Risks
Poisonings with marsh tea due to abusive application, e.g., abortion, are frequently reported.

The essential oil, when taken internally, causes severe irritation of the gastrointestinal tract with vomiting and diarrhea, as well as irritation and damage to the kidneys and lower urinary tract.

Described also are heavy perspiration, pain in muscle and joints, excitation of the central nervous system with narcotic intoxication (a "high") followed by paralysis.

No data are available concerning the toxicity of small amounts of marsh tea herb.

Contraindications
Pregnancy.

Evaluation
Since the effectiveness of marsh tea preparations is not documented, a therapeutic application cannot be justified because of the risks.

Actions
Irritation of skin and mucous membranes.
Experimentally:
  Inhibited motility
Prolongation of sleeping time after administration of barbiturates and alcohol
Antitussive
Antiinflammatory

Mentzelia
Mentzeliae cordifoliae summitatidis/stipitidis et radix
Mentzelia cordifolia Zweigspitzen, -Stengel und -Wurzel
Published September 24, 1993

Name of Drug
Mentzeliae cordifoliae summitatidis, stipitidis et radix, mentzelia branch tips, stems and roots.

Composition of Drug
Mentzelia branch tips, stems and roots in a mixture of an unknown ratio.

The herb consists of the dried branch tips, stems and roots of *Mentzelia cordifolia* Dombey [Fam. Loasaceae] in an unknown ratio of composition.

Pharmacological Properties, Pharmacokinetics, Toxicology

1. Uses
a) Uses as a result of evaluation: None.
b) Claimed uses which have been negatively evaluated:
Preparations of mentzelia branch tips, stems, and roots are used for general disturbances of the gastrointestinal system, gastritis, gastrointestinal catarrh, nervous gastric disorders and digestive symptoms, hyperacidity, gastric spasms, feeling of fullness, pressure on the stomach, upset stomach, gastric irritation due to alcohol abuse, innate digestive weakness and gastric pain.

The effectiveness for the claimed applications is not documented.

Risks
None known.

Evaluation
Since the effectiveness for the claimed uses is not documented, a therapeutic application cannot be recommended.

Milk Thistle herb
Cardui mariae herba
Mariendistelkraut
Published March 11, 1992

Name of Drug
Cardui mariae herba, milk thistle herb.

Composition of Drug
Milk thistle herb consists of the fresh or dried, above-ground parts of *Silybum marianum* (L.) Gaertner [Fam. Asteraceae], as well as preparations thereof.

Uses
Preparations of milk thistle herb are used for maintaining health, for stimulation and functional disorders of liver and gallbladder, for jaundice, gallbladder colics, diseases of the spleen and pleurisy.

The effectiveness for the claimed applications is not documented.

Risks
None known.

Evaluation
Since the effectiveness for the claimed uses is not documented, a therapeutic application cannot be recommended.
[**Ed. note:** A standardized preparation of Milk Thistle fruits is listed in the **Approved Herbs** section.]

Monkshood

Aconiti tuber, herba
Blauer Eisenhut
Published October 15, 1987

Name of Drug
Aconiti tuber, monkshood tuber, blue monkshood root, aconite root.
Aconiti herba, monkshood herb, blue monkshood herb, aconite.

Composition of Drug
Monkshood tuber consists of fresh or dried tubers and roots of *Aconitum napellus* L. [Fam. Ranunculaceae] harvested in autumn after flowering, as well as their preparations.

Monkshood herb consists of the dried herb of *A. napellus* L. collected at the beginning of the flowering season, as well as their preparations.

The herb contains alkaloids. The principal alkaloid is aconitine.

Uses
Preparations of Monkshood are used for pain, facial paralysis, ailments of the joints, arthritis, gout, rheumatic complaints, inflammation, pleurisy, pericarditis sicca, fever, skin and mucosal diseases, and for disinfection and wound treatment.

In combinations, preparations of Monkshood are also used as prophylaxis for diseases of the respiratory tract, cardiac and circulatory system and gastrointestinal tract, for loss of appetite, allergic disorders, strengthening of the immune system, for conditions of nervous excitement, sleep disorders, depression, spasms, eclampsia, epilepsy, mood changes, as a remedy to increase circulation after frostbite, for contractions, treatment of scar tissue, insertion into the tooth root canal, anesthesia of mucous membranes, prophylaxis of caries, hair loss and dandruff.

The effectiveness of Monkshood for most of the claimed applications has not been documented. However, Monkshood has been indicated as effective for neuralgia.

Risks
Because of the limited therapeutic range, intoxications can occur within the range of therapeutic dosage. Manifestations of intoxication include paresthesia, vomiting, dizziness, muscle spasms, hypothermia, bradycardia and rhythmic disorders of the heart, and paralysis of the respiratory system.

Evaluation
Because of the existing risks within the therapeutic range of Monkshood, its administration cannot be justified.

Mountain Ash berry
Sorbi aucupariae fructus
Ebereschenbeeren
Published July 6, 1988

Name of Drug
Sorbi aucupariae fructus, mountain ash berry.

Composition of Drug
Mountain ash berry consists of the fresh or dried fruit, or fruit cooked and dried thereafter, of *Sorbus aucuparia* L. s.l. [Fam. Rosaceae], as well as preparations thereof.

Uses
Mountain ash berry and its preparations are used for kidney diseases, for diabetes, arthritis, disorders of the uric acid metabolism, for dissolution of uric acid deposits, for catarrh, internal inflammations, vitamin C deficiency, for alkalization of the blood, increase of metabolism, and for "blood purification."

The effectiveness of the claimed applications is not verified.

Risks
None known.
Note: Fresh mountain ash berry contains parasorbic acid, which causes local irritation. During the drying process, the compound is largely degraded. It is fully destroyed upon cooking.

Evaluation
Since the effectiveness of mountain ash berry for the claimed applications is not documented, a therapeutic use cannot be recommended.

Mugwort
Artemisiae vulgaris herba, radix
Beifuß
Published July 6, 1988

Name of Drug
Artemisiae vulgaris herba, mugwort herb.
Artemisiae vulgaris radix, mugwort root.

Composition of Drug
Mugwort herb consists of the above-ground parts of *Artemisia vulgaris* L., as well as preparations thereof.

Mugwort root consists of the underground parts of *A. vulgaris* L. [Fam. Asteraceae], as well as preparations thereof.

Uses
Mugwort herb is used in complaints and problems involving the gastrointestinal tract, such as colic, diarrhea, constipation, cramps, weak digestion, to stimulate secretion of gastric juice and bile, as a laxative in cases of obesity and "for the liver," also against worm infestations, and for hysteria, epilepsy, persistent vomiting, convulsions in children, menstrual problems and irregular periods, to promote circulation and to act as a sedative.

The root is used for asthenic states as a tonic, and in combination with other remedies for psychoneuroses, neurasthenia, depression, hypochondria, autonomic neuroses, general irritability and restlessness, insomnia, and anxiety states.

The efficacy of mugwort for the listed indications has not been substantiated.

Risks
An abortifacient action has been reported. Allergic reactions are possible in previously sensitized subjects.

Evaluation
Since the effectiveness for the claimed applications is not verified, a therapeutic administration is not recommended.

Muira Puama
Ptychopetali lignum
Potenzholz
Published October 15, 1987

Name of Drug
Ptychopetali lignum, muira puama wood.

Composition of Drug
Muira puama consists of the wood from the trunk and/or roots of *Ptychopetalum olacoides* Bentham and/or *P. unicatum* Anselmino [Fam. Olacaceae], as well as preparations thereof.

Uses
Muira puama is used for the prevention of sexual disorders and as an aphrodisiac. The effectiveness of the claimed applications has not been documented.

Risks
None known.

Evaluation
The administration of muira puama preparations cannot be recommended, since the effectiveness has not been documented.

Night-blooming Cereus
Seleniceri grandiflori flos, herba
Königin der Nacht
Published February 1, 1990

Name of Drug
Selenicerei grandiflori flos, night-blooming cereus flower.
Selenicerei grandiflori herba, night-blooming cereus herb.

Composition of Drug
The fresh or dried flowers or the fresh or dried, above-ground parts of *Selenicereus grandiflorus* (L.) Britton et Rose [Fam. Cactaceae], as well as preparations thereof.

Uses
Preparations of *S. grandiflorus* are used for nervous cardiac disorders, angina pectoris, stenocardia, and urinary ailments.

The effectiveness for the claimed applications is not documented.

Risks
None known.

Evaluation
Since the effectiveness for the claimed uses has not been documented, a therapeutic application cannot be recommended.

Action
Stabilizing arrhythmia on isolated frog heart.

Nutmeg
Myristicae semen, aril
Muskatnußbaum
Published September 18, 1986

Name of Drug
Myristicae semen, nutmeg seed.
Myristicae aril, mace.

Composition of Drug
Nutmeg consists of the dried seed, separated from the aril and coat, of *Myristica fragrans* Houttuyn [Fam. Myristicaceae], as well as preparations thereof. Mace consists of the dried aril of *M. fragrans* Houttuyn, as well as preparations thereof.

The spice contains essential oil.

Uses
Nutmeg and/or Mace is used for ailments and complaints of the gastrointestinal tract, such as diarrhea, gastric spasms, intestinal catarrh and flatulence.

The claimed efficacies have not been sufficiently documented.

Risks
Intake of 5 g causes a series of psychic disturbances manifesting themselves in a range from mild changes of consciousness to intense hallucinations.

With ingestion of 9 teaspoons of Nutmeg powder per day, an atropine-like effect was observed.

When taken in larger amounts, the herb has abortifacient action.

Safrole, contained in the essential oil, shows mutagenic and carcinogenic effects.

No mutagenic effects are known for nutmeg essential oil.

Evaluation
Since the effectiveness of Nutmeg preparations is not sufficiently demonstrated, a therapeutic application cannot be justified because of the risks involved.

There are no concerns for its use as an aroma or flavor corrigent.

Actions
Antispasmodic
MAO inhibition
Inhibits prostaglandin synthesis

Nux Vomica
Strychni semen
Brechnußsamen
Published September 18, 1986

Name of Drug
Strychni semen, nux vomica, strychnos seed, poison nut, Quaker buttons.

Composition of Drug
Nux vomica consists of the seeds of *Strychnos nux-vomica* L. [Fam. Loganiaceae], as well as preparations thereof.

Uses
Nux vomica and its preparations are used in combinations for diseases and conditions of the gastrointestinal tract, organic and functional disorders of the heart and circulatory system, diseases of the eye, nervous conditions, depression, migraine, climacteric complaints, in geriatrics, for Sympatalgien, diseases and conditions of the respiratory tract, Raynaud's disease, secondary anemia, and a tonic and appetite-stimulating remedy.

The effectiveness of most of the claimed actions is not documented.

Risks
Nux vomica alkaloids, especially strychnine, act on the central nervous system as spastic poison. At low dosage, the spinal cord is selectively affected. Strychnine is antagonistic to the inhibitory transmitter glycine, leading to heightened convulsive response of the muscles; external irritations or substances with stimulating actions on the central nervous system can initiate convulsions. A therapeutically useful action exists at sub-convulsive dosage. Strychnine accumulates during extended administration. This occurs especially if liver damage exists.

Evaluation
Since the effectiveness of most claimed applications is not documented, the therapeutic use of nux vomica and its preparations, even as bitter principle and tonic, is not justifiable due to the risks.

Oat herb
Avenae herba
Haferkraut
Published October 15, 1987

Name of Drug
Avenae herba, oat herb, wild oat herb.

Composition of Drug
Oat herb consists of the fresh or dried above-ground parts of *Avena sativa* L. [Fam. Poaceae], harvested during flowering season, as well as preparations thereof.

Uses
Oat herb preparations are used for acute and chronic anxiety, stress and excitation, neurasthenic and pseudoneurasthenic syndromes, skin diseases, connective tissue deficiencies, weakness of the bladder, and as a tonic and roborant.

In combinations, wild oat herb preparations are used also for diseases and ailments of the heart and circulatory system and the respiratory system, for metabolic diseases and disorders, diseases and discomforts due to old age, various forms of anemia, hypothyroidism, neuralgia and neuritis, hematoma, pulled muscle, sexual disorders, tobacco abuse, spasms, as a lactagogue and to increase performance capacity.

The effectiveness for the claimed applications is not documented.

Risks
None known.

Evaluation
Since the effectiveness of oat herb preparations is not documented, the therapeutic administration cannot be recommended.

Oats
Avenae fructus
Haferfrüchte
Published May 5, 1988

Name of Drug
Avenae fructus, oats.

Composition of Drug
Oats consists of the ripe, dried fruits of *Avena sativa* L. [Fam. Poaceae], as well as preparations thereof.

Uses
Oat preparations are used for diseases and complaints of the gastric intestinal tract and in combination with physical weakness and fatigue; for neurasthenia and syndrome of neurasthenia, diabetes, consequences of nicotine abuse and in tonics.

The claimed effectiveness has not been substantiated.

Risks
Allergic reaction to oat gluten is possible in rare cases.

Evaluation
Since the efficacy for the claimed uses has not been demonstrated, a therapeutic application of oat preparation cannot be justified.

Oleander leaf
Oleandri folium
Oleanderblätter
Published July 6, 1988; Revised March 2, 1989, and February 1, 1990

Name of Drug
Oleandri folium, oleander leaf.

Composition of Drug
Oleander leaf consists of the leaves of *Nerium oleander* L. [Fam. Apocynaceae], as well as preparations thereof.

Uses
Oleander leaf is used for diseases and functional disorders of the heart, as well as for skin diseases. The effectiveness for the claimed applications is not sufficiently proven.

Risks
Accidental intake of parts of Oleander leaf and the consumption of Oleander leaf tea led to poisonings, sometimes with fatal outcome.

Evaluation
Adequate data for the effectiveness, as well as pharmacokinetics and kinetics of efficacy of oleander leaf preparations, are not available.

A correlation is not given for the chemically determined amount of oleandrin and the biological efficacy of the herb. An indication concerning applications and required dosage is, therefore, not possible.

Since the effectiveness of Oleander leaf preparations is not adequately documented, and considering that there is no correlation between the content of individual glycosides and the efficacy of the herb, a therapeutic administration of oleander leaf is not justifiable.

Note: Benefit and risk of fixed combinations of [herbs containing] cardiac glycosides must be documented and examined specifically for each preparation.

Actions
Positively inotropic
Negatively chronotropic

Olive leaf
Oleae folium
Olivenblätter
January 17, 1991

Name of Drug
Oleae folium, olive leaf.

Composition of Drug
Olive leaf consists of the fresh or dried leaf of *Olea europaea* L. s.l. [Fam. Oleaceae], as well as preparations thereof.

Uses
Preparations of Olive leaf are used as an antihypertensive and diuretic. The effectiveness of olive leaf for the claimed applications is not sufficiently documented.

Risks
None known.

Evaluation
Since the effectiveness of the drug and its preparations for the claimed uses is not documented, a therapeutic application for hypertonia cannot be justified.

Actions
In animal experiments:
    Antispasmodic
    Bronchodilator
    Coronary dilator
    Hypotensive
    Antiarrhythmic and arrhythmogenic
    Antipyretic
    Hypoglycemic
    Diuretic

Olive oil
Olivae oleum
Olivenöl
Published September 21, 1991

Name of Drug
Olivae oleum, olive oil.

Composition of Drug
Olive oil consists of the fatty oil of the ripe drupes of *Olea europaea* L. s.l. [Fam. Oleaceae], obtained by cold-pressed or other suitable mechanical procedures, as well as preparations thereof.

Uses
Preparations of Olive oil are used for cholangiitis, cholecystitis, cholelithiasis, icterus, flatulence, meteorism, lack of bacteria in the intestines, Roemheld syndrome, as a depurative, mild laxative, for spastic constipation, as an intestinal lubricant, as well as externally for wound dressing, and for minor burns and psoriasis.

In combinations, preparations of Olive oil are used for the prevention and therapy of stretch marks due to pregnancy (ointment), for wounds, burns and muscle tears, for firming the breasts (dragee, soft gelatin capsule), for ringing and pain of the ears (ear drops) and as nose drops.

The effectiveness of the claimed applications is not documented.

Risks
In rare cases, applications on the skin can cause allergic reactions.

Evaluation
The therapeutic use of Olive oil for gallstones cannot be justified, because of the risk of triggering gallbladder colic.

Since the effectiveness for the other claimed uses is not documented, a therapeutic application cannot be recommended.

Action
Cholecystokinetic

Oregano
Origani vulgaris herba
Dostenkraut
Published July 6, 1988

Name of Drug
Origani vulgaris herba, oregano.

Composition of Drug
Oregano consists of the above-ground parts of *Origanum vulgare* L. [Fam. Lamiaceae], as well as preparations thereof.

Uses
Oregano is used for ailments and difficulties of the respiratory tract, coughing, bronchial catarrh, as an expectorant and for antispasmodic relief of coughing. It is used for disturbances of the gastrointestinal tract, bloating, stimulation of gall excretion and digestion, and an appetite-stimulating and antispasmodic agent.

Oregano is also used for disorders and afflictions of the urinary tract, abdominal diseases, painful menstruation, as a diuretic, for arthritis, scrofulosis, as a sedative and diaphoretic.

Oregano is also used in gargles and baths.

The claimed efficacy for this herb has not been documented.

Risks
None known.

Evaluation
Since efficacy has not been documented, a therapeutic use of this herb cannot be recommended.

Orris root
Iridis rhizoma
Schwertlilienwurzelstock
Published November 25, 1993

Name of Drug
Iridis rhizoma, orris root.

Composition of Drug
Orris root consists of the carefully peeled and dried rhizome of *Iris germanica* L., *I. pallida* Lamarck (var. *dalmatica*), or *I. florentina* L. [Fam. Iridaceae], as well as preparations thereof.

[**Ed. note:** The herb identified here as *Iris florentina* is more properly identified as the cultivar *I. germanica* var. *florentina* (L.) Dykes.]

Pharmacological Properties, Pharmacokinetics, Toxicology
None known.

Clinical Data

1. Uses
a) Uses as a result of evaluation:
   None.
b) Claimed uses that have been negatively evaluated:
   Preparations of orris root are used as "blood-purifying," "stomach-strengthening" and "gland-stimulating" remedies, for increased activity of the kidneys, and for skin diseases.

In combinations, preparations of orris root are used internally for headache, toothache, muscle and joint pain, migraine, neuralgia, acute and chronic catarrhs of the respiratory tract, bronchitis, bronchial asthma, cough, mucous congestion, nasal catarrh, hoarseness, for better blood supply of the bronchi and mucous membranes, smoker's catarrh, for interval therapy of asthmatics, for the care of heart, nerves and stomach, as a sedative, for nervous disturbances of cardiovascular function, for difficulties in falling asleep and sleep disorders, loss of appetite, gastrointestinal disturbances, sluggishness of the bowels, feeling of fullness, bloating, ailments of gallbladder, liver and pancreas, diabetes, for the relief of irritations caused by inflammatory diseases of the urinary tract, skin diseases, as well as topically for tumors, swelling of the lymph glands, uric acid sedimentation, kyphosis, keloid formation, for rheumatic discomforts, and for burns and cuts.

The effectiveness for the claimed applications is not documented.

2. Risks
None known.

Evaluation
Since the effectiveness for the claimed uses is not documented, a therapeutic application cannot be recommended. There is no objection to its use as an aroma or flavor corrigent.

Papain
Papainum crudum
Papain
Published August 25, 1994

Name of Drug
Papainum crudum, papain.

Composition of Drug
Raw papain is latex from *Carica papaya* L. (pawpaw) [Fam. Caricaceae] that has been dried using various methods; where necessary it is decontaminated mechanically or by filtration.

Papain is the enzyme mixture extracted using various means from raw papain; it contains, along with papain (EC 3.4.22.2), chymopapain A and B and papaya peptidase A.

Pharmacological Properties, Pharmacokinetics, Toxicology
There is no extensive, satisfactory scientific experimental material available on the effects of raw papain/papain. The results on the analgesic and antiinflammatory effects are contradictory. Experiments have shown that papain has an edema-reducing effect. The fibrinogenous effect has not been sufficiently proven.

On the basis of animal experiments papain is said to demonstrate an absorption rate of 3 - 4 percent when taken orally. There is no research material available on the human pharmacokinetics of the drug. There is no extensive, satisfactory scientific experimental material available on the toxicology of papain/raw papain. Papain is not embryo-toxic or teratogenic; there are positive results in the case of raw papain.

There is no material available on the mutagenicity and carcinogenicity of papain.

Clinical Data

1. Uses
a) Indications established through research: None.
b) Reported indications for therapeutic use and grounds for rejection:
Infestation with ascarids, oxyurids, and trichocephalus nematodes.

Papain/raw papain is used in combination in preparations for the treatment of inflammatory conditions of the mouth, throat and pharynx and of the upper respiratory tract; for influenza-type infections; loss of appetite; satiety; flatulence; Roemheld syndrome; putrefying-fermenting dyspepsias; enzyme deficiency; gastrointestinal digestion complaints; inflammations and ulcers in the gastro-duodenal area; pancreas excretion insufficiency; dyskinesia of the liver and of the gallbladder ducts; chronic constipation; congestion of the liver; viral infections; anal thrombosis; concomitant therapy of malignant tumors; metastases; relapse prophylaxis; side effects of radiation treatment; lymphatic congestion following surgery and radiation treatment; palliative treatment of tumor patients; carcinomas, sarcomas, Hodgkin's disease, leukemia; circulatory complaints, arteriosclerosis, vascular disease, thrombophlebitis, thrombosis, hemorrhoids, varicose ulcers, poorly healing wounds, burns, abscesses, fistulas, traumatory edema, hematoma, acute and chronic inflammations, bronchitis, adnexitis, urethritis, rheumatic and degenerative complaints; conditions of aging, exhaustion, and exhaustion syndrome, in convalescence; vitamin, mineral and metabolic substance deficiency, metabolic illnesses, dyscrasia, neurosthenia, neuritis, physical and mental exhaustion and depression. The efficacy of the drug in the above conditions is insufficiently proven with the exception of some effect of papain in the treatment of traumatory and postoperative edema.

There are other more effective substances available for the treatment of worm infestation.

2. Risks
An increase in the tendency to bleed in people with clotting disorders cannot be excluded. Allergic reactions may occur.

Evaluation
Due to the insufficiently proven efficacy of its use in the treatment of worm infestation and the risks associated, as well as the availability of treatment alternatives, the use of raw papain/papain cannot be recommended.

The efficacy of Papain in combination with other drugs used in the treatment of inflammations, edema and swelling following trauma and surgery needs to be specifically proven. Various experiment-based studies as well as clinical research indicate that Papain may be effective in high doses (daily dose = 1500 mg corresponding to 2520 FIP units).

Papaya leaf
Caricae papayae folium
Melonenbaumblätter
Published October 15, 1987

Name of Drug
Caricae papayae folium, papaya leaf.

Composition of Drug
Papaya leaf consists of fresh or dried leaf of *Carica papaya* L. [Fam. Caricaceae], harvested before fruit development, as well as preparations thereof.

Uses
Papaya leaf preparations are used singly or in combinations for prophylaxis and therapy of diseases and discomforts of the gastrointestinal tract, for infections with intestinal parasites, as an anthelmintic for oxyurids, strongyloides, ascarides, ancylostoma, such as *Necator americanus*, and other nematodes, and also for a sedative and diuretic.

The effectiveness for the claimed applications has not been documented.

Risks
None known.

Evaluation
The therapeutic administration cannot be recommended, since the effectiveness of papaya leaf is not documented, and other, guaranteed herbs are available for the treatment of intestinal infections, particularly those by nematodes.

Paprika (Cayenne) species low in capsaicin
Capsici fructus
capsicinarme Paprika-Arten
Published April 27, 1989

Name of Drug
Capsici fructus, capsaicin-low paprika species.

Composition of Drug
Paprika consists of fresh or dried fruits of various low capsaicin-containing *Capsicum* species [Fam. Solanaceae], as well as preparations thereof.

Uses
Low capsaicin-containing paprika preparations are used internally for disturbances of the digestive system, stomach and intestinal problems, and as a supportive remedy for heart and circulatory functions.

The effectiveness for the claimed application is not documented.

Risks
Rare hypersensitivity reactions (urticaria).

Evaluation
Since efficacy has not been documented, a therapeutic use of low capsaicin-containing paprika preparation cannot be recommended.

Parsley seed
Petroselini fructus
Petersilienfrüchte
Published March 2, 1989

Name of Drug
Petroselini fructus, parsley fruit, parsley seed.

Composition of Drug
Parsley seed consists of the dried ripe fruits of *Petroselinum crispum* (Miller) Nyman ex A. W. Hill [Fam. Apiaceae], as well as preparations thereof.

Uses
Parsley seed is used for ailments and complaints of the gastrointestinal tract, as well as the kidney and lower urinary tract, and for stimulating digestion.

The claimed efficacy has not been sufficiently documented.

Risks
Large doses of parsley seed essential oil and of the phenylpropane derivative it contains, apiol, bring about vascular congestion and increased contractility of the smooth muscle of the bladder, intestines, and especially the uterus.

Parsley seed and oil are therefore often used to bring about abortion.

After taking parsley seed preparations, the renal epithelium becomes irritated or damaged; cardiac arrhythmias have also been described.

Large doses of apiol can lead to fatty liver, emaciation, extensive mucosal bleeding, and inflammatory hemorrhagic infiltration of the gastrointestinal tract, hemoglobulinuria, methemoglobulinuria, and anuria.

In animal experiments, myristicin, present in the essential oil, has been shown to be bound to mouse-liver DNA. No hepatocarcinogenic effects have been observed with either myristicin or apiol.

The toxicological risk of aqueous extracts [i.e., teas] from parsley seeds is less, because of the smaller essential oil content.

Evaluation
Since the efficacy of parsley seed and preparations thereof is not documented, a therapeutic application cannot be justified because of high risks.

Pasque flower
Pulsatillae herba
Küchenschellenkraut
Published November 30, 1985

Name of Drug
Pulsatillae herba, pasque flower, pulsatilla.

Composition of Drug
Pasque flower herb consists of the dried, above-ground parts of *Pulsatilla vulgaris* Miller and/*or P. pratensis* (L.) Miller [Fam. Ranunculaceae], as well as preparations thereof.

The herb contains protoanemonin which is degraded to an unknown extent during the drying process, as well as ranunculin and its degradation products (e.g., anemonin, anemoninic acid, anemonic acid).

Uses
Based on existing evidence, the claimed applications are:
Diseases and functional disorders of genital organs, inflammatory and infectious diseases of skin and mucosa, diseases and functional disorders of the gastrointestinal tract and the urinary tract. Neuralgia, migraine, and general restlessness are not documented from the phytotherapeutic viewpoint.

Risks
Use of preparations from fresh plants, as well as preparations with protoanemonin, produces severe irritations on skin and mucosa with itching, rashes and pustules (ranunculus dermatitis).

Internal use in higher dosages results in irritation to the kidneys and urinary tract.

Use in pregnancy is absolutely contraindicated.

Actions
In animal experiments, after absorption, protoanemonin causes first stimulation, then paralysis of the central nervous system.

Irritations occur in the kidney and the urinary tract. These may be caused by the alkylating action of protoanemonin. This effect may be connected to the observed inhibition of caryokinase and mitosis.

The ingestion of protoanemonin-containing plants by grazing animals has been observed to lead to abortion and teratogenic effects.

The anti-infectious action of the herb is based on protoanemonin.

Peony
Paeoniae flos, radix
Pfingstrose
Published May 5, 1988

Name of Drug
Paeoniae flos, peony flower.
Paeoniae radix, peony root.

Composition of Drug
Peony flower consists of the petals of *Paeonia officinalis* L. emend. Willdenow s. l. and/or *P. mascula* (L.) Miller s.l. [Fam. Paeoniaceae], as well as preparations thereof.

Peony root consists of the dried secondary roots of *P. officinalis* L. emend. Willdenow s.l. and/or *P. mascula* (L.) Miller s.l., as well as preparations thereof.

Uses
Peony flower is used for diseases of the skin and mucous membranes, fissures, anal fissures associated with hemorrhoids, gout, arthritis, also for ailments of the respiratory tract, and in combinations for nervous conditions, heart trouble and gastritis. The effectiveness of peony flower for the claimed applications is not verified.

Peony root is used for spasms of various kinds and origins, in combinations as a supplement for arthritis, diseases of the gastrointestinal tract, for the heart and circulatory system, neurasthenia and neurasthenic symptoms, neuralgia, migraine, allergic complaints, and as a tonic.

The effectiveness of peony root for the claimed applications is not documented.

Risks
None known.

Evaluation
Since the efficacy of peony preparations is not documented, the therapeutic administration cannot be recommended.

There are no objections to the use of peony flower as a brightening agent for tea mixtures.

Periwinkle
Vincae minoris herba
Immergrünkraut
Published September 18, 1986

Name of Drug
Vincae minoris herba, small periwinkle.

Composition of Drug
Periwinkle herb consists of the aboveground parts of *Vinca minor* L. [Fam. Apocynaceae], as well as preparations thereof.

Uses
Periwinkle is used for circulatory disorders, cerebral circulatory impairment, support for the metabolism of the brain and its improved oxygen supply, prophylaxis of memory and concentration impairment, improvement of memory and thinking capacity, mental productivity, prevention

of premature aging of brain cells, for geriatric support, as a sedative and as a blood pressure-lowering remedy, for catarrhs, feebleness, and for improvement of the immune function, for diarrhea, vaginal flux, throat ailments, tonsillitis and angina, sore throat, intestinal inflammation, toothache, dropsy, as a diuretic and blood-purifying remedy, for promotion of wound healing, as a hemostatic remedy, and a bitter principle.

The effectiveness for the claimed applications has not been adequately documented.

Risks
In animal experiments, administration of periwinkle caused destruction of blood components, manifested as leukocytopenia, lymphocytopenia, and lowering of the α, α_2-, and γ-globulin level, all presumably due to a suppression of the immune system.

The vincamine content in the herb is low and fluctuates greatly. Vincamine, as a pure substance, is available for therapeutic administration.

Evaluation
Since the effectiveness of periwinkle for most claimed applications is not sufficiently documented, adequate levels of vincamine in the plasma cannot be obtained with periwinkle herb and its preparations, and the suspicion of blood modifications in humans could not be removed, the therapeutic application of this herb and its preparations is not justifiable.

Petasites leaf
Petasitidis hybridus, Petasitidis folium
Pestwurz, Pestwurzblätter
Published July 27, 1990

Name of Drug
Petasitidis hybridus, petasites.
Petasitidis folium, petasites leaf.

Composition of Drug
Petasites consists of the whole plant of *Petasites* species [Fam. Asteraceae], as well as preparations thereof.

Petasites leaf consists of the leaves of *Petasites* species, as well as preparations thereof.

Uses
Petasites leaf or its preparations are used for nervous cramp-like states and such states associated with pain, colic, headaches, and to stimulate the appetite. Combined with other herbs petasites is used for complaints and disorders of the respiratory tract, chills, for liver, bile, and pancreas disorders, to strengthen the nerves, promote sleep, and to prevent internal restlessness. ·

The effectiveness for the claimed uses is not documented.

Risks
Petasites contains in all plant parts greatly varying amounts of toxic pyrrolizidine alkaloids (PA), which are known to damage organs, especially the liver. In animal experiments, PA have been shown to have carcinogenic effects brought about by a genotoxic mechanism.

Evaluation
In consideration of the risks, and lack of documentation for the effectiveness of the herb for the claimed applications, a therapeutic application cannot be justified.

Pimpinella herb
Pimpinellae herba
Bibernellkraut
Published June 1, 1990

Name of Drug
Pimpinellae herba, pimpinella herb.

Composition of Drug
Pimpinella herb consists of the above-ground parts of *Pimpinella saxifraga* L. s.l. and/or *P. major* (L.) Hudson s.l. [Fam. Apiaceae], as well as preparations thereof.

Uses
Preparations of pimpinella herb are used for lung ailments, for stimulation of gastrointestinal activity, and, externally, for varicose veins.

The effectiveness for the claimed applications is not documented.

Risks
None known.

Evaluation
Since the effectiveness for the claimed uses is not documented, a therapeutic application cannot be recommended.

Raspberry leaf
Rubi idaei folium
Himbeerblätter
Published October 15, 1987

Name of Drug
Rubi idaei folium, raspberry leaf.

Composition of Drug
Raspberry leaf consists of the leaf of *Rubus idaeus* L. [Fam. Rosaceae], as well as preparations thereof.

Uses
Raspberry leaf is used for disorders of the gastrointestinal tract, the respiratory tract, the cardiovascular system, and the mouth and throat, and also for skin rashes and inflammation, influenza, fever, menstrual problems, diabetes, vitamin deficiency, as a diaphoretic, diuretic, and choleretic, and also to "purify the skin and blood."

The effectiveness of raspberry leaves for the foregoing indications has not been documented.

Risks
None known.

Evaluation
Since the efficacy has not been documented, a therapeutic application cannot be recommended.

Rhododendron, Rusty-leaved

Rhododendri ferruginei folium
Rostrote Alpenrosenblätter
Published September 1, 1990

Name of Drug
Rhododendri ferruginei folium, rusty-leaved rhododendron.

Composition of Drug
Rusty-leaved rhododendron consists of the dried leaves of *Rhododendron ferrugineum* L. [Fam. Ericaceae] and preparations thereof.

Uses
Rusty-leaved rhododendron leaves are used exclusively in combination preparations in the treatment of hypertonia, muscle and joint rheumatism, arthroses, hardening of muscles; muscular pain, weak connective tissue; neuralgia, sensitivity to weather change, sciatica, trigeminus neuralgia, migraine, headaches, intercostal neuralgia, gout, lithiasis, and in geriatric drugs for disorders and complaints associated with aging.

The efficacy of the drug in the above-named areas has not been proven.

Risks
Rhododendron species can contain toxic diterpene with an andromedic basic structure. There is contradictory evidence on the occurrence of andromeda derivatives in rhododendron. Reports of grazing animals being poisoned by rhododendron indicate that compounds of these groups do occur in the leaves. Symptoms of acute grayanotoxine poisoning are a drop in blood pressure, bradycardia, cramps, cardiac arrest, and cessation of breathing. Chronic toxicity of the compounds in animals is relatively minimal. In humans, the following poisoning symptoms were reported after eating honey (among other foodstuffs) containing grayanotoxine: Vomiting, diarrhea, pains and cramps in the gastrointestinal tract, joint pains, impaired balance, difficulty in breathing, sensitivity of the central nervous system; paralysis, as well as burning and itching of the skin and mucous membrane.

If the drug is taken over a long period there is also danger of intoxication with hydroquinone because of the arbutin contained in the drug. There are no reports of serious instances of poisoning of patients used to taking it as an infusion in folk medicine (daily dose 5 - 6 g).

Evaluation
Due to the insufficiently proven efficacy of the drug and its pharmaceutical preparations as well as the associated risks, therapeutic use cannot be recommended.

Rose Hip
Rosae pseudofructus
Hagebuttenschalen
Published September 1, 1990

Name of Drug
Rosae pseudofructus, rose hip.

Composition of Drug
Rose hip consists of the ripe, fresh or dried seed receptacle of various species of the genus *Rosa* L. [Fam. Rosaceae], freed from seeds and attached trichomes, as well as preparations thereof.

Uses
Preparations of rose hips are used for the prevention and treatment of colds, chills, and influenza-type infections, infectious diseases, for the prevention and treatment of vitamin C deficiencies, to increase resistance, gastric-juice deficiency, bowel disorders, to aid digestion, for gallstones, biliary complaints and colic, complaints and disorders of the lower urinary tract, edema, for "strengthening the kidneys," as a diuretic, for arthritis, rheumatic disorders, and as an eyewash.

The activity in most of the aforementioned indications has not been substantiated. The activity in treating or preventing possible vitamin C deficiency is questionable in view of the herb's low vitamin C content that rapidly declines with storage.

Risks
None known.

Evaluation
Since the effectiveness for some claims is not sufficiently documented and for others not at all, a therapeutic application cannot be recommended, if only because of the rapidly decreasing vitamin C content.

The consumption of rose hip preparations as a vitamin C-containing food is primarily assigned to the food industry. There is no objection to its use as a taste enhancer in tea mixtures.

Rose Hip and seed
Rosae pseudofructus cum fructibus
Hagebutten
Published September 1, 1990

Name of Drug
Rosae pseudofructus cum fructibus, rose hip and seed.

Composition of Drug
Rose hip and seed consist of the ripe, fresh or dried " fruit" of various species of the genus *Rosa* L. [Fam. Rosaceae], freed from seeds and attached trichomes, as well as preparations thereof.

Uses
Preparations of rose hip and seed are used for prevention and treatment of colds and influenza-like infections, infectious diseases, prophylaxis and therapy of vitamin C deficiencies, fever, for increase in the immune mechanism during general exhaustion, gastric spasms, gastric acid deficiency, prevention of inflammation of the gastric mucosa and gastric ulcers, as a

"stomach tonic," for intestinal diseases, for diarrhea, as prophylaxis of intestinal catarrhs, as a laxative, for gallstones, gallbladder discomforts and ailments, diseases and discomforts of the lower urinary tract, dropsy, as a "tonic for the kidneys," as a diuretic, for gout, metabolic disorders of the uric acid metabolism, arthritis, sciatica, diabetes, inadequate peripheral circulation, as an astringent, for lung ailments, and as an eye rinse.

The effectiveness of the herb for most of its claimed applications is not documented. The effectiveness for therapy and prophylaxis of possible vitamin C deficiency is questionable because of the low and rapidly decreasing content of vitamin C.

Risks
None known.

Evaluation
Since the effectiveness of the herb for some claims is not sufficiently documented and, for other claims, not documented at all, a therapeutic application cannot be recommended. The consumption of rose hip preparations as a vitamin C-containing food is primarily assigned to the food industry.

There is no objection to the use of the herb as a flavor corrigent in tea mixtures.

Rose Hip seed
Rosae fructus
Hagebuttenkerne
Published September 1, 1990

Name of Drug
Rosae fructus, rose hip seed.

Composition of Drug
Rose hip consists of the ripe, dried seed of various species of the genus *Rosa* L. [Fam. Rosaceae], as well as preparations thereof.

Uses
Preparations of rose hip seed are used for diseases and ailments of the kidney and lower urinary tract, for dropsy (hydrops), as a diuretic, for arthritic conditions, rheumatism, gout, sciatica, for colds, as a laxative, for diseases with fever, as an astringent, for vitamin C deficiency, and for "blood purification."

The effectiveness for the claimed applications is not documented.

Risks
None known.

Evaluation
Since the effectiveness is not documented, a therapeutic application cannot be recommended.

Rue
Rutae folium, herba
Raute
Published March 2, 1989

Name of Drug
Rutae folium, rue leaf.
Rutae herba, rue herb.

Composition of Drug
Rue leaf consists of the dried leaf of *Ruta graveolens* L. ssp. *vulgaris* Willkomm [Fam. Rutaceae], as well as preparations thereof.

Rue herb consists of the dried, aboveground parts of *R. graveolens* L. ssp. *vulgaris* Willkomm, as well as preparations thereof.

Uses
Preparations of rue herb and/or leaf are used for menstrual disorders and discomforts, as a uterine stimulant and for abortion; furthermore for loss of appetite and dyspeptic complaints, circulatory disorders, arteriosclerosis, palpitation of the heart, for nervousness, hysteria, fever, pleurisy, headache, neuralgic afflictions, toothache, weakness of the eyes and respiratory complaints. It is also used internally and externally for ailments and discomforts of arthritic conditions, for dislocations, sprains, injuries of the bone, for skin diseases, and as an antispasmodic, diuretic and inflammatory agent.

The effectiveness for the claimed applications is not verified.

Risks
Rue oil can cause contact dermatitis in humans.

Furthermore, phototoxic reactions causing dermatoses have been described. Severe liver and kidney damage is also documented.

The herb contains furanocoumarins which have phototoxic and mutagenic actions.

Deaths of pregnant women have been reported upon usage of rue for abortion.

Therapeutic dosages can cause the following side effects:

Melancholic moods, sleep disorders, tiredness, dizziness, and spasms.

The juice of fresh leaves can lead to painful irritations of the stomach and intestines, fainting, sleepiness, low pulse, abortion, swelling of the tongue and clammy skin.

Evaluation
A therapeutic administration must be declined since the effectiveness for the claimed applications is not documented, and because of the unfavorable ratio of benefit to risk.

Rupturewort
Herniariae herba
Bruchkraut
Published September 18, 1986

Name of Drug
Herniariae herba, rupturewort.

Composition of Drug
Rupturewort consists of the dried, above-ground parts of *Herniaria glabra* L. and/or *Herniaria hirsuta* L. [Fam. Caryophyllaceae], as well as preparations thereof.

Uses
Rupturewort is used for the treatment and alleviation of conditions and disorders involving the kidneys and urinary tract or the respiratory tract, and in neuritis and neural catarrh, in arthritis and rheumatism, and for "purifying the blood."

Efficacy in the indicated areas of use has not been adequately demonstrated.

Risks
None known.

Evaluation
Since the effectiveness for the claimed uses is not sufficiently documented, a therapeutic application cannot be recommended.

Action
Mildly antispasmodic

Saffron
Croci stigma
Safran
Published April 23, 1987

Name of Drug
Croci stigma, saffron.

Composition of Drug
Saffron consists of the stigmata, usually connected by a short piece of pistil, of *Crocus sativa* L. [Fam. Iridaceae], as well as preparations thereof.

Uses
Saffron is used as a sedative, for spasms and asthma.

The effectiveness of the herb for its claimed applications has not been documented.

Risks
Presently, no risks have been documented for a maximum daily dosage of 1.5 g. The lethal dosage is 20 g; the abortifacient dosage is 10 g.

From the administration of saffron as an abortifacient, the following effects have been observed:

Severe purpura after ingestion of 5 g of saffron (suspended in milk) with pitch black necrosis of the nose and a thrombocytopenia of 24,000, hypothrobinemia of 41 percent and severe collapse with uremia.
Additionally: bleeding of the uterus, bloody diarrhea, hematuria, bleeding from the nose, lips and eyelids, vertigo, dizziness, numbness. Yellowing of the sclera, skin and mucous membranes, a condition that may falsely imply icterus.

Sandalwood, Red
Santali lignum rubrum
Rotes Sandelholz
Published October 15, 1987

Name of Drug
Santali lignum rubrum, red sandalwood.

Composition of Drug
Red sandalwood consists of the heartwood of the trunk of *Pterocarpus santalinus* L. f. [Fam. Fabaceae], freed from sapwood, as well as preparations thereof.

Uses
Red sandalwood is used for ailments and complaints of the gastrointestinal tract, as a diuretic, astringent, for "blood purification" and for cough.

Risks
None known.

Evaluation
The therapeutic administration of red sandalwood cannot be recommended, since its effectiveness has not been documented.

Sarsaparilla root
Sarsaparillae radix
Sarsaparillewurzel
Published September 1, 1990

Name of Drug
Sarsaparillae radix, sarsaparilla root.

Composition of Drug
Sarsaparilla root consists of the dried root of *Smilax* species, such as *Smilax aristolochiaefolii* Miller, *S. regelii* Kill. et C.V. Morton and *S. febrifuga* Knuth [Fam. Smilacaceae], as well as preparations thereof.

Uses
Preparations of sarsaparilla root are used for skin diseases, psoriasis and its sequelae, rheumatic complaints, kidney diseases, and as a diuretic and diaphoretic.
   The claimed efficacy has not been documented.

Risks
Taking sarsaparilla preparations leads to gastric irritation and temporary kidney impairment [diuresis]. The absorption of simultaneously administered substances, for example digitalis glycosides or bismuth, is increased. The elimination of other substances (e.g., hypnotics) is accelerated. This can cause an uncontrolled condition of increased or decreased action of herbs taken simultaneously.

Evaluation
Since the efficacy for psoriasis has not been documented, a therapeutic application cannot be justified because of the risks.

[**Ed. note:** Contrary to the undocumented claims of gastric irritation due to saponin content of sarsaparilla root, we can find nothing in the scientific literature that substantiates this assertion. It is well known that many commonly consumed vegetables contain saponins and sarsaparilla root is a common ingredient in soft drinks, e.g., root beer and many herbal teas. Therefore, we disagree with the Commission that potential gastric irritation is a problem associated with the ingestion of this herb in normal quantities.]

Sarsaparilla, German

Caricis rhizoma
Sandriedgraswurzelstock
Published June 1, 1990

Name of Drug
Caricis rhizoma, German sarsaparilla.

Composition of Drug
German sarsaparilla consists of the dried, underground parts of *Carex arenaria* L. [Fam. Cyperaceae], as well as preparations thereof.

Uses
Preparations of German sarsaparilla are used for the prevention of gout, arthritis, inflammations of the joints, for skin ailments and as a diaphoretic and diuretic.

The effectiveness of the claimed application is not documented.

Risks
Based on the saponin content, local irritations could occur.

Evaluation
Since the effectiveness for the claimed uses is not documented, a therapeutic application cannot be recommended.

Scotch Broom flower

Cytisi scoparii flos
Besenginsterblüten
Published January 17, 1991

Name of Drug
Cytisi scoparii flos, Scotch broom flower.

Composition of Drug
Scotch Broom flower consists of the blossoms of *Cytisus scoparius* (L.) Link (syn. *Sarothamnus scoparius* (L.) Wimm. ex W.D.J. Koch), as well as preparations thereof.

Pharmacological Properties, Pharmacokinetics, Toxicology
The drug can contain more than 2 percent tyramine. It contains small amounts of alkaloids; the main alkaloid is sparteine. Tyramine acts indirectly as a sympathomimetic drug, a vasoconstrictive and hypertensive effect. Sparteine has a negative inotropic and negative chronotropic

effect. Because of the very small sparteine concentration, certain effects cannot be expected upon administration of the herb.

Clinical Data

Clinical data reported by physicians and other materials of medical experiences concerning the use of Scotch Broom flower are not available.

1. Components of the Following Drug Combinations

Combinations containing up to 5 components:
　　None.
Combinations containing more than 5 components:
Primary use, cardiovascular system:
a) Scotch broom flower, night-blooming cereus, spigelia anthelmia, lily-of-the-valley, hawthorn leaf and flower, arnica (whole plant).
b) Scotch broom flower, valerian root, hawthorn flower, horsetail, silver weed, lemon balm, hawthorn berry.
c) Scotch broom flower, yarrow herb and flower, hops, mistletoe, sandy everlasting flower, rosemary leaf.
d) Scotch broom flower, camphor, hawthorn berry, lily-of-the-valley, night-blooming cereus flower, pheasant's eye herb, bugleweed herb, bitter candy tuft, american wormseed (*Chenopodium anthelminticum*).
e) Scotch broom flower, arnica flower, valerian root, lovage root, hawthorn flower, yarrow herb, mistletoe, pheasant's eye herb, hedge hyssop, oleander leaf.
f) Scotch broom flower, hawthorn flower, valerian root, pheasant's eye herb, hops, St. John's Wort, 13 homeopathic components.
g) Scotch broom flower, arnica flower, valerian root, lovage root, linden flower, hawthorn flower and leaf, red sandalwood, lemon balm, hops, mistletoe, sandy everlasting flower, calendula flower, rosemary leaf, lavender flower, pheasant's eye herb, sunflower ray flower, yarrow flower.
h) Scotch broom flower, belladonna leaf, valerian root, hawthorn flower, lemon balm, St. John's Wort, mistletoe, arnica root, lily-of-the-valley, strophanthus seed, extracts fermented by yeast.
i) Scotch broom flower, bishop's weed fruit, 8 homeopathic components.

Primary use, kidney:
j) Scotch broom flower, hawthorn flower, birch leaf, seed-free bean shells, horsetail herb, rupturewort, meadowsweet flower.
k) Scotch broom flower, European goldenrod herb, birch leaf, horsetail, restharrow root, white willow bark, boldo leaf, Java tea leaf, spearmint leaf, Tinnevelly senna fruit.
l) Scotch broom flower, European goldenrod herb, birch leaf, horsetail, restharrow root, white willow bark, boldo leaf, Java tea leaf, spearmint leaf, senna fruit.
m) Scotch broom flower, uva ursi leaf, juniper berry, European goldenrod herb, birch leaf, restharrow root, madder root, rupturewort, Java tea leaf, boldo leaf, heather.

Other indications:
n) Scotch broom flower, caraway seed, senna leaf, juniper berry, birch leaf, walnut leaf, horsetail, ground Ivy (*Glechoma hederacea*), stinging nettle leaf, calendula flower, veronica herb.
o) Scotch broom flower, uva ursi leaf, birch leaf, blackberry leaf, yarrow herb and flower, hops, rosemary leaf, lady's woundwort flower (*Anthyllis vulneraria*), stinging nettle leaf, raspberry leaf, strawberry leaf, cowslip flower without calyx.
p) Scotch broom flower and herb, ivy leaf, tormentilla root, marsh tea, rue leaf, pine sprout tips, heart's ease herb, knotweed, hops, meadowsweet flower, peony flower, moneywort, lithium sali-

cylate, magnesium salicylate, rubidium chloride and bromide.
q) Scotch broom flower, uva ursi leaf, buckthorn bark, peppermint leaf, wormwood herb, birch leaf, cornflower blossom, horsetail, sweet flag (*Acorus calamus*), calendula herb, barberry root bark, chicory herb, boldo leaf, oat straw.
r) Scotch broom flower, buckthorn bark, elderberry flower, senna leaf, birch leaf, kelp, watercress herb, bogbean leaf, chicory, small bindweed (*Convolvulus arvense*), parsley root.
s) Scotch broom flower, buckthorn bark, chamomile flower, peppermint leaf, senna leaf, licorice root, thyme, juniper berry, red sandalwood, birch leaf, dandelion, yarrow herb, couch grass, horsetail, restharrow root, mistletoe, rosemary leaf, watercress herb, hawthorn leaf and flower, small bindweed herb, motherwort, parsley root, raspberry leaf, heather blossom, calendula flower, soapwort herb (*Saponaria officinalis*).

2. Claimed Uses of the Above Combinations

a) Coronary insufficiency, arrhythmia, regulation of high blood pressure, geriatric heart, interval and post treatment with digitalis and strophanthus tinctures, functional cardiac disorders.
b) Favorable influence on cardiac action and stimulation of blood circulation, strengthening of the heart muscle and blood vessels, considerably decreases the risk of circulatory disorders and arteriosclerosis.
c) Adjuvant for nervous cardiac disorders.
d) Hypotonic symptomatic complex with dizziness, sensitivity to changes in the weather, delayed convalescence.
e) Supportive therapy for cardiovascular disorders.
f) Cardiac and circulatory remedy with sedative action.
g) Cardiac and circulatory insufficiency.
h) Cardiogenic hypertonia, chronic latent cardiac insufficiency, cardiac support during convalescence.
i) Cardiac irregularity, hypotonia.
j) Supportive therapy for edema.
k) Diseases of the urinary tract, functional stimulation of kidneys, disinfecting, antiinflammatory, gravel and stone formation.
l) Supportive therapy for the function of kidney and bladder.
m) Nephrolithiasis, nephritis, cystitis, pyelitis, dropsy, bacteriuria.
n) Supportive therapy for skin eczema and allergic skin reactions.
o) Stimulation for the self-purification of the skin, due to a better circulation, removal of water from the tissue, purification of the body, for skin blemishes, pimples, pustules, whelk, and blackheads.
p) Arthritis of the muscles and joints, arthritis urica, as a supplement for relieving pain due to spondylosis.
q) Flux of liver and gall, gallstones, gall gravel.
r) Supportive treatment of general obesity.
s) Support of all organic functions.

3. Risks
Contraindication:
Therapy with MAO-inhibitors.
High blood pressure.

Side Effects
None known.

Precautions While Using This Medicine
None known.

Interactions with Other Drugs
The administration of the drug and simultaneous therapy with MAO-inhibitors can cause a blood pressure crisis because of its tyramine content.

Dosage and Mode of Administration
The drug is used in tea mixtures and extract preparations.

Overdosage
None known.

Special Precautions
None known.

Effects on Operators of Vehicles and Machinery
None known.

Evaluation
Based on the insufficiently documented effectiveness and possible interactions, a therapeutic application is not justifiable. There is no objection to using this drug as brightening agent up to 1 percent in tea mixtures.

[Ed. note: This herb is an Unapproved Component Characteristic and belongs in Chapter 6. However, this misplacement in the Unapproved Herbs section was discovered only after this book was paginated, just prior to press time.]

Senecio herb
Senecionis herba
Fuchskreuzkraut
Published July 27, 1990

Name of Drug
Senecionis herba, senecio herb.

Composition of Drug
Senecio herb consists of the above-ground parts of *Senecio nemorensis* ssp. *fuchsii* C. Gmelin [Fam. Asteraceae], as well as preparations thereof.

Uses
Senecio herb is used for diabetes mellitus, hemorrhage, high blood pressure, for spasms, and as a uterine stimulant.

The effectiveness for diffuse mucosal hemorrhages is not sufficiently verified.

The effectiveness for the other claimed uses is not documented.

Risks
Senecio herb contains varying amounts of toxic pyrrolizidine alkaloids (PA) which are known to have organotoxic, in particular hepatotoxic, effects. Carcinogenic activity, operating through a genotoxic mechanism, has been demonstrated in animal experiments.

In addition to being an ineffective remedy for diabetes mellitus, use of the herb represents a considerable health risk.

Evaluation
The therapeutic administration of senecio herb is not justifiable because of its insufficient or undocumented effectiveness and the presence of toxic pyrrolizidine alkaloids.

Action
Shortening of hemorrhage.

Soapwort herb, Red
Saponariae rubrae herba
Seifenkraut
Published April 27, 1989

Name of Drug
Saponariae rubrae herba, soapwort herb.

Composition of Drug
Soapwort herb consists of the dried, above-ground parts of *Saponaria officinalis* L. [Fam. Caryophyllaceae], as well as preparations thereof.

Uses
Red soapwort preparations are used as an expectorant for cough and other diseases of the respiratory tract, as an emetic, laxative, for ailments of the gastrointestinal tract, for liver and kidney diseases, as a diuretic, a diaphoretic, for metabolic modifications.

Externally, soapwort preparations are used for compresses, baths and washing of lichen, skin rashes and other afflictions of the skin.

The effectiveness for the claimed applications is not sufficiently substantiated.

Risks
At higher concentrations, triterpene saponins from *S. officinalis* cause irritation of mucous membranes. Higher dosages used for external application may also lead to irritations.

Evaluation
Since the effectiveness for the claimed applications is not sufficiently documented, and especially since the dosage indications are missing, a therapeutic administration for the respiratory tract and skin cannot be recommended.

The use for the other applications is not justifiable.

Spinach leaf
Spinaciae folium
Spinatblätter
Published May 5, 1988

Name of Drug
Spinaciae folium, spinach.

Composition of Drug
Spinach consists of the fresh or dried leaf of *Spinacia oleracea* L. [Fam. Chenopodiaceae], as well as preparations thereof.

Uses
Spinach preparations are used for ailments and complaints of the gastrointestinal tract, as a blood-generating remedy, to stimulate growth in children, as an appetite stimulant, for fatigue, and for supporting convalescence.

The claimed applications have not been sufficiently documented.

Risks
None known.

Evaluation
Since the efficacy has not been documented, a therapeutic application cannot be recommended.

Strawberry leaf
Fragariae folium
Erdbeerblätter
Published February 1, 1990

Name of Drug
Fragariae folium, strawberry leaf.

Composition of Drug
Strawberry leaf consists of the dried leaf of *Fragaria* species, mainly *F. vesca* L. s.l. and *F. viridis* Duchesne [Fam. Rosaceae], as well as preparations thereof.

Uses
Preparations of strawberry leaf are used externally as compresses for rashes, and internally for catarrhs of the gastrointestinal tract, diarrhea, intestinal sluggishness, liver disease, jaundice, catarrhs of the respiratory tract, gout, arthritis, nervous tension, kidney ailments involving gravel and stones, as a diuretic, supportive for heart and circulatory ailments, for fever, for night perspiration, as well as for blood purification, for stimulation of the metabolism, for anemia, as a tonic, as an inhibitor of menstruation, and a support for "natural weight loss."

Activity in the indications listed has not been adequately demonstrated.

Risks
Strawberry leaf can cause allergic reactions in persons with a sensitivity to strawberries.

Evaluation
Since the effectiveness for the claimed applications has not been sufficiently documented, a therapeutic application cannot be recommended. The use of the herb as a filler in tea mixtures is acceptable. In fact, the use of strawberry leaf for teas or tea-like products is to be considered a food additive.

Sweet Woodruff
Galii odorati herba
Waldmeisterkraut
Published October 15, 1987

Name of Drug
Galii odorati herba, sweet woodruff herb.

Composition of Drug
Sweet woodruff herb consists of fresh or dried above-ground parts of *Galium odoratum* (L.) Scopoli [Fam. Rubiaceae], as well as preparations thereof.

Uses

Sweet woodruff herb is used for prophylaxis and therapy of diseases and discomforts of the respiratory tract, gastrointestinal tract, liver and gallbladder, as well as the kidney and urinary tract, also for circulatory disorders, venous complaints, weak veins, hemorrhoids, as an antiinflammatory and for dilation of the blood vessels. Furthermore, as sedative for sleep disorders, for inducing sleep, for spasms, abdominal discomforts, skin diseases, for wound treatment, as a diaphoretic, as a remedy for strengthening the nervous system and heart function, and for blood purification.

The effectiveness for the claimed applications has not been documented.

Risks

None known.

Evaluation

The therapeutic administration of sweet woodruff herb cannot be recommended, since the effectiveness is not documented.

Tansy flower and herb
Chrysanthemi vulgaris flos/herba
Rainfarn
Published July 6, 1988

Name of Drug

Chrysanthemi vulgaris flos, tansy flower.
Chrysanthemi vulgaris herba, tansy herb.

Composition of Drug

Tansy flower consists of the inflorescence of *Chrysanthemum vulgare* (L.) Bernhardi ([preferred] syn. *Tanacetum vulgare* L.) [Fam. Asteraceae], well as preparations thereof in effective dosage.

Tansy herb consists of the above-ground parts of *C. vulgare* (L.) Bernhardi ([preferred] syn. *T. vulgare* L.), as well as preparations thereof in effective dosage.

Uses

Tansy preparations are used as an anthelmintic, for migraine, neuralgia, rheumatism, meteorism and loss of appetite.

The effectiveness for the claimed applications has not been demonstrated.

Risks

Tansy contains an essential oil which usually includes thujone. Thujone possesses neurotoxic properties.

Abuse of large amounts of this herb or its essential oil to induce abortion caused the following symptoms of intoxication: vomiting, abdominal pain, gastroenteritis, reddening of the face, severe clonic-tonic spasms after loss of consciousness, greatly accelerated breathing, and irregular heart beat. Mydriasis and pupillary rigidity, bleeding of the uterus, under certain circumstances abortion, kidney damage, liver damage.

The lethal dosage of the essential oil for humans is 15 - 30 g.

Uncontrolled usage of tansy, depending on the quality of the herb, can result in the absorption of thujone in toxic amounts, even at normal dosages.

Studies of the toxicity of thujone-free chemotypes are not available.

Evaluation
Since the effectiveness of tansy preparations for the claimed uses has not been documented, a therapeutic application cannot be justified because of the risks involved.

Verbena herb
Verbenae herba
Eisenkraut
Published February 1, 1990

Name of Drug
Verbenae herba, verbena herb.

Composition of Drug
Verbena herb consists of the aboveground parts of *Verbena officinalis* L. [Fam. Verbenaceae], as well as preparations thereof.

Uses
Preparations of verbena are used for diseases and ailments of the oral and pharyngeal mucosa, such as angina, sore throats, diseases of the respiratory tract, such as cough, asthma, and whooping cough, also pain, spasms, exhaustion, nervous conditions, digestive disorders, liver and gallbladder diseases, jaundice, diseases and ailments of the kidneys and lower urinary tract, menopausal complaints, irregular menstruation, for lactation during nursing, furthermore, for arthritic conditions, gout, metabolic disorders, anemia, dropsy, and externally for poorly healing wounds, abscesses and burns.

The effectiveness for the claimed applications is not documented.

Risks
None known.

Evaluation
Since effectiveness of the claimed applications has not been documented, therapeutic application of the herb cannot be recommended.

Because of its secretolytic action, it is possible that the herb can contribute positively to the activity of established combinations for use in catarrhs of the upper respiratory tract. However, the contribution to such preparations must be specifically determined.

Action
Secretolytic

Veronica herb
Veronicae herba
Ehrenpreiskraut
Published June 1, 1990

Name of Drug
Veronicae herba, veronica herb, speedwell.

Constituents of Drug
Veronica herb consists of the aboveground parts of *Veronica officinalis* L. [Fam.

Scrophulariaceae], as well as preparations thereof.

Uses
Veronica herb preparations are used for diseases and discomforts of the respiratory tract, gastrointestinal tract, liver, kidney and lower urinary tract, for gout, arthritis and rheumatic complaints, diseases of the spleen, scrofulosis, nervous irritation, for "blood purification," promotion of metabolism, as an appetite stimulant and tonic, also as a diaphoretic. In addition, veronica herb preparations are used externally for perspiration of the feet, stimulation of wound healing, chronic skin conditions, and itching.

The effectiveness for the claimed applications is not verified.

Risks
None known.

Evaluation
Since the effectiveness for the claimed applications is not documented, a therapeutic administration cannot be recommended.

Walnut hull
Juglandis fructus cortex
Walnußfrüchtschalen
Published June 1, 1990

Name of Drug
Juglandis fructus cortex, walnut hull.

Composition of Drug
Walnut hull consists of the pericarps of *Juglans regia* L. [Fam. Juglandaceae], as well as preparations thereof.

Uses
Walnut hull preparations are used for catarrhs of the gastrointestinal tract, skin diseases, abscesses, inflammation of the eyes, in combinations for diabetes, gastritis, for "blood purification," blood poisoning, and anemia.

The effectiveness for the claimed applications is not documented.

Risks
Fresh walnut hull contains the napthoquinone derivative juglone. The juglone content of the dried walnut hulls has been insufficiently investigated. Juglone acts as a mutagen in various model systems. Application of juglone-containing walnut preparations onto the skin and mucous membranes leads to yellow to brown discoloration. The topical, daily use of juglone-containing preparations of walnut bark is tied to an increased occurrence of cancer of the tongue and leukoplakia of the lips.

Evaluation
Since the effectiveness for the claimed uses is not documented and risks are known, the application of walnut hull preparations cannot be justified.

White Dead Nettle herb
Lamii albi herba
Weißes Taubnesselkraut
Published July 14, 1993

Name of Drug
Lamii albi herba, white dead nettle herb.

Composition of Drug
White dead nettle herb consists of the dried above-ground parts of *Lamium album* L. [Fam. Lamiaceae], gathered during flowering season, as well as preparations thereof.

Pharmacological Properties, Pharmacokinetics, Toxicology
Not known.

Clinical Data

1. Uses
Preparations of white dead nettle herb are used as supporting treatment for gastrointestinal discomforts, such as irritation of the gastric mucosa, feeling of fullness, flatulence, and for strengthening the intestines.

In combinations, preparations of white dead nettle herb are used for nervousness, nervous unrest and irritation, for sleep disorders, as a tonic, for relaxation and stimulation, during menopause, for all kinds of female ailments, menstrual disorders, "blood purification," metabolic stimulation, support of gallbladder and liver function, tendency to gallbladder gravel, as an appetite stimulant, for neutralization of gastric hyperacidity, stimulation of digestion, flatulence, stimulation of pancreatic function, regulation of the blood lipid level, irrigation therapy for inflammatory and spastic bladder trouble, functioning capacity of the prostate, stimulation of cardiovascular system and blood circulation, dizziness, flickering of the eyes, tinnitus, increased blood supply to the heart, increased heart capacity, improvement of lymph flow and stimulation of lymph production, strengthening of the respiratory tract, dissolution of mucus, improvement in vitality and general weakness, especially after diseases and surgery.

2. Risks
None known.

Evaluation
Since the effectiveness for the claimed uses is not documented, a therapeutic application cannot be recommended.

Yohimbe bark
Yohimbehe cortex
Yohimbeherinde
Published October 15, 1987; Revised February 1, 1990

Name of Drug
Yohimbehe cortex, yohimbe bark.

Composition of Drug
Yohimbe bark consists of the dried bark of the trunk and/or branches of *Pausinystalia yohimbe* (K. Schumann) Pierre ex Beille

[syn. *Corynanthe yohimbi* Schumann] [Fam. Rubiaceae], as well as preparations thereof.

The bark contains alkaloids. The main alkaloid is yohimbine.

Uses
Yohimbe bark is used for sexual disorders, as an aphrodisiac, and for feebleness and exhaustion.

The effectiveness of this herb and its preparations for the claimed applications is not documented.

Risks
Therapeutic administration of yohimbine can cause nervous excitation, tremor, sleeplessness, anxiety, increased blood pressure, and tachycardia, as well as nausea and vomiting. In case of existing liver and kidney diseases, yohimbe preparations should not be used.

Interactions with psychopharmacological herbs have been reported. Corresponding observations for preparations are not documented.

Evaluation
The therapeutic administration of yohimbe bark and its preparations is not recommended because of insufficient proof of efficacy and the unforeseeable correlation between risk and benefit.

Zedoary rhizome
Zedoariae rhizoma
Zitwerwurzelstock
Published July 6, 1988

Name of Drug
Zedoariae rhizoma, zedoary rhizome.

Composition of Drug
Zedoary rhizome consists of the dried rhizome of *Curcuma zedoaria* (Christmann) Roscoe [Fam. Zingiberaceae], as well as preparations thereof.

Uses
Zedoary rhizome is used as a stomachic for digestive debility, colic and spasms.

The effectiveness for the claimed applications is not documented.

Risks
None known.

Evaluation
Since the effectiveness for the claimed applications is not documented, a therapeutic use of this herb cannot be recommended.

Chapter 6

Unapproved Component Characteristics

Aspen bark and leaf
Populi cortex/-folium
Pappelrinde/-blätter
Published August 29, 1992

Name of Drug
Populi cortes, folium. Aspen bark leaf.

Composition of Drug
Aspen bark consists of the fresh or dried bark of *Populus* species [Fam. Salicaceae], rich in salicin, particularly P. *tremula* or P. *tremuloides*, as well as preparations thereof.

Aspen leaf consists of the fresh or dried leaf of *Populus* species, rich in salicin, particularly P. *tremula* or P. *tremuloides*, as well as preparations thereof.

Pharmacological Properties, Pharmacokinetics, Toxicology
There are no pharmacological data available for the single drugs.

The following results are documented for extracts made from a mixture of aspen bark and aspen leaf (1:2).

[In herb preparations] the extract ratio is not always given:

- The "phenylchinon writhing-test" in mice was initiated by administration of 6.3 ml aspen extract/kg of body weight through a stomach tube, an average latency of 8.7 minutes and a 42.8 percent inhibition of writhing was observed.
- The "brewer's yeast inflammation-pain test" in rats, initiated by administration of 6.34 ml aspen extract/kg body weight through a stomach tube, resulted in a 45 percent increase of the pain wave after 4 hours.
- In the dextran-edema test and the carrageenan-edema test in rats, after administration of 3.15 and 6 ml aspen extract/kg body weight through a stomach tube, no significant differences from the control animals were observed. Following administration of 360 mg of aspen dry extract/kg of body weight, the carrageenan-edema-test showed a 12.3 and 13.5 percent volume reduction of the paws after 6 and 8 hours, respectively.
- The cotton-pellet test in rats, initiated by administration of 3 ml aspen extract/kg body weight through a stomach tube, showed no significant differences from the control.
- Compared to the control, significant inhibition of the synthesis of prostaglandin E2, I2 and D2 in the perfused rabbit ear was observed after administration of 2 ml and 10 ml of aspen extract/ml.
- In the sensitized, perfused lung of guinea pig, 0.997 mg aspen dry extract/g and 0.334 mg fluidextract/ml inhibited the release of histamine by 43 percent and 76 per-

cent, of leukotrienes by 83 percent and 78.25 percent, and of prostaglandin E2 by 77 percent and 55 percent, respectively.

Clinical Data

Clinical experiments are available only for rheumatic disorders. In clinical experiments the reduction of pain and swelling due to inflammation is demonstrated by a combination product containing aspen bark and leaf, goldenrod and ash bark.

1. Component of the Following Drug Combinations

a) Aspen leaf, aspen bark, saw palmetto fruit, stinging nettle root.
b) Aspen leaf, aspen bark, stinging nettle root.
c) Aspen leaf, pumpkin seed flour, globulin from pumpkin seed flour, goldenrod herb.
d) Aspen bark and leaf, goldenrod herb, ash bark.

2. Claimed Uses of the Above Combinations

a) Early state of benign prostate enlargement, geriatric prostate with difficulties of voiding the bladder, pre- and post-operative treatment of prostatectomy, chronic inflammation of the prostate, prostate disorders with congestion, nervous prostate disorders, nervous bladder and atony of the bladder sphincter without organic reason for both men and women.
b) Early state of benign prostate enlargement, geriatric prostate with difficulties of voiding the bladder, pre- and post-treatment of prostatectomy, chronic inflammation of the prostate, prostate disorders with congestion, nervous prostate disorders, nervous bladder and atony of the bladder sphincter without organic reason for both men and women.
c) Therapeutic agent for prostate diseases, prostate hypertrophy with difficulty with urination disorders and formation of residual urine in the bladder, nervous bladder.
d) Acute and sub-acute rheumatic ailments, lumbago, sciatica, neuralgia.

3. Risks
None known.

4. Contraindications
Hypersensitivity to salicylate.

5. Side Effects
In very rare cases, allergic reactions may occur.

6. Precautions
Use for prostate discomforts:
Note: This medication relieves only the discomfort of an enlarged prostate, without eliminating the enlargement.
A physician should be consulted at regular intervals.

7. Use During Pregnancy and Lactation
None known.

8. Interaction with Other Drugs
None known.

9. Dosage and Mode of Administration

The dosage depends on the respective amount of the drugs in the specific combinations; this amount must be documented for each preparation. No scientific knowledge is available to document the necessary dosage for the effectiveness of the drug.

For the two combinations for rheumatic ailments the dosage is given as 130 mg 3 - 4 times daily. The dosage for the combinations for prostate discomfort is 60 mg 2 - 4 times daily. The dosage in other preparations cannot be ascertained, because the drug/extract ratio is not known.

10. Overdosage
None known.

11. Special Precautions
None known.

12. Effects on Drivers and Operators of Machinery
None known.

Evaluation
Because of the pharmacological properties of the salicylate-containing drug, a positive contribution for the effectiveness in the combinations cannot be assumed, since the effective dosage cannot be attained with the extract. Empirical observations by physicians prescribing the single drug are not available.

Basil oil
Basilici aetheroleum
Basilikumöl
Published March 18, 1992

Name of Drug
Basilici aetheroleum, basil oil.

Composition of Drug
Basil oil is the essential oil of the dried, above-ground parts of *Ocimum basilicum* L. [Fam. Lamiaceae], obtained by water steam distillation, as well as preparations thereof.

Pharmacological Properties, Pharmacokinetics, Toxicology
In vitro antimicrobial.

Clinical Data
Medicinal and/or clinical reports and other material of empirical medicine for the use of basil oil are not available.

1. Component of the Following Drug Combinations
Combinations containing up to 5 components:
a) Basil oil, rosemary oil, cinnamon oil, peppermint oil.
b) Basil oil, rosemary oil, cinnamon oil, peppermint oil, 1 homeopathic component.

Combinations containing more than 5 components:
c) Basil oil, juniper berry oil, licorice root, glycyrrhizic acid, horsetail herb, restharrow root, angelica oil, echinacea root, uva ursi leaf, white willow bark, birch leaf, couch grass, Virginian wild black cherry herb.
d) Basil oil, anise oil, lemon oil, eucalyptus oil, fennel oil, clove oil, peppermint oil, juniper berry oil, citronella oil, guaiazulene, bergamot oil, Siberian pine oil, rosemary oil, mugo pine oil, orange peel oil, thyme oil, sage oil, Maltese orange oil, Chinese cinnamon oil, wintergreen oil, sassafras root oil, spearmint oil, absinthe oil, nutmeg oil, wild thyme oil, mint oil, 1 homeopathic component.
e) Basil oil, camphor, lemon oil, eucalyptus oil, lavender oil, menthol, peppermint oil, citronella oil, bergamot oil, rosemary oil, mugo pine oil,

white spruce oil, cineol, thyme oil, sage oil, spearmint oil, terpineol, myrrh oil, garlic oil, castor oil, orange oil.

2. Claimed Uses of the Above Combinations

a) Wound treatment, rheumatic discomforts, colds, bruises, painful joints, irrigation therapy.
b) Maintenance and stimulation of sexual capacity, prevention of sexual fatigue in male and female, prevention of frigidity in male and female.
c) Supportive treatment for infections of the lower urinary tract, as well as inflammations of kidneys, bladder and urethra.
d) Nasal catarrh, temporary shortness of breath, fatigue, cough, congestion, muscle pain, nerve pain, pain in the limbs (neuralgia), lumbago, sprains, dislocations, contusions, heartburn, flatulence, bad breath, insect bites, body odor, headaches, travel fatigue, inflammation, oral hygiene, air quality improvement, foot baths, bath additive.
e) Supportive therapy for massages used as warm-up procedures of the muscles before sports activities and particularly exertions in order to prevent muscle sprains and muscle spasms and their consequences, and for massages of hardened muscle parts.

3. Risks

Basil oil contains up to 85 percent estragole. Estragole, after metabolic activation, shows a mutagenic effect. Animal experiments point to a carcinogenic effect, which needs further investigation.

4. Contraindications

Due to the high estragole content, basil oil preparations should not be used during pregnancy, nursing, by infants and small children, or over extended periods of time.

5. Side Effects

None known.

6. Precautions While Using this Medicine

None known.

7. Use During Pregnancy

Not to be used during pregnancy and lactation.

8. Interactions with Other Drugs

None known.

9. Dosage and Mode of Administration

None known.

10. Overdosage

None known.

11. Special Precautions

None known.

12. Effects on Operators of Vehicles and Machinery

None known.

Evaluation

Since the effectiveness for the claimed uses is not documented, and because of the risks, a therapeutic application cannot be justified.

California Poppy
Eschscholziae californica
Kalifornischer Goldmohn
Published September 21, 1991

Name of Drug
Eschscholziae californica, California Poppy.

Composition of Drug
California Poppy consists of the above-ground parts of *Eschscholzia californica* Chamisso [Fam. Papaveraceae], as well as preparations thereof.

Pharmacological Properties, Pharmacokinetics, Toxicology
The drug contains alkaloids. Its principal alkaloid is cryptopine. Cryptopine, at a concentration of 1:1,000,000, should have a stimulating action on the uterus in guinea pigs.

In mice, an intraperitoneal application of tincture (equivalent to 130 mg drug/kg of body weight) produces a reduction in spontaneous motility, as well as a prolongation of pentobarbital-induced sleep.

Using the jejunum of the rat as testing system, the addition of tincture (equivalent to 1.75 mg of drug/ml) prevents spasms induced by administration of $BaCl_2$.

Clinical Data

1. Component of the Following Drug Combinations
Combinations containing up to 5 components:
a) California Poppy herb, valerian root, St. John's Wort, passionflower herb, hollowroot-birthwort.

Combinations containing more than 5 components:
b) California Poppy herb, lemon balm leaf, night-blooming cereus, yohimbe bark, horned poppy herb, 2 homeopathic drugs.
c) California Poppy herb, valerian root, buckthorn bark, mallow flower, peppermint leaf, garden sage leaf, cornflower flower, lemon balm leaf, hibiscus leaf, hops, squill, sweet clover, rosemary leaf, lavender flower, passionflower herb, hawthorn leaf with flower, rose flower, oat straw.

2. Claimed Uses of the Above Combinations
a) Reactive, agitated and masked depressions, melancholy, neurasthenia, neuropathy, organ neurosis.
b) Vegetative-dystonic disturbances, imbalances, foehn illness, vasomotor dysfunction, vegetative-endocrine syndrome, constitutional lability of the nervous system, vasomotor cephalgia, sensitivity to changes of the weather.
c) Sleep-inducing and sedating tea.

3. Risks
Use during pregnancy and lactation: Experiments pertaining to the use during pregnancy are not available. Based on its pharmacological activity, this drug should be avoided during pregnancy.

Evaluation
Medical and/or clinical reports and other material of empirical medicine concerning the phytotherapeutic application of California Poppy is not available. Since the effectiveness for the claimed uses is not documented, a therapeutic application cannot be recommended.

Cocoa seed
Cacao semen
Kakaosamen
Published February 27, 1991

Name of Drug
Cacao semen, cocoa seed.

Composition of Drug
Cocoa seed consists of the seeds of *Theobroma cacao* L. [Fam. Sterculiaceae], as well as preparations thereof. The seeds are freed from the testae, fermented and lightly roasted.

Pharmacological Properties, Pharmacokinetics, Toxicology
Cocoa seed can cause constipation due to its tannin content. The seeds contain methylxanthines, primarily theobromine. The action of methylxanthines is diuretic, broncholytic, vasodilator, stimulatory to the heart muscle action, mildly muscle relaxing.

Clinical Data
Medical and clinical reports and various other empirical information on the application of cocoa seeds are not available.

1. Component in the Following Drug Combinations
Combinations with up to 5 ingredients:
a) Cocoa seed, white clay, oak bark, apple.

Combinations with more than 5 ingredients:
b) Cocoa seed, fennel, colt's foot leaf, linden flower, peppermint leaf, licorice root, thyme, rose hip, cornflower, sunflower ray florets.
c) Cocoa seed, arnica flower, colt's foot leaf, salvia leaf, plantain leaf, quebracho bark, cornflower, horsetail herb, cat's foot flower, calendula flower, Iceland moss, horehound herb, eucalyptus leaf, woundwort flower, elecampane root, red poppy petal, flores acaciae robiniae, star anise fruit, flores althaeae, flores malvae arboreae, sassafras root bark.
d) Cocoa seed, licorice root, cornflower, bladderwrack, horsetail herb, cat's foot bark, marshmallow leaf, woundwort flower, red poppy petal, flores acaciae robiniae, carrageenan, flores althaeae, red clover flower.

2. Claimed Uses of the Above Combinations
a) Infectious disease in the intestine, diarrhea.
b) Bronchial expectorant, diaphoretic.
c) Asthma, bronchial asthma, breathing difficulties, asthmatic symptoms, irritating cough, pulmonary congestion.
d) For goiter and struma, regulates the function of endocrine glands, especially the thyroid, ease of breathing.

Risks
None known.

Contraindications
Allergic disposition to cocoa products.

Side Effects
Cocoa and cocoa products can cause allergic skin reactions and migraine headaches.

Use During Pregnancy and Lactation
Methylxanthines enter into the milk ducts; the concentration of methylxanthines in the mother's milk equals that of blood

plasma levels. Effects and side effects in nursed infants have not been studied.

Dosage
No dosage information is available.

Mode of Administration
Ground drug used for infusions as well as other galenical forms for oral use.

Evaluation
Since the effectiveness for the claimed uses has not been documented, a therapeutic application cannot be recommended.

There is no concern for its use as additive ingredient, e.g., as a flavor corrigent.

Echinacea Purpurea root
Echinaceae purpureae radix
Purpursonnenhutwurzel
Published August 29, 1992

Name of Drug
Echinaceae purpureae radix, echinacea purpurea root, purple coneflower root.

Composition of Drug
Echinacea purpurea root, consisting of fresh or dried root of *Echinacea purpurea* (L.) Moench [Fam. Asteraceae], as well as preparations thereof.

Pharmacological Properties, Pharmacokinetics, Toxicology
Animal Experiment: In the carbon clearance test, alcoholic root extracts show a rate increase in the elimination of carbon particles.
In vitro:
>Alcoholic extracts show an increase in phagocytic elements when tested in granulocyte smears.

Acute toxicity of *E. purpurea* root extract was measured on NMRI-mice using oral application. The toxicity was greater than 3000 mg/kg body weight. More information concerning the kind of extract is not given. Extrapolation to the herb [i.e., above-ground parts] or other preparations is not possible.

Clinical Data

1. Component in the Following Drug Combinations
Combinations with up to 5 components:
a) Echinacea purpurea root, coneflower root, arborvitae tips, indigo weed rhizome.
b) Echinacea purpurea root, ß-sitosterol, α-tocopherol acetate.
c) Echinacea purpurea root, witch hazel leaves, horse chestnut seeds, esculin.
d) Echinacea purpurea root, 1 homeopathic preparation.
e) Echinacea purpurea root, onion, pumpkin seed, poplar buds, pareira root.
f) Echinacea purpurea root, onion, pumpkin seed, poplar buds, pareira root.

Combinations with more than 5 components:
g) Echinacea purpurea root, peppermint leaves, turmeric root, buckthorn bark, milk thistle fruit, dandelion whole plant, tetterwort, madder root.
h) Echinacea purpurea root, fennel, caraway, coriander fruit, hawthorn leaves, hawthorn flowers, hawthorn herb, mistletoe, melissa, eleuthero ginseng root.

i) Echinacea purpurea root, hawthorn flowers, valerian root, lily-of-the-valley herb, arnica flowers, large-flowered cereus flowers, arborvitae tips.

2. Claimed Uses of Above Combinations

a) Nonspecific irrigation therapy, prophylaxis and therapy for infectious diseases, common infections (virus, influenza), leukopenia after radiation therapy or cytostatic therapy, support of anti-infectious chemotherapy.
b) Prostatic syndrome (hypertrophy, adenoma), disturbances of bladder functions, disturbances of micturition, chronic inflammation of bladder lining.
c) Varicose symptoms, ulcus cruris, thrombophlebitis, varicose veins, edema, hemorrhoids, varicose stasis, paresthesia, dysmenorrhea.
d) Disturbances of hair growth, loss of hair, hair damage, for improved sheen and elasticity of the hair, seborrhea, brittleness of nails.
e) Prostatitis syndrome, irritated bladder condition in men and women, abacterial chronic and recurrent prostatitis, bacterial chronic and recurrent prostatitis–needed in combination with a targeted antibacterial therapy, vegetatively fixed prostatitis, catarrhal adnexitis, symptomatic therapy for radiation-damaged bladder, support of antibiotic therapy of acute bacterial prostatitis by removal of inflamed and vegetative components of this disease form, and by its additive antibacterial effect.
f) Functional, hormonal, radiogenic micturition disturbances, cystitis, infections of the bladder, prophylaxis and therapy of infections in the urinary system after urologic and gynecologic surgery.
g) Diseases of the liver-gall-system, recidivous prophylaxis for gallstones, cholecystitis, cholangiitis, gall spasms, postcystectomic syndrome, posthepatic syndrome, hypotonic-asthenic dyskinesia.
h) For stress symptoms, fatigue, unrest, tiredness, exhaustion, convalescence.
i) For coronary circulation problems, inflammation of the peri- and endocardium, neurosis of the circulatory system.

3. Risks

In case of tendency for allergies, especially from *Asteraceae*, and during pregnancy, no parenteral application to be used.
Warning: The metabolic condition of diabetics can decline upon parenteral application.

Contraindications

External:
    None known.
Oral use:
    Progressive systemic diseases such as tuberculosis, leukosis, collagenosis, multiple sclerosis, AIDS, HIV infection, and other autoimmune diseases.

Side Effects

Oral and External:
    None known.
Parenteral use:
    Depending upon dosage, chills, short-term fever reactions, nausea and vomiting may occur. In single cases, allergic reactions of the immediate type are possible.

Special Precautions for Use

None known.

Usage During Pregnancy and Lactation

No parenteral application during pregnancy.

Interference with Other Drugs
None known.

Dosage and Form of Administration
No dosage information submitted. Form of application: cut or ground herb for tea or other galenical preparations.

Overdosage
None known.

Special Warnings
None.

Effects on Operators of Vehicles and Machinery
None.

Evaluation
Since the effectiveness for the claimed applications is not documented, therapeutic use cannot be recommended. The application of parenteral preparations is not justifiable because of various risks.
[**Ed. note:** *Echinacea purpurea* leaf is an approved herb. See Introduction page 61 for a discussion of the approvals and rejections of *Echinacea* preparations.]

Horse Chestnut bark and flower
Hippocastani cortex/-flos
Roßkastanienrinde/-blüten
Published November 25, 1993

Name of Drug
Hippocastani cortex, horse chestnut bark. Hippocastani flos, horse chestnut flower.

Composition of Drug
Horse chestnut bark consists of the fresh or dried bark of *Aesculus hippocastanum* L. [Fam. Hippocastanaceae], harvested in the spring or autumn from 3 - 5-year-old branches, as well as preparations thereof. Horse chestnut flower consists of the fresh or dried flowers of *A. hippocastanum* L., as well as preparations thereof.

Pharmacological Properties, Pharmacokinetics, Toxicology
Not known.

Clinical Data

1. Combination Partner
Preparations of horse chestnut bark/flower are combined with the following ingredients: yarrow, pheasant's eye herb, aesculin, aloe, mandrake root, horehound herb, arnica flower and root, arnica, Artemisia abrotanum e foliis, eyebright herb, uva ursi leaf, blessed thistle herb, Scotch broom herb, birch leaf, stinging nettle, blackberry leaf, rupturewort, watercress herb, calcium fluoratum, calcium sulfuricum, calendula, camphor, carrageen, citron peel, Collinsonia canadensis, echinacea, echinacea angustifolia herb , strawberry leaf, fumatory herb, buckthorn bark, fennel, ferrum phosphoricum, psyllium seed, silverweed herb, ginkgo leaf, goldenrod herb, guaiac wood, rose hip, witch hazel leaf/bark, heparin, motherwort herb, shepherd's purse herb, elderberry flower, hops, Indian nard root*, St. John's Wort, chamomile, cleavers, night-blooming cereus flower, mullein leaf/flower, cornflower flower, buckthorn berries, lavender flower, linseed, lemon grass, lovage root, linden flower, dandelion flower/whole plant,

lycopodium clavatum, meadowsweet flower, lily-of-the-valley leaf, mallow flower, milk thistle seed, wall pepper (sedum), scilla bulb (squill), lemon balm leaf, masterwort root, mistletoe herb/fruit, oleander leaf, Java tea leaf, parsley seed, peppermint leaf/herb, peony petals/root, Jamaican dogwood root bark, bitter orange fruit, pyridoxine hydrochloride, couch grass root, rhatany tincture, rue leaf, calendula petals/whole flower, rosemary leaf, horse chestnut leaf/seed, sandy everlasting flower, rutosid, brewer's yeast, seed-free bean pods, horsetail herb, yarrow flower/herb, blackthorn flower, Chinese pagoda tree flower buds, ergot, celery root, senna leaf/fruit, sunflower ray flower/whole flower stands, sweet clover herb, viola herb, strychnos seed, licorice root, sulfur, centaury herb, thiamine chloride hydrochloride, tormentil root, knotweed herb, walnut leaf, white willow bark, hawthorn berry, hawthorn leaf, hawthorn leaf with flower, hawthorn flower, white dead nettle flower, elderberry fruit, sweet woodruff herb, mullein, zincum aceticum, zinc oxide.

2. Claimed Uses for the Above Named Combinations

Hemorrhoids, ease of defecation, anal fissures, anal eczema, for progressive shrinking of hemorrhoidal nodes, proctitis, pruritus ani, prevention of embolism of varices and thrombosis, strengthening of the veins, stimulation of blood circulation, improvement of circulatory functions, promotion and support of cardiac function, circulation and blood flow, ringing in the ears, for a more active balance of heart and circulation stress, low and high blood pressure, circulatory disturbances in feet and legs, varicose veins, phlebectasia, angioneurosis, endoangiitis obliterans, leg edema, brachyalgia, ulcus cruris, relief of discomforts of varicose veins, supportive for thrombosis, thrombophlebitis, paresthesia, prophylaxis of thrombosis, static edema, mild cardiac insufficiency, especially in old age after infectious diseases, dizziness, psychogenic disturbances of blood flow through the heart muscle.

Also, stimulant, foehn discomforts, fatigue, disinclination for work, conditions of anxiety, sleeplessness, overweight, immobility, uric acid diathesis, supportive therapy for acute and chronic kidney or bladder diseases, dropsy, atherosclerosis, supportive for mild hemorrhages, especially of the gums, congestion in the liver, cholangiitis, cholecystitis, pancreatitis, blockage of the portal circulation.

3. Risks
None known.

Evaluation
Since the effectiveness for the claimed uses is not documented, a therapeutic application cannot be recommended.

*[**Ed. note:** "Indian nard root" is mentioned with reference to three different plants:
   1. *Nardostachys jatamansi* [Fam. Valerianaceae].
   2. *Vetiveria zizanioides* [Fam. Poaceae].
   3. *Cymbopogon jwarancusa* [Fam. Poaceae].]
[**Ed. note:** There is an approved monograph for Horse Chestnut seed extract in the **Approved Herbs** section.]

Mistletoe berry
Visci albi fructus
Mistelfrüchte
Published July 14, 1993

Name of Drug
Visci albi fructus, mistletoe berry.

Composition of Drug
Mistletoe berry consists of the fresh or dried fruit of *Viscum album* L. [Fam. Viscaceae], as well as preparations thereof.

Pharmacological Properties, Pharmacokinetics, Toxicology
None known.

Clinical Data

1. Components of the Following Drug Combinations
Combinations containing up to 5 components:
1) Mistletoe berry, mistletoe herb.
2) Mistletoe berry, mistletoe herb.
3) Mistletoe berry, mistletoe herb.
4) Mistletoe berry, mistletoe herb, hawthorn berry, garlic, rutoside.
5) Mistletoe berry, mistletoe herb, 3 chemically defined components.

Combinations containing more than 5 components:
6) Mistletoe berry, mistletoe herb, valerian root, chamomile, peppermint leaf, blackberry leaf, yarrow herb, lemon balm leaf, hops, lavender flower, rose hip seed, heather, ripe poppy seed capsules.
7) Mistletoe berry, mistletoe herb, valerian root, silver weed, rosemary, wormwood, oregano, cleavers, wood betony.
8) Mistletoe berry, mistletoe herb, walnut leaf, couch grass, white willow bark, silver weed, rosemary, shepherd's purse, tormentil root, fumatory, masterwort, meadowsweet flower, horse chestnut flower.
9) Mistletoe berry, mistletoe herb, hawthorn flower, hawthorn leaf, lemon balm leaf, rosemary.
10) Mistletoe berry, mistletoe herb, birch leaf, horsetail herb, Indian snakeroot, rutoside, three homeopathic components.
11) Mistletoe berry, mistletoe herb, hawthorn flower, berry and leaf, blackberry leaf, yarrow, St. John's Wort, silver weed, lemon balm leaf.
12) Mistletoe berry, mistletoe herb, hawthorn flower, cola nut, ginseng root, royal jelly, 2 chemically defined components.
13) Mistletoe berry, mistletoe herb, valerian root, licorice, birch leaf, cornflower, restharrow root, parsley fruit, cat's foot flower, calendula flower, maté leaf, hawthorn leaf with flower, motherwort, woundwort flower, red poppy petals, acaciae robiniae flos, marshmallow flower, red clover flower.
14) Mistletoe berry, mistletoe herb, buckthorn bark, senna leaf, chamomile, licorice root, cornflower flower, dandelion root and herb, yarrow herb, stinging nettle, cat's foot flower, calendula flower, shepherd's purse, witch hazel leaf, yarrow flower, woundwort flower, red poppy petals, acaciae robiniae flos, marshmallow flower, red clover flower.
15) Mistletoe berry, mistletoe herb, valerian root, chamomile, senna leaf, birch leaf, cornflower flower, yarrow herb, rue leaf (ruta graveolens), cat's foot flower, calendula flower, shepherd's purse, heather, hawthorn leaf with

flower, witch hazel leaf, yarrow flower, woundwort flower, absinthe herb, red poppy petals, acaciae robiniae flos, marshmallow flower, red clover flower.
16) Mistletoe berry, mistletoe herb, uva ursi leaf, gentian root, fennel seed, caraway seed, sage leaf, thyme, juniper berry, dandelion herb with root, lemon balm leaf, rosemary, lavender flower, sweet flag rhizome, marjoram herb, chamomile, arnica root, agrimony, peppermint herb, elderberry, eyebright herb, cloves, nutmeg, wood betony.
17) Mistletoe berry, mistletoe herb, sage leaf, mullein, plantain leaf, St. John's Wort, horsetail grass, lemon balm leaf, calendula flower, rosemary, lavender flower, cowslip flower, watercress, eyebright herb, wild thyme, oregano, wood sanicle.

2. Claimed Uses of the Above Combinations

1) Blood pressure regulation.
2) Internal bleeding, epilepsy, arteriosclerosis, pulmonary bleeding, infantile convulsions, gout, hysteria, circulatory system regulation, elimination, blood purification, for massive loss of blood.
3) High blood pressure, circulatory disorders, improvement of vitality.
4) Prophylaxis for the care of the cardiovascular and nervous systems.
5) Mild to moderate high blood pressure, arteriosclerosis.
6) Sedating.
7) Epilepsy, sedating, antispasmodic.
8) Tonic for the blood circulatory system.
9) Tonic for the blood circulatory system and general arteriosclerosis.
10) Hypertension, essential hypertonia, supportive for renal hypertonia, arteriosclerosis, vertigo, neurasthenia, depression.
11) Tonic for the cardiovascular system.
12) Increase in physical and mental stamina.
13) Cardiotonic.
14) Constipation, intestinal fermentation, hemorrhoids, itching of the anus, varices, circulatory disorders.
15) Female disorders, such as menstrual disorders, poor blood circulation, menopausal discomforts, stagnation of blood, hot flashes, headaches.
16) Purification of the body, prevention of progressive aging.
17) Nervous heart trouble, headaches, sleep disorders.

3. Risks

Poisonings of children after consumption of mistletoe berry have been observed.

Dosage and Mode of Administration

There are no data available for dosage of this herb in combination.

Evaluation

Since the effectiveness for the claimed uses is not documented, a therapeutic application cannot be recommended.

Mistletoe stem
Visci albi stipites
Mistelstengel
Published June 29, 1994

Name of Drug
Visci albi stipites, mistletoe stem

Composition of Drug
Mistletoe stem consists of the fresh or dried stems of *Viscum album* L. [Fam. Viscaceae] and preparations thereof.

Pharmacological Properties, Pharmacokinetics, Toxicology
None known.

Clinical Data

1. Combination Partners
The drug and its preparations are combined with the following drugs or substances:

disodium salt, aloe, ammi visnaga berries (bishop's weed), angelica root, anise, arnica flowers, belladonna (potencies)*, valerian root, barium carbonate (potencies), barium chlorate (potencies), blessed thistle, berberis root, broom, birch leaves, bladderwrack, stinging nettle, calcium lactate-pentahydrate, cola seed, hawthorn (potencies), cyanocobalamin, foxglove (potencies), carline thistle, marshmallow, gentian root, frangula, fennel, dried magnesium sulphate, glycerol-1(2) dihydrogen phosphate mixture from iron (iii) salts, witch hazel bark, motherwort (herba leonuri cardiacae), hop cones, hyperoside, St. John's Wort, potassium- sodium (r,r)-tartrate times 4 H$_2$O, potassium-hydroaspartate, potassium sulphate, calamus root, poppy flowers, garlic, coriander, cornflower petals, lavender flowers, dandelion plant, magnesium-hydroaspartate dihydrite, magnesium peroxide, fructus cardui mariae, masterwort stem, balm leaves, mistletoe, nicotinamide, agrimonia, parsley root, peppermint leaves, phenobarbital, rue, *vomitoria* (potencies), rauvolfia root, retinol, rhubarb root, marigold flowers, robinia flowers, rosemary leaves, horse chestnut seeds, cudweeds, rutin, seedless garden bean pods, horsetail, yarrow, pagoda tree flower buds, celandine, sulphur, *selenicereus grandiflorus* (potencies), senna leaves, senna pods, *spigelia anthelmia* (potencies), centaury, aneurin (vitamin B1), dried brewer's yeast, troxerutin, mistletoe (potencies), whitethorn berries, whitethorn leaves with flowers, whitethorn flowers, meadow clover leaves, anthyllis flowers, cinnamon bark.

[**Ed. note:** "Potencies" refers to homeopathic preparations of a substance.]

2. Reported Indications for Therapeutic Use in the Above Combinations
For its calming effect; in the treatment of mental and physical exhaustion; as a tranquilizer against nervous conditions such as agitation, anxiety and increased excitability; for menopausal symptoms; sleeplessness; exam nerves; stage fright; hot flashes; blood rushes to the head; inner nervousness; to calm and strengthen the heart in the case of nervous heart irregularities; in the treatment of high and low blood pressure; in the early stages of treatment of arteriosclerosis, for muzziness, headaches, buzzing in the ears, dizziness, mood swings; latent cardiac insufficiency, presbycardia, functional heart and circulatory complaints, cor nervosa; prophylaxis and treatment of arteriosclerosis, vascular disease, circulatory disorders, hypertonia,

hardening of the arteries, circulatory and metabolic disorders of the heart, myocardial insufficiency, cardiac arrhythmia, cardiasthenia during and after infectious diseases, prophylaxis and treatment after cardiac arrest, nervous heart conditions, heart palpitations during states of agitation, anxiety, apprehension and tension; heart complaints during menopause; weather-dependent heart complaints, unstable blood pressure, nervousness, tendency to dizzy spells, pressure headaches, shortness of breath, weak spells, circulatory complaints, varicose veins, hemorrhoids, venous congestion, lazy bowel, cholelithiasis, cholecystitis, icterus, hepatitis, dyspepsia, constipation.

There is no evidence of the efficacy of mistletoe stem in any of the given combinations.

3. Risks
None known.

Evaluation
Since the efficacy of combinations has not been sufficiently documented in the above-named areas, therapeutic use of mistletoe stem cannot be recommended.

[**Ed. note:** Scotch Broom flower on page 373 belongs here.]

Sweet Violet root and herb
Violae odoratae rhizoma/herba
Märzveilchen
Published June 17, 1994

Name of Drug
Violae odoratae rhizoma; sweet violet root.
Violae odoratae herba; sweet violet herb.

Composition of Drug
Sweet violet root, consisting of the dried root of *Viola odorata* L. [Fam. Violaceae] and pharmaceutical preparations thereof.

Sweet violet herb, consisting of the dried above-ground parts of *V. odorata* L. and pharmaceutical preparations thereof.

Pharmacological Characteristics, Pharmacokinetics, Toxicology
The drug is said to contain saponins. Saponins can have an expectorant effect and irritate the mucous membrane when used in higher doses. There are no studies available on preparations of the drug.

Clinical Data

1. Combination Partners
The drug and preparations thereof are combined with the following drugs and substances:

acidum arsenicosum (potencies)*, ambra grisca (potencies), white horehound (herba marrubi), angelica root, anise, arnica, arnica root, *avena sativa* (potencies), valerian root, base bismuth nitrate, mugwort, erigeron, pimpernel root, bitter milkwort (complete plant), fenugreek seeds, stinging nettle, butetamat dihydrogencitrate, *caulophyllum thalictroides* (potencies), *chamaelirium luteum* (potencies), *chelidonium majus* (potencies), quinine bark, *cimicifuga racemosa* (potencies), condurango bark, *convallaria majalis* (potencies), *crataegus* (potencies), *crocus sativus* (potencies), cyclamen (potencies), *delphinium staphisagria*, marshmallow root, gentian root, ephedrine hydrochloride, fumaria, eucalyptus leaves, frangula, fennel, lady's mantle, galanga stem, *tormentilla anserina*, garden sorrel, woodbine, smooth sumach, goldenrod, grindelia, lignum vitae, oat straw, heather flowers, autumn-Helen flower, elderflower, hop cones, *hydrastis canadensis* (potencies), carob, St. John's Wort, potassium monohydrophosphate, calamus root, chamomile flowers, chestnut leaves, burdock root, coriander berries, caraway, lavender flowers, toadflax, *lilium lancifolium* (potencies), lungwort, filipendula, magnesium-hydrophosphate trihydrate, magnesium peroxide, balm leaves, nutmeg seeds, naja naja (potencies), cloves, agrimony, passionflower plant, pepsin, peppermint leaves, dogwood, bitter orange peel/flowers, quassia wood, rhubarb root, rosemary, sage leaves, wood sage, seedless garden bean pods, sand sedge, sarsaparilla root, sassafras root wood, sour cherry stems, horsetail, yarrow plant/flowers, cowslip flowers, black currant leaves, *senecio aureus* (potencies), senna leaves, sundew, star anise, pansy plant, *strychnos nux-vomica* (potencies), licorice root, *centaurium erythraea*, thyme, turnera diffusa (potencies), *vitex agnus castus* (potencies), juniper berries, woodruff plant, walnut leaves, water fennel berries, willow bark, white dead nettle flowers, wormwood, yohimbe bark, cedar wood, stachys, cinnamon bark, aspen leaves.

*[Ed. note: "Potencies" refers to homeopathic preparations made of the particular ingredient.]

2. Claimed Uses of the Above Combinations

Acute and chronic bronchitis, bronchial asthma, acute and chronic catarrh of the respiratory organs, cold symptoms of the upper respiratory tract: hoarseness, coughing, mucous congestion, bronchial inflammation, late "flu" symptoms, chesty cough, spastic cough, whooping cough, emphysema, dust-damaged lung. It is said to strengthen the bronchi and to soothe coughs and the respiratory organs.

Urinary incontinence with various causes: senile incontinence, irritable bladder, enuresis nocturna, prostate conditions. In the treatment of insomnia, to improve deep sleep; to calm and relax nerves, in the treatment of physical and mental exhaustion; in the treatment of climacteric complaints such as hot flashes, metabolic imbalances, insomnia, depressions, irritability, anxiety states; gastrointestinal complaints, abdominal pain, gallbladder complaints, gastric catarrh, intestinal catarrh, enteritis, duodenitis, digestion problems caused by incorrect diet, flatulence, heartburn, loss of appetite.

Supports metabolism, detoxifies the blood.

Is used in the treatment of skin impurities and skin disorders.

3. Risks

None known.

Evaluation

Due to the insufficiently proven efficacy of the drug and its pharmaceutical preparations as well as the associated risks, therapeutic use cannot be recommended.

The traditional use of sweet violet root as an expectorant for the respiratory tract is well documented.

Yellow Jessamine root
Gelsemii rhizoma
Gelsemiumwurzelstock
Published September 21, 1991

Name of Drug
Gelsemii rhizoma, yellow jessamine root.

Composition of Drug
Yellow Jessamine root consists of the rhizome with roots of *Gelsemium sempervirens* (L.) Aiton [Fam. Loganiaceae], as well as preparations thereof.

Pharmacological Properties, Pharmacokinetics, Toxicology
Animal experiments showed the following effects:

Gelsemium tincture/fluidextract: vasodilating, blood pressure lowering, bronchodilating; decreasing the vagus tone with resulting increase of heart frequency; paralyzing to the central nervous system, first the motor, then the sensory centers; curare-like effects on the voluntary nerves; atropine-like effect on the nervous system; elevated reflex irritability; inhibiting the absorption of dopamine, nor-adrenalin and serotonin in synaptic-somatic preparations of the rat brain and in a chloralized dog; an ECG showed bradycardia and conductivity disorders, potentiation of the analgesic effect of salicylamide and phenacetin. Pharmacological experiments for the total extract are not available.

Toxicology
see **Overdosage**.

Clinical Data
Clinical data reported by physicians and other material of medicinal experiences concerning the use of yellow jessamine root for phytotherapy are not available.

1. Component of the Following Drug Combinations
Combinations containing up to 5 components:
a) Yellow jessamine root, monkshood tuber, elderberry juice.
b) Yellow jessamine root, atropine sulfate, colloidal silver, angelica root, linseed.
c) Yellow jessamine root, hawthorn, oleander, Scotch broom herb.
d) Yellow jessamine root, papaverine hydrochloride, propyl phenazone, inositol nicotinate, ergotamine tartrate.
e) Yellow jessamine root, St. John's Wort, dehydrocholic acid, phenazone-citric acid-caffeine mixture.

Combinations with more than 5 components:
f) Yellow jessamine root, deadly nightshade extract, magnesium peroxide, sodium hydrogen carbonate, bismuth subnitrate, precipitated calcium carbonate.
g) Yellow jessamine root, sodium bromide, lavender flower, hops, angelica herb, American crampbark, sweet woodruff, wormwood herb.
h) Yellow jessamine root, St. John's Wort, valerian root, silverweed herb, rosemary leaf, hops, lavender flower, lemon balm herb.
i) Yellow jessamine root, fennel oil, caraway oil, peppermint oil, citronella oil, L-sparteine sulfate, night-blooming cereus flower, pheasant's eye herb, squill.
j) Yellow jessamine root, fennel oil, caraway oil, peppermint oil, citronella oil, L-sparteine sulfate, night-blooming cereus flower, pheasant's eye herb.
k) Yellow jessamine root, foxglove, phosphorus, hawthorn flower, hops,

night-blooming cereus flower, pheasant's eye herb, squill, West Indian lemongrass oil, lily-of-the-valley herb, valerian root.
l) Yellow jessamine root, *Silybum marianum, Kalmia latifolia, Selenicerus grandiflorus, Strychnos nux vomica, Veratrum album*, squill.
m) Yellow jessamine root, St. John's Wort, hawthorn berry, ginseng root, blessed thistle, arnica root, lily-of-the-valley herb, lemon balm herb.
n) Yellow jessamine root, sage leaf, thyme fluidextract, mullein, plantain herb, greater pimpernel root, white willow bark, bitter milkwort–entire plant, chestnut leaf, sundew herb, heart's ease herb, red soapwort root, hempnettle, elecampane root, cowslip flower without calyx, eryngo, anise, codeine phosphate hemi-hydrate, licorice juice.
o) Yellow jessamine root, allyl-mustard oil, *Chamomilla recutita, Citrullus colocynthis, Aconitum napellus*, ammonium bromatum, *Veratrum album*, atropinum sulfuricum, cuprum sulfuricum, *Passiflora incarnata*, St. John's Wort flower oil, cayenne, *Laricifomes officinalis*.

2. Claimed Applications of the Above Combinations
a) Neuralgic pain, particularly headache, migraine and sensitivity to weather changes.
b) Gastric disorders, nervous gastric irritations, sensation of fullness, burning, pressure in the stomach area, supportive treatment for gastric and duodenal ulcers, pylorospasm in infants.
c) Sedating cardiac and circulatory agent.
d) Migraine, migraine-like headaches, spasms of the intestinal tract, spasms of the gallbladder area, menstrual discomforts.
e) Migraine, migraine-like headaches, spasms of the gallbladder and intestinal area, menstrual discomforts.
f) Gastritis, gastroenteritis, colitis, hyperacidity, gastric and duodenal ulcers.
g) Neurasthenia, anxiety neurosis, insomnia.
h) Nervous ailments, nervousness, neurasthenia, depression.
i) Extrasystole, stenocardia, tachycardia, geriatric heart, thyrotoxicosis, spastic migraine, sedative, Roemheld symptoms.
j) Influence on heart function, palpitation, prophylaxis for overexertion, care of geriatric heart condition.
k) Coronary and circulatory disorders, arrhythmia, elevated blood pressure, heart tonic.
l) Heart remedy, circulatory agent, for minor heart therapy.
m) Low blood pressure, variations in blood pressure.
n) Cough, influenza infections, colds.
o) Muscular pain, sports injuries, spasmodic conditions.

3. Risks
Because of the narrow therapeutic range, numerous intoxications have occurred, some with fatal consequences.

Contraindications
Cardiac insufficiency.

Use During Pregnancy and Lactation
Information not available.

Interaction with Other Drugs
Animal experiments show that in combination with salicylamide and phenacetin, analgesic effects are potentiated.

Dosage and Mode of Administration
No data are available for the dosage of the combination products. For the prescription of yellow jessamine tincture or fluidextract the following information is given:
Yellow jessamine tincture (*Erg. B. 6*):
    mean single dosage:
    0.3 g (=18 drops)

maximum single dosage: 1 g
maximum daily dosage: 3 g
Yellow jessamine fluidextract:
single dosage: 1 - 3 drops

Overdosage

Described characteristic symptoms of overdosage are:

Dizziness, loss of speech, inability to move the tongue and to swallow, dryness of the mouth, paralysis of the eyelids, visual disturbances or double vision, enlargement of the pupils, tremor of the limbs, weakness or rigidity of the muscles, dropping of the lower jaw.

Evaluation

A therapeutic administration is not justifiable because of insufficiently documented effectiveness, narrow therapeutic range and frequently reported poisonings with occasional fatal results.

Chapter 7

Unapproved Fixed Combinations

Fixed combinations of Belladonna with drugs in homeopathic preparations
Published September 24, 1993

Name of Drug
Fixed combinations of Belladonna, *Atropa belladonna* L. [Fam. Solanaceae], with drugs in homeopathic preparations.

Apis mellifica
Arnica montana
Calcium carbonicum
Chamomilla recutita
Chelidonium majus
Gelsemium sempervirens
Hamamelis virginiana
Lycopus virginicus

Composition of Drug
Fixed combinations of Belladonna are available with the following compounds prepared according to homeopathic regulations:

(B. Anz. No. 190a of October 10, 1985)
(B. Anz. No. 217a of November 22, 1985)
(B. Anz. No. 44 of March 3, 1990)
(B. Anz. No. 217a of November 22, 1985)
(B. Anz. No. 190a of October 10, 1985)
(B. Anz. No. 217a of November 22, 1985)
(B. Anz. No. 29a of February 12, 1986)
(B. Anz. No. 29a of February 12, 1986)

This list of components will be supplemented according to the development of preparations.

Pharmacological Properties, Pharmacokinetics, Toxicology
For Belladonna (*Atropa belladonna*) and the drugs of homeopathic preparations, refer to the respective monographs.
[**Ed. note:** Homeopathic preparations are regulated in Germany by Commission D, not Commission E. Thus, they are not included in this publication.]

Clinical Data

1. Uses
The following indications are claimed for combination preparations:
 Hemorrhoids.
 Disturbances of gall production and gall secretion, disturbances of liver function, spasms in the area of the

bile ducts, gastritis, duodenitis, supportive therapy for ulcus ventriculi and duodeni, gastroenteritis, colitis, digestive problems, especially constipation caused by liver insufficiency.

Angina, stomatitis, periarthritis, conservative treatment and pre-treatment of abscesses, panaritium, furuncles, adjuvant for pleurisy.

Sleeping disorders, vegetative dystonia, psychosexual disturbances, climacteric complaints, thyrotoxicosis, neurasthenia.

The effectiveness of the combinations for the claimed uses has not been documented.

2. Risks

The harmlessness of these combination products is specified by the data given for the homeopathic preparations in the individual monographs.

The following risks are valid for Belladonna:
Do not use in case of tachycardiac arrhythmia, prostate edema with residual urine, narrow-angle glaucoma, acute edema of the lungs, mechanical stenoses of the gastrointestinal tract, megacolon.

3. Side Effects

Dry mouth, decrease of perspiration gland function, accommodation disturbances, reddening and dryness of the skin, hyperthermia, tachycardia, difficulties in urination, hallucinations and spastic conditions, especially when overdosed.

The anticholinergic action of the drug can be enhanced by tricyclic antidepressants, amantadine and quinidine.

Evaluation

The indicated uses of the components are listed in their respective monographs. Concerning the combinations of Belladonna with homeopathically prepared drugs, no data are available from which a positive contribution to the effectiveness of these drug combinations can be deduced. According to the evaluation results of the homeopathic preparations, these neither contribute to the effectiveness nor to the tolerance of Belladonna-containing medicines.

The combination of Belladonna, an alkaloid drug with narrow dosage limitations and high toxicity, with other compounds is not recommended. The therapeutic principle of homeopathy generally does not agree with that of phytotherapy. Therefore, fixed combinations of homeopathic and phytotherapeutic preparations are not sensible.

Approval of such combination products cannot be recommended.

Fixed combinations of Belladonna with other drugs
Published September 24, 1993

Name of Drug
Fixed combinations of Belladonna [*Atropa belladonna*] with other drugs.

Composition of Drug
Fixed combinations of Belladonna are available with the following drugs:

Pheasant's Eye herb	(B. Anz. No. 85 of May 5, 1988)
Aloe	(B. Anz. No. 154 of August 21, 1985)
Horehound herb	(B. Anz. No. 22a of February 1, 1990)
Arnica flower	(B. Anz. No. 228 of December 5, 1984)
Valerian root	(B. Anz. No. 90 of May 15, 1985)
Pimpinella root	(B. Anz. No. 101 of June 1, 1990)
Monkshood	(B. Anz. No. 193a of October 15, 1987)
Stinging Nettle root	(B. Anz. No. 173 of September 18, 1986)
Nux Vomica	(B. Anz. No. 173 of September 18, 1986)
Camphor	(B. Anz. No. 228 of December 5, 1984)
Turmeric root	(B. Anz. No. 223 of November 30, 1985)
Ivy leaf	(B. Anz. No. 122 of July 6, 1988)
Gentian root	(B. Anz. No. 223 of November 30, 1985)
Eucalyptus leaf	(B. Anz. No. 177a of September 24, 1986)
Eucalyptus oil	(B. Anz. No. 177a of September 24, 1986)
Buckthorn bark	(B. Anz. No. 228 of December 5, 1984)
Witch Hazel leaf and bark	(B. Anz. No. 154 of August 21, 1985)
Henbane leaf	(B. Anz. No. 85 of May 5, 1988)
St. John's Wort	(B. Anz. No. 228 of December 5, 1984)
Coffee Charcoal	(B. Anz. No. 85 of May 5, 1988)
Chamomile flower, German	(B. Anz. No. 228 of December 5, 1984)
Caraway seed	(B. Anz. No. 22a of February 1, 1990)
Blessed Thistle fruit	(B. Anz. No. 50 of March 13, 1986)
Mistletoe herb	(B. Anz. No. 228 of December 5, 1984)
Agrimony	(B. Anz. No. 50 of March 13, 1986)
Paprika (Cayenne)	(B. Anz. No. 22a of February 1, 1990)
Peppermint leaf	(B. Anz. No. 223 of November 30, 1985)
Peppermint oil	(B. Anz. No. 50 of March 30, 1986)
Bitter Orange peel	(B. Anz. No. 193a of October 15, 1987)
Primrose root	(B. Anz. No. 122 of July 6, 1988)
Rhubarb root	(B. Anz. No. 228 of December 5, 1984)
Horse Chestnut seed	(B. Anz. No. 228 of December 5, 1984)
Sandy Everlasting	(B. Anz. No. 122 of July 6, 1988)
Saw Palmetto Berry	(B. Anz. No. 43 of March 2, 1989)
Sage leaf	(B. Anz. No. 90 of May 15, 1985)
Yarrow	(B. Anz. No. 22a of February 1, 1990)
Celandine herb	(B. Anz. No. 90 of May 15, 1985)
Senna leaf	(B. Anz. No. 228 of December 5, 1984)
Jimsonweed leaf and seed	(B. Anz. No. 22a of February 1, 1990)

Plantain	(B. Anz. No. 223 of November 30, 1985)
Licorice root	(B. Anz. No. 90 of May 15, 1985)
Thyme	(B. Anz. No. 228 of December 5, 1984)
Uzara root	(B. Anz. No. 164 of September 1, 1990)
Hawthorn	(B. Anz. No. 1 of January 3, 1984)
Soapwort root, White	(B. Anz. No. 101 of June 1, 1990)
Wormwood	(B. Anz. No. 228 of December 5, 1984)

This list of components will be supplemented according to the development of preparations.

Pharmacological Properties, Pharmacokinetics, Toxicology

For Belladonna and the other herbs, refer to the respective monographs.

Clinical Data

1. Uses

The following indications are claimed for the combination preparations:

a) Bronchitis, asthma, acute and chronic diseases of the respiratory tract and lung, emphysema of the lung, tuberculosis of the lung, influenza-like infections, dust lung, whooping cough, smoker's cough, fever with eruptive children's diseases, and as an antitussive and expectorant.

b) Hemorrhoids, anal fissures, spasms of the anal sphincter, cryptitis, mucosal prolapse, and for pre-and post-operative treatment of surgery in the anal area.

c) Disturbances of gall production and gall secretion, disturbances of liver functions, icterus, spasms in the area of the bile ducts, cholangiitis, cholelithiasis, dyspepsia, hyperacidity of the stomach, severe spasms of acute and chronic gastric disorders, gastritis, duodenitis, supportive in the treatment of ulcus ventriculi et duodeni, gastroenteritis, colitis, digestive disorders, bloating and feeling of fullness, especially constipation caused by liver insufficiency, loss of appetite, acute and chronic constipation, reconstitution of damaged intestinal flora with concurrently desired laxative effect, colic, and gastrocardiac symptomatic complex.

d) Angina, stomatitis, periarthritis, conservative treatment and pre-treatment of abscesses, panaritium, furuncles, and as an adjuvant for pleurisy.

e) Sleeping disorders, vegetative dystonia, psychosexual disturbances, discomforts due to foehn, neurovegetative misregulations of all origins, especially disorders of the cardiovascular system and the digestive organs, hormonal based difficulties during puberty, menopause, for hyperfunction of the thyroid during the course of infectious diseases, conditions of anxiety and stress, depression, thyrotoxicosis, neurasthenia, migraine, as a day-time sedative, in preparation for surgery, for hyperhydrosis, enuresis nocturna, vegetative neuroses, cardiac and vascular neuroses, Ménière's disease, dizziness, nausea and vomiting of various origins, headaches, and difficulty in concentrating.

f) Tachycardia, over-excitability of the conduction system, extrasystole, vascular spasms, functional problems at hypertonia, angina pectoris, geriatric heart.

g) Arteriosclerosis.

h) Prostate edema, prostatitis, nervous bladder, residual urine, difficulties in urination, increased frequency in urination, cystitis, tenesmus, parametritis, adnexitis.

i) Rheumatic ailments, sciatica, lumbago, gout, neuralgia, muscle strain, sprains, pain in the limbs and joints, hallux valgus, swelling of the big toe joint.

The effectiveness of the combinations for the claimed uses has not been documented.

2. Risks

The safety of these combination products is specified by the data given in the individual monographs.

The following risks are valid for Belladonna:

Do not use in case of tachycardiac arrhythmia, prostate edema with residual urine, narrow-angle glaucoma, acute edema of the lungs, mechanical stenoses of the gastrointestinal tract, and megacolon.

3. Side Effects

Dry mouth, decrease of perspiratory gland function, accommodation disturbances, reddening and dryness of the skin, hyperthermia, tachycardia, difficulties in urination, hallucinations and spastic conditions, especially when overdosed.

The anticholinergic action of the drug can be enhanced by tricyclic anti-depressants, amantadine and quinidine.

Evaluation

The uses of the individual components are listed in their respective monographs. Concerning the combinations of Belladonna with other drugs, no data are available from which a positive contribution to the effectiveness of these drug combinations can be deduced. According to the evaluation results of the other mentioned drugs, these neither contribute to the effectiveness nor to the tolerance of deadly nightshade-containing medicines.

The combination of Belladonna, an alkaloid drug with narrow dosage limitations and high toxicity, with other compounds is not recommended. Poisonings with this herb have been reported. There is no rationale for the additions in the fixed combinations. The risks of side effects and overdosing must be rated higher than the usefulness. Some of the combinations claim uses such as tachycardia and prostate edema with residual urine, which are contraindications for Belladonna. There are neither clinical nor pharmacological data available for the evaluation of fixed combinations with Belladonna for spasms and colic-like pain in the area of the gastrointestinal tract and bile ducts. Furthermore, there are respective monopreparations of Belladonna available as therapy for these symptoms.

Approval for such combination products cannot be recommended.

Fixed combinations of Lily-of-the-valley herb and Squill

Published July 14, 1993

Name of Drug

Fixed combinations of lily-of-the-valley herb and squill.

Composition of Drug

Fixed combinations consisting of:
Lily-of-the-valley herb corresponding to *DAB* 10; squill corresponding to *DAB* 10;
as well as their preparations.

Pharmacological Properties, Pharmacokinetics, Toxicology

The leading glycoside of lily-of-the-valley leaf is convallatoxin; of squill, proscillaridin A.

The actions of cardiac glycosides on the heart are:
a) positive inotropic (increasing contractile strength and velocity while delaying relaxation);
b) negative chronotropic (decreasing the time or rate of contraction);
c) negative dromotropic (decreasing stimulus conduction);
d) positive bathmotropic (increasing stimulation of the ventricular muscle).

Pharmacokinetics

Convallatoxin:

For convallatoxin an absorption rate of 10 percent and a subsidence rate of 40 - 50 percent are given. The absorption rate is believed to be increased by saponins contained in the herb. No information is available concerning its metabolism in humans. A renal/biliary excretion is assumed. Binding to plasma proteins lies between 16 and 23 percent.

Recent investigations, particularly for the substance reacting in combination, are not available.

Proscillaridin A:

Proscillaridin A is absorbed at a rate of 20 - 30 percent; the half-life value is 45 - 50 hours. The plasma protein binding is about 85 percent. Proscillaridin A is eliminated after biliary conjugation with glucuronic and sulfuric acid. There is evidence for an entero-hepatic circulation. Recent information pertaining to the substance in the combination is not available. Pharmacodynamic and pharmacokinetic studies with the fixed combination of lily-of-the-valley herb and squill are not available.

A "sub-additive" effect on guinea pigs is described for the toxicity of proscillaridin A and convallatoxin. The transferability of these data to the herbs is not clear.

Pertaining to the cumulative effect and pharmacokinetics affecting patients at risk, e.g., patients with kidney insufficiency, there are no data available for the herbs and their fixed combination.

Clinical Data

1. Uses

Preparations of the fixed combination of lily-of-the-valley and squill are used for mild and moderate forms of heart insufficiency, also for diminished kidney capacity, geriatric heart, chronic cor pulmonale, continuation of digitalis therapy (interval treatment), hypertonia, neurocirculatory disturbances, such as tachycardia, feeling of oppression, as a diuretic with mainly cardiac target, and for functional heart symptoms.

There is no useful information available for the claimed uses. The effectiveness for the claimed applications is not documented.

2. Risks

Not to be used in case of therapy with digitalis glycosides, digitalis intoxication, hypercalcemia, potassium deficiency, bradycardia, ventricular tachycardia.

Since no investigations for the use by children are available, the application is contraindicated.

Caution if conduction disturbances exist and i.v. calcium therapy is applied.

Side effects that may occur: nausea, vomiting, gastric disturbances, irregular pulse and cardiac dysrhythmia.

Increase in effectiveness, and thus also side effects, occurs with simultaneous administration of quinidine, calcium, saluretics, laxatives and long-term therapy with glucocorticoids. One case report exists of an Adam-Stokes seizure. More information is not available.

Evaluation

Positive monographs are available for the individual herbs.

Sufficiently validated information concerning the dosage of the herb in the combination products, as well as the ratio of the herbs to each other, is not available. Because of the inadequate pharmacodynamic and pharmacokinetic study, as well as inadequate clinical study pertaining to the fixed combination, effectiveness and safety of preparations of lily-of-the-valley herb and squill cannot be evaluated.

Without further investigation, the risk of the combination cannot be evaluated. Cardiac glycosides have a comparatively narrow therapeutic range, making respective investigations necessary, especially if a prolonged therapy is required. The risks are not biased to the fixed combination as compared to the individual herbs. No scientific information is available for the effectiveness of this medicinal combination.

Fixed combinations of Pheasant's Eye herb and Lily-of-the-valley herb

Published July 14, 1993

Name of Drug

Fixed combinations of pheasant's eye herb and lily-of-the-valley herb.

Composition of Drug

Fixed combinations consisting of:
Pheasant's eye corresponding to DAB 10;
Lily-of-the-valley herb corresponding to DAB 10; as well as their preparations.

Pharmacological Properties, Pharmacokinetics, Toxicology

The leading glycoside of pheasant's eye herb is cymarin, of lily-of-the-valley leaf is convallatoxin.

The actions of cardiac glycosides on the heart are:
a) positive inotropic (increasing contractile strength and velocity while delaying relaxation);
b) negative chronotropic (decreasing the time or rate of contraction);
c) negative dromotropic (decreasing stimulus conduction);
d) positive bathmotropic (increasing stimulation of the ventricular muscle).

Pharmacokinetics

Cymarin:
The indication for the absorption of cymarin lies between 15 and 47 percent. The half-life of elimination is given as 13 - 23 hours. Elimination of cymarin occurs mainly by renal discharge. The subsidence rate is 50 percent.

Recent investigations, particularly of cymarin's actions in combinations, are not available.

Convallatoxin:
For convallatoxin an absorption rate of 10 percent and a subsidence rate of 40 - 50 percent are given. The absorption rate is supposedly increased by saponins contained in the herb. No information is available concerning its metabolism in humans. A

renal/biliary excretion is assumed. The binding to plasma proteins lies between 16 and 23 percent.

Pharmacodynamic and pharmacokinetic studies with the fixed combination of pheasant's eye herb and lily-of-the-valley herb are not available. Pertaining to the cumulative effect and pharmacokinetics affecting patients at risk, e.g., patients with kidney insufficiency, there are no data available for the herbs and their fixed combinations.

Clinical Data

1. Uses

Preparations of the fixed combinations of pheasant's eye herb and lily-of-the-valley herb are used for heart problems, vascular problems, circulatory ailments, decompensated geriatric heart function, stress and hypertonic heart function, mild to moderate heart muscle insufficiency, for myocardia, as a tonic for the cardiovascular system after coronary infarction, continuation treatment after digitalis therapy, for functional heart and circulatory disturbances, nervous heart (cardiac neurosis), mild irregular heart action, support of the cardiovascular system prior to and after surgery, treatment of pressure and sensation of constriction in the heart area, improvement of blood and oxygen supply of the heart, for declining heart capacity, strengthening of the heart muscle and for a more efficient cardiac capacity.

There is no useful information available for the claimed uses.

The effectiveness for the claimed applications is not documented.

2. Risks

Not to be used in case of therapy with digitalis glycosides, digitalis intoxication, hypercalcemia, potassium deficiency, bradycardia, ventricular tachycardia.

Since no investigations for the use by children are available, the application is contraindicated.

Caution if nervous conduction disturbances exist and i.v. calcium therapy is applied.

Side effects which may occur: nausea, vomiting, gastric disturbances, irregular pulse and cardiac dysrhythmia.

Increase in effectiveness, and thus also side effects, occur with simultaneous administration of quinidine, calcium, saluretics, laxatives and long-term therapy with glucocorticoids.

Evaluation

Positive monographs are available for the individual herbs.

Sufficient validated information concerning the dosage of the herb in the combination products, as well as the ratio of the herbs to each other, is not available.

Because of the inadequate pharmacodynamic and pharmacokinetic study, as well as inadequate clinical study pertaining to the fixed combination, effectiveness and safety of preparations of pheasant's eye herb and lily-of-the-valley herb cannot be evaluated.

Without further study, the risks of the combination cannot be evaluated. Cardiac glycosides have a comparatively narrow therapeutic range, making respective investigations necessary, especially if a prolonged therapy is demanded. The risks are not biased to the fixed combination as compared to the individual herbs. No scientific information is available for the effectiveness of this medicinal combination.

Fixed combinations of Pheasant's Eye herb and/or Lily-of-the-valley herb and/or Squill and/or Oleander leaf with herbs that do not contain cardiac glycosides

Published July 14, 1993

Name of Drug

Fixed combinations of Pheasant's Eye herb and/or Lily-of-the-valley herb and/or Squill and/or Oleander leaf with herbs which do not contain cardiac glycosides.

- Elecampane root
- Anise seed
- Arnica flower
- Uva Ursi leaf
- Valerian root
- Blessed Thistle herb
- Scotch Broom herb
- Pimpinella root
- Birch leaf
- Bogbean leaf
- Monkshood
- Boldo leaf
- Stinging Nettle herb and leaf
- Blackberry leaf
- Rupturewort
- Cola nut
- Dill seed
- Verbena
- Ephedra
- Buckthorn bark
- Fennel seed
- Silverweed
- Yellow Jessamine root
- Ginseng root
- Goldenrod
- Guaiac wood
- Rose Hip
- Rose Hip seed
- Witch Hazel leaf and bark
- Spiny Restharrow root
- Motherwort herb
- Elder flower

Components of Drug

Fixed combinations of Pheasant's Eye and/or Lily-of-the-valley herb and/or Squill and/or Oleander leaf are available with the following herbs not containing cardiac glycosides:

- (B. Anz. No. 85 of May 5, 1988)
- (B. Anz. No. 122 of July 6, 1988)
- (B. Anz. No. 228 of December 5, 1984)
- (B. Anz. No. 228 of December 5, 1984)
- (B. Anz. No. 90 of May 15, 1985)
- (B. Anz. No. 193a of October 15, 1987)
- (B. Anz. No. 11 of January 17, 1991)
- (B. Anz. No. 101 of June 1, 1990)
- (B. Anz. No. 50 of March 13, 1986)
- (B. Anz. No. 22a of February 1, 1990)
- (B. Anz. No. 193a of October 15, 1987)
- (B. Anz. No. 76 of April 23, 1987)
- (B. Anz. No. 76 of April 23, 1987)
- (B. Anz. No. 22a of February 1, 1990)
- (B. Anz. No. 173 of September 18, 1986)
- (B. Anz. No. 127 of July 12, 1991)
- (B. Anz. No. 193a of October 15, 1987)
- (B. Anz. No. 22a of February 1, 1990)
- (B. Anz. No. 11 of January 17, 1991)
- (B. Anz. No. 228 of December 5, 1984)
- (B. Anz. No. 74 of April 19, 1991)
- (B. Anz. No. 223 of November 30, 1985)
- (B. Anz. No. 178 of September 21, 1991)
- (B. Anz. No. 11 of January 17, 1991)
- (B. Anz. No. 193a of October 15, 1987)
- (B. Anz. No. 76 of April 23, 1987)
- (B. Anz. No. 164 of September 1, 1990)
- (B. Anz. No. 164 of September 1, 1990)
- (B. Anz. No. 154 of August 21, 1985)
- (B. Anz. No. 76 of April 23, 1987)
- (B. Anz. No. 50 of March 13, 1985)
- (B. Anz. No. 50 of March 13, 1985)

Hops	(B. Anz. No. 228 of December 5, 1984)
St. John's Wort	(B. Anz. No. 228 of December 5, 1984)
Chamomile flower, German	(B. Anz. No. 228 of December 5, 1984)
Pine sprouts	(B. Anz. No. 173 of September 18, 1986)
Night-blooming Cereus	(B. Anz. No. 22a of February 1, 1990)
Cornflower	(B. Anz. No. 43 of March 2, 1989)
Madder root	(B. Anz. No. 173 of September 18, 1986)
Caraway seed	(B. Anz. No. 22a of February 1, 1990)
Pumpkin seed	(B. Anz. No. 223 of November 30, 1985)
Lavender flower	(B. Anz. No. 228 of December 5, 1984)
Lovage root	(B. Anz. No. 101 of June 1, 1990)
Dandelion root and herb	(B. Anz. No. 228 of December 5, 1984)
Meadowsweet	(B. Anz. No. 43 of March 2, 1989)
Marjoram	(B. Anz. No. 226 of December 2, 1992)
Mallow flower	(B. Anz. No. 43 of March 2, 1989)
Milk Thistle seed	(B. Anz. No. 50 of March 13, 1986)
Maté	(B. Anz. No. 85 of May 15, 1988)
Lemon Balm	(B. Anz. No. 228 of December 5, 1984)
Mistletoe herb	(B. Anz. No. 228 of December 5, 1984)
Java Tea	(B. Anz. No. 50 of March 13, 1986)
Passionflower herb	(B. Anz. No. 223 of November 30, 1985)
Parsley seed	(B. Anz. No. 43 of March 2, 1989)
Parsley herb and root	(B. Anz. No. 43 of March 2, 1989)
Peppermint leaf	(B. Anz. No. 223 of November 30, 1985)
Primrose root	(B. Anz. No. 122 of July 6, 1988)
Rue	(B. Anz. No. 43 of March 2, 1989)
Serpent wood root	(B. Anz. No. 173 of September 18, 1986)
Rosemary leaf	(B. Anz. No. 223 of November 30, 1985)
Horse Chestnut seed	(B. Anz. No. 228 of December 5, 1984)
Saw Palmetto berry	(B. Anz. No. 43 of March 2, 1989)
Sage leaf	(B. Anz. No. 90 of May 15, 1985)
Kidney bean pods (without seeds)	(B. Anz. No. 50 of March 13, 1990)
Sandalwood, Red	(B. Anz. No. 193a of October 15, 1987)
Horsetail herb	(B. Anz. No. 173 of September 18, 1986)
Yarrow	(B. Anz. No. 22a of February 1, 1990)
Celandine, herb	(B. Anz. No. 90 of May 15, 1985)
Senna	(B. Anz. No. 228 of December 5, 1984)
Echinacea Angustifolia root	(B. Anz. No. 162 of August 29, 1992)
Asparagus root	(B. Anz. No. 127 of July 12, 1991)
Heart's Ease herb	(B. Anz. No. 50 of March 13, 1986)
Licorice root	(B. Anz. No. 90 of May 15, 1985)
Kelp	(B. Anz. No. 101 of June 1, 1990)
Tormentil root	(B. Anz. No. 85 of May 5, 1988)
Juniper berry	(B. Anz. No. 228 of December 5, 1984)
Walnut leaf	(B. Anz. No. 101 of June 1, 1990)
White Willow bark	(B. Anz. No. 228 of December 5, 1984)
Wormwood	(B. Anz. No. 228 of December 5, 1984)
Bugleweed	(B. Anz. No. 22a of February 1, 1990)

This list of components will be supplemented according to the progress of the Commission's work.

Pharmacological Properties, Pharmacokinetics, Toxicology

For pheasant's eye herb, lily-of-the-valley-herb, squill, oleander and the other herbs that do not contain cardiac glycosides, refer to the respective monographs.

Clinical Data

1. Uses

The following indications are claimed for these combination preparations:
a) Mild forms of heart insufficiency, even with diminished kidney capacity, geriatric heart, athletic heart, cardiac dropsy, chronic cor pulmonale, myodegeneration of the heart, nervous heart, cardiac- and vasoneurosis, as a tonic for the heart during starvation (hunger) or fasting cures, as a tonic for the cardiac and circulatory system, for heart damage caused by tobacco, anginal discomforts, improvement of coronary blood supply, rhythmic disturbances, as a supplement to digitalis and strophanthin therapies, and for inflammation of the heart muscle and heart lining.
b) Feeling of ill health due to low blood pressure (dizziness, disturbances of sight, decrease in physical and mental capacity, vegetative dystonia, depression), hypotonic regulatory disorders, during and after infectious diseases, circulatory disturbances, and high blood pressure, especially during menopause.
c) Varicose symptoms, phlebectasia, angioneurosis, brachyalgia, endangiitis obliterans, ulcer of the leg, hemorrhoids.
d) Stimulation of kidney function, fluid removal during heart and kidney ailments, disturbances of the metabolism, e.g., high values of uric acid and overweight, dropsy, supporting treatment of catarrhs of the bladder and renal pelvis, cystitis, pyelonephritis, prevention of urinary gravel and urinary calculi, for renal, cardiac, hepatogenic or static edema, ascites, "bladder and kidney congestion," liver congestion, urine retention, reduction of residual urine, urination disorders, prostatitis, and hypertrophy of the prostate.
e) Supportive to treatment of obesity.
f) Arteriosclerosis.
g) Anxiety, sleeping disorders due to nervous palpitation, symptoms of "manager disease," vegetative dystonia.
h) Neuralgia, skin diseases, allergies, "disorders of secretions."

No useful information is available pertaining to the claimed applications.

The effectiveness of the combinations for the claimed uses has not been documented.

2. Risks

The harmlessness of these combination preparations pertains to the herbs without cardiac glycosides, as specified by the data given in the individual monographs. Interactions between the herbs containing cardiac glycosides and the other herbs have not been investigated.

Pheasant's eye herb, lily-of-the-valley herb, squill, and oleander leaf contain cardiac glycosides.

The following risks apply:

Not to be used during therapy with digitalis glycosides, digitalis intoxication, hypercalcemia, potassium deficiency, bradycardia, ventricular tachycardia. Since studies regarding the use by children are not available, the administration is contraindicated.

Caution in cases of conduction disturbances and during i.v. calcium therapy. Side effects that may occur: nausea, vomiting and cardiac dysrhythmia.

Increased effectiveness, and thus also of side effects, occurs with simultaneous administration of quinidine, calcium, saluretics, laxatives, and, during long-term therapy, with glucocorticoids.

Evaluation

The indicated uses of the component herbs are listed in their respective monographs.

Concerning the combinations of pheasant's eye herb and/or lily-of-the-valley herb and/or squill and/or oleander leaf with herbs which do not contain cardiac glycosides, no data are available from which a positive contribution to the effectiveness of these drug combinations can be deduced. According to the evaluation results [of investigations] of the herbs not containing cardiac glycosides, these neither contribute to the effectiveness nor to the tolerance of pheasant's eye herb and/or lily-of-the-valley herb and/or squill and/or oleander leaf-containing medicines.

The combination of pheasant's eye herb and/or lily-of-the-valley herb and/or squill and/or oleander leaf, being drugs containing cardiac glycosides with narrow dosage ranges and high toxicity, with other compounds is not to be recommended. Permission of such combination products cannot be recommended.

Fixed combinations of Pheasant's Eye herb and/or Lily-of-the-valley herb and/or Squill and/or Oleander leaf with chemically defined drugs

Published July 14, 1993

Name of Drug

Fixed combinations of Pheasant's Eye herb and/or Lily-of-the-valley herb and/or Squill and/or Oleander leaf with chemically defined drugs.

Thiamine hydrochloride
Ascorbic acid
Camphor
Camylofine
Caffeine
Vitamin D3
Dehydrocholic acid
Dehydroxypropyl theophyllin (Diprophyllin)
Ephedrine hydrochloride
Folic acid
Nitroglycerin

Composition of Drug

Fixed combinations of Pheasant's Eye herb and/or Lily-of-the-valley herb and/or Squill and/or Oleander leaf are available with the following chemically defined compounds:

(*B. Anz.* No. 131 of July 21, 1987)
(*B. Anz.* No. 18 of January 28, 1992)
(*B. Anz.* No. 228 of December 5, 1984)
(*B. Anz.* No. 149 of August 11, 1989)
(*B. Anz.* No. 209 of November 8, 1988)
(*B. Anz.* No. 147 of August 10, 1988)
(*B. Anz.* No. 147 of August 10, 1988)
Prepublication

Prepublication
(*B. Anz.* No. 45 of March, 1987)
(*B. Anz.* No. 43 of March 2, 1990)

Guaiazulene	(B. Anz. No. 128 of July 13, 1990)
Potassium chloride	(B. Anz. No. 103 of June 8, 1991)
Potassium citrate	(B. Anz. No. 103 of June 8, 1991)
Magnesium sulfate	(B. Anz. No. 118 of June 29, 1990)
Nicotinamide	(B. Anz. No. 148 of August 10, 1989)
Antipyrine (Phenazone)	(B. Anz. No. 145 of August 5, 1989)
Procaine	(B. Anz. No. 198 of October 23, 1991)
Proscillaridin	(B. Anz. No. 43 of March 2, 1990)
Proxyphylline	Prepublication
Theobromine-Na-salicylate	(B. Anz. No. 30 of February 13, 1993)
Verapamil	(B. Anz. No. 43 of March 2, 1990)
Vitamin B2	(B. Anz. No. 46 of March 8, 1988)
Vitamin B12	(B. Anz. No. 59 of March 29, 1989)

This list of components will be supplemented according to the progress of the Commission's work.

Pharmacological Properties, Pharmacokinetics, Toxicology

For pheasant's eye herb, lily-of-the-valley herb, squill, oleander leaf, and chemically defined drugs refer to the respective individual monographs.

Clinical Data

1. Uses

For the combination preparations, the following indications are claimed:

a) Cardiac and circulatory insufficiency, even with diminished kidney output, angina pectoris, coronary insufficiency, rhythmic disturbances of the heart, extrasystole, tachycardia, mild forms of bradycardia, endocarditis, myodegeneration of the heart, functional disorders of the heart, especially with added nervous overtones, such as of old age, after infectious diseases, during menopause, weather changes, delayed convalescence, by uncommon physical and psychological stress, geriatric heart, increased demand on the heart muscle, e.g., balneological treatments, hypotonic symptoms with dizziness, tendency to collapse, cardiac stenosis, acute cardiac neuralgia, nocturnal tachycardia, especially after abuse of alcohol and tobacco, as a tonic and stimulant for heart and circulation, peripheral and cerebral disturbances of blood flow, for interval treatment and as an adjuvant of digitalis and strophanthin therapy, digitalis intolerance, thyrotoxicosis, chronic cor pulmonale, prevention of arteriosclerosis, high blood pressure, post-treatment of severe high blood pressure with cardiac decompensation, for prevention and post-treatment of coronary infarction.

b) For treatment of symptoms of chronic venous insufficiency, varicosis, syndromes occurring after thrombosis, concomitant treatment of trophic changes, e.g., varicose ulcers.

c) Potassium and magnesium deficiency.

d) Bronchial asthma, cardiac asthma, acute, chronic bronchitis, especially with severe spasms of the bronchial muscles, spasms connected with emphysema of the lungs, allergic reactions, congestion of the respiratory tract, adjuvant for pertussis.

e) Edema, as a diuretic, acute and chronic diseases of the kidneys and the efferent urinary tract, such as acute and

chronic interstitial nephritis, nephrosis, nephrosclerosis, pyelonephritis, nephrolithiasis, cystitis, difficulties of urination, for the ease of the discharge of stones, for the prevention of ascending infections of users of catheters, treatment of infections resistant to antibiotics and sulfonamide.
f) For gastrointestinal discomforts, such as pressure, spasms of unknown origin, feeling of fullness, bloating, heartburn, Roemheld's syndrome, as a laxative, for loss of appetite.
g) Gallbladder and liver ailments.
h) For spasms of the muscles and organs.
i) For conditions of anxiety and excitation, depression, mental stress, vegetative dystonia, spastic migraine, as a sedative, sleeplessness due to nervously caused circulatory disturbances, difficulty in falling asleep and staying asleep, nervousness, "vaso- and psychoneurosis", menopausal disorders, and decrease in vitality.
j) Impaired function of the glands, disturbances of development and growth, disinterest in school, and difficulty in learning.

There is no worthwhile information available for the support of the claimed applications.

The effectiveness of the combinations for the claimed uses is not documented.

2. Risks

For the safety of these combination preparations, the information given in the individual monographs of the chemically defined compounds is adequate.

Interactions between the cardiac glycosides and the chemically defined substances have not been studied.

Pheasant's eye herb, lily-of-the-valley herb, squill and oleander leaf are classified under the cardiac glycosides. The following risks apply:

Not to be used during therapy with digitalis glycosides, digitalis intoxication, hypercalcemia, potassium deficiency, bradycardia, ventricular tachycardia.

Since there are no investigations for the application in children, the use is contraindicated.

Caution in cases of disturbances of conduction and during i.v. calcium therapy.

Side effects which may occur:
nausea, vomiting, and cardiac arrhythmia.

Effectiveness and, therefore, also side effects are increased with simultaneous administration of quinidine, calcium, saluretics, laxatives and long-term therapy with glucocorticoids.

Evaluation

Effectiveness for the individual components of the above-mentioned fixed combinations is documented for the indications specified in the respective monographs for the individual herbs and chemically defined drugs.

Regarding the combination of pheasant's eye herb and/or lily-of-the-valley herb and/or squill and/or oleander leaf with chemically defined drugs, no information is available from which a positive contribution to the effectiveness of this medicinal combination can be deduced. According to the results of the investigation by the Commission, the listed drugs neither contribute to the effectiveness, nor to the tolerance of the pheasant's eye herb and/or lily-of-the-valley herb and/or squill and/or oleander leaf containing medicines.

The combination of pheasant's eye herb and/or lily-of-the-valley herb and/or squill and/or oleander leaf as cardiac glycoside medication cannot be recommended because of the narrow dosage range and high toxicity. Fixed combinations of plant pharmaceutics with cardiac glycosides and chemically defined substances, especially those with a narrow therapeutic range, are not reasonable. Permission of such combinations cannot be recommended.

Part Three

Therapeutic Indexes

8. Uses and Indications of Approved Herbs	419
9. Contraindications of Approved Herbs	433
10. Side Effects of Approved Herbs	443
11. Side Effects of Unapproved Herbs	451
12. Pharmacological Actions of Approved Herbs	459
13. Pharmacological Actions of Unapproved Herbs	471
14. Interactions of Herbs with Conventional Drugs	475
15. Duration of Administration for Approved Herbs	483

Chapter 8

Uses and Indications of Approved Herbs

This chapter, condensed from the monographs, provides information on the appropriate use of herbs. It links medical indications and uses cited in the text and the approved herbs found to be effective in their treatment. However, some of the herbs listed here may have been found effective for treatment of minor symptoms or for prevention of a condition of disease, or in some cases as adjuvant (secondary) therapy. For example, Psyllium seed husk is used as an adjuvant therapy for anal fissures — a mild laxative to soften the stool but not directly beneficial to the anal fissures themselves. Herbs in approved fixed combinations are abbreviated as F.C.

The information is prepared as a guide for health professionals, researchers and consumers but should not be considered as a suggestion for self-medication. It is essential to refer to the complete monograph in order to view the role the herb may provide for each indication as well as any contraindications and side effects.

A guide of indications by medical category is included to help identify the types of indications listed in this chapter. Immediately following this guide, the herbs are listed alphabetically under each indication.

Indication Guide by Medical Category

Cardiovascular
Arterial Occlusive Disease
Atherosclerosis
Cardiac Insufficiency
Cardiac Symptoms
Circulatory Disorders
Cor pulmonale
Geriatric Vascular Changes
Hypercholesteremia
Hyperemia
Hypertension
Phlebitis
Post-thrombic Syndrome
Tachycardia

Dermatological
Acne
Ano-genital Irritation
Burns
Eczema
Frostbite
Furunculosis
Gums, Inflamed
Insect Bites
Irrigation, Mouth
Itching
Milk Scall
Rubefacient
Seborrhea
Skin, Bacterial Infections
Skin Injury or Irritation

Endocrinology, Reproductive System, Obstetrics/ Gynecology, Prostate
Breast Pain
Dysmenorrhea
Fatigue
Lactation, Poor
Leukorrhea
Menorrhagia
Menopausal Symptoms
Menstrual Disorders
Metrorrhagia
Pancreas, Exocrine Insufficiency
Pelvic Cramps
Premenstrual Syndrome (PMS)
Prostatitis
Urination, Diminished, Associated with BPH Stages 1 and 2

Gastrointestinal
Anal fissures
Appetite, Loss of
Bloating, Feeling of Abdominal Fullness
Bowel, Irritable (see Colon, Irritable)
Colon, Irritable (Irritable Bowel Syndrome)
Constipation
Diarrhea
Diverticulitis
Dyspepsia
Flatulence
Emetic
Gargle/Mouthwash
Gastric Mucosa, Inflammation of
Gastrointestinal Disorders
Hemorrhoids
Inflammation, Gastrointestinal Tract
Nervous Stomach
Pain, Gastrointestinal
Purgative
Rectum, Post-surgical Care of

Hematology, Lymphatic, Cancer
Blood, Superficial Effusion of
Condyloma
Familial Mediterranean Fever
Hematoma
Malignant Tumors

Immunology, AIDS, Infectious Diseases
Convalescence
Debility
Fever
Free Radical Deactivation

Liver and Gallbladder
Biliary Dyskinesia
Biliary Spasm
Cholelithiasis
Gallbladder Disorders
Hepatitis
Liver Cirrhosis
Liver Disease

Neurology, Psychiatry
Anesthesia, Topical
Anxiety
Depression
Headache
Insomnia (see Sleep Disturbances)
Locomotor System, Degenerative Disorders of
Memory
Mental Concentration
Mood Disturbance
Motion Sickness
Nervous System Disorder
Neuralgia
Perspiration, Excessive
Restlessness
Sleep Disturbances

RESPIRATORY
(Lower and Upper Respiratory Tract Including Ears, Nose, Throat, Sinuses)
- Asthma
- Bronchial Secretion, Excessive
- Bronchospasm
- Catarrh, Upper Respiratory Tract
- Colds and Flu
- Cough
- Inflammation, Oral or Pharyngeal
- Influenza
- Mucous Membrane, Irritation
- Nose Bleed
- Respiratory Catarrh
    (see Catarrh, Upper Respiratory Tract)
- Respiratory Infection, Chronic
- Sinusitis

RHEUMATOLOGICAL, ORTHOPEDIC, MUSCLES, CONTUSIONS
- Arthrosis
- Arthritis
- Bruises, Contusions
- Dislocations, Bone
- Edema, Post-traumatic
- Gout
- Injuries
- Joint Pain
- Leg Cramps
- Ligaments, Pulled
- Muscle Pain
- Muscle Spasm
- Prostheses, Bruises Caused by
- Rheumatism

URINARY TRACT SYSTEM
(Kidney, Ureter, Bladder)
- Bladder Irritation
- Diuretic
- Dysuria
- Kidney Capacity, Diminished
- Kidney Stones and Gravel

Herb Guide by Indication

Acne
   Yeast, Medicinal

Anal Fissures
   Manna
   Psyllium seed, Blonde (secondary)
   Psyllium seed husk, Blonde (secondary)

Anesthesia, Topical
   Cloves

Ano-genital Irritation
   Chamomile flower, German
   Oak bark

Anxiety
   Hops
   Indian snakeroot
   Kava Kava
   Passionflower herb
   St. John's Wort
   Valerian root

Appetite, Loss of
   Angelica root
   Bitter Orange peel
   Blessed Thistle herb
   Bogbean leaf
   Centaury herb
   Chicory
   Cinchona bark
   Cinnamon bark
   Cinnamon bark, Chinese
   Condurango bark
   Coriander seed
   Dandelion herb
   Dandelion root with herb
   Devil's Claw root
   F.C. of Angelica root, Gentian root, and Bitter Orange peel
   F.C. of Angelica root, Gentian root, and Fennel
   F.C. of Angelica root, Gentian root, and Wormwood
   F.C. of Angelica root, Gentian root, Wormwood, and Peppermint oil
   F.C. of Ginger root, Gentian root, and Wormwood
   F.C. of Peppermint leaf, Caraway seed, Chamomile flower, and Fenugreek seed
   Galangal
   Gentian root
   Horehound herb
   Iceland Moss
   Onion
   Orange peel
   Pollen
   Soy Phospholipid
   Wormwood
   Yarrow
   Yeast, Medicinal

Arterial Occlusive Disease
   Ginkgo Biloba Leaf Extract

Arthrosis
   White Mustard seed

Arthritis
   Hay flower
   Mistletoe herb
   White Mustard seed

Asthma
   Ephedra

Atherosclerosis
   Onion

Biliary Dyskinesia
   Absinth
   Dandelion root with herb
   Radish
   Wormwood

Biliary Spasm
   Belladonna
   Celandine herb

Fumitory
Peppermint leaf
Peppermint oil
Scopolia root

Bladder Irritation
Pumpkin seed

Bloating, Feeling of Abdominal Fullness
Angelica root
Caraway oil
Caraway seed
Cinnamon bark
Cinnamon bark, Chinese
Dandelion herb
F.C. of Peppermint leaf and Caraway seed
F.C. of Peppermint leaf and Fennel seed
F.C. of Peppermint leaf, Caraway seed, and Chamomile flower
F.C. of Peppermint leaf, Caraway seed, and Fennel seed
F.C. of Peppermint leaf, Caraway seed, Chamomile flower, and Bitter Orange peel
F.C. of Peppermint leaf, Caraway seed, Fennel seed, and Chamomile flower
F.C. of Peppermint leaf, Fennel seed, and Chamomile flower
F.C. of Peppermint oil and Caraway oil
F.C. of Peppermint oil and Fennel oil
F.C. of Peppermint oil, Caraway oil, and Chamomile flower
F.C. of Peppermint oil, Caraway oil, and Fennel oil
F.C. of Peppermint oil, Caraway oil, Fennel oil, and Chamomile flower
F.C. of Peppermint oil, Fennel oil, and Chamomile flower
Fennel oil
Fennel seed
Gentian root

Blood, Superficial Effusion of
Sweet Clover

Bowel, Irritable
(see Colon, Irritable)

Breast Pain
Bugleweed

Bronchial Secretion, Excessive
Turpentine oil, Purified

Bronchitis
Ivy leaf
Thyme

Bronchospasm
Ephedra

Bruises, Contusions
Arnica flower (external)
Comfrey herb and leaf (external)
Comfrey root (external)
Peruvian Balsam (external)
St. John's Wort (external)
Sweet Clover (external)

Burns
Peruvian Balsam
St. John's Wort (external)

Cardiac Insufficiency
Hawthorn leaf with flower
Lily-of-the-valley herb
Pheasant's Eye herb
Squill

Cardiac Symptoms
Motherwort herb

Catarrh, Upper Respiratory Tract
Anise seed
Camphor
Coltsfoot leaf
Eucalyptus leaf
Eucalyptus oil
F.C. of Anise oil and Iceland Moss
F.C. of Anise seed, Linden flower, and Thyme
F.C. of Anise seed, Marshmallow root, Iceland Moss, and Licorice root
F.C. of Anise seed, Marshmallow root, Primrose root, and Sundew
F.C. of Camphor, Eucalyptus oil, and Purified Turpentine
F.C. of Eucalyptus oil, Primrose root and Thyme

F.C. of Gumweed herb, Primrose root and Thyme
F.C. of Ivy leaf, Licorice root, and Thyme
F.C. of Licorice root, Primrose root, Marshmallow root, and Anise seed
F.C. of Marshmallow root, Fennel seed, Iceland Moss, and Thyme
F.C. of Marshmallow root, Primrose root, Licorice root, and Thyme oil
F.C. of Primrose root and Thyme
F.C. of Primrose root, Marshmallow root, and Anise seed
F.C. of Primrose root, Sundew, and Thyme
F.C. of Sundew and Thyme
Fennel oil
Fennel seed
Fir Needle oil
Fir Shoots, Fresh
Gumweed herb
Hempnettle herb
Horseradish
Ivy leaf
Knotweed herb
Larch Turpentine
Licorice root
Mint oil
Mullein flower
Nasturtium
Niauli oil
Peppermint oil
Pimpinella root
Pine needle oil
Pine sprout
Plantain
Primrose flower
Primrose root
Radish
Sanicle herb
Senega Snakeroot
Soapwort root, Red
Soapwort root, White
Star Anise seed
Thyme
Thyme, Wild
Tolu Balsam
Turpentine oil, Purified
Watercress
White Dead Nettle flower
White Mustard seed (external)

Cholelithiasis
Bishop's Weed fruit (secondary)
Petasites root
Radish

Circulatory Disorders
Butcher's Broom
Camphor
Ginkgo Biloba Leaf Extract
Lavender flower
Pheasant's Eye herb
Rosemary leaf
Scotch Broom herb

Cirrhosis, Hepatic
Milk Thistle fruit

Colds and Flu
Echinacea Pallida root
Echinacea Purpurea herb
Elder flower
Ephedra
F.C. of Anise oil, Fennel oil, Licorice root, and Thyme
F.C. of Anise oil, Primrose root, and Thyme
F.C. of Anise seed, Ivy leaf, Fennel seed and Licorice root
F.C. of Anise seed, Marshmallow root, Eucalyptus oil, and Licorice root
F.C. of Eucalyptus oil, Primrose root and Thyme
F.C. of Gumweed herb, Primrose root and Thyme
F.C. of Ivy leaf, Licorice root, and Thyme
F.C. of Marshmallow root, Fennel seed, Iceland Moss, and Thyme
F.C. of Primrose root and Thyme
F.C. of Star Anise seed and Thyme
F.C. of Thyme and White Soapwort root
Linden flower
Meadowsweet

Colon, Irritable (Irritable Bowel Syndrome)
Flaxseed
Peppermint oil
Psyllium seed husk, Blonde
Psyllium seed, Black
Psyllium seed, Blonde

Condyloma
Mayapple root and resin (external)

Constipation
Aloe
Buckthorn bark
Buckthorn berry
Cascara Sagrada bark
F.C. of Senna leaf and Blonde Psyllium seed husk
F.C. of Senna leaf, Peppermint oil, and Caraway oil
Flaxseed
Manna
Psyllium seed husk, Blonde
Psyllium seed, Black
Psyllium seed, Blonde
Rhubarb root
Senna leaf
Senna pod

Convalescence
Eleuthero (Siberian Ginseng) root
Ginseng root

Cor pulmonale
Lily-of-the-valley herb

Cough
Coltsfoot leaf
F.C. of licorice root, Primrose root, Marshmallow root, and Anise seed
F.C. of Primrose root, Marshmallow root, and Anise seed
Iceland Moss
Linden flower
Mallow flower
Mallow leaf
Marshmallow leaf
Marshmallow root
Sundew

Debility
Eleuthero (Siberian Ginseng) root
Ginseng root
Pollen

Depression
Ginkgo Biloba Leaf Extract (secondary)
St. John's Wort

Diarrhea
Agrimony
Bilberry fruit
Blackberry leaf
Coffee Charcoal
Jambolan bark
Lady's Mantle
Oak bark
Potentilla
Psyllium seed husk, Blonde
Psyllium seed, Blonde (secondary)
Tormentil root
Uzara root

Dislocations, Bone
Arnica flower

Diuretic
Dandelion root with herb

Diverticulitis
Flaxseed

Dysmenorrhea
Black Cohosh root
Potentilla

Dyspepsia
Angelica root
Anise seed
Artichoke leaf
Bitter Orange peel
Blessed Thistle herb
Bogbean leaf
Boldo leaf
Caraway oil
Caraway seed
Cardamom seed
Centaury herb
Chicory
Cinchona bark
Cinnamon bark

Cinnamon bark, Chinese
Cloves
Coriander seed
Dandelion herb
Dandelion root with herb
Devil's Claw root
Dill seed
F.C. of Angelica root, Gentian root and Bitter Orange peel
F.C. of Angelica root, Gentian root, and Caraway seed
F.C. of Angelica root, Gentian root, and Wormwood
F.C. of Angelica root, Gentian root, Wormwood, and Peppermint oil
F.C. of Anise oil, Fennel oil, and Caraway oil
F.C. of Anise seed, Fennel seed, and Caraway seed
F.C. of Caraway oil and Fennel oil
F.C. of Caraway oil, Fennel oil and Chamomile flower
F.C. of Caraway seed and Fennel seed
F.C. of Caraway seed, Fennel seed, and Chamomile flower
F.C. of Dandelion root with herb, Celandine herb, and Wormwood
F.C. of Dandelion root with herb, Peppermint leaf, and Artichoke leaf
F.C. of Ginger root, Gentian root, and Wormwood
F.C. of Javanese Turmeric root, Celandine herb, and Wormwood
F.C. of Javanese Turmeric root, Peppermint leaf, and Wormwood
F.C. of Milk Thistle fruit, Peppermint leaf, and Wormwood
F.C. of Peppermint leaf and Caraway seed
F.C. of Peppermint leaf and Fennel seed
F.C. of Peppermint leaf, Caraway seed, and Chamomile flower
F.C. of Peppermint leaf, Caraway seed, and Fennel seed
F.C. of Peppermint leaf, Caraway seed, Chamomile flower, and Bitter Orange peel
F.C. of Peppermint leaf, Caraway seed, Fennel seed, and Chamomile flower
F.C. of Peppermint leaf, Chamomile flower, and Caraway seed
F.C. of Peppermint leaf, Fennel seed, and Chamomile flower
F.C. of Peppermint oil and Caraway oil
F.C. of Peppermint oil and Fennel oil
F.C. of Peppermint oil, Caraway oil, and Chamomile flower
F.C. of Peppermint oil, Caraway oil, and Fennel oil
F.C. of Peppermint oil, Caraway oil, Fennel oil, and Chamomile flower
F.C. of Peppermint oil, Fennel oil, and Chamomile flower
F.C. of Turmeric root and Celandine herb
Fennel oil
Fennel seed
Galangal
Gentian root
Ginger root
Haronga bark and leaf
Horehound herb
Juniper berry
Lemon Balm
Milk thistle
Mistletoe herb
Radish
Rosemary leaf
Sage leaf
Sandy Everlasting
St. John's Wort
Star Anise seed
Turmeric root
Turmeric root, Javanese
Wormwood
Yarrow

Dysuria
Kidney Bean pods (without seeds)

Eczema
Woody Nightshade stem

Edema, Post-traumatic
Arnica flower
Horsetail herb

Emetic
  Bryonia root

Familial Mediterranean Fever
  Autumn Crocus

Fatigue
  Cola nut
  Eleuthero (Siberian Ginseng) root
  Ginseng root
  Maté

Fever
  White Willow bark

Flatulence
  Angelica root
  Caraway oil
  Cinnamon bark
  Cinnamon bark, Chinese
  Dandelion herb
  F.C. of Angelica root, Gentian root, and Wormwood
  F.C. of Peppermint leaf and Caraway seed
  F.C. of Peppermint leaf and Fennel seed
  F.C. of Peppermint leaf, Caraway seed, and Chamomile flower
  F.C. of Peppermint leaf, Caraway seed, and Fennel seed
  F.C. of Peppermint leaf, Caraway seed, Chamomile flower, and Bitter Orange peel
  F.C. of Peppermint leaf, Caraway seed, Fennel seed, and Chamomile flower
  F.C. of Peppermint leaf, Fennel seed, and Chamomile flower
  F.C. of Peppermint oil and Caraway oil
  F.C. of Peppermint oil and Fennel oil
  F.C. of Peppermint oil, Caraway oil, and Chamomile flower
  F.C. of Peppermint oil, Caraway oil, and Fennel oil
  F.C. of Peppermint oil, Caraway oil, Fennel oil, and Chamomile flower
  F.C. of Peppermint oil, Fennel oil, and Chamomile flower
  Fennel oil
  Fennel seed
  Gentian root

  Horehound herb
  Mint oil
  Poplar bud

Free Radical Deactivation
  Ginkgo Biloba Leaf Extract

Frostbite
  Peruvian Balsam
  Poplar bud

Furunculosis
  Arnica flower
  Larch turpentine
  Yeast, Medicinal

Gallbladder Disorders
  F.C. of Dandelion root with herb, Celandine herb, and Wormwood
  Fumitory
  Mint oil
  Peppermint leaf

Gargle/Mouthwash
  Chamomile flower, German

Gastric Mucosa, Inflammation of
  Marshmallow root

Gastrointestinal Disorders
  F.C. of Dandelion root with herb, Celandine herb, and Artichoke leaf
  Lavender flower
  Mint oil
  Peppermint oil

Geriatric Vascular Changes
  Garlic
  Hawthorn leaf with flower
  Onion

Gout
  Autumn Crocus

Gums, Inflamed
  Chamomile flower, German

Headache
  White Willow bark

Hematoma
  Arnica flower
  Sweet Clover

Hemorrhoids
Butcher's Broom
Manna
Peruvian Balsam
Poplar bud
Psyllium seed husk, Blonde (secondary)
Psyllium seed, Blonde (secondary)
Senna leaf
Sweet Clover
Witch Hazel leaf and bark

Hepatitis
Soy Phospholipid

High Cholesterol/Hypercholesteremia
Garlic
Soy Lecithin
Soy Phospholipid

Hoarseness
Coltsfoot leaf

Hyperemia
Horseradish

Hyperlipidemia
Garlic

Hypertension
Indian Snakeroot

Inflammation, Gastrointestinal Tract
Chamomile flower, German
Marshmallow root

Inflammation, Oral or Pharyngeal
Agrimony
Arnica flower
Bilberry fruit
Blackberry leaf
Blackthorn berry
Calendula flower
Chamomile flower, German
Cloves
Coffee Charcoal
Coltsfoot leaf
Iceland Moss
Jambolan bark
Knotweed herb
Mallow flower
Mallow leaf
Marshmallow leaf
Marshmallow root
Myrrh
Oak bark
Peppermint oil
Plantain
Potentilla
Rhatany root (external)
Rose flower
Sage leaf (external)
Tormentil root
Usnea
White Dead Nettle flower (external)

Influenza
Echinacea Pallida root
Echinacea Purpurea herb

Injuries
Arnica flower (external)
St. John's Wort (external)

Insect Bites
Arnica flower

Insomnia
(see Sleep Disturbances)

Irrigation Therapy
Asparagus root
Birch leaf
Couch Grass
Goldenrod
Horsetail herb
Java Tea
Lovage root
Spiny Restharrow root
Stinging Nettle herb and leaf

Irrigation, Mouth
Mallow flower

Itching
Butcher's Broom
Horse Chestnut seed
Oat straw
Sweet Clover

Joint Inflammation, Degenerative
Mistletoe herb

Joint Pain
    Arnica flower (external)
    F.C. of Camphor, Eucalyptus oil, and
        Purified Turpentine oil (external)

Kidney Capacity, Diminished
    Squill

Kidney Stones and Gravel
    Asparagus root
    Birch leaf
    Bishop's Weed fruit
    Couch Grass leaf
    F.C. of Birch, Goldenrod, and Java tea
    Goldenrod
    Horsetail herb
    Java tea
    Lovage root
    Parsley herb and root
    Petasites root
    Spiny restharrow root
    Stinging Nettle herb and leaf

Lactation, Poor
    Chaste Tree fruit

Leg Cramps
    Butcher's Broom
    Horse Chestnut seed
    Sweet Clover

Leukorrhea
    White Dead Nettle flower

Ligaments, Pulled
    Comfrey root

Liver Cirrhosis
    Milk Thistle fruit

Liver Disease
    Milk Thistle fruit
    Soy Phospholipid

Locomotor System, Degenerative Disorders of
    Devil's Claw root

Lymphatic Congestion
    Sweet Clover

Malignant Tumors
    Mistletoe herb

Memory
    Ginkgo Biloba Leaf Extract

Menopausal Symptoms
    Black Cohosh root
    Chaste Tree fruit

Menorrhagia
    Shepherd's Purse

Menstrual Disorders
    Chaste Tree fruit

Mental Concentration
    Eleuthero (Siberian Ginseng) root
    Ginkgo Biloba Leaf Extract
    Ginseng root

Metrorrhagia
    Shepherd's Purse

Milk Scall
    Heart's Ease herb

Mood Disturbance
    Hops
    Lavender flower

Motion Sickness
    Ginger root

Mucous Membrane, Irritation
    Chamomile flower, German
    Jambolan bark
    Mallow flower
    Mallow leaf
    Marshmallow leaf
    Marshmallow root
    Peppermint oil
    Plantain
    Witch Hazel leaf and bark

Muscle Pain
    Camphor
    Fir Needle oil
    F.C. of Camphor, Eucalyptus oil, and
        Purified Turpentine
    Kava Kava
    Nasturtium
    Peppermint oil (external)
    Pine Sprouts (external)
    St. John's Wort (external)

Muscle, Pulled
Comfrey root

Muscle Spasm
Paprika

Nervous Stomach
F.C. of Licorice root and German Chamomile flower
Lavender flower

Nervous System Disorder
Bugleweed

Neuralgia
Cajeput oil
Fir Needle oil (external)
Fir shoots, Fresh
Larch Turpentine
Mint oil (external)
Monkshood
Peppermint oil (external)
Pine needle oil (external)
Pine Sprouts (external)
Turpentine oil, Purified

Nose Bleed
Shepherd's Purse (external)

Pain, Gastrointestinal
Belladonna

Pancreas, Insufficiency
Haronga bark and leaf

Pelvic Cramps
Yarrow

Perspiration, Excessive
Sage leaf
Walnut leaf

Phlebitis
Arnica flower
Sweet Clover

Post-thrombic Syndrome
Horse Chestnut seed
Sweet Clover

Premenstrual Syndrome (PMS)
Black Cohosh root
Chaste Tree fruit
Yarrow

Prostatitis
Aspen bark and leaf

Prostheses, Bruises Caused by
Peruvian Balsam (external)

Purgative
F.C. of Senna leaf, Peppermint oil, and Caraway oil
Senna

Rectum, Post-surgical Care of
Manna (secondary)
Psyllium seed, Blonde (secondary)

Respiratory Catarrh
(see Catarrh, Upper Respiratory Tract)

Respiratory Infection, Chronic
Chamomile flower, German
Echinacea Purpurea herb

Restlessness
F.C. of Passionflower herb, Valerian root, and Lemon Balm
F.C. of Valerian root, Hops, and Lemon Balm
F.C. of Valerian root, Hops, and Passionflower herb
Hops
Kava Kava
Lavender flower
Passionflower herb
Valerian root

Retinal Lesion and Edema
Ginkgo Biloba Leaf Extract

Rheumatism
Arnica flower
Birch leaf (secondary)
Cajeput oil
Camphor
Eucalyptus oil
Fir Needle oil
Guaiac wood
Larch Turpentine

Pine Needle oil (external)
Rosemary leaf
Stinging Nettle herb and leaf
Turpentine oil, Purified
White Willow bark

Roborant
Pollen

Rubefacient
Cajeput oil

Seborrhea
Heart's Ease herb (external)
Oat straw

Sinusitis
Bromelain

Skin, Bacterial Infections
Chamomile flower, German

Skin Injury or Irritation
Agrimony
Bryonia root
Chamomile flower, German
Jambolan bark
Oak bark (external)
Oat straw
Plantain (external)
Poplar bud
Shepherd's Purse
Walnut leaf
White Dead Nettle flower
Witch Hazel leaf and bark

Sleep Disturbances
F.C. of Passionflower herb, Valerian root, and Lemon Balm
F.C. of Valerian root and Hops
F.C. of Valerian root, Hops, and Lemon Balm
F.C. of Valerian root, Hops, and Passionflower herb
Hops
Lavender flower
Lemon Balm
Valerian root

Sore Throat
Agrimony
Arnica flower

Bilberry fruit
Blackberry leaf
Blackthorn berry
Calendula flower
Cloves
Coffee Charcoal
Coltsfoot leaf
Iceland Moss
Jambolan bark
Knotweed herb
Mallow flower
Mallow leaf
Marshmallow leaf
Oak bark

Spasms
Chamomile flower, German
Paprika
Petasites root

Spasm, Gastrointestinal
Angelica root
Belladonna
Boldo leaf
Caraway oil
Caraway seed
Celandine herb
Chamomile flower, German
Cinnamon bark
Cinnamon bark, Chinese
F.C. of Angelica root, Gentian root, and Caraway seed
F.C. of Licorice root, Peppermint leaf, and German Chamomile flower
Fumitory
Henbane leaf
Peppermint leaf
Scopolia root

Sprains
Comfrey herb and leaf
Comfrey root

Stress
Kava Kava

Sunburn
Poplar bud

Swelling, Legs
Butcher's Broom

Swelling, Post-operative or Post-traumatic
  Bromelain
  Butcher's Broom
  Horse Chestnut seed

Sympatheticotonia
  Indian Snakeroot

Tachycardia
  Indian Snakeroot
  Motherwort herb

Thrombophlebitis
  Sweet Clover

Thrush
  White Dead Nettle flower

Thyroid, Overactive
  Bugleweed
  Motherwort herb

Tinnitus
  Ginkgo Biloba Leaf Extract

Tonic
  Eleuthero (Siberian Ginger) root
  Ginseng root

Ulcers, Gastrointestinal
  F.C. of Licorice root and German Chamomile flower
  F.C. of Licorice root, Peppermint leaf, and Chamomile flower
  Licorice root

Ulcers, Skin
  Peruvian Balsam
  Echinacea Purpurea herb

Ulcus Cruris
  Calendula flower
  Peruvian Balsam

Urinary Disorders
  Parsley herb and root

Urinary Infection or Inflammation
  Asparagus root
  Birch leaf
  Couch Grass
  Echinacea Purpurea herb
  F.C. of Birch leaf, Goldenrod, and Java tea
  F.C. of Uva Ursi leaf, Goldenrod, and Java tea
  Horseradish
  Horsetail herb
  Java tea
  Lovage root
  Nasturtium
  Sandalwood, White (secondary)
  Spiny Restharrow root
  Stinging Nettle herb and leaf
  Uva Ursi leaf (secondary)

Urinary Spasm
  Scopolia root

Urination, Diminished, Associated with BPH Stages 1 and 2
  Pumpkin seed
  Saw Palmetto berry
  Stinging Nettle root

Urination, Diminished, Associated with Prostate Adenoma
  Pumpkin seed
  Saw Palmetto berry
  Stinging Nettle root

Varicose Veins/Varicosis
  Horse Chestnut seed
  Witch Hazel leaf and bark

Venous Insufficiency
  Butcher's Broom (secondary)
  Horse Chestnut seed
  Sweet Clover

Vertigo
  Ginkgo Biloba Leaf Extract

Whooping Cough
  Thyme

Wounds
  Calendula flower
  Echinacea Purpurea herb
  Hay flower
  Horsetail herb
  Peruvian Balsam

Chapter 9

Contraindications of Approved Herbs

This chapter, condensed from the monographs, provides contraindications cited in the text with the herbs which should be avoided with particular conditions or diseases.

It is essential to refer to the complete monograph before making any therapeutic judgements. For example, the contraindication listed in the Anise seed monograph is "allergy to anise and anethole" but this chapter lists Anise seed under "Allergy/Hypersensitivity" without specifying an allergy to a particular constituent of the herb.

A guide of contraindications by medical category is included to help identify the types of contraindications listed in this chapter. Immediately following this guide, the herbs are listed alphabetically under each contraindication.

Contraindication Guide by Medical Category

Cardiovascular
- Cardiac Arrhythmias (Either Tachycardia or Bradycardia)
- Cardiac Glycosides, Treatment with
- Cardiac Insufficiency
- Digitalis Glycosides, Treatment with
- Hypertension
- Hypokalemia
- Pheochromocytoma
- Pulmonary Edema

Dermatological
- Burns
- Collagenosis
- Exanthemas, Urticarial
- Irrigation Therapy with Concurrent Edema
- Skin Injury

Endocrinology, Reproductive System, Obstetrics/Gynecology, Prostate
- Children/Infants
- Diabetes Mellitus
- Hypercalcemia
- Lactation
- Pancreatitis
- Pheochromocytoma
- Potassium Deficiency
- Pregnancy
- Progressive, Systemic Diseases
- Prostate Adenoma
- Thyroid Enlargement
- Thyroid, Low-Functioning
- Thyrotoxicosis

Gastrointestinal
- Abdominal Pain of Unknown Origin
- Appendicitis
- Colitis, Ulcerative

Crohn's Disease
Esophageal Stenosis
Gastrointestinal Inflammation
Gastrointestinal Stenosis
Ileus
Intestinal Inflammation
Intestinal Obstruction
Megacolon
Ulcers, Gastric and Duodenal

HEMATOLOGY, LYMPHATIC, CANCER
Pheochromocytoma

IMMUNOLOGY, AIDS, INFECTIOUS DISEASES
AIDS
Allergy/Hypersensitivity
Autoimmune Diseases
HIV
Hypersensitivity
 (see Allergy/Hypersensitivity)
Infection, Chronic-Progressive
Infectious Diseases
Leukosis
Tuberculosis

LIVER AND GALLBLADDER
Bile Duct Inflammation
Bile Duct Obstruction
Cholestatic Liver Disorders
Cirrhosis of the Liver
 (see also Liver Disease)
Gallbladder Empyema
Gallbladder Inflammation
Gallstones
Liver Disease

NEUROLOGY, PSYCHIATRY
Anxiety
Cerebral Circulation, Impaired
Depression
Hypertonia
Multiple Sclerosis
Restlessness

OPHTHALMOLOGY
Glaucoma

RESPIRATORY
(Lower and Upper Respiratory Tract Including Ears, Nose, Throat, Sinuses)
Asthma
Pulmonary Edema
Respiratory Inflammation
Whooping Cough

URINARY TRACT SYSTEM
(Kidney, Ureter, Bladder)
Kidney Disease (Inflammation)
Kidney Insufficiency
Renal Inflammation or Disease

Herb Guide by Contraindication

Abdominal Pain of Unknown Origin
Aloe
Buckthorn bark
Buckthorn berry
Cascara Sagrada bark
F.C. of Senna leaf and Blonde Psyllium seed husk
F.C. of Senna leaf, Peppermint oil, and Caraway oil
Rhubarb root
Senna leaf
Senna pod

AIDS
Echinacea Pallida root
Mistletoe herb
Woody Nightshade stem

Allergy/Hypersensitivity
Anise seed
Arnica flower
Artichoke leaf
Black Cohosh root
Blessed Thistle herb
Bromelain
Chicory
Cinchona bark
Cinnamon bark
Cinnamon bark, Chinese
Dandelion herb (rare)
Echinacea Purpurea herb (injectible)
F.C. of Camphor, Eucalyptus oil, and Purified Turpentine oil
F.C. of Licorice root, Primrose root, Marshmallow root, and Anise seed
F.C. of Primrose root, Marshmallow root, and Anise seed
Ginkgo Biloba Leaf Extract
Larch Turpentine
Meadowsweet
Mistletoe herb
Paprika
Peruvian Balsam
Pollen
Poplar bud
Primrose flower
Turpentine oil, Purified
Yarrow

Anxiety
Ephedra

Appendicitis
Aloe
Buckthorn bark
Buckthorn berry
Cascara Sagrada bark
F.C. of Senna leaf and Blonde Psyllium seed husk
F.C. of Senna leaf, Peppermint oil, and Caraway oil
Rhubarb root
Senna leaf
Senna pod

Asthma
Fir Needle oil
Pine Needle oil

Autoimmune Diseases
Echinacea Pallida root
Woody Nightshade stem

Bile Duct Inflammation
Eucalyptus leaf
Eucalyptus oil

Bile Duct Obstruction
Artichoke leaf
Boldo leaf
Dandelion herb
Dandelion root with herb
Eucalyptus leaf
Eucalyptus oil
F.C. of Angelica root, Gentian root, Wormwood, and Peppermint oil

F.C. of Dandelion root with herb, Celandine herb, and Artichoke leaf
F.C. of Dandelion root with herb, Celandine herb, and Wormwood
F.C. of Dandelion root with herb, Peppermint leaf, and Artichoke leaf
F.C. of Javanese Turmeric root, Celandine herb, and Wormwood
F.C. of Javanese Turmeric root, Peppermint leaf, and Wormwood
F.C. of Peppermint oil and Caraway oil
F.C. of Peppermint oil and Fennel oil
F.C. of Peppermint oil, Caraway oil, and Chamomile flower
F.C. of Peppermint oil, Caraway oil, and Fennel oil
F.C. of Peppermint oil, Caraway oil, Fennel oil, and Chamomile flower
F.C. of Peppermint oil, Fennel oil, and Chamomile flower
F.C. of Turmeric root and Celandine herb
Haronga bark and leaf
Kava Kava
Mint oil
Peppermint oil
Sandy Everlasting
Turmeric root
Turmeric, Javanese

Burns
Camphor
F.C. of Camphor, Eucalyptus oil, and Purified Turpentine oil

Cardiac Arrhythmias (Either Tachycardia or Bradycardia)
Belladonna
F.C. of Pheasant's eye fluidextract, Lily-of-the-valley powdered extract, Squill powdered extract, and Oleander leaf powdered extract
Henbane leaf
Scopolia root

Cardiac Glycosides, Treatment with
Uzara root

Cardiac Insufficiency
F.C. of Pheasant's Eye fluidextract, Lily-of-the-valley powdered extract, Squill powdered extract, and Oleander leaf powdered extract
Oak bark

Cerebral Circulation, Impaired
Ephedra

Children/Infants
Aloe
Buckthorn bark
Buckthorn berry
Cajeput oil
Camphor
Cascara Sagrada bark
Eucalyptus leaf
Eucalyptus oil
F.C. of Anise oil, Fennel oil, and Caraway oil
F.C. of Anise oil, Fennel oil, Licorice root, and Thyme
F.C. of Camphor, Eucalyptus oil, and Purified Turpentine oil
F.C. of Caraway oil and Fennel oil
F.C. of Peppermint oil and Fennel oil
F.C. of Peppermint oil, Caraway oil, and Fennel oil
F.C. of Peppermint oil, Caraway oil, Fennel oil, and Chamomile flower
F.C. of Peppermint oil, Fennel oil, and Chamomile flower
F.C. of Senna leaf and Blonde Psyllium seed husk
F.C. of Senna leaf, Peppermint oil, and Caraway oil
Fennel oil
Horseradish
Mint oil (external)
Nasturtium
Peppermint oil (external)
Rhubarb root
Senna leaf
Senna pod
Watercress

Cholestatic Liver Disorders
F.C. of Anise seed, Ivy leaf, Fennel seed, and Licorice root
F.C. of Ivy leaf, Licorice root, and Thyme (above 100 mg glycyrrhizin)

F.C. of Licorice root, Peppermint leaf, and German Chamomile flower
F.C. of Licorice root, Primrose root, Marshmallow root, and Anise seed
F.C. of Marshmallow root, Primrose root, Licorice root, and Thyme oil (above 100 mg glycyrrhizin)
F.C. of Licorice root and German Chamomile flower
Licorice root

Cirrhosis of the Liver (see also Liver Disease)
F.C. of Anise seed, Ivy leaf, Fennel seed and Licorice root
F.C. of Licorice root and German Chamomile flower
F.C. of Licorice root, Peppermint leaf, and German Chamomile flower
F.C. of Licorice root, Primrose root, Marshmallow root, and Anise seed
Licorice root

Collagenosis
Echinacea Pallida root
Echinacea Purpurea herb
Woody Nightshade stem

Colitis, Ulcerative
Aloe
Buckthorn bark
Buckthorn berry
Cascara Sagrada bark
F.C. of Senna leaf and Psyllium seed husk, Blonde
F.C. of Senna leaf, Peppermint oil, and Caraway oil
Rhubarb root
Senna leaf
Senna pod

Crohn's Disease
Aloe
Buckthorn bark
Buckthorn berry
Cascara Sagrada bark
F.C. of Senna leaf and Psyllium seed husk, Blonde
F.C. of Senna leaf, Peppermint oil, and Caraway oil
Rhubarb root
Senna leaf
Senna pod

Depression
Indian snakeroot
Kava Kava

Diabetes Mellitus
Blackthorn flower
Echinacea Purpurea herb (injectible)
F.C. of Senna leaf and Psyllium seed husk, Blonde
Psyllium seed, Blonde
Psyllium seed husk, Blonde

Digitalis Glycosides, Treatment with
F.C. of Pheasant's Eye fluidextract, Lily-of-the-valley, powdered extract, Squill powdered extract, and Oleander powdered extract
Lily-of-the-valley herb
Pheasant's Eye herb
Squill

Edema, Due to Cardiac or Renal Insufficiency
Couch Grass

Esophageal Stenosis
Psyllium seed, Black
Psyllium seed, Blonde

Exanthemas, Urticarial
Chaste Tree fruit

Gallbladder Empyema
Dandelion herb
Dandelion root with herb
F.C. of Dandelion root with herb, Celandine herb, and Artichoke leaf
F.C. of Dandelion root with herb, Celandine herb and Wormwood
F.C. of Dandelion root with herb, Peppermint leaf, and Artichoke leaf
Haronga bark and leaf

Gallbladder Inflammation
F.C. of Angelica root, Gentian root, Wormwood, and Peppermint oil
F.C. of Peppermint oil and Caraway oil

F.C. of Peppermint oil and Fennel oil
F.C. of Peppermint oil, Caraway oil, and Chamomile flower
F.C. of Peppermint oil, Caraway oil, and Fennel oil
F.C. of Peppermint oil, Caraway oil, Fennel oil, and Chamomile flower
F.C. of Peppermint oil, Fennel oil, and Chamomile flower
Mint oil
Niauli oil
Peppermint oil

Gallstones
Artichoke leaf
Boldo leaf
Cardamom seed
Chicory
Dandelion herb
Dandelion root with herb
Devil's Claw root
F.C. of Angelica root, Gentian root, Wormwood, and Peppermint oil
F.C. of Dandelion root with herb, Celandine herb and Wormwood
F.C. of Dandelion root with herb, Peppermint leaf, and Artichoke leaf
F.C. of Javanese Turmeric root, Celandine herb, and Wormwood
F.C. of Javanese Turmeric root, Peppermint leaf, and Wormwood
F.C. of Milk Thistle fruit, Peppermint leaf, and Wormwood
F.C. of Peppermint leaf and Caraway seed
F.C. of Peppermint leaf and Fennel seed
F.C. of Peppermint leaf, Caraway seed, and Chamomile flower
F.C. of Peppermint leaf, Caraway seed, and Fennel seed
F.C. of Peppermint leaf, Caraway seed, Chamomile flower, and Bitter Orange peel
F.C. of Peppermint leaf, Caraway seed, Fennel seed, and Chamomile flower
F.C. of Peppermint leaf, Fennel seed, and Chamomile flower
F.C. of Peppermint oil and Fennel oil
F.C. of Peppermint oil, Caraway oil, and Chamomile flower
F.C. of Peppermint oil, Caraway oil, and Fennel oil
F.C. of Peppermint oil, Caraway oil, Fennel oil, and Chamomile flower
F.C. of Peppermint oil, Fennel oil, and Chamomile flower
F.C. of Turmeric root and Celandine herb
Ginger root
Haronga bark and leaf
Peppermint leaf
Peppermint oil
Radish
Turmeric root
Turmeric, Javanese

Gastrointestinal Inflammation
Eucalyptus leaf
Eucalyptus oil
F.C. of Anise seed, Marshmallow root, Eucalyptus oil, and Licorice root
F.C. of Eucalyptus oil, Primrose root and Thyme
Niauli oil

Gastrointestinal Stenosis
Belladonna
F.C. of Senna leaf and Psyllium seed husk, Blonde
Henbane leaf
Psyllium seed, Black
Psyllium seed, Blonde
Psyllium seed husk, blonde
Scopolia root

Glaucoma
Belladonna
Ephedra
Henbane leaf
Scopolia root

HIV
Echinacea Pallida root
Mistletoe herb
Woody Nightshade stem

Hypersensitivity
(see Allergy/Hypersensitivity)

Hypercalcemia
F.C. of Pheasant's Eye fluid extract, Lily-of-the-valley powdered extract, Squill powdered extract, and Oleander powdered extract.

Hypertonia
F.C. of Anise seed, Ivy leaf, Fennel seed, and Licorice root
F.C. of Anise seed, Marshmallow root, Eucalyptus oil, and Licorice root (above 100 mg glycyrrhizin)
F.C. of Anise seed, Marshmallow root, Iceland Moss, and Licorice root (above 100 mg glycyrrhizin)
F.C. of Ivy leaf, Licorice root, and Thyme (above 100 mg glycyrrhizin)
F.C. of Licorice root and German Chamomile flower
F.C. of Licorice root, Peppermint leaf, and German Chamomile flower
F.C. of Licorice root, Primrose root, Marshmallow root, and Anise seed
F.C. of Marshmallow root, Primrose root, Licorice root, and Thyme oil (above 100 mg glycyrrhizin)
Licorice root
Oak bark

Hypertension
Eleuthero root
Ephedra

Hypokalemia
F.C. of Anise seed, Ivy leaf, Fennel seed, and Licorice root
F.C. of Anise seed, Marshmallow root, Eucalyptus oil, and Licorice root (above 100 mg glycyrrhizin)
F.C. of Anise seed, Marshmallow root, Iceland Moss, and Licorice root (above 100 mg glycyrrhizin)
F.C. of Ivy leaf, Licorice root, and Thyme (above 100 mg glycyrrhizin)
F.C. of Licorice root and German Chamomile flower
F.C. of Licorice root, Peppermint leaf, and German Chamomile flower
F.C. of Licorice root, Primrose root, Marshmallow root, and Anise seed
F.C. of Marshmallow root, Primrose root, Licorice root, and Thyme oil (above 100 mg glycyrrhizin)
Flaxseed
Licorice root
Lily-of-the-valley herb
Pheasant's Eye

Ileus
Blackthorn flower
Dandelion herb
Dandelion root with herb
F.C. of Anise seed, Marshmallow root, Eucalyptus oil, and Licorice root (above 100 mg glycyrrhizin)
F.C. of Anise seed, Marshmallow root, Iceland Moss, and Licorice root
F.C. of Dandelion root with herb, Celandine herb, and Artichoke leaf
F.C. of Dandelion root with herb, Celandine herb, and Wormwood
F.C. of Dandelion root with herb, Peppermint leaf, and Artichoke leaf
F.C. of Ivy leaf, Licorice root, and Thyme
F.C. of Marshmallow root, Primrose root, Licorice root, and Thyme oil
F.C. of Senna leaf and Psyllium seed husk, Blonde
F.C. of Senna leaf, Peppermint oil, and Caraway oil
Flaxseed
Haronga bark and leaf
Psyllium seed husk, Blonde
Psyllium seed, Blonde
Senna leaf

Infants
(see Children/Infants)

Infection, Chronic-Progressive
Mistletoe herb
F.C. of Anise seed, Marshmallow root, Eucalyptus oil, and Licorice root (above 100 mg glycyrrhizin)
F.C. of Ivy leaf, Licorice root, and Thyme (above 100 mg glycyrrhizin)
F.C. of Marshmallow root, Primrose root, Licorice root, and Thyme oil (above 100 mg glycyrrhizin)

Infectious Diseases
Oak bark

Intestinal Inflammation
Aloe
Buckthorn bark
Buckthorn berry
Cascara Sagrada bark
Eucalyptus leaf
Eucalyptus oil
F.C. of Camphor, Eucalyptus oil, and Purified Turpentine
F.C. of Senna leaf and Psyllium seed husk, Blonde
F.C. of Senna leaf, Peppermint oil, and Caraway oil
Niauli oil
Rhubarb root
Senna leaf
Senna pod

Intestinal Obstruction
Aloe
Buckthorn bark
Buckthorn berry
Cascara Sagrada bark
Belladonna
Rhubarb root
Senna leaf
Senna pod

Irrigation Therapy with Concurrent Edema
Birch leaf
Couch Grass
F.C. of Birch leaf, Goldenrod, and Java tea
F.C. of Uva Ursi leaf, Goldenrod, and Java tea
Goldenrod
Horsetail herb
Lovage root
Spiny Restharrow root
Stinging Nettle herb and leaf

Kidney Disease (Inflammation)
Asparagus root
Juniper berry
Parsley herb and root
Sandalwood, White
Watercress

Kidney Insufficiency
F.C. of Anise seed, Ivy leaf, Fennel seed, and Licorice root
F.C. of Anise seed, Marshmallow root, Eucalyptus oil, and Licorice root (above 100 mg glycyrrhizin)
F.C. of Anise seed, Marshmallow root, Iceland Moss, and Licorice root (above 100 mg glycyrrhizin)
F.C. of Ivy leaf, Licorice root, and Thyme (above 100 mg glycyrrhizin)
F.C. of Marshmallow root, Primrose root, Licorice root, and Thyme oil (above 100 mg glycyrrhizin)
Licorice root

Lactation
Aloe
Buckthorn bark
Buckthorn berry
Cascara Sagrada bark
Coltsfoot leaf
F.C. of Senna leaf, Peppermint oil, and Caraway oil
Kava Kava
Petasites root
Indian snakeroot
Rhubarb root
Senna leaf
Uva Ursi

Leukosis
Echinacea Pallida root
Echinacea Purpurea herb
Woody Nightshade stem

Liver Disease
Boldo leaf
Eucalyptus leaf
Eucalyptus oil
F.C. of Angelica root, Gentian root, Wormwood, and Peppermint oil
F.C. of Anise seed, Marshmallow root, Eucalyptus oil, and Licorice root (above 100 mg glycyrrhizin)
F.C. of Anise seed, Marshmallow root, Iceland Moss, and Licorice root (above 100 mg glycyrrhizin)
F.C. of Eucalyptus oil, Primrose root and Thyme

CONTRAINDICATIONS OF APPROVED HERBS — PREGNANCY

F.C. of Peppermint oil and Caraway oil
F.C. of Peppermint oil and Fennel oil
F.C. of Peppermint oil, Caraway oil, and Chamomile flower
F.C. of Peppermint oil, Caraway oil, and Fennel oil
F.C. of Peppermint oil, Caraway oil, Fennel oil, and Chamomile flower
F.C. of Peppermint oil, Fennel oil, and Chamomile flower
Haronga bark and leaf
Mint oil
Niauli oil
Peppermint oil

Megacolon
Belladonna
Henbane leaf

Multiple Sclerosis
Echinacea Pallida root
Echinacea Purpurea herb
Woody Nightshade stem

Pancreatitis
Haronga bark and leaf

Pheochromocytoma
Ephedra
Indian snakeroot

Potassium Deficiency
Lily-of-the-valley herb
Pheasant's Eye
Squill

Pregnancy
Aloe
Autumn crocus
Black Cohosh root
Buckthorn bark
Buckthorn berry
Cascara Sagrada bark
Chaste Tree fruit
Cinchona bark
Cinnamon bark
Coltsfoot leaf
Comfrey herb and leaf
Comfrey root
Echinacea Purpurea herb (injectable)
F.C. of Angelica root, Gentian root, and Fennel seed
F.C. of Anise oil, Fennel oil, and Caraway oil
F.C. of Anise oil, Fennel oil, Licorice root, and Thyme
F.C. of Anise seed, Fennel seed and Caraway seed
F.C. of Anise seed, Ivy leaf, Fennel seed, and Licorice root
F.C. of Anise seed, Marshmallow root, Eucalyptus oil, and Licorice root (above 100 mg glycyrrhizin)
F.C. of Anise seed, Marshmallow root, Iceland Moss, and Licorice root (above 100 mg glycyrrhizin)
F.C. of Caraway oil and Fennel oil
F.C. of Caraway oil, Fennel oil and Chamomile flower
F.C. of Caraway seed and Fennel seed
F.C. of Caraway seed, Fennel seed, and Chamomile flower
F.C. of Ivy leaf, Licorice root, and Thyme (above 100 mg glycyrrhizin)
F.C. of Licorice root, Peppermint leaf and German Chamomile flower
F.C. of Licorice root, Primrose root, Marshmallow root, and Anise seed
F.C. of Marshmallow root, Fennel seed, Iceland Moss, and Thyme
F.C. of Marshmallow root, Primrose root, Licorice root, and Thyme oil (above 100 mg glycyrrhizin)
F.C. of Peppermint leaf and Fennel seed
F.C. of Peppermint leaf, Caraway seed, and Fennel seed
F.C. of Peppermint leaf, Caraway seed, Fennel seed, and Chamomile flower
F.C. of Peppermint leaf, Fennel seed, and Chamomile flower
F.C. of Peppermint oil and Fennel oil
F.C. of Peppermint oil, Caraway oil, and Fennel oil
F.C. of Peppermint oil, Caraway oil, Fennel oil, and Chamomile flower
F.C. of Peppermint oil, Fennel oil, and Chamomile flower
F.C. of Senna leaf, Peppermint oil, and Caraway oil

Fennel oil
Fennel seed
Ginger root
Indian snakeroot
Juniper berry
Kava Kava
Licorice root
Mayapple root and resin
Parsley herb and root
Petasites root
Rhubarb root
Sage leaf
Senna leaf
Uva Ursi leaf

Progressive Systemic Diseases
Echinacea Pallida root
Echinacea Purpurea herb
Woody Nightshade stem

Prostate Adenoma
Belladonna
Ephedra
Henbane leaf
Scopalia root

Pulmonary Edema
Belladonna
Henbane leaf

Renal Inflammation or Disease
Asparagus root
F.C. of Licorice root and German Chamomile flower
F.C. of Licorice root, Peppermint leaf, and German Chamomile flower
F.C. of Licorice root, Primrose root, Marshmallow root, and Anise seed
Horseradish
Juniper berry
Licorice root
Lovage root
Sandalwood, White
Watercress

Respiratory Inflammation
Larch Turpentine

Restlessness
Ephedra

Skin Injury
Camphor (external)
Comfrey root (external)
F.C. of Camphor, Eucalyptus oil, and Purified Turpentine oil (external)
Oak bark (external)
Paprika (external)

Thyroid Enlargement
Bugleweed

Thyroid, Low-Functioning
Bugleweed

Thyrotoxicosis
Ephedra

Tuberculosis
Echinacea Pallida root
Echinacea Purpurea herb
Mistletoe herb
Woody Nightshade stem

Ulcers, Gastric and Duodenal
Cola nut
Devil's Claw root
F.C. of Angelica root, Gentian root and Bitter Orange peel
F.C. of Angelica root, Gentian root, and Fennel seed
F.C. of Angelica root, Gentian root, Wormwood and Peppermint oil
F.C. of Ginger root, Gentian root, and Wormwood
Gentian root
Horseradish
Indian snakeroot
Nasturtium
Rhubarb root
Watercress

Whooping Cough
Fir Needle oil
Pine Needle oil

CHAPTER 10

SIDE EFFECTS OF APPROVED HERBS

This chapter, condensed from the monographs, lists potential adverse side effects of specific approved herbs. The listing of a particular herb to a corresponding side effect does not necessarily constitute a clear correlation of the herb with the effect; it means that it may be produced under certain conditions in some individuals. It is essential to refer to the complete monograph before making any therapeutic judgements. Side effects are sometimes only observed "in rare cases" and/or "in sensitive individuals." For example, nausea and vomiting are listed here as possible side effects of Uva Ursi. However, the monograph clarifies that "nausea and vomiting may occur in persons with sensitive stomachs." Thus, inclusion of a particular herb under a corresponding side effect should not be interpreted as an inevitable result of using the herb.

A guide of side effects by medical category is included to help identify the types of side effects listed in this chapter. Immediately following this guide, the herbs are listed alphabetically under each side effect.

SIDE EFFECT GUIDE BY MEDICAL CATEGORY

CARDIOVASCULAR
Angina
Cardiac Arrhythmia
Chills
Edema
Heart Function, Disorders of
Hypertension
Orthostatic Circulatory Disturbance
Pulse Irregularity
Tachycardia

DERMATOLOGICAL
Alopecia
Dermatitis
Eczema
Hives
Itching
Perspiration, Decreased

Photosensitization
Skin Allergy
Skin Alteration
Skin Damage
Skin Dryness
Skin Irritation
Skin, Reddening of the
Skin, Vesicles and Necrosis of the

ENDOCRINOLOGY, REPRODUCTIVE SYSTEM, OBSTETRICS/ GYNECOLOGY, PROSTATE
Electrolyte Imbalance
Menstruation, Early Post-partum Return of
Mineralocorticoid Effects
Potassium Deficiency
Sodium Retention

Thyroid Enlargement
Water Retention

Gastrointestinal
Abdominal Pain
Allergic Reactions, Gastrointestinal Tract
Cramps
Diarrhea
Dry Mouth
Flatulence
Gastrointestinal Disturbance
Intestinal Sluggishness
Laxative
Nausea
Vomiting

Hematology, Lymphatic, Cancer
Agranulocytosis
Aplastic Anemia
Leukopenia
Thrombocytopenia

Immunology, AIDS, Infectious Diseases
Allergy, General
Fever/Hyperthermia

Liver and Gallbladder
Jaundice/Yellow Skin

Neurology, Psychiatry
Convulsions
Dependency
Hallucination
Headache
Irritability
Nerve Damage
Poisoning, Central Nervous System
Restlessness
Sleep Disorder

Ophthalmology
Accommodation Disturbance, Ocular
Glaucoma

Respiratory
(Lower and Upper Respiratory Tract Including Ears, Nose, Throat, Sinuses)
Allergic Reactions, Respiratory Tract
Bronchospasm Increase
Mucous Membrane Irritation

Rheumatological, Orthopedic, Muscles, Contusions
Myopathy
Muscle Spasm

Urinary Tract System
(Kidney, Ureter, Bladder)
Albuminuria
Hematuria
Kidney Inflammation
Myoglobinuria
Poisoning, Renal
Urination, Difficulties in

Herb Guide by Side Effect

Abdominal Pain
  Autumn Crocus

Accommodation Disturbance, Ocular
  Belladonna
  Henbane leaf
  Kava Kava
  Scopolia root

Agranulocytosis
  Autumn Crocus

Albuminuria
  Aloe
  Buckthorn bark
  Buckthorn berry
  Cascara Sagrada bark
  Rhubarb root
  Senna leaf
  Senna pod

Allergic Reactions, Gastrointestinal Tract
  Anise seed
  F.C. of Anise oil and Iceland Moss
  F.C. of Anise oil, Fennel oil, Licorice root, and Thyme
  F.C. of Anise oil, Primrose root and Thyme
  F.C. of Anise seed, Fennel seed, and Caraway seed
  F.C. of Anise seed, Ivy leaf, Fennel seed, and Licorice root
  F.C. of Anise seed, Marshmallow root, Eucalyptus oil, and Licorice root
  F.C. of Anise seed, Marshmallow root, Iceland Moss, and Licorice root
  F.C. of Anise seed, Marshmallow root, Primrose root, and Sundew

Allergic Reactions, Mucosa
  Cinnamon bark
  Cinnamon bark, Chinese
  Rhatany root

Allergic Reactions, Respiratory Tract
  Anise seed
  F.C. of Angelica root, Gentian root, and Fennel seed
  F.C. of Anise oil and Iceland Moss
  F.C. of Anise oil, Fennel oil, Licorice root, and Thyme
  F.C. of Anise oil, Primrose root and Thyme
  F.C. of Anise seed, Fennel seed, and Caraway seed
  F.C. of Anise seed, Ivy leaf, Fennel seed, and Licorice root
  F.C. of Anise seed, Marshmallow root, Eucalyptus oil, and Licorice root
  F.C. of Anise seed, Marshmallow root, Iceland Moss, and Licorice root
  F.C. of Anise seed, Marshmallow root, Primrose root, and Sundew
  F.C. of Caraway oil and Fennel oil
  F.C. of Caraway oil, Fennel oil and Chamomile flower
  F.C. of Caraway seed and Fennel seed
  F.C. of Caraway seed, Fennel seed, and Chamomile flower
  F.C. of Marshmallow root, Fennel seed, Iceland Moss, and Thyme
  F.C. of Peppermint leaf and Fennel seed
  F.C. of Peppermint leaf, Caraway seed, and Fennel seed
  F.C. of Peppermint leaf, Caraway seed, Fennel seed, and Chamomile flower
  F.C. of Peppermint leaf, Fennel seed, and Chamomile flower
  F.C. of Peppermint oil and Fennel oil
  F.C. of Peppermint oil, Caraway oil, and Fennel oil
  F.C. of Peppermint oil, Caraway oil, Fennel oil, and Chamomile flower
  F.C. of Peppermint oil, Fennel oil, and Chamomile flower
  Fennel oil

Allergic Reactions, Skin
  Anise seed
  Chicory
  Cinnamon bark
  Cinnamon bark, Chinese
  F.C. of Angelica root, Gentian root, and Fennel seed
  F.C. of Anise oil and Iceland Moss
  F.C. of Anise oil, Fennel oil, Licorice root, and Thyme
  F.C. of Anise oil, Primrose root and Thyme
  F.C. of Anise seed, Ivy leaf, Fennel seed, and Licorice root
  F.C. of Anise seed, Marshmallow root, Eucalyptus oil, and Licorice root
  F.C. of Anise seed, Marshmallow root, Iceland Moss, and Licorice root
  F.C. of Anise seed, Marshmallow root, Primrose root, and Sundew
  F.C. of Caraway oil and Fennel oil
  F.C. of Caraway oil, Fennel oil and Chamomile flower
  F.C. of Caraway seed and Fennel seed
  F.C. of Caraway seed, Fennel seed, and Chamomile flower
  F.C. of Marshmallow root, Fennel seed, Iceland Moss, and Thyme
  F.C. of Peppermint leaf and Fennel seed
  F.C. of Peppermint leaf, Caraway seed, and Fennel seed
  F.C. of Peppermint leaf, Caraway seed, Fennel seed, and Chamomile flower
  F.C. of Peppermint leaf, Fennel seed, and Chamomile flower
  F.C. of Peppermint oil and Fennel oil
  F.C. of Peppermint oil, Caraway oil, and Fennel oil
  F.C. of Peppermint oil, Caraway oil, Fennel oil, and Chamomile flower
  F.C. of Peppermint oil, Fennel oil, and Chamomile flower
  Fennel oil
  Hay flower
  Larch turpentine (topical)
  Parsley herb and root
  Peruvian Balsam

Allergy, General
  Anise seed
  Asparagus root
  Bromelain
  Cinchona bark
  Echinacea Purpurea herb
  Fennel oil
  Fenugreek seed
  Garlic
  Ginkgo Biloba Leaf Extract
  Hay flower
  Kava Kava
  Larch Turpentine
  Mistletoe herb
  Peruvian Balsam
  Poplar bud
  Psyllium seed, Black
  Psyllium seed, Blonde
  Psyllium seed husk, Blonde
  Rhatany root

Alopecia
  Autumn Crocus

Angina
  Mistletoe herb

Aplastic Anemia
  Autumn Crocus

Bronchospasm Increase
  Fir Needle oil
  Pine Needle oil

Cardiac Arrhythmia
  Ephedra
  Lily-of-the-valley herb
  Squill

Chills
  Mistletoe herb

Convulsions
  Sage leaf

Cramps
  Aloe
  Buckthorn bark
  Buckthorn berry
  Cascara Sagrada bark
  Rhubarb root

Senna leaf
Senna pod

Dependency
Ephedra

Dermatitis
Arnica flower

Diarrhea
Autumn Crocus
Bromelain
Cajeput oil
Eucalyptus leaf
Eucalyptus oil
F.C. of Eucalyptus oil, Primrose root and Thyme
Niauli oil
Soy Phospholipid
Squill

Dry Mouth
Belladonna
Henbane leaf
Scopolia root

Eczema
Arnica flower
Camphor

Edema
Licorice root

Electrolyte Imbalance
Aloe
Buckthorn bark
Buckthorn berry
Cascara Sagrada bark
Rhubarb root
Senna leaf
Senna pod

Excitability
Cola nut

Fever
Belladonna
Cinchona bark
Echinacea Purpurea herb (injectible)
Mistletoe herb
Scopolia

Flatulence
Manna
Yeast, Medicinal

Gastrointestinal Disturbance
Black Cohosh root
Bromelain
Butcher's Broom
Cajeput oil
Cola nut
Dandelion root with herb
Eucalyptus leaf
Eucalyptus oil
F.C. of Angelica root, Gentian root, Wormwood, and Peppermint oil
F.C. of Eucalyptus oil, Primrose root and Thyme
F.C. of Gumweed herb, Primrose root and Thyme
F.C. of Javanese Turmeric root, Celandine herb, and Wormwood
F.C. of Javanese Turmeric root, Peppermint leaf, and Wormwood
F.C. of Peppermint oil and Caraway oil
F.C. of Peppermint oil, Caraway oil, and Chamomile flower
F.C. of Peppermint oil, Caraway oil, Fennel oil, and Chamomile flower
F.C. of Primrose root and Thyme
F.C. of Primrose root, Sundew, and Thyme
Garlic
Ginkgo Biloba Leaf Extract
Gumweed herb
Horse chestnut seed
Horseradish
Indian Snakeroot
Mint oil
Pollen
Potentilla
Primrose flower
Primrose root
Saw Palmetto berry
Senega Snakeroot
Soapwort root, Red
Soapwort root, White
Soy Phospholipid
Squill
Stinging Nettle root

Tormentil root
Turmeric
Turmeric, Javanese
Watercress

Glaucoma
Scopolia root

Hallucination
Belladonna

Headache
Ephedra
F.C. of Angelica root, Gentian root, and Fennel seed
Gentian root
Ginkgo Biloba Leaf Extract
Mistletoe herb
Sweet Clover
Yeast, Medicinal

Heart Function, Disorders of
Aloe
Buckthorn bark
Cascara Sagrada bark
Rhubarb
Senna leaf

Hematuria
Aloe
Buckthorn bark
Buckthorn berry
Cascara Sagrada bark
Rhubarb root
Senna leaf
Senna pod

Hives
Chaste Tree fruit
Paprika

Hypertension
Ephedra
Licorice root

Hyperthermia
Belladonna
Scopalia root

Intestinal Flora Changes
Garlic

Intestinal Sluggishness
Aloe
Buckthorn bark
Buckthorn berry
Cascara sagrada bark

Irritability
Ephedra

Itching
Chaste Tree fruit
Sandalwood, White

Kidney Inflammation
Juniper berry

Laxative
Milk Thistle fruit

Leukopenia
Autumn Crocus

Menstruation, Early Post-partum Return of
Chaste Tree fruit

Mineralocorticoid Effects
F.C. of Anise oil, Fennel oil, Licorice root, and Thyme (above 100 mg glycyrrhizin)
F.C. of Anise seed, Marshmallow root, Eucalyptus oil, and Licorice root (above 100 mg glycyrrhizin)
F.C. of Anise seed, Marshmallow root, Iceland Moss, and Licorice root (above 100 mg glycyrrhizin)
F.C. of Ivy leaf, Licorice root, and Thyme (above 100 mg glycyrrhizin)
F.C. of Marshmallow root, Primrose root, Licorice root, and Thyme oil (above 100 mg glycyrrhizin)
Licorice root

Mucous Membrane Irritation
Cloves
Fir Needle oil
Pine Needle oil

Muscle Spasm
Belladonna

Myoglobinuria
F.C. of Anise seed, Marshmallow root, Eucalyptus oil, and Licorice root (above 100 mg glycyrrhizin)
F.C. of Anise seed, Marshmallow root, Iceland Moss, and Licorice root (above 100 mg glycyrrhizin)
Licorice root

Myopathy
Autumn Crocus

Nausea
Autumn Crocus
Butcher's Broom
Echinacea Purpurea herb (injectible)
Ephedra
Eucalyptus leaf
Eucalyptus oil
F.C. of Eucalyptus oil, Primrose root and Thyme
F.C. of Gumweed herb, Primrose root and Thyme
F.C. of Primrose root and Thyme
F.C. of Primrose root, Sundew, and Thyme
Lily-of-the-valley herb
Manna
Niauli oil
Primrose flower
Primrose root
Sandalwood, White
Squill
Uva Ursi

Nerve Damage
White Mustard seed

Orthostatic Circulatory Disturbance
Mistletoe herb

Perspiration, Decreased
Belladonna
Scopolia root

Photosensitization
Angelica root
Bitter Orange peel
F.C. of Angelica root, Gentian root, and Bitter Orange peel
F.C. of Angelica root, Gentian root, and Fennel seed
F.C. of Angelica root, Gentian root, Wormwood, and Peppermint oil
F.C. of Peppermint leaf, Caraway seed, Chamomile flower, and Bitter Orange peel
Haronga bark and leaf
St. John's Wort

Poisoning, Central Nervous System
Turpentine oil, Purified

Poisoning, Renal
Turpentine oil, Purified

Potassium Deficiency
Aloe
Buckthorn bark
Buckthorn berry
Cascara Sagrada bark
Licorice root
Rhubarb root
Senna leaf
Senna pod

Pulse Irregularity
Squill

Restlessness
Cola nut
Ephedra

Skin Allergy
Cinchona bark
Poplar bud

Skin Alteration
Autumn Crocus

Skin Damage
White Mustard seed

Skin Dryness
Belladonna

Skin Irritation
Fir Needle oil
Pine Needle oil

Skin, Reddening
  Belladonna
  Scopalia root

Skin, Vesicles and Necrosis
  Arnica flower

Sleep Disorder
  Cola nut
  Ephedra

Sodium Retention
  Licorice root

Tachycardia
  Belladonna
  Ephedra
  Henbane leaf
  Scopolia root

Thrombocytopenia
  Cinchona bark

Thyroid Enlargement
  Bugleweed

Urination, Difficulties in
  Belladonna
  Ephedra
  Henbane leaf
  Scopolia root

Vomiting
  Autumn Crocus
  Echinacea Purpurea herb (injectible)
  Ephedra
  Eucalyptus leaf
  Eucalyptus oil
  F.C. of Eucalyptus oil, Primrose root and Thyme
  Lily-of-the-valley herb
  Niauli oil
  Squill
  Uva Ursi leaf

Water Retention
  Licorice root

Yellow Skin
  Kava Kava

Chapter 11

Side Effects of Unapproved Herbs

This chapter, condensed from the monographs, lists potential adverse side effects of unapproved herbs. The listing of a particular herb under a corresponding side effect does not necessarily constitute a clear correlation of the herb with the effect; it means that it may be produced under certain conditions in some individuals. It is essential to refer to the complete herb monograph before making any therapeutic judgements.

A guide of side effects by medical category is included to help identify the types of side effects listed in this chapter. Immediately following this guide, the herbs are listed alphabetically under each side effect.

Side Effect Guide by Medical Category

Cardiovascular
Bradycardia
Cardiac Arrest
Cardiac Arrhythmia
Cardiac Insufficiency
Hypertension
Hypotension
Tachycardia
Vascular Congestion

Dermatological
Allergic Skin Reactions
Clammy Skin
Depigmentation of skin
Dermatitis
    (see Allergic Skin Reactions)
Irritation, Skin
Perspiration
Photosensitization
Skin Discoloration
Swelling of Tongue
Urticaria

Endocrinology, Reproductive System, Obstetrics/Gynecology, Prostate
Abortion
Bleeding of the Uterus
Hyperthyroidism
Hypoglycemia
Hypothermia
Uterine Contraction, Stimulates

Gastrointestinal
Abdominal Pain
Constipation
Cramps
Diarrhea
Gastroenteritis
Gastrointestinal Tract, Irritation
Gastrointestinal Tract, Disturbance
    with Nausea
Nausea
Poisoning
Weight Loss

HEMATOLOGY, LYMPHATIC, CANCER
Methemoglobinuria

IMMUNOLOGY, AIDS, INFECTIOUS DISEASES
Allergic Mucosa Reactions
Allergies
Chills
Fever
Leukocytopenia
Lymphocytopenia

LIVER AND GALLBLADDER
Bilirubinuria
Cholestatic Icterus/Jaundice
Hepatotoxic

NEUROLOGY, PSYCHIATRY
Anaphylactic shock
Anxiety
Central Nervous System, Excitation
Central Nervous System, Sensitivity
Confusion
Dizziness
Fainting
Flushed Face
Hallucination
Headache
Headache, Migraine
Impaired Balance
Intoxication
Lethargy
Melancholic Moods
Nervous Excitation
Numbness
Organotoxic
Psychic Disturbances
Restlessness
Sleep Disorder
Tremor
Vertigo

OPHTHALMOLOGY
Eye Irritation
Blindness
Mydriasis
Pupillary Rigidity
Visual Disturbances

RESPIRATORY
(Lower and Upper Respiratory Tract Including Ears, Nose, Throat, Sinuses)
Alveolitis
Bleeding from the Nose, Lips, & Eyelids
Bleeding of the Mucous Membranes
Dyspnea
Irritation, Mucous Membrane
Nose Bleed
Paralysis, Respiratory System
Pseudoallergic Reaction
Respiratory Insufficiency
Rhinitis

RHEUMATOLOGICAL, ORTHOPEDIC, MUSCLES, CONTUSIONS
Muscle Spasm
Spasms, Clonic-tonic
Colic
Convulsions
Pain in Muscles and Joints
Paralysis

URINARY TRACT SYSTEM
(Kidney, Ureter, Bladder)
Albuminuria
Anuria
Diuresis
Hematuria
Hemoglobinuria
Kidney Damage
Kidney Irritation
Nephritis
Urinary Tract Irritation

Herb Guide by Side Effect

Abdominal Pain
Rhododendron, Rusty-leaved
Tansy

Abortion
Bryonia root
Marsh Tea
Mugwort
Nutmeg
Parsley seed
Rue
Saffron
Tansy

Albuminuria
Male Fern

Allergic Mucosa Reactions
Cinnamon flower

Allergic Skin Reactions
Asparagus herb
Cinnamon flower
Cocoa
Elecampane root
Liverwort herb
Olive oil
Pasque flower
Rhododendron, Rusty-leaved
Rue

Allergies
Aspen bark and leaf
Bladderwrack
Celery
Chamomile, Roman
Echinacea Angustifolia herb and root (parenteral use)
Echinacea Pallida herb (parenteral use)
Echinacea Purpurea root (parenteral use)
Ginkgo Biloba leaf
Kelp
Lemongrass, Citronella oil
Mugwort
Oats
Papain
Strawberry leaf

Alveolitis
Lemongrass, Citronella oil

Anaphylactic Shock
Celery
Chamomile, Roman

Anuria
Parsley seed

Anxiety
Yohimbe bark

Bilirubinuria
Male Fern

Bleeding from the Nose, Lips, & Eyelids
Saffron

Bleeding of the Mucous Membranes
Parsley seed

Bleeding of the Uterus
Saffron
Tansy

Blindness
Male Fern

Bradycardia
Delphinium
Monkshood
Rhododendron, Rusty-leaved

Cardiac Arrest
Delphinium
Rhododendron, Rusty-leaved

Cardiac Arrhythmia
Male Fern
Monkshood

Parsley seed
Tansy

Cardiac Insufficiency
Male Fern

Central Nervous System, Excitation
Marsh Tea
Nux Vomica

Central Nervous System, Sensitivity
Rhododendron, Rusty-leaved

Chills
Echinacea Angustifolia herb and root (parenteral use)
Echinacea pallida herb (parenteral use)

Cholestatic Icterus/Jaundice
Bishop's Weed

Clammy Skin
Rue

Colic
Bryonia root

Confusion
Male Fern

Constipation
Cocoa seed

Convulsions
Bryonia root
Male Fern
Nux Vomica

Cramps
Elecampane root
Rhododendron, Rusty-leaved

Depigmentation of Skin
Marjoram

Dermatitis
(see Allergic Skin Reactions)

Diarrhea
Barberry
Bryonia root
Elecampane root
Male Fern
Marsh Tea
Rhododendron, Rusty-leaved
Saffron
Turpentine oil, Sulfurated

Diuresis
Sarsaparilla root

Dizziness
Bryonia root
Male Fern
Monkshood
Rue
Saffron

Dyspnea
Barberry
Male Fern

Eye Irritation
Barberry

Fainting
Rue

Fever
Echinacea Angustifolia herb and root (parenteral use)
Echinacea Pallida herb (parenteral use)
Echinacea Purpurea root (parenteral use)

Flushed Face
Tansy

Gastroenteritis
Tansy

Gastrointestinal Tract, Disturbance with Nausea
Barberry

Gastrointestinal Tract, Irritation
Marsh Tea
Rue
Sarsaparilla

Hallucination
Nutmeg

Headache
  Cocoa
  Male Fern

Headache, Migraine
  Cocoa

Hematuria
  Saffron
  Turpentine oil, Sulfurated

Hemoglobinuria
  Parsley seed

Hepatotoxic
  Borage
  Coltsfoot
  Hound's Tongue
  Madder root
  Petasites leaf
  Rue
  Senecio herb
  Tansy

Hypertension
  Yohimbe bark

Hyperthyroidism
  Bladderwrack
  Kelp

Hypoglycemic
  Goat's Rue herb

Hypotension
  Delphinium flower
  Rhododendron, Rusty-leaved
  Rue

Hypothermia
  Monkshood

Impaired Balance
  Rhododendron, Rusty-leaved

Intoxication
  Bilberry leaf
  Marsh Tea
  Monkshood
  Tansy
  Yellow Jessamine root

Irritation, Mucous Membrane
  Elecampane
  Liverwort
  Pasque flower
  Soapwort

Irritation, Skin
  Barberry
  Buchu leaf
  Liverwort herb
  Mountain Ash berry
  Pasque flower
  Sarsaparilla, German
  Soapwort

Kidney Damage
  Bryonia root
  Marsh Tea
  Parsley seed
  Rue
  Tansy

Kidney Irritation
  Barberry
  Liverwort herb
  Marsh Tea
  Parsley seed
  Pasque flower

Lethargy
  Barberry

Leukocytopenia
  Periwinkle

Lymphocytopenia
  Periwinkle

Melancholic Moods
  Rue

Methemoglobinuria
  Parsley seed

Muscle Spasm
  Male Fern
  Monkshood
  Rue

Mydriasis
  Tansy

Nausea
  Barberry
  Bryonia root
  Echinacea Angustifolia herb and root
     (parenteral use)
  Echinacea Pallida herb (parenteral use)
  Echinacea Purpurea root
     (parenteral use)
  Elecampane root
  Male Fern
  Marsh Tea
  Monkshood
  Rhododendron, Rusty-leaved
  Tansy
  Yohimbe

Nephritis
  Barberry

Nervous Excitation
  Bryonia root
  Yohimbe

Nose Bleed
  Barberry

Numbness
  Saffron

Organotoxic
  Borage
  Coltsfoot
  Petasites leaf
  Senecio herb

Pain in Muscles and Joints
  Marsh Tea
  Rhododendron, Rusty-leaved

Paralysis
  Elecampane root
  Marsh Tea
  Rhododendron, Rusty-leaved

Paralysis, Respiratory System
  Barberry
  Delphinium
  Monkshood

Paresthesia
  Monkshood

Perspiration
  Marsh Tea

Photosensitization
  Angelica herb
  Angelica seed
  Bishop's Weed fruit
  Celery
  Rue

Poisoning
  Hyssop oil
  Jimsonweed leaf and seed
  Lemongrass, Citronella oil
  Male Fern
  Marsh Tea
  Mistletoe berry
  Nux Vomica
  Oleander leaf
  Rhododendron, Rusty-leaved

Pseudoallergic Reaction
  Bishop's Weed fruit

Psychic Disturbances
  Nutmeg
  Rue

Pupillary Rigidity
  Tansy

Respiratory Insufficiency
  Male Fern
  Rhododendron, Rusty-leaved

Restlessness
  Yohimbe

Rhinitis
  Chamomile, Roman

Skin Discoloration
  Saffron
  Walnut hull

Sleep Disorder
  Rue
  Yohimbe

Spasms, Clonic-tonic
  Hyssop oil
  Tansy

Swelling of Tongue
  Rue

Tachycardia
  Yohimbe

Tremor
  Male Fern
  Yohimbe

Urinary Tract Irritation
  Liverwort herb
  Marsh Tea
  Pasque flower
  Turpentine oil, Sulfurated

Urticaria
  Paprika species low in capsaicin

Uterine Contraction, Stimulates
  Male Fern

Vascular Congestion
  Parsley seed

Vertigo
  Saffron

Visual Disturbances
  Male Fern

Weight Loss
  Parsley seed

Chapter 12

Pharmacological Actions of Approved Herbs

This chapter, condensed from the monographs, provides a list of pharmacological actions of approved herbs. In some cases, the pharmacological actions listed were demonstrated in in vitro experiments or in vivo studies (on animals) but have not been confirmed in human clinical trials. Their inclusion is intended to help health professionals understand the potential activity, risks, and/or benefits of the herb. It is essential to refer to the complete herb monograph before making any therapeutic judgements.

A guide of pharmacological actions by medical category is included to help identify the types of actions listed in this chapter. Immediately following this guide, the herbs are listed alphabetically under each pharmacological action.

Pharmacological Action Guide by Medical Category

Cardiovascular
Antihypertensive
Cholesterol Lowering
Chronotropic, Negatively
Chronotropic, Positively
Circulatory Stimulant
Circulatory/Vascular Tonic
Coronary Artery Flow, Increases
Hyperemic
Inotropic, Positively
Lipid-Lowering
Myocardial Circulation, Increases
Roborant
Venous Pressure, Lowers
Venous Tonic

Dermatological
Absorbent
Anti-exudative
Antiperspirant
Astringent
Callus Formation
Deodorant
Granulatory
Skin Irritation, Decreases
Skin Irritation, Stimulates
Skin Metabolism, Stimulates
Wound Healing

Endocrinology, Reproductive System, Obstetrics/Gynecology, Prostate
Antiandrogenic
Antigonadotropic
Antithyrotropic
Blood Sugar Regulation
Blood Supply, Increase
Corpus Luteum-Like Effects
Endurance, Increased
Estrogen Receptor Site Binding

Glycogenolytic
Luteinizing Hormone Suppression
Prolactin Level, Decreases
Tyrosinase Inhibiting
Uterine Contraction, Stimulates

GASTROINTESTINAL
Antiemetic
Antiflatulent
Carminative
Gastric Juices, Stimulates
Gastric Ulcers, Accelerate Healing of
Laxative
Lipolytic
Motility, Inhibiting
Motility, Stimulating
Pancreatic Exocrine Secretion, Stimulates
Peristalsis, Regulation of
Salivation, Increases
Secretion of Gastric Juices
Secretolytic
Secretomotory
Smooth Muscle Contraction
Spasmolytic

HEMATOLOGY, LYMPHATIC, CANCER
Antichemotactic
Cytotoxic
Fibrinolytic Activity, Increases
Hemostatic
Leucocyte Increase
Lymphocyte Increase
Mitosis Inhibitor
Platelet Aggregation, Inhibits
Prothrombin Time, Increases
Spleen Cell Increase
Thrombocyte Aggregation, Inhibits

IMMUNOLOGY, AIDS, INFECTIOUS DISEASES
Antibacterial
Antifungal
Antimicrobial
Antiparasitic
Antiseptic
Antiviral
Immunomodulation
Phagocytosis, Stimulates
Pyretic
T-Cell Production
Temperature Elevation

LIVER AND GALLBLADDER
Cholagogue
Cholecystokinetic
Choloretic
Hepatoprotective

NEUROLOGY, PSYCHIATRY
Acetylcholinesterase Inhibitor
Analgesic
Anesthesia, Topical
Anti-anxiety
Anticholinergic
Anticonvulsant
Antidepressant
Antiphlogistic
Antipyretic
Antispasmodic
Bathmotropic, Negatively
Central Nervous System, Stimulant
Dromotropic, Positively
MAO Inhibitor
Muscarine-like
Musculotropic
Nerve Damaging
Papaverine-like
Parasympatholytic
Salivation, Increases
Sedative
Soporific
Sympathomimetic
Tonus, Increases

Respiratory
(Lower and Upper Respiratory Tract Including Ears, Nose, Throat, Sinuses)
- Analeptic, Respiratory
- Anti-irritant
- Antitussive
- Bronchial Secretion, Increased
- Bronchial Secretion, Reduced
- Bronchoantispasmodic
- Demulcent
- Expectorant
- Mucociliary Activity, Increases
- Mucous Membrane Irritant
- Oral-pharyngeal Anti-irritant

Rheumatological, Orthopedic, Muscles, Contusions
- Anti-edematous
- Cytostatic
- Electrolyte-like Reaction on Capillary Wall

Urinary Tract System
(Kidney, Ureter, Bladder)
- Diuretic
- Kaliuretic
- Natriuretic
- Residual Urine, Reduces
- Urinary Flow, Increases

Herb Guide by Pharmacological Action (Approved Herbs)

Absorbent
  Coffee Charcoal

Acetylcholinesterase Inhibitor
  Knotweed herb

Analeptic, Respiratory
  Camphor
  Cola nut
  Maté

Analgesic
  Arnica flower
  Devil's Claw root
  White Willow bark

Anesthestic, Topical
  Cloves

Antiandrogenic
  Saw Palmetto berry

Anti-anxiety
  Kava Kava

Antibacterial
  Anise seed
  Chamomile flower, German
  Cinnamon bark
  Cinnamon bark, Chinese
  Cloves
  Dill seed
  Ephedra
  F.C. of Anise oil, Fennel oil, and Caraway oil
  F.C. of Anise seed, Fennel seed, and Caraway seed
  F.C. of Peppermint oil and Caraway oil
  F.C. of Peppermint oil and Fennel oil
  F.C. of Peppermint oil, Caraway oil, and Chamomile flower
  F.C. of Peppermint oil, Caraway oil, and Fennel oil
  F.C. of Peppermint oil, Caraway oil, Fennel oil, and Chamomile flower
  F.C. of Peppermint oil, Fennel oil, and Chamomile flower
  Galangal
  Garlic
  Gumweed herb
  Mint oil
  Onion
  Peppermint oil
  Peruvian Balsam
  Plantain
  Poplar bud
  Sage leaf
  Sandalwood, White
  Thyme
  Uva Ursi leaf
  White Mustard seed
  Yarrow
  Yeast, Medicinal

Antichemotactic
  Autumn Crocus

Anticholinergic
  Belladonna
  Henbane leaf
  Scopolia root
  Woody Nightshade stem

Anticonvulsant
  Kava Kava

Antidepressant
  St. John's Wort

Anti-edematous
  Bromelain
  Sweet Clover

Antiemetic
  Ginger root

Anti-exudative
Horse Chestnut seed
Saw Palmetto berry

Antiflatulent
Lavender flower

Antifungal
Cinnamon bark
Cinnamon bark, Chinese
Cloves
Garlic
Sage leaf

Antigonadotropic
Bugleweed

Antihypertensive
Lily-of-the-valley herb
Onion
Squill

Antiinflammatory
Calendula flower
Cola nut
Comfrey herb and leaf
Comfrey root
St. John's Wort
Turmeric root
Witch Hazel leaf and bark

Anti-irritant
Marshmallow leaf
Mullein flower
Plantain

Antiperspirant
Sage leaf

Antimicrobial
Caraway oil
Caraway seed
Couch Grass
Fennel oil
Horseradish
Iceland Moss
Radish
Usnea
Uva Ursi
Thyme, Wild
Woody Nightshade stem

Antimycotic
Garlic

Antiparasitic
Peruvian Balsam

Antiphlogistic
Arnica flower
Autumn Crocus
Butcher's Broom
Chamomile flower, German
Devil's Claw root
Cola nut
Goldenrod
Galangal
White Willow bark
Woody Nightshade stem

Antipyretic
Mint oil
Peppermint oil
White Willow bark

Antiseptic
Arnica flower
Cloves
Fenugreek seed
Fir Needle oil
Fir Shoots, Fresh
Larch Turpentine
Peruvian Balsam
Pine Needle oil
Pine Sprouts
Turpentine oil, Purified

Antispasmodic
Angelica root
Anise seed
Boldo leaf
Caraway oil
Caraway seed
Celandine herb
Chamomile flower, German
Cloves
Dill seed
Eucalyptus leaf
Eucalyptus oil
Fennel oil
Fennel seed
Fumitory

Galangal
Ginger root
Goldenrod
Ivy leaf
Java tea
Kava Kava
Licorice root
Lovage root
Mint oil
Peppermint leaf
Peppermint oil
Petasites root
Rosemary leaf
Yarrow
Star Anise seed
Thyme, Wild

Antithyrotropic
Bugleweed

Antitussive
Ephedra
Sundew

Antiviral
Cloves
Cardamom seed
Oak bark
Sage leaf

Appetite Stimulant
Dandelion root with herb
Devil's Claw root
F.C. of Angelica root, Gentian root, and Bitter Orange peel
F.C. of Angelica root, Gentian root, and Fennel seed
F.C. of Angelica root, Gentian root, and Wormwood
F.C. of Ginger root, Gentian root, and Wormwood
Pollen
Wormwood

Astringent
Agrimony
Bilberry fruit
Blackberry leaf
Blackthorn berry
Coffee Charcoal
Jambolan bark

Knotweed herb
Lady's Mantle
Myrrh
Oak bark
Plantain
Potentilla
Rhatany root
Rose flower
Sage leaf
Walnut leaf
Witch Hazel leaf and bark
Woody Nightshade stem
Yarrow

Bathmotropic, Negatively
Hawthorn leaf with flower

Blood Sugar Regulation
Psyllium seed husk, Blonde

Blood Supply, Increase
Rosemary leaf (external)

Bronchial Secretion, Increased
Camphor
Elder flower
Gentian root

Bronchial Secretion, Reduced
Turpentine oil, Purified

Bronchoantispasmodic
Camphor
F.C. of Sundew and Thyme
Sundew
Thyme

Callus Formation
Comfrey root

Carminative
F.C. of Caraway oil and Fennel oil
F.C. of Caraway oil, Fennel oil and Chamomile flower
F.C. of Caraway seed and Fennel seed
F.C. of Javanese Turmeric root, Peppermint leaf, and Wormwood
F.C. of Milk Thistle fruit, Peppermint leaf, and Wormwood
F.C. of Peppermint leaf and Caraway seed

F.C. of Peppermint leaf and Fennel seed
F.C. of Peppermint leaf, Caraway seed, and Chamomile flower
F.C. of Peppermint leaf, Caraway seed, and Fennel seed
F.C. of Peppermint leaf, Caraway seed, Fennel seed, and Chamomile flower
F.C. of Peppermint oil and Caraway oil
F.C. of Peppermint oil and Fennel oil
F.C. of Peppermint oil, Caraway oil, and Chamomile flower
F.C. of Peppermint oil, Caraway oil, and Fennel oil
F.C. of Peppermint oil, Caraway oil, Fennel oil, and Chamomile flower
F.C. of Peppermint oil, Fennel oil, and Chamomile flower
Lemon Balm
Mint oil
Peppermint leaf
Peppermint oil

Central Nervous System, Stimulant
Ephedra

Cholagogue
Angelica root
Cardamom seed
Ginger
Mint oil
Peppermint oil

Cholecystokinetic
Haronga bark
Turmeric root

Cholesterol Lowering
Psyllium seed, Blonde
Psyllium seed husk, Blonde

Choloretic
Artichoke leaf
Boldo leaf
Chicory
Dandelion root with herb
Devil's Claw
F.C. of Javanese Turmeric root, Peppermint leaf, and Wormwood
F.C. of Milk Thistle fruit, Peppermint leaf, and Wormwood

Haronga bark and leaf
Horehound herb
Peppermint leaf
Sandy Everlasting
Turmeric root
Turmeric, Javanese
Yarrow

Chronotropic, Negatively
Squill

Chronotropic, Positively
Belladonna
Cola nut
Hawthorn
Maté
Scopolia root
Shepherd's Purse herb

Circulatory Stimulant
Pine Sprouts

Circulatory/Vascular Tonic
Camphor
Horse Chestnut seed
Lily-of-the-valley herb

Coronary Artery Flow, Increases
Hawthorn leaf with flower
Rosemary leaf

Corpus Luteum-Like Effects
Chaste Tree fruit

Cytostatic
Celandine herb

Cytotoxic
Soapwort root, White

Demulcent
Iceland Moss
Mallow flower
Mallow leaf
Marshmallow root

Deodorant
Chamomile flower, German

Diaphoretic
Elder flower
Linden flower

Diuretic
  Asparagus root
  Birch leaf
  Butcher's Broom
  Cola nut
  Dandelion root with herb
  Goldenrod
  Horsetail herb
  Java tea
  Juniper berry
  Kidney Bean pods (without seeds)
  Maté
  Spiny Restharrow root

Dromotropic, Positively
  Belladonna
  Hawthorn leaf with flower
  Scopolia root

Electrolyte-like Reaction on Capillary Wall
  Butcher's Broom

Endurance, Increased
  Eleuthero (Siberian Ginseng) root

Estrogen Receptor Site Binding
  Black Cohosh root

Expectorant
  Anise seed
  Eucalyptus leaf
  Eucalyptus oil
  F.C. of Anise oil, Primrose root and Thyme
  F.C. of Eucalyptus oil, Primrose root and Thyme
  F.C. of Ivy leaf, Licorice root, and Thyme
  F.C. of Primrose root and Thyme
  Ivy leaf
  Licorice root
  Mullein flower
  Primrose flower
  Primrose root
  Senega Snakeroot
  Soapwort root, Red
  Star Anise seed
  Thyme

Fibrinolytic Activity, Increases
  Garlic

Gastric Juices, Stimulates
  Angelica root
  Blessed Thistle herb
  Bogbean leaf
  Boldo leaf
  Centaury herb
  Cinchona bark
  Cola nut
  Condurango bark
  Gentian root
  Ginger root
  Haronga bark

Gastric Ulcers, Accelerate Healing of
  Licorice root

Glycogenolytic
  Maté

Granulatory
  Calendula flower
  Peruvian Balsam
  Poplar bud

Hemostatic
  Witch Hazel leaf and bark

Hepatoprotective
  Soy Phospholipid
  Milk Thistle fruit

Hyperemic
  Camphor
  Eucalyptus oil
  Fenugreek seed
  Fir Needle oil
  Fir Shoots, Fresh
  Hay flower (external)
  Horseradish
  Larch Turpentine
  Paprika
  Pine Needle oil
  Turpentine oil, Purified

Immunomodulation
  Celandine herb
  Echinacea Purpurea herb
  Eleuthero (Siberian Ginseng) root
  Mistletoe herb

Inotropic, Positively
Ginger root
Hawthorn leaf with flower
Lily-of-the-valley herb
Maté
Pheasant's Eye herb
Rosemary leaf
Shepherd's Purse
Squill

Kaliuretic
Lily-of-the-valley herb

Laxative
Aloe
Buckthorn bark
Buckthorn berry
Cascara Sagrada bark
Flaxseed
Manna
Rhubarb root
Senna leaf
Senna pod

Leucocyte Increase
Echinacea Purpurea herb

Lipid-Lowering
Garlic
Onion
Soy Lecithin

Lipolytic
Cola nut
Maté

Luteinizing Hormone Suppression
Black Cohosh root

Lymphocyte Increase
Eleuthero (Siberian Ginseng) root

MAO Inhibitor
St. John's Wort

Mitosis Inhibitor
Autumn Crocus

Motility, Inhibiting (Intestinal)
Passionflower herb
Uzara root

Motility, Stimulating (Intestinal)
Aloe
Buckthorn bark
Buckthorn berry
Cascara Sagrada bark
Cinnamon bark
Cinnamon bark, Chinese
Cola nut
Fennel oil
Fennel seed
Ginger root
Radish

Mucociliary Activity, Increased
Fennel seed

Mucous Membrane Irritant
Ivy leaf
Soapwort root, White
Woody Nightshade stem

Muscarine-Like
Shepherd's Purse

Musculotropic
Chamomile flower, German

Myocardial Circulation, Increases
Hawthorn leaf with flower

Natriuretic
Lily-of-the-valley herb

Nerve Damaging
Paprika

Oral-pharyngeal Anti-irritant
Mallow leaf

Pancreatic Exocrine Secretion, Stimulates
Haronga bark and leaf

Papaverine-like
Celandine herb

Parasympatholytic
Belladonna
Henbane leaf
Scopalia root

Peristalsis, Regulation of
Psyllium seed, Black
Psyllium seed, Blonde

Phagocytosis, Stimulates
Echinacea Pallida root
Echinacea Purpurea herb
Marshmallow root
Yeast, Medicinal

Platelet Aggregation, Inhibits
Garlic

Prolactin Level, Decreases
Bugleweed
Chaste Tree fruit

Prothrombin Time, Increases
Garlic

Pyretic
Echinacea Purpurea herb

Residual Urine, Reduces
Stinging Nettle root

Roborant
Gentian root

Salivation, Increases
Blessed Thistle herb
Bogbean leaf
Cinchona bark
Condurango bark
Ginger root
Gentian root

Secretion of Gastric Juices
Angelica root
Gentian root

Secretolytic
Fennel seed
Fenugreek seed
Fir Needle oil
Fir shoots, Fresh
Ginger root
Licorice root
Mint oil
Peppermint oil
Pine needle oil
Pine Sprouts
Primrose flower
Primrose root
Senega snakeroot

Secretomotory
Eucalyptus leaf
Eucalyptus oil
Sage leaf
Radish

Sedative
F.C. of Passionflower herb, Valerian root, and Lemon Balm
F.C. of Valerian root, Hops, and Lemon Balm
F.C. of Valerian root, Hops, and Passionflower herb
Kava Kava
Henbane leaf
Lavender flower
Lemon Balm
Valerian root

Skin Irritation, Decreases
Marshmallow leaf
Marshmallow root

Skin Irritation, Stimulates
Ivy leaf
Paprika
Rosemary leaf
White Mustard seed

Skin Metabolism, Stimulates
Chamomile flower, German

Smooth Muscle Contraction
Juniper berry

Soporific
F.C. of Anise oil, Fennel oil, Licorice root, and Thyme
F.C. of Anise seed, Ivy leaf, Fennel seed, and Licorice root
F.C. of Anise seed, Marshmallow root, Iceland Moss, and Licorice root
F.C. of Anise seed, Marshmallow root, Primrose root, and Sundew
F.C. of Birch leaf, Goldenrod, and Java tea

F.C. of Camphor, Eucalyptus oil,
    and Purified Turpentine oil
F.C. of Dandelion root with herb,
    Celandine herb, and Wormwood
F.C. of Dandelion root with herb,
    Peppermint leaf, and Artichoke leaf
F.C. of Eucalyptus oil and Pine
    Needle oil
F.C. of Eucalyptus oil, Primrose root
    and Thyme
F.C. of Ginger root, Gentian root,
    and Wormwood
F.C. of Ivy leaf, Licorice root, and
    Thyme
F.C. of Javanese Turmeric root,
    Celandine herb, and Wormwood
F.C. of Javanese Turmeric root,
    Peppermint leaf, and Wormwood
F.C. of Licorice root and German
    Chamomile flower
F.C. of Licorice root, Peppermint leaf,
    and German Chamomile flower
F.C. of Licorice root, Primrose root,
    Marshmallow root, and Anise seed
F.C. of Passionflower herb, Valerian
    root, and Lemon Balm
F.C. of Valerian root, Hops, and
    Lemon Balm
F.C. of Valerian root, Hops, and
    Passionflower herb
Hops flower
Valerian root

Spasmolytic
Sandalwood, White

Spleen Cell Increase
Echinacea Purpurea herb

Sympathomimetic
Ephedra

T-Cell Production
Ginseng root

Temperature Elevation
Echinacea Purpurea herb

Thrombocyte Aggregation, Inhibits
Onion

Tonus, Increase
Potentilla

Tyrosinase Inhibiting
Uva Ursi leaf

Urinary Flow, Increases
Stinging Nettle root

Uterine Contraction, Stimulates
Shepherd's Purse herb

Venous Pressure, Lowers
Lily-of-the-valley herb
Squill

Venous Tonic
Butcher's Broom
Lily-of-the-valley herb
Pheasant's Eye herb

Wound Healing
Calendula flower
Chamomile flower, German
Poplar bud
Sweet Clover

Chapter 13

Pharmacological Actions of Unapproved Herbs

This chapter, condensed from the monographs, provides a list of actions of unapproved herbs. In some cases, the pharmacological actions listed were demonstrated in in vitro experiments or in vivo studies (on animals) but have not been confirmed in human clinical trials. Their inclusion is intended to help health professionals understand the potential activity, risks, and/or benefits of the herb. It is essential to refer to the complete herb monograph before making any therapeutic judgements.

A guide of pharmacological actions by medical category is included to help identify the types of actions listed in this chapter. Immediately following this guide, the herbs are alphabetically listed under each pharmacological action.

Pharmacological Action Guide by Medical Category

Cardiovascular
- Antiarrhythmic
- Arrhythmia, Stabilizes
- Arrhythmogenic
- Chronotropic, Negatively
- Coronary Dilator
- Heart Muscle Stimulant
- Hypotensive
- Vasodilator

Dermatological
- Anti-exudative
- Phototoxic

Endocrinology, Reproductive System, Obstetrics/Gynecology, Prostate
- Abortifacient
- Glycine Antagonist
- Hypoglycemic
- Prostaglandin Synthesis, Inhibits
- Teratogenic Effects

Gastrointestinal
- Constipating
- Emetic
- Laxative
- Motility, Inhibiting

Hematology, Lymphatic, Cancer
- Antihemorrhagic
- Carcinogenic
- Mutagenic

Immunology, AIDS, Infectious Diseases
Anti-infectious
Antimicrobial

Liver and Gallbladder
Cholecystokinetic
Hepatotoxic

Neurology, Psychiatry
Analgesic
Antipyretic
Central Nervous System Paralysis
MAO Inhibitor
Sedative

Respiratory (Lower and Upper Respiratory Tract Including Ears, Nose, Throat, Sinuses)
Antitussive
Bronchodilator
Mucosal Irritation
Secretolytic

Rheumatological, Orthopedic, Muscles, Contusions
Antiinflammatory
Antispasmodic
Inotropic, Positively

Urinary Tract System (Kidney, Ureter, Bladder)
Diuretic

Herb Guide by Pharmacological Action (Unapproved Herbs)

Abortifacient
Mugwort
Pasque flower
Rue
Tansy

Analgesic
Ash bark and leaf

Antiarrhythmic
Olive leaf

Anti-exudative
Ash bark and leaf

Antihemorrhagic
Senecio herb

Anti-infectious
Pasque flower

Antiinflammatory
Marsh Tea

Antimicrobial
Basil herb

Antiphlogistic
Ash bark and leaf
Marsh Tea
Nutmeg

Antipyretic
Olive leaf

Antispasmodic
Nutmeg
Olive leaf
Rupturewort
Turpentine oil, Sulfurated

Antitussive
Marsh Tea

Arrhythmia, Stabilizes
Night-blooming Cereus

Arrhythmogenic
Olive leaf

Bronchodilator
Olive leaf
Yellow Jessamine root

Carcinogenic
(Includes herbs for which only an identifiable chemical component may be carcinogenic.)
Basil herb
Borage
Madder root
Nutmeg
Senecio herb
Walnut hull

Central Nervous System Paralysis
Pasque flower

Cholecystokinetic
Olive oil
Turpentine oil, Sulfurated

Chronotropic, Negatively
Oleander leaf
Rue

Constipating
Cocoa

Coronary Dilator
Olive leaf

Diuretic
Asparagus herb
Celery
Cocoa
Olive leaf

Emetic
Bryonia root

Glycine Antagonist
Nux Vomica

Heart Muscle Stimulant
Cocoa seed

Hepatotoxic
Borage
Petasites leaf
Senecio herb
Tansy

Hyperemic
Turpentine oil, Sulfurated

Hypoglycemic
Olive leaf

Hypotensive
Olive leaf

Inotropic, Positively
Oleander leaf

Laxative
Bryonia root
Colocynth

MAO Inhibitor
Nutmeg

Motility, Inhibiting
Marsh Tea

Mucosal Irritation
Marsh Tea
Soapwort herb, Red

Mutagenic
Rue

Phototoxic
Celery
Rue

Prostaglandin Synthesis, Inhibits
Nutmeg

Secretolytic
Verbena herb

Skin Irritation
Marsh Tea
Turpentine oil, Sulfurated

Teratogenic Effects
Pasque flower

Vasodilator
Cocoa seed
Yellow Jessamine root

Chapter 14

Interactions of Herbs with Conventional Drugs

This chapter, condensed from the monographs, summarizes the possible antagonistic or synergistic interactions an herb may have with conventional pharmaceutical medicines. The interactions are divided into two parts: (1) by the herb with the corresponding drugs and (2) by drug and other substance with the corresponding herbs. It is essential to refer to the complete herb monograph before making any therapeutic judgments.

Interactions by Herb

Monopreparations

Aloe
Chronic use/abuse can increase loss of serum potassium, thereby potentiating cardiac glycosides and antiarrhythmic agents. Potassium deficiency can be increased by simultaneous use of thiazide diuretics, corticosteroids, and licorice root.
Note: Similar data applies to all other approved stimulant laxatives: cascara sagrada bark, buckthorn bark and berry, rhubarb root, and senna leaf and fruits. Also, the reader should note that the aloe referred to in the monograph is "drug aloe" (made from the inner leaf) not the aloe gel from which numerous drinks are made and marketed in the U.S. Ingestion of aloe gel does not produce a significant laxative effect nor does it produce the drug interactions noted here.

Belladonna leaf and root
Increased anticholinergic effect by tricyclic anti-depressants, amantadine and quinidine.

Bromelain
Increased tendency for bleeding with simultaneous administration of anti-coagulants and inhibitors of thrombocytic aggregation. Increased plasma and urine levels of tetracyclines.

Buckthorn bark/berry
Chronic use/abuse can increase loss of serum potassium thus potentiating cardiac glycosides and antiarrhythmic agents. Potassium deficiency can be increased by simultaneous use of thiazide diuretics, corticosteroids, and licorice root.
Note: Two separate monographs

Bugleweed
None known. No simultaneous administration of thyroid preparations. Interferes with diagnostic procedures with radioactive isotopes.

Cascara Sagrada bark
Chronic use/abuse can increase loss of serum potassium thus potentiating cardiac glycosides and antiarrhythmic agents. Potassium deficiency can be increased by simultaneous use of thiazide diuretics, corticosteroids, and licorice root.

Chaste Tree fruit
Interactions unknown. Animal experiments show evidence of dopaminergic effect; therefore, a reciprocal weakening of the effect can occur in cases of ingestion of dopamine-receptor antagonists.

Cinchona bark
Increases the effect of anticoagulants if given simultaneously.

Coffee Charcoal
Due to the high absorption capacity of coffee charcoal, the absorption of other, simultaneously administered drugs can be influenced.

Cola nut
Strengthening of the action of psychoaneleptic drugs and caffeine-containing beverages.

Ephedra
In combination with: Cardiac glycosides or halothane: disturbance of heart rhythm. Guanethidine: enhancement of the sympathomimetic effect. MAO-inhibitors: greatly raising the sympathomimetic action of ephedrine. Secale alkaloid derivatives or oxytocin: development of hypertension.

Eucalyptus leaf and oil
None known for leaf. Oil induces liver enzyme system involved in detoxification process so the effects of other drugs can be weakened and/or shortened.
Note: Two separate monographs

Flaxseed
Mucilage may negatively affect absorption of other drugs.

Henbane leaf
Enhancement of anticholinergic action by tricyclic antidepressants, amantadine, antihistamines, phenothiazines, procainamide, and quinidine.

Indian Snakeroot
These drugs taken with Indian snakeroot produce the following reactions: Digitalis glycosides: bradycardia; barbiturates: mutual potentiation; levodopa: reduced effectiveness, but undesired extra pyramidal motor symptoms can be increased; sympathomimetics (e.g. cough/cold medications, and appetite suppressants): initial strong blood pressure increase.

Kava Kava
Possible potentiation of effectiveness for substances acting on CNS, e.g., alcohol, barbiturates and psychopharmacological agents.

Licorice root
Potassium loss due to other drugs, e.g. thiazide diuretics, can be increased, resulting in increased sensitivity to digitalis glycosides.

Lily-of-the-valley herb
Increased effectiveness and side effects of simultaneously administered quinidine, calcium, saluretics, laxatives, and extended therapy with glucocorticoids.

Marshmallow leaf and root
None known. Absorption of other drugs taken simultaneously may be delayed.
Note: Two separate monographs

Niauli oil
High cineol content causes induction of enzymes involved in liver detoxification, so the effect of other drugs can be reduced and/or shortened.

Oak bark
Absorption of alkaloids and other alkaline drugs may be reduced or inhibited.

Pheasant's Eye herb
Enhanced effectiveness and side effects of simultaneous intake of quinidine, calcium, saluretics, laxatives, and extended therapy with glucocorticoids.

Psyllium Seed, Blonde
Psyllium Seed Husk, Blonde
Intestinal absorption of other medication taken at the same time may be delayed. Possible reduction of insulin dosage in insulin-dependent diabetics.
Note: Two separate monographs

Rhubarb root
With long-term use/abuse, due to loss in potassium, an increase in effectiveness of cardiac glycosides and an effect on antiar-

rhythmics is possible. Potassium deficiency can be increased by simultaneous application of thiazide diuretics, corticoadrenal steroids or licorice root.

Sarsaparilla root (Unapproved)
Absorption of simultaneously administered substances is increased, e.g., digitalis glycosides or bismuth. Elimination of other substances, e.g., hypnotics, is accelerated. This can increase or decrease the action of herbs taken simultaneously.

Scopolia root
Increased effectiveness of simultaneously administered tricyclic antidepressants, amantadine, and quinidine.

Scotch Broom herb
Due to the tyramine content, application of the drug can cause a blood pressure crisis by simultaneous administration of MAO-inhibitors.

Senna pod/leaf
Chronic use/abuse can increase loss of serum potassium thus potentiating cardiac glycosides and antiarrhythmic agents. Potassium deficiency can be increased by simultaneous use of thiazide diuretics, corticosteroids, and licorice root.
Note: Two separate monographs

Squill
Increased effectiveness and side effects by simultaneously administered quinidine, calcium, salduretics, and laxatives and extended therapy with glucocorticoids.

Uva Ursi leaf
Should not be administered with any substances that cause acidic urine as this reduces the antibacterial effect.

White Willow bark
Because of the bark's active constituents, interactions like those encountered with salicylates may arise, although there was no case of this reported in the scientific literature available at the time the monograph was published (May 12, 1984).

Yeast, Brewer's
Simultaneous intake of MAO inhibitors can cause an increase in blood pressure.

Yeast, Brewer's/Hansen CBS 5926
The simultaneous intake of brewer's yeast and antimycotics can influence the activity of brewer's yeast.
Warning: Simultaneous intake of MAO-inhibitors may cause increased blood pressure.

Fixed Combinations

The following interactions pertain to approved fixed combinations and are usually consistent with interactions listed above for a particular ingredient in the combination.

Anise oil, Fennel oil, Licorice root, and Thyme
For a daily dosage up to 100 mg glycyrrhizin:
  None known.
At a dosage above 100 mg glycyrrhizin:
  Loss of potassium can be increased through other drugs, e.g., thiazide and loop diuretics. Sensitivity to digitalis glycosides increased through loss of potassium.

Anise seed, Marshmallow root, Eucalyptus oil, and Licorice root
For a daily dosage up to 100 mg glycyrrhizin:

Eucalyptus oil causes the induction of the enzyme system in the liver responsible for the break-down of foreign materials. The effect of other medications may, therefore, be reduced and/or shortened.

At a dosage above 100 mg glycyrrhizin: Loss of potassium can be increased through other drugs, e.g., thiazide and loop diuretics. Sensitivity to digitalis glycosides is increased through loss of potassium. Eucalyptus oil causes the induction of the enzyme system in the liver responsible for the break-down of foreign materials. The effect of other medications may, therefore, be reduced and/or shortened.

Warning: The absorption of other, simultaneously taken medications, can be delayed.

Anise seed, Marshmallow root, Iceland Moss, and Licorice root

For a daily dosage up to 100 mg glycyrrhizin:
    None known.

Warning: The absorption of other, simultaneously taken, medications may be delayed.

At a dosage above 100 mg glycyrrhizin:
    Loss of potassium can be increased through other drugs, e.g., thiazide and loop diuretics. Sensitivity to digitalis glycosides is increased through loss of potassium.

Warning: The absorption of other, simultaneously taken medications can be delayed.

Eucalyptus oil, Primrose root, and Thyme

Eucalyptus oil induces the enzyme system responsible for the break-down of foreign substances in the liver. The effectiveness of other medications may, therefore, be diminished and/or shortened.

Ivy leaf, Licorice root, and Thyme

For a daily dosage up to 100 mg glycyrrhizin:
    None known.

For a daily dosage of more than 100 mg glycyrrhizin:
    Loss of potassium through other medications can be increased, e.g., thiazide and loop diuretics. The sensitivity toward digitalis glycosides increases with loss of potassium.

Licorice root and German Chamomile flower

For a daily dosage up to 100 mg of glycyrrhizin:
    None known.

For a daily dosage of more than 100 mg of glycyrrhizin:
    Loss of potassium due to other medications, e.g., thiazide and loop diuretics, can be intensified. Loss of potassium increases the sensitivity to digitalis glycosides.

Licorice root, Peppermint leaf, and German Chamomile flower

Increased loss of potassium due to other medication, e.g., thiazide and loop diuretics, and increased sensitivity to digitalis glycosides.

Licorice root, Primrose root, Marshmallow root, and Anise seed

For daily dosages below 100 mg glycyrrhizin:
    No interactions known.

For daily dosages above 100 mg glycyrrhizin:
    Increased loss of potassium due to other medications, e.g., thiazide and loop diuretics, and increased sensitivity to digitalis glycosides. Possible delay in absorption of other, simultaneously administered drugs.

Marshmallow root, Fennel seed, Iceland Moss, and Thyme

    None known.

Warning: The absorption of other, simultaneously taken drugs can be delayed.

Marshmallow root, Primrose root, Licorice root, and Thyme oil

For a daily dosage up to 100 mg glycyrrhizin:

None known.

Warning: The absorption of other, simultaneously taken drugs can be delayed.

For a daily dosage of more than 100 mg glycyrrhizin:

Loss of potassium through other medications can be increased, e.g., thiazide and loop diuretics. The sensitivity toward digitalis glycosides increases with loss of potassium.

Warning: The absorption of other, simultaneously taken medication can be delayed.

Pheasant's Eye fluidextract, Lily-of-the-valley powdered extract, Squill powdered extract, and Oleander leaf powdered extract

Increased effectiveness and side effects of simultaneously administered quinidine, calcium, saluretics, laxatives, and long-term therapy with glucocorticoids.

Primrose root, Marshmallow root, and Anise seed

Absorption of other simultaneously administered medicines can be delayed.

Senna leaf and Blonde Psyllium seed husk

Chronic use/abuse can increase loss of serum potassium thus potentiating cardiac glycosides and antiarrhythmic agents. Potassium deficiency can be increased by simultaneous use of thiazide diuretics, corticosteroids, and licorice root.

Note: Reduction in insulin dosage may be necessary in insulin-dependent diabetics.

Senna leaf, Peppermint oil, and Caraway oil

Chronic use/abuse can increase loss of serum potassium thus potentiating cardiac and antiarrhythmic agents. Potassium deficiency can be increased by simultaneous use of thiazide diuretics, corticosteroids, and licorice root.

Uva Ursi, Goldenrod, and Java tea

Should not be given simultaneously with medicines intended to acidify urine.

Interactions by Drug or Other Substance

Alcohol
Kava Kava

Alkaline drugs
Oak bark

Alkaloids
Oak bark

Amantadine
Belladonna leaf and root
Henbane leaf
Pheasant's Eye herb
Scopolia root

Antiarrythmic agents
Aloe

Buckthorn bark/berry
Cascara Sagrada bark
Senna pod and leaf

Anticoagulants
Bromelain
Cinchona bark

Antihistamines
Henbane leaf

Barbiturates
Indian Snakeroot
Kava Kava

Caffeine-containing beverages
Cola nut

Calcium
  Lily-of-the-valley
  Pheasant's Eye herb
  Squill

Cardiac glycosides
  Aloe
  Buckthorn bark/berry
  Cascara Sagrada bark
  Ephedra
  Senna pod and leaf

Corticosteroids
  Aloe
  Buckthorn bark/berry
  Cascara Sagrada bark
  Senna pod and leaf

Digitalis glycosides
  Indian Snakeroot
  Licorice root

Dopamine receptor agonists
  Chaste Tree fruit (shown in animal experiments only)

Glucocorticoids
  Lily-of-the-valley herb
  Pheasant's Eye herb
  Squill

Guanethidine
  Ephedra

Halothane
  Ephedra

Laxatives
  Lily-of-the-valley herb
  Pheasant's Eye herb
  Squill

Levodopa
  Indian Snakeroot

Licorice root
  Aloe
  Buckthorn bark/berry
  Cascara Sagrada bark
  Senna pod and leaf

MAO inhibitors
  Ephedra
  Yeast, Brewer's
  Yeast, Brewer's/Hansen CBS 5926

Oxytocin
  Ephedra

Phenothiazines
  Henbane leaf

Procainamide
  Henbane leaf

Psychoanaleptic drugs
  Cola nut

Psychopharmacological agents
  Kava Kava

Quinidine
  Belladonna leaf and root
  Henbane leaf
  Lily-of-the-valley herb
  Pheasant's Eye herb
  Scopolia root
  Squill

Radioactive isotopes
  Bugleweed

Saluretics
  Lily-of-the-valley herb
  Pheasant's Eye herb
  Squill

Secale alkaloid derivatives
  Ephedra

Sympathomimetics
  Indian Snakeroot

Tetracycline
  Bromelain

Thiazide diuretics
  Aloe
  Buckthorn bark/berry
  Cascara Sagrada bark
  Licorice root
  Senna pod and leaf

Thrombocytic aggregation inhibitors
 Bromelain

Thyroid preparations
 Bugleweed

Tricyclic antidepressants
 Belladonna leaf and root
 Henbane leaf
 Scopolia root

Urine-acidifying agents
 Uva Ursi leaf

Chapter 15

Duration of Administration for Approved Herbs

In general, most of the Approved Herbs are relatively safe to take without limiting the length of use. However, responsible therapeutic use of some herbs sometimes requires that they be used for only a specified period of time. This is necessitated for a variety of factors, including, for example, concern regarding laxative dependence and intestinal sluggishness for stimulant laxatives. Nine herbs are limited to 3 to 4 days use if diarrhea persists. In some cases the reason for limiting the duration of administration is not mentioned in the monographs.

Herb	Limitation/Duration of Use
Aloe	Not more than 1 - 2 weeks without medical advice.
Autumn Crocus	In treatment for gout in 3 days.
Bilberry fruit	If diarrhea persists for more than 3- 4 days, consult a physician.
Black Cohosh	Not more than 6 months.
Blackberry leaf	If diarrhea persists for more than 3- 4 days, consult a physician.
Bromelain	8 -10 days.
Buckthorn bark	Not more than 1 - 2 weeks without medical advice.
Buckthorn berry	Not more than 1 - 2 weeks without medical advice.
Cascara Sagrada bark	Not more than 1 - 2 weeks without medical advice.
Coffee Charcoal	If diarrhea persists for more than 3 - 4 days, consult a physician.
Coltsfoot leaf	Not longer than 4 - 6 weeks per year.
Comfrey herb and leaf	Not longer than 4 - 6 weeks per year.
Comfrey root	Not longer than 4 - 6 weeks per year.
Echinacea pallida root	Not longer than 8 weeks.
Echinacea Purpurea herb	Not longer than 8 weeks (external and internal); not longer than 3 weeks (parenteral).
Eleuthero	Generally up to 3 months; a repeated course is feasible.
Ephedra	Short-term only.
Fennel oil	Should not consumed for extended period (several weeks).

Herb	Limitation/Duration of Use
Fennel seed	Should not be used for prolonged period (several weeks) without consulting a physician or pharmacist.
Ginkgo Biloba Leaf Extract	Depending on indication: a. cognitive: at least 8 weeks; b. intermittent claudication: not less than 6 weeks; c. vertigo and tinnitus: use for more than 6 - 8 weeks has no therapeutic value.
Ginseng root	Generally up to 3 months.
Hawthorn leaf with flower	6 weeks minimum.
Jambolan bark	If diarrhea persists for more than 3 - 4 days, consult a physician.
Kava Kava	Not more than 3 months without medical advice.
Lady's Mantle	If diarrhea persists for more than 3 - 4 days, consult a physician.
Licorice root	Not longer than 4 - 6 weeks without medical advice. OK for flavoring up to daily intake of 100 mg glycyrrhizin.
Manna	Laxatives should not be used for extended time without consulting a physician.
Oak bark	If diarrhea persists for more than 3 - 4 days, consult a physician; other applications: not more than 2 - 3 weeks.
Onion	If onion preparations are used over several months, the daily maximum amount of diphenylamine is 0.035 g.
Paprika	Externally: Not more than 2 days with 14 day interval for application in same location.
Peruvian Balsam	No longer than 1 week.
Petasites root	No longer than 4 - 6 weeks per year.
Psyllium seed, Blonde	If diarrhea persists for more than 3 - 4 days, consult a physician.
Psyllium seed Husk, Blonde	If diarrhea persists for more than 3 - 4 days, consult a physician.
Rhatany root	Not more than 2 weeks without medical advice.
Rhubarb root	Not more than 2 weeks without medical advice.
Sandalwood, White	Not more than 6 weeks without medical advice.
Senna leaf	Not more than 2 weeks without medical advice.
Senna pod	Not more than 2 weeks without medical advice.
Uva Ursi	Medication containing arbutin should not be taken for longer than a week or 5 times a year without consulting a physician.
Uzara root	If diarrhea persists for more than 3 - 4 days, consult a physician.
White Mustard seed	Up to 2 weeks.

Part Four

Chemical and Taxonomic Indexes

16. Chemical Glossary and Index   487

17. Taxonomic Cross-Reference
    By English Common Name   499
    By Botanical Name   516
    By Pharmacopeial Name   533

Chapter 16

Chemical Glossary and Index

This chapter, condensed from the monographs, is divided into two parts: (1) definitions of the chemical classifications listed in the monographs and (2) an index of herbs by compound (e.g., 1,8-cineol) or class of compounds (e.g., tannins). Despite the wealth of information available on the chemical constituents of Commission E herbs, the monographs are primarily intended as a therapeutic guide, and include only primary compounds that are believed to contribute to the plant drug's overall efficacy.

In some cases, a compound is mentioned due to safety concerns. For example, the Nutmeg (Unapproved) monograph lists safrole, potentially hepatotoxic in relatively small doses, but does not mention myristicin, a psychoactive chemical in Nutmeg which produces adverse effects only when taken in excessive dosage (Hocking, 1997).

Within each monograph, chemical constituents are found generally in the Composition of Drug section. However, they are sometimes mentioned in the Contraindication or Side Effects section.

Glossary of Chemical Group Classifications

1. Polysaccharides (glycans)
The monographs refer to the specialized fructan polysaccharide inulin, found in Chicory, and the various forms of cellulose found in Flaxseed.

2. Simple nitrogen-containing compounds (excluding alkaloids)
Over fifteen thousand chemical compounds containing nitrogen are found in plants. Many of the nitrogen-containing compounds give plants a pungent odor. Chemical by-products of the amino acids, the **decarboxylation amines** also have pungent odors. Some **amines**, such as ephedrine (Ephedra), have very important effects in human physiology. The **glucoinolates** contain not only nitrogen, but sulfur, characteristic of **mustard oils** (Radish, Watercress, White Mustard seed). The **glucosinolates** or **mustard oil glycosides** are a group of bound toxins that release volatile, bad-smelling, acrid mustard oils when the herb is crushed.

Plants, like all living organisms, contain the **purine** and **pyrimidine** bases of the nucleic acids RNA and DNA. The **purine** and **pyrimidine** bases consist of a five-carbon sugar bound to an amino acid. Among the purines are the stimulants caffeine and theobromine, the methylxanthines.

Plants, like animals, can string together large numbers of amino acids to form **proteins**. The **glycoprotein** bromelain (Pineapple) has a molecular weight of approximately 33,000 and acts as an enzyme.

3. Alkaloids
Alkaloids are also nitrogen-containing compounds. Because of their pharmacological sig-

nificance, most authors consider the alkaloids separately from other nitrogen-containing compounds found in plants. The alkaloids possess a nitrogen atom as part of a heterocyclic ring. The alkaloids possess an array of structural diversity and physiological activity unrivaled by any other group of natural products. In nature, the alkaloids serve herbs to protect them from herbivores, as is also the case with the few animals possessing alkaloid substances, such as fire ants, ladybirds, and toads.

The **diterpenoid alkaloids** are found primarily in nontherapeutic herbs, notably herbs from the plant family Ranunculaceae (Monkshood, Delphinium). **Aconitum** species (e.g. Monkshood), used extensively in Chinese traditional medicine, are among the most poisonous plants known. A 2 - 5 mg dose of the pure alkaloid can be fatal in humans.

The **indole alkaloids** are derived from the amino acid tryptophan. The indole nucleus is common to all members of the group. Among the more notorious indole alkaloids are the **ergot alkaloids**, most familiar to the general public through their synthetic derivative LSD, and the more than 90 alkaloids obtained from the Madagascar periwinkle, (*Catharanthus roseus*)including vinblastine and vincristine, used in treating childhood leukemia and Hodgkin's disease, respectively. The alkaloid constituents of Yohimbe and Indian Snakeroot are also among the indole alkaloids.

The same family containing the famous alkaloid morphine also contains the alkaloid boldine found in boldo leaf. The **isoquinoline alkaloids** are derived from the amino acids phenylalanine and/or tyrosine. The **quinoline alkaloids** are characteristic of the Rue family (Rutaceae). This family includes the remedy quinine, derived from Cinchona bark.

A consistent disqualifier for therapeutic use of herbs considered by Commission E is the presence of **pyrrolizidine alkaloids (PAs)**, chemically distinguished by two fused, five-membered rings. The pyrrolizidine or **Senecio** alkaloids are hepatotoxins and can cause liver damage, producing the characteristic syndrome veno-occlusive disease (VOD).

The **tropane alkaloids** are characteristic of the nightshades (Solanaceae), and consist of a bridged eight-membered (3-2-1)-azabicyclic. The tropane alkaloids include hyoscyamine (atropine is *dl* form), belladonine, and hyscine.

4. Phenolics

The phenolics contain an aromatic ring with one or more hydroxyl (-OH) groups. This group includes arbutin, hydroquinone, khellin, myristicin, and usnic acid, as well as the flavonoids. The flavonoids are more complicated phenolics formed by the union of an aromatic (hydroxycinnamyl coenzyme A ester) and aliphatic (malonyl coenzyme A) group. The flavonoids include the anthocyanins, red-to-blue flower pigments, and tannins, which are distinguished by their ability to bind to protein. The tannins include both flavonoids and simpler phenolics based on gallic acid, the gallotannins and ellagitannins. Phenolics contribute color, taste, and flavor to foods and are pharmacologically significant for their antiinflammatory and hepatoprotective properties.

The coumarins are all derived from the parent compound coumarin, or 1,2-benzopyrone, which has the odor of freshly mowed hay. The coumarins found in Commission E herbs are the simple hydroxycoumarins (e.g., umbelliferone in arnica) and the furanocoumarins (angelicin in Angelica, bergapten in numerous herbs, pimpinellin). The furanocoumarins are phototoxic to some of the animals that consume them, as well as to light-skinned humans.

The flavones and flavonols are found as co-pigments (usually not giving a color by themselves) with anthocyanins, in plant saps and exudates, and in the leaves of higher plants. The principal flavone is the free radical scavenger, antiinflammatory, and antibacterial agent quercetin, which has a methylated derivative isorhamnetin. The only other common flavonol aglycones in addition to quercetin are kaempferol and myricetin. Rutin, found in Hawthorn and Rue, is important in the treatment of capillary fragility. Vitexin, found in Hawthorn and Chaste Tree fruit, is regarded as a potent inhibitor of free radical action (inhibits peroxidases) with a particular potency in thyroid tissue.

Lignans are found mainly in woody tissues. Lignans are of pharmacological interest because of their antitumor and antiviral activity, such as that of podophyllotoxin (Mayapple).

Phenols and phenolic acids are universal in higher plants. Typically the phenolic acids are found in bound form, as in the cases of p-hydroxybenzoic acid, vanillic acid, and gallotannin. Very few phenols are found in free form in plants; among these free agents are hydroquinone and the better known tetrahydrocannabinol (from marijuana, not listed by Commission E). A general characteristic of all phenolics is their antimicrobial activity. Other phenolic compounds reduce swelling and inflammation, such as salicin and salicylic acid (White Willow).

The phenylpropanoids contain the basic structure of phenol plus a three-carbon chain as a side group. The most common members of this group are the hydroxycinnamic acids, p-coumaric acid, ferulic acid, caffeic acid, and caffeic acid's ester, chlorogenic acid. This group includes curcumurin (Turmeric), estragole (Basil, Goldenrod, and Chrysanthemum), eugenol (Cloves), anethole (Anise and Fennel), and myristicin (Nutmeg).

The yellow, orange, and red pigments found in bark, heartwood, or root are typically quinones. Quinones all contain two carbonyl groups in conjugation with two carbon-carbon double bonds. The largest group of plant quinones are the anthraquinones including the purgative agents aloe-emodin, chrysophanol, emodin, and physcion. Dimeric anthraquinones include sennoside A (Senna) and hypericin (St. John's wort). Also included in this group are aloin (Aloe), cascaroside A (Cascara Sagrada), frangulins A and B (Buckthorn), and juglone (Walnut).

Tannins have the ability to lock to proteins. Some tannins, for instance, cross-link proteins in animal skin to form the water-insoluble copolymers known as leather. Plant tissues high in tannin, for instance oak leaf, are largely avoided by most herbivores because of their astringent taste.

Condensed tannins are formed by the linking of catechin units into chains. Most condensed tannins are procyanidins. The hydrolyzable tannins (soluble in acid) include gallotannins and ellagitannins. Condensed tannins have been approved in medical practice for the treatment of wounds and burns. Hydrolyzable tannins exhibit antiviral effects.

5. Terpenoids

The **terpenoids** are classified in terms of multiples of five carbons. The terpenoids are all derived from the 5-carbon precursor isoprene. Two 5-carbon compounds condense to form the C10 intermediate, geranyl pyrophosphate. This compound is the immediate precursor of the **monoterpenoids** and **monoterpene lactones,** known as **iridoids.** Geranyl pyrophosphate can condense with another 5-carbon unit of isopentenyl pyrophosphate to produce the 15-carbon intermediate, farnesyl pyrophosphate. This 15-carbon compound is the starting point for the 15-carbon **sesquiterpenoids** and **sesquiterpene lactones.** The 15-carbon intermediate can join with another isopentenyl pyrophospate residue to produce the 20-carbon **diterpenoids.** Alternatively, two 15-carbon groups can condense to a single 30-carbon group, the **triterpenoids.** Finally, two molecules of geranygeranyl pyrophosphate, C20, may condense tail-to-tail to produce a C40 intermediate, phytoene, which is the precursor of the yellow **carotenoid** pigments.

The **monoterpenoids** include linalool (Lavender), nerol, and citronellol. From the monoterpenoid-terpineol are derived limonene (Juniper), terpinolen, and 1,8-cineol.

Likewise interrelated are α-pinene, ß-pinene, borneol, α-thujone, and ß-thujone (Sage and Wormwood). Monoterpenoids can be classified according to their functional groups: limonene is an unsaturated hydrocarbon, linalool an alcohol, cintronellal an aldehyde, and carvone an unsaturated ketone — all based on the p-menthane skeleton. Monoterpenoids are typically odoriferous, as exemplified by camphor (Camphor, Lavender, Sage).

The **sesquiterpene lactones** are biologically very active, many of them associated with allergic reactions of the skin. The majority of naturally occurring sesquiterpene lactones have been identified in plants of the composite family, Asteraceae, as in these compounds found in Commission E herbs:

> absinthin or absinthiin (Wormwood); achillin or santolin (Yarrow), alantolactone and isoalantolactone, together known as helenin (Elecampane); artabsin (Wormwood); and cnicin (Blessed Thistle).

The **diterpenoids** are 20-carbon compounds derived from geranylgeraniol. This group includes the bitter constituent of Ginkgo, ginkgolide A (a diterpene lactone), as well as marrubiin (Horehound).

The **triterpenoid saponins** are a group of plant glycosides in which water-soluble sugars are attached to a steroid (C27) or triterpenoid (C30). These chemicals form foams in water and cause red blood cells to disintegrate. Among the triterpenoid saponins in Commission E herbs are aescin (Horse Chestnut seed), avenacin A-1 (Oats), the ginsenosides (Ginseng), saponoside D (Soapwort), senegin (Senega Snakeroot), soya saponin I and A1 (soybean). The steroid saponins are 27-carbon compounds related to the cardiac glycosides and include asparagoside A (Asparagus), avenacoside A and its derivative 26 y-desglucoavenacoside A (Oats), capsicoside A (Paprika), and ruscogenin and its glycosides ruscosides A and B (Butcher's Broom).

The **cardenolides** and **bufadienolides** are 23-carbon and 24-carbon steroids derived from triterpenoids. The cardenolides are potent heart poisons which in small doses are useful in controlling congestive heart failure. A typical cardenolide is digoxin, obtained from foxglove. Cardiac glycosides occur principally in the families Apocynaceae and Asclepiadaceae. Cardiac glycosides are found also among the Scrophulariaceae (foxglove) and Liliaceae (Squill).

The **bufadienolides** were originally identified in toad venoms. The bufadienolides differ from the cardenolides by the presence of a six-membered rather than five-membered carbon ring. Bufadienolides are found in squill.

The cardenolide/bufadienolide group includes adonitoxin (Pheasant's Eye), convallatoxin (Lily-of-the-valley), digoxin (Foxglove), scillaren (Squill), and veradigin (Pheasant's Eye).

HERB GUIDE BY CHEMICAL CONSTITUENTS REFERENCED IN THE MONOGRAPHS

Absinthin
Wormwood

Aconitine
Monkshood

Aglycones
Aloe
Buckthorn bark
Calendula flower
Cascara Sagrada bark
Rhubarb
Senna leaf
Senna pod

Agnuside
Chaste Tree fruit

Alantolactone
  Elecampane root

Albumin
  Flaxseed

Alkaloids
  Boldo leaf
  California Poppy
  Celandine herb
  Delphinium flower
  Ergot
  Henbane leaf
  Jimsonweed leaf
    and seed
  Motherwort herb
  Nux Vomica
  Scopolia root

Allantoin
  Comfrey herb and leaf
  Comfrey root

Alliin
  Garlic
  Onion

Aloe-emodin
  Aloe
  Senna leaf
  Senna pod

Aloin
  Aloe

Amarogentin
  Gentian

Amines, biogenic
  Hawthorn leaf with
    flower

Anabsin
  Wormwood

Anabsinthin
  Wormwood

Andromeda derivatives
  Rhododendron,
    Rusty-leaved

Anethole
  Fennel oil
  Anise seed

Anthocyanins
  Bilberry
  Potentilla
  Squill

Anthranoids
  Aloe
  Buckthorn bark
  Buckthorn berry
  Cascara sagrada bark
  Rhubarb root
  Senna leaf
  Senna pod

Apigenin
  Chamomile, German

Apigenin-7-glucoside
  Chamomile, German

Apiol
  Parsley seed

Arbutin
  Uva Ursi leaf
  Marjoram
  Rhododendron,
    Rusty-leaved

Artabsin
  Wormwood

Artubiin
  Wormwood

Ascaridol
  Boldo leaf

Ascorbic acid
  Wormwood

Astragalin
  Arnica flower

Atropine
  Belladonna

Aucubin
  Chaste Tree fruit
  Plantain

Benzoic acid
  Peruvian Balsam
  Tolu Balsam

Benzyl esters
  Peruvian Balsam
  Tolu Balsam

Benzyl isothiocyanate
  Nasturtium

Berberine
  Barberry

Bilobalide
  Ginkgo Biloba Leaf
    Extract

α-Bisabolol
  Chamomile, German

Bisabolol oxides
  Chamomile, German

Bitter principles
  Artichoke leaf
  Bitter Orange peel
  Blessed Thistle herb
  Bogbean leaf
  Chicory
  Condurango bark
  Dandelion herb
  Dandelion root with
    herb
  Devil's Claw root
  Elecampane root
  Gentian root
  Hops
  Horehound herb
  Iceland Moss
  Lemon Balm
  Motherwort herb
  Orange peel
  Sage leaf
  Wormwood

Boldine
  Boldo leaf

2-Bornanone
  Camphor

Bufenolide
 Motherwort herb
 Squill

Cadinene
 Juniper berry

Caffeic acid
 Arnica
 Bugleweed

Caffeine
 Cola nut
 Maté

Caffeoylquinic acid
 Artichoke leaf

Calcium salts
 Licorice root
 Stinging Nettle herb
  and leaf

Camphor
 Lavender flower
 Sage
 Sage bath

Capsaicinoids
 Paprika

Cardenolide glycosides
 Uzara root

Cardiac glycosides
 Lily-of-the-valley herb
 Pheasant's eye

Carnosol
 Sage bath

Carotenoids
 Calendula flower
 Caraway

Carvacrol
 Thyme, Wild

Carvone
 Dill seed

d-Carvone
 Caraway oil

Caryophyllene
 Juniper berry

Cascaroside A
 Cascara Sagrada bark

Castin
 Chaste Tree fruit

Catapol
 Plantain

Catechins
 Hawthorn leaf with
  flower

Catechin derivatives
 Witch Hazel bark

Cellulose
 Flaxseed

Chelidonine
 Celandine herb

Chlorogenic acid
 Arnica

Chrysophanol
 Aloe
 Buckthorn bark
 Cascara Sagrada bark

Chymopapain A & B
 Papain

Cineol
 Cajeput oil
 Niauli oil
 Sage leaf

1,6-cineol
 Sage bath

1,8-cineol
 Cardamom seed
 Eucalyptus leaf
 Eucalyptus oil
 Lavender flower

Cinnamic acid
 Peruvian Balsam
 Tolu Balsam

Benzyl esters
 Tolu Balsam

Citral A
 Lemon Balm

Citral B
 Lemon Balm

Citronellal
 Lemon Balm

Cnicin
 Blessed Thistle

Colchicine
 Autumn Crocus

Condurangin
 Condurango bark

Convallatoxin
 Lily-of-the-valley herb

o-coumaric acid
 Sweet Clover

Coumarin
 Angelica root
 Licorice root
 Sweet Clover

Coumarin derivatives
 Angelica root
 Arnica flower
 Eleuthero (Siberian
  Ginseng) root
 Licorice root
 Lovage root
 Passionflower herb
 Sweet Clover

Cryptopine
 California Poppy

Cucurbitacin
 Colocynth

Cucurbitin
 Pumpkin seed

Curcumin
 Turmeric root

Cynarin
  Arnica flower
  Artichoke leaf

Depside ellagitannins
  Witch Hazel bark

Dicinnamoylmethane derivatives
  Turmeric root
  Turmeric, Javanese

11,13-dihydrohelenalin
  Arnica flower

Dihydrosamidine
  Bishop's weed

1,8-dihydroxyanthracene derivatives
  Aloe
  Buckthorn bark
  Buckthorn berry
  Cascarda Sagrada bark
  Haronga bark and leaf
  Onion
  Rhubarb root

Diterpenes
  Sage leaf

Elemene
  Juniper berry

Ellagitannin
  Witch Hazel bark

Emodin
  Aloe
  Buckthorn berry
  Senna leaf
  Senna pod

Emodin-physcion
  Buckthorn bark

Ephedrine
  Ephedra

Epicatechins
  Hawthorn leaf with flower

(-)-Epicatechol
  Hawthorn leaf with flower

Escin
  Horse Chestnut seed

Essential oil
  Angelica root
  Anise seed
  Basil herb
  Birch leaf
  Bitter Orange peel
  Cajeput oil
  Calendula flower
  Caraway seed
  Cardamom seed
  Chamomile, German
  Cinnamon bark
  Cloves
  Coriander seed
  Couch Grass
  Dill seed
  Elecampane root
  Eucalyptus leaf
  Fennel seed
  Fir shoots, fresh
  Galangal
  Garlic
  Ginger root
  Gumweed herb
  Hops flower
  Java tea
  Larch Turpentine
  Lovage root
  Marsh root
  Marsh Tea
  Meadowsweet
  Nutmeg
  Onion
  Orange peel
  Passionflower herb
  Peppermint leaf
  Pimpinella root
  Pine Sprouts
  Poplar bud
  Radish
  Rosemary leaf
  Sage leaf
  Sage bath
  Sandalwood, White
  Spiny Restharrow root
  Star Anise seed
  Tansy
  Thyme, Wild
  Tolu Balsam
  Turmeric, Javanese
  Valerian root
  Witch Hazel leaf
  Yarrow

Esters
  Mint oil
  Peppermint oil
  Peruvian Balsam
  Tolu Balsam

Estragole
  Basil herb
  Basil oil

Estragon
  Fennel oil
  Fennel seed

Eupatorin
  Java tea

Fatty oil
  Chaste Tree fruit
  Flaxseed
  Saw Palmetto berry

Fenchone
  Fennel oil

Fiber
  Flaxseed

Flavanone derivatives
  Licorice root

Flavone derivatives
  Chamomile, German

Flavones
  Ginkgo Biloba Leaf Extract
  Hawthorn leaf with flower
  Sage leaf
  Wormwood

Flavonoids
Agrimony
Arnica flower
Birch leaf
Boldo leaf
Bugleweed
Chaste Tree fruit
Galangal
Goldenrod
Hawthorn leaf with flower
Heart's Ease
Horsetail
Lady's Mantle
Lemon Balm
Licorice root
Linden flower
Meadowsweet
Passionflower herb
Pheasant's Eye herb
Poplar bud
Potentilla
Sandy Everlasting
Squill
Spiny Restharrow root
Sweet Clover
Uva Ursi
Witch Hazel leaf

Flavonoid glycosides
Bilberry
Fumitory
Ginkgo Biloba Leaf Extract
Juniper berry
Pheasant's Eye herb
Sage leaf

Flavonols
Hawthorn leaf with flower

Furanocoumarins
Angelica seed and herb
Angelica root
Bishop's Weed fruit
Celery
Rue

Galegin
Goat's Rue herb

Gallic acid
Potentilla
Witch Hazel bark

Gallotannins
Witch Hazel leaf

Gentiobiose
Gentian root

Gentiopicroside
Gentian root

Ginkgolic acids
Ginkgo Biloba Leaf Extract

Ginkgolides
Ginkgo Biloba Leaf Extract

Ginsenosides
Ginseng root

Glucans
Yeast, Brewer's
Yeast, Brewer's/ Hansen CBS 5926

Glucofrangulin A
Buckthorn bark
Buckthorn berry

Glycosides
Motherwort herb
Squill
Stinging Nettle herb
Uzara root

ß-Glycosides
Aloe
Buckthorn bark
Buckthorn berry
Cascara Sagrada bark
Rhubarb
Senna leaf
Senna pod
Squill

Glycyrrhizic acid
Licorice root

Grayanotoxine
Rhododendron, Rusty-leaved

Guaiazulene
Guaiac wood

Guaiene
Guaiac wood

ß-Hamamelitannins
Witch Hazel bark

γ-Hamamelitannins
Witch Hazel bark

Harunganin
Haronga bark

Helenalin
Arnica flower

Hemicellulose
Flaxseed

Hydrocinnamic acid
Bugleweed

Hydroquinone derivatives
Uva Ursi leaf

Hydroxyquinone
Marjoram

Hyoscyamine
Belladonna
Henbane leaf
Jimsonweed leaf and seed
Scopolia root

L-Hyoscyamine
Jimsonweed leaf and seed
Scopolia root

Hypericin
Haronga leaf
St. John's Wort

Hyperoside
Birch leaf
Hawthorn leaf with flower

Inulin
Chicory

Iodine
Kelp

Iridoid glycosides
Plantain

Isoflavonoids
Spiny Restharrow root

Isoflavanone derivatives
Licorice root

Isoquercetin
Arnica flower

Isoquinoline
Fumitory

Isorhamnetin
Ginkgo Biloba Leaf Extract

Juglone
Sundew
Walnut hull

Kaempferol
Ginkgo Biloba Leaf Extract

Kava pyrone
Kava Kava

Ketones
Mint oil
Peppermint oil

Khellin
Bishop's Weed fruit

Lactucopricin (Taraxacin)
Dandelion root with herb

Lichenic acid
Usnea

Lignans
Eleuthero (Siberian Ginger) root

Lignin
Flaxseed

Ligustilide
Lovage root

Limonene
Juniper berry

Linalool
Lavender flower

Linalyl acetate
Lavender flower

Linamarin
Flaxseed

Linolenic acid esters
Flaxseed

Linustatin
Flaxseed

Lithospermic acid
Bugleweed

Lucidin
Madder root

Luteolin-7-glucoside
Arnica flower

Madagascin
Haronga bark

Maltol
Passionflower herb

Mannans
Yeast, Brewer's
Yeast, Brewer's/ Hansen CBS 5926

Mannitol
Manna

Matricin
Chamomile, German

Melilotin
Sweet Clover

Melilotoside
Sweet Clover

Menthol
Mint oil
Peppermint oil

Menthone
Mint oil
Peppermint oil

Menthyl acetate
Mint oil
Peppermint oil

2-Methyl-3-butanol
Hops

Methyl xanthines
Cocoa
Cocoa seed
Cola nut

Mineral salts
Stinging Nettle herb and leaf

Monoterpenes
Lemon Balm
Valerian root

Mucilage
Coltsfoot leaf
Iceland Moss
Linden flower
Mallow flower
Marshmallow leaf
Plantain
Psyllium husk, Blonde
White Dead Nettle flower

Mucopolysaccharides
Comfrey root
Mullein flower

Mustard oil
Horseradish
Watercress
White Mustard seed

Mustard oil glycosides
Horseradish
Radish
Watercress
White Mustard seed

Myrcene
Juniper berry

Myristicin
Parsley seed

Napthoquinone derivatives
Sundew

Neoruscogenin
Butcher's Broom

ß-Ocimene
Lavender flower

Oligomeric procyanidins
Hawthorn leaf with flower

Oil
Soy Phospholipid

Ononin
Spiny Restharrow root

Papayapeptidase A
Papain

Parasorbic acid
Mountain Ash berry

Pentosan
Chicory

Peptides
Onion

Petasin
Petasites root

Phenol carbonic acid
Arnica flower

Phenol glycosides
Goldenrod
Meadowsweet
Poplar bud

Phenols
Thyme

3-sn-phosphatidylcholine
Soy Lecithin
Soy Phospholipid

Phosphatidylethanolamine
Soy Lecithin
Soy Phospholipid

Phosphatidylinositic acid
Soy Phospholipid

Phosphatidylinositol
Soy Lecithin

Phosphoglycerides
Soy Phospholipid

Phospholipids
Soy Lecithin
Soy Phospholipid

Physcion
Cascara Sagrada bark

Phytoalexins
Kidney Bean pod (without seeds)

Phytosterols
Dandelion root with herb
Licorice root
Potentilla
Pumpkin seed
Saw Palmetto berry

Pinene
Juniper berry

α-Pinene
Juniper berry

ß-Pinene
Juniper berry

Podophyllotoxin
Mayapple

Polysaccharides
Saw Palmetto berry

Potassium salts
Java tea
Licorice root
Stinging nettle herb and leaf

Proazulene
Yarrow

Proscillaridin A
Squill

Protoanemonin
Liverwort herb
Pasque flower

Pseudoephedrine
Ephedra

Pseudohypericin
Haronga leaf

Pungent principles
Galangal
Ginger root

Pyranocoumarins
Bishop's Weed fruit

Pyrrolizidine alkaloids
Borage flower and herb
Coltsfoot
Coltsfoot leaf
Comfrey herb and leaf
Comfrey root
Hound's Tongue
Petasites root
Senecio herb

γ-Pyrones
Bishop's Weed fruit

Quercetin
Ginkgo Biloba Leaf Extract
Hawthorn leaf with flower

Quercetin glycosides
Ginkgo Biloba Leaf Extract
Hawthorn leaf with flower

Quinidine
Cinchona bark

Quinine
Cinchona bark

Ranunculin
Pasque flower

Reserpine
Indian Snakeroot

Resin
Guaiac wood
Juniper berry
Pine Sprouts
Rosemary

Rhein Anthrone
Senna leaf
Senna pod

Rosmarinic acid
Comfrey herb and leaf
Sage bath

Ruscin
Butcher's Broom

Ruscocide
Butcher's Broom

Ruscogenin
Butcher's Broom

Rutin
Hawthorn leaf with flower
Rue

Sabinene
Juniper berry

Salicin
White Willow bark

Samidine
Bishop's Weed fruit

Saponins
Artichoke leaf
Birch leaf
Couch Grass
Goldenrod
Guaiac wood
Hempnettle herb
Indian Snakeroot
Ivy leaf
Mullein flower
Pimpinella root
Primrose flower
Primrose root
Sanicle herb
Sarsaparilla, German
Senega Snakeroot
Soapwort herb, Red
Soapwort root, Red
Soapwort root, White
Sweet Violet root and herb
White Dead Nettle flower

Scillaren A
Squill

Scopolamine
Belladonna
Henbane leaf
Scopolia root

L-Scopolamine
Jimsonweed leaf and seed

Scopoletin
Arnica
Stinging Nettle root

Scutellarein tetramethyl ether
Java tea

Selenium
Pumpkin seed

Sennosides
Senna leaf
Senna pod

Sesquiterpene lactones
Arnica
Dandelion herb
Elecampane root
Wormwood

Sesquiterpene lactones, helenaloid
Arnica

Sesquiterpenes
Lemon Balm
Petasites root
Valerian root

Silicic acid
Horsetail herb
Knotweed herb
Oat straw
Stinging Nettle herb and leaf

Silybin
Milk Thistle fruit

Silybinin
Milk Thistle fruit

Silychristin
Milk Thistle fruit

Silydianine
Milk Thistle fruit

Sinensetin
Java tea

ß-Sitosterol
Stinging Nettle root

Sparteine
Scotch Broom flower

Stachydrine
Motherwort herb

Steroid alkaloids
Woody Nightshade

Steroid saponins
Butcher's Broom
Woody Nightshade

Steroids
Sage leaf

Strychnine
Nux Vomica

Tannins
Agrimony
Bilberry
Birch leaf
Blackberry leaf

Blackthorn berry
Coltsfoot leaf
Eucalyptus leaf
Hempnettle herb
Horehound herb
Jambolan bark
Juniper berry
Knotweed herb
Lady's Mantle
Lavender flower
Lemon Balm
Linden flower
Oak bark
Peppermint leaf
Plantain
Potentilla
Rhatany root
Rose flower
Sage leaf
Uva Ursi leaf
Walnut leaf
White Dead Nettle flower
Witch Hazel leaf and bark
Woody Nightshade stem
Wormwood

Taraxagin
Dandelion root with herb

Terpene alcohols
Juniper berry

Terpene lactones
Ginkgo Biloba Leaf Extract

α-Terpineol
Cardamom seed

4-Terpineol
Juniper berry

Terpinyl acetate
Cardamom seed

Theobromine
Cola nut

Thujone
Juniper berry
Sage leaf
Sage bath
Tansy
Wormwood

Thymol
Arnica flower
Thyme
Thyme, Wild
Wormwood

ß-Tocopherol
Pumpkin seed

γ-Tocopherol
Pumpkin seed

Tormentoside
Potentilla

Triterpenes
Sage leaf

Triterpene glycosides
Black Cohosh root
Calendula flower
Horse Chestnut seed

Triterpenoids
Dandelion root with herb

Triterpenylic acid
Lemon Balm

Tyramine
Scotch Broom flower

Umbelliferone
Arnica flower

Valerenic acid
Valerian root

Vincamine
Periwinkle

Visnadin
Bishop's Weed fruit

Visnagin
Bishop's Weed fruit

Vitamin B complex
Yeast, Brewer's
Yeast, Brewer's/ Hansen CBS 5926

Vitamin C
Rose Hip
Rose Hip and seed

Vitexin
Bishop's Weed fruit
Chaste Tree fruit
Hawthorn leaf with flower
Passionflower herb

Vitexin rhamnose
Hawthorn leaf with flower

Volatile oils
Arnica flower
Bitter Orange flower
Chaste Tree fruit
Juniper berry
Turmeric root
Wormwood

Wax
Juniper berry

Yohimbine
Yohimbe bark

Chapter 17

Taxonomic Cross-Reference

By English Common Name

English	Botanical	Plant Family	Pharmacopeial	German
Aconite herb	Aconitum napellus	Ranunculaceae	Aconiti herba	Blauer Eisenhutkraut
Aconite tuber	Aconitum napellus	Ranunculaceae	Aconiti tuber	Blauer Eisenhutwurzel
Agrimony	Agrimonia eupatoria	Rosaceae	Agrimoniae herba	Odermennigkraut
Agrimony	Agrimonia procera	Rosaceae	Agrimoniae herba	Odermennigkraut
Aloe	Aloe vera	Liliaceae	Aloe barbadensis	Aloe
Aloe	Aloe barbadensis	Liliaceae	Aloe barbadensis	Aloe
Aloe	Aloe ferox	Liliaceae	Aloe capensis	Kap-Aloe
Alpine Lady's Mantle herb	Alchemilla alpina	Rosaceae	Alchemillae alpinae herba	Frauenmantelkraut
Angelica herb	Angelica archangelica	Apiaceae	Angelicae herba	Angelikakraut
Angelica root	Angelica archangelica	Apiaceae	Angelicae radix	Angelikawurzel
Angelica seed	Angelica archangelica	Apiaceae	Angelicae fructus	Angelikafrüchte
Anise	Pimpinella anisum	Apiaceae	Anisi fructus	Anis
Arnica flower	Arnica montana	Asteraceae	Arnicae flos	Arnikablüten
Arnica flower	Arnica chamissonis	Asteraceae	Arnicae flos	Arnikablüten
Artichoke leaf	Cynara scolymus	Asteraceae	Cynarae folium	Artischokenblätter
Ash bark	Fraxinus excelsior	Oleaceae	Fraxini cortex	Esche
Ash leaf	Fraxinus excelsior	Oleaceae	Fraxini folium	Esche
Asparagus herb	Asparagus officinalis	Liliaceae	Asparagi herba	Spargelkraut
Asparagus root	Asparagus officinalis	Liliaceae	Asparagi rhizoma	Spargelwurzelstock
Aspen bark	Populus spp.	Salicaceae	Populi cortex	Pappelrinde
Aspen bark	Populus tremula	Salicaceae	Populi cortex	Pappelrinde
Aspen bark	Populus tremuloides	Salicaceae	Populi cortex	Pappelrinde
Aspen leaf	Populus spp.	Salicaceae	Populi folium	Pappelblätter
Aspen leaf	Populus tremuloides	Salicaceae	Populi folium	Pappelblätter
Aspen leaf	Populus tremula	Salicaceae	Populi folium	Pappelblätter
Autumn Crocus	Colchicum autumnale	Liliaceae	Colchicum, Colchicum autumnale	Herbstzeitlose

English	Botanical	Plant Family	Pharmacopeial	German
Barberry	*Berberis vulgaris*	Berberidaceae	Berberis vulgaris	*Berberitze*
Barberry	*Berberis vulgaris*	Berberidaceae	Berberidis fructus	*Berberitze*
Barberry bark	*Berberis vulgaris*	Berberidaceae	Berberidis cortex	*Berberitze*
Barberry root	*Berberis vulgaris*	Berberidaceae	Berberidis radix	*Berberitze*
Barberry root bark	*Berberis vulgaris*	Berberidaceae	Berberidis radicis cortex	*Berberitzenrinde*
Basil herb	*Ocimum basilicum*	Lamiaceae	Basilici herba	*Basilikumkraut*
Basil oil	*Ocimum basilicum*	Lamiaceae	Basilici aetheroleum	*Basilikumöl*
Belladonna leaf	*Atropa belladonna*	Solanaceae	Belladonnae folium	*Tollkirsche*
Belladonna root	*Atropa belladonna*	Solanaceae	Belladonnae radix	*Tollkirschewurzel*
Bilberry fruit	*Vaccinium myrtillus*	Ericaceae	Myrtilli fructus	*Heidelbeeren*
Bilberry leaf	*Vaccinium myrtillus*	Ericaceae	Myrtilli folium	*Heidelbeerblätter*
Birch leaf	*Betula pendula*	Betulaceae	Betulae folium	*Birkenblätter*
Birch leaf	*Betula pubescens*	Betulaceae	Betulae folium	*Birkenblätter*
Bishop's Weed fruit	*Ammi daucoides*	Apiaceae	Ammeos visnagae fructus	*Ammi-visnaga-Früchte*
Bishop's Weed fruit	*Ammi visnaga*	Apiaceae	Ammeos visnagae fructus	*Ammi-visnaga-Früchte*
Bitter Orange flower	*Citrus aurantium*	Rutaceae	Aurantii flos	*Pomeranzenblüten*
Bitter Orange flower oil	*Citrus aurantium*	Rutaceae	Aurantii flos aetheroleum	*Pomeranzenblütenöl*
Bitter Orange peel	*Citrus aurantium*	Rutaceae	Aurantii pericarpium	*Pomeranzenschale*
Black Cohosh root	*Cimicifuga racemosa*	Ranunculaceae	Cimicifugae racemosae rhizoma	*Cimicifugawurzelstock*
Blackberry leaf	*Rubus fruticosus*	Rosaceae	Rubi fruticosi folium	*Brombeerblätter*
Blackberry root	*Rubus fruticosus*	Rosaceae	Rubi fruticosi radix	*Brombeerwurzel*
Blackthorn berry	*Prunus spinosa*	Rosaceae	Pruni spinosae fructus	*Schlehdornfrüchte*
Blackthorn flower	*Prunus spinosa*	Rosaceae	Pruni spinosae flos	*Schlehdornblüten*
Bladderwrack	*Ascophyllum nodosum*	Fucaceae	Fucus	*Tang*
Bladderwrack	*Fucus vesiculosus*	Fucaceae	Fucus	*Tang*
Blessed Thistle herb	*Cnicus benedictus*	Asteraceae	Cnici benedicti herba	*Benediktenkraut*
Blue Mallow flower	*Malva sylvestris*	Malvaceae	Malvae flos	*Malvenblüten*
Blue Monkshood herb	*Aconitum napellus*	Ranunculaceae	Aconiti herba	*Blauer Eisenhutkraut*
Blue Monkshood tuber	*Aconitum napellus*	Ranunculaceae	Aconiti tuber	*Blauer Eisenhutwurzel*
Blueberry	*Vaccinium myrtillus*	Ericaceae	Myrtilli fructus	*Heidelbeeren*
Blueberry leaf	*Vaccinium myrtillus*	Ericaceae	Myrtilli folium	*Heidelbeerblätter*
Bogbean	*Menyanthes trifoliata*	Menyanthaceae	Menyanthis folium	*Bitterkleeblätter*

English	Botanical	Plant Family	Pharmacopeial	German
Boldo leaf	*Peumus boldus*	Monimiaceae	Boldo folium	*Boldoblätter*
Borage flower	*Borago officinalis*	Boraginaceae	Boraginis flos	*Boretsch*
Borage herb	*Borago officinalis*	Boraginaceae	Boraginis herba	*Boretsch*
Brewer's Yeast	*Candida utilis*	Cryptococcaeae	Faex medicinalis	*Medizinische Hefe*
Brewer's Yeast	*Saccaromyces cerevisiae*	Saccharomycetaceae	Faex medicinalis	*Medizinische Hefe*
Brewer's Yeast/ Hansen CBS 5926	*Saccaromyces cerevisiae*	Saccharomycetaceae	Saccharomyces cerevisiae	*Trokenhefe aus Saccharomyces cerevisiae*
Bromelain	*Ananas comosus*	Bromeliaceae	Bromelainum	*Ananas*
Broom flower, Scotch	*Cytisus scoparius*	Fabaceae	Cytisi scoparius flos	*Besenginsterblüten*
Broom flower, Scotch	*Sarothamnus scoparius*	Fabaceae	Cytisi scoparius flos	*Besenginsterblüten*
Broom herb, Scotch	*Cytisus scoparius*	Fabaceae	Cytisi scoparius herba	*Besenginsterkraut*
Broom herb, Scotch	*Sarothamnus scoparius*	Fabaceae	Cytisi scoparius herba	*Besenginsterkraut*
Bryonia root	*Bryonia cretica*	Cucurbitaceae	Bryoniae radix	*Zaunrübenwurzel*
Bryonia root	*Bryonia alba*	Cucurbitaceae	Bryoniae radix	*Zaunrübenwurzel*
Buchu leaf	*Agathosma betulina*	Rutaceae	Barosmae folium	*Buccoblätter*
Buchu leaf	*Barosma betulina*	Rutaceae	Barosmae folium	*Buccoblätter*
Buckthorn bark	*Frangula alnus*	Rhamnaceae	Frangulae cortex	*Faulbaumrinde*
Buckthorn bark	*Rhamnus frangula*	Rhamnaceae	Frangulae cortex	*Faulbaumrinde*
Buckthorn berry	*Rhamnus catharticus*	Rhamnaceae	Rhamni cathartici fructus	*Kreuzdonnbeeren*
Bugleweed	*Lycopus europaeus*	Lamiaceae	Lycopi herba	*Wolfstrappkraut*
Bugleweed	*Lycopus virginicus*	Lamiaceae	Lycopi herba	*Wolfstrappkraut*
Burdock root	*Arctium lappa*	Asteraceae	Bardanae radix	*Klettenwurzel*
Burdock root	*Arctium minus*	Asteraceae	Bardanae radix	*Klettenwurzel*
Burdock root	*Arctium tomentosum*	Asteraceae	Bardanae radix	*Klettenwurzel*
Butcher's Broom rhizome	*Ruscus aculeatus*	Liliaceae	Rusci aculeati rhizoma	*Mäusedornwurzelstock*
Cajeput oil	*Melaleuca leucodendra*	Myrtaceae	Cajuputi aetheroleum	*Cajuputöl*
Calendula flower	*Calendula officinalis*	Asteraceae	Calendulae flos	*Ringelblumenblüten*
Calendula herb	*Calendula officinalis*	Asteraceae	Calendulae herba	*Ringelblumenkraut*
California Poppy	*Eschscholzia californica*	Papaveraceae	Eschscholziae	*Kalifornischer Goldmohn*
Camphor	*Cinnamomum camphora*	Lauraceae	Camphora	*Campher*
Cape aloe	*Aloe ferox*	Liliaceae	Aloe capensis	*Kap-Aloe*
Caraway oil	*Carum carvi*	Apiaceae	Carvi aetheroleum	*Kümmelöl*
Caraway seed	*Carum carvi*	Apiaceae	Carvi fructus	*Kümmel*
Cardamom	*Elettaria cardamomum*	Zingiberaceae	Cardamomi fructus	*Kardamomen*

English	Botanical	Plant Family	Pharmacopeial	German
Cascara Sagrada bark	*Rhamnus purshiana*	Rhamnaceae	Rhamni purshianae cortex	*Amerikanische Faulbaumrinde*
Cascara Sagrada bark	*Frangula purshiana*	Rhamnaceae	Rhamni purshianae cortex	*Amerikanische Faulbaumrinde*
Cat's Ear flower	*Antennaria dioica*	Asteraceae	Antennariae dioicae flos	*Katzenpfötchenblüten*
Cat's Foot flower	*Antennaria dioica*	Asteraceae	Antennariae dioicae flos	*Katzenpfötchenblüten*
Cayenne (Paprika)	*Capsicum frutescens*	Solanaceae	Capsicum	*Paprika*
Cayenne (Paprika) species low in capsaicin	*Capsicum* spp.	Solanaceae	Capsicum	*capsaicinarme Paprika-Arten*
Celandine herb	*Chelidonium majus*	Papaveraceae	Chelidonii herba	*Schöllkraut*
Celery	*Apium graveolens*	Apiaceae	Apium graveolens	*Sellerie*
Celery herb	*Apium graveolens*	Apiaceae	Apii herba	*Selleriekraut*
Celery root	*Apium graveolens*	Apiaceae	Apii radix	*Selleriewurzel*
Celery seed	*Apium graveolens*	Apiaceae	Apii fructus	*Selleriefrüchte*
Centaury herb	*Centaurium minus*	Gentianaceae	Centaurii herba	*Tausendgüldenkraut*
Centaury herb	*Centaurium umbellatum*	Gentianaceae	Centaurii herba	*Tausendgüldenkraut*
Centaury herb	*Erythraea centaurium*	Gentianaceae	Centaurii herba	*Tausendgüldenkraut*
Ceylon Citronella grass	*Cymbopogon nardus*	Poaceae	Cymbopoginis nardi herba	*Cymbopogon-Arten*
Chamomile, German	*Matricaria recutita*	Asteraceae	Matricariae flos	*Kamilenblüten*
Chamomile, German	*Chamomilla recutita*	Asteraceae	Matricariae flos	*Kamilenblüten*
Chamomile, Roman	*Chamaemelum nobile*	Asteraceae	Chamomillae romanae flos	*Römishe Kamillenblüten*
Chamomile, Roman	*Anthemis nobilis*	Asteraceae	Chamomillae romanae flos	*Römishe Kamillenblüten*
Chaste Tree fruit	*Vitex agnus castus*	Verbenaceae	Agni casti fructus	*Keuschlammfrüchte*
Chestnut leaf	*Castanea sativa*	Fagaceae	Castaneae folium	*Kastanienblätter*
Chestnut leaf	*Castanea vesca*	Fagaceae	Castaneae folium	*Kastanienblätter*
Chestnut leaf	*Castanea vulgaris*	Fagaceae	Castaneae folium	*Edelkastanienblätter*
Chicory	*Cichorium intybus*	Asteraceae	Cichorium intybus	*Wegwarte*
Cinchona bark	*Cinchona pubescens*	Rubiaceae	Cinchonae cortex	*Chinarinde*
Cinchona bark	*Cinchona succirubra*	Rubiaceae	Cinchonae cortex	*Chinarinde*
Cinnamon	*Cinnamomum verum*	Lauraceae	Cinnamomi ceylanici cortex	*Zimtrinde*
Cinnamon	*Cinnamomum zeylanicum*	Lauraceae	Cinnamomi ceylanici cortex	*Zimtrinde*
Cinnamon flower	*Cinnamomum aromaticum*	Lauraceae	Cinnamomi flos	*Zimtblüten*
Cinnamon flower	*Cinnamomum cassia*	Lauraceae	Cinnamomi flos	*Zimtblüten*

English	Botanical	Plant Family	Pharmacopeial	German
Cinnamon bark, Chinese	Cinnamomum aromaticum	Lauraceae	Cinnamomi cassiae cortex	Chinesischer Zimt
Cinnamon bark, Chinese	Cinnamomum cassia	Lauraceae	Cinnamomi cassiae cortex	Chinesischer Zimt
Citronella	Cymbopogon citratus	Poaceae	Cymbopogon species	Cymbopogon-Arten
Citronella	Cymbopogon nardus	Poaceae	Cymbopogon species	Cymbopogon-Arten
Citronella	Cymbopogon winterianus	Poaceae	Cymbopogon species	Cymbopogon-Arten
Cloves	Syzygium aromaticum	Myrtaceae	Caryophylli flos	Gewürznelken
Cloves	Jambosa caryophyllus	Myrtaceae	Caryophylli flos	Gewürznelken
Cloves	Eugenia caryophyllata	Myrtaceae	Caryophylli flos	Gewürznelken
Cocklebur	Agrimonia eupatoria	Rosaceae	Agrimoniae herba	Odermennigkraut
Cocklebur	Agrimonia procera	Rosaceae	Agrimoniae herba	Odermennigkraut
Cocoa	Theobroma cacao	Sterculiaceae	Cacao testes	Kakaoschalen
Cocoa seed	Theobroma cacao	Sterculiaceae	Cacao semen	Kakaosamen
Coffee charcoal	Coffea arabica	Rubiaceae	Coffeae carbo	Kaffeekohle
Coffee charcoal	Coffea canephora	Rubiaceae	Coffeae carbo	Kaffeekohle
Coffee charcoal	Coffea liberica	Rubiaceae	Coffeae carbo	Kaffeekohle
Coffee charcoal	Coffea spp.	Rubiaceae	Coffeae carbo	Kaffeekohle
Cola nut	Cola nitida	Sterculiaceae	Colae semen	Kolasamen
Cola nut	Cola spp.	Sterculiaceae	Colae semen	Kolasamen
Colocynth	Citrullus colocynthis	Cucurbitaceae	Colocynthidis fructus	Koloquinthen
Coltsfoot flower	Tussilago farfara	Asteraceae	Farfarae flos	Huflattichblüten
Coltsfoot herb	Tussilago farfara	Asteraceae	Farfarae herba	Huflattichkraut
Coltsfoot leaf	Tussilago farfara	Asteraceae	Farfarae folium	Huflattichblätter
Coltsfoot root	Tussilago farfara	Asteraceae	Farfarae radix	Huflattichwurzel
Comfrey herb	Symphytum officinale	Boraginaceae	Symphyti herba	Beinwellkraut
Comfrey leaf	Symphytum officinale	Boraginaceae	Symphyti folium	Beinwellblätter
Comfrey root	Symphytum officinale	Boraginaceae	Symphyti radix	Beinwellwurzel
Condurango bark	Marsdenia condurango	Asclepiadaceae	Condurango cortex	Condurangorinde
Coriander	Coriandrum sativum	Apiaceae	Coriandri fructus	Koriander
Corn Poppy	Papaver rhoeas	Papaveraceae	Rhoeados flos	Klatschmohnblüten
Cornflower	Centaurea cyanus	Asteraceae	Cyani flos	Kornblume
Couch grass	Agropyron repens	Poaceae	Graminis rhizoma	Queckenwurzelstock
Curaçao aloe	Aloe vera	Liliaceae	Aloe barbadensis	Curaçao-Aloe
Curaçao aloe	Aloe barbadensis	Liliaceae	Aloe barbadensis	Curaçao-Aloe
Cymbopogon	Cymbopogon spp.	Poaceae	Cymbopogon species	Cymbopogon-Arten

English	Botanical	Plant Family	Pharmacopeial	German
Damiana herb	*Turnera diffusa*	Turneraceae	Turnerae diffusae herba	*Damianakraut*
Damiana leaf	*Turnera diffusa*	Turneraceae	Turnerae diffusae folium	*Damianablätter*
Dandelion herb	*Taraxacum officinale*	Asteraceae	Taraxaci herba	*Löwenzahnkraut*
Dandelion root with herb	*Taraxacum officinale*	Asteraceae	Taraxaci radix cum herba	*Löwenzahn-wurzel mit Kraut*
Deadly Nightshade leaf	*Atropa belladonna*	Solanaceae	Belladonnae folium	*Tollkirsche*
Deadly Nightshade root	*Atropa belladonna*	Solanaceae	Belladonnae radix	*Tollkirschewurzel*
Delphinium flower	*Delphinium consolida*	Ranunculaceae	Delphinii flos	*Ritterspornblüten*
Devil's Claw root	*Harpagophytum procumbens*	Pedaliaceae	Harpagophyti radix	*Südafrikanische Teufelskrallenwurzel*
Dill herb	*Anethum graveolens*	Apiaceae	Anethi herba	*Dillkraut*
Dill seed	*Anethum graveolens*	Apiaceae	Anethi fructus	*Dillfrüchte*
Echinacea Angustifolia herb	*Echinacea angustifolia*	Asteraceae	Echinaceae angustifoliae herba	*schmalblättriges Sonnenhutkraut*
Echinacea Angustifolia root	*Echinacea angustifolia*	Asteraceae	Echinaceae angustifoliae radix	*schmalblättriges Sonnenhutwurzel*
Echinacea Pallida herb	*Echinacea pallida*	Asteraceae	Echinaceae pallidae herba	*Blasses Kegelblumenkraut*
Echinacea Pallida root	*Echinacea pallida*	Asteraceae	Echinaceae pallidae radix	*Echinacea-pallida Wurzel*
Echinacea Purpurea herb	*Echinacea purpurea*	Asteraceae	Echinaceae purpureae herba	*Purpursonnenhutkraut*
Echinacea Purpurea root	*Echinacea purpurea*	Asteraceae	Echinaceae purpureae radix	*Purpursonnenhutwurzel*
Elder flower	*Sambucus nigra*	Caprifoliaceae	Sambuci flos	*Holunderblüten*
Elecampane	*Inula helenium*	Asteraceae	Helenii radix	*Alantwurzelstock*
Eleuthero root	*Acanthopanax senticosus*	Araliaceae	Eleurherococci radix	*Eleutherococcus-senticosus-Wurzel*
Eleuthero root	*Eleutherococcus senticosus*	Araliaceae	Eleurherococci radix	*Eleutherococcus-senticosus-Wurzel*
English plantain	*Plantago lanceolata*	Plantaginaceae	Plantaginis lanceolatae herba	*Spitzwegerichkraut*
Ephedra	*Ephedra sinica*	Ephedraceae	Ephedrae herba	*Ephedrakraut*
Ephedra	*Ephedra shennungiana*	Ephedraceae	Ephedrae herba	*Ephedrakraut*
Ergot	*Claviceps purpurea*	Clavicipitaceae	Secale cornutum	*Mutterkorn*
Eucalyptus leaf	*Eucalyptus globulus*	Myrtaceae	Eucalypti folium	*Eucalyptusblätter*
Eucalyptus oil	*Eucalyptus fructicetorum*	Myrtaceae	Eucalypti aetheroleum	*Eucalyptusöl*
Eucalyptus oil	*Eucalyptus globulus*	Myrtaceae	Eucalypti aetheroleum	*Eucalyptusöl*
Eucalyptus oil	*Eucalyptus polybractea*	Myrtaceae	Eucalypti aetheroleum	*Eucalyptusöl*
Eucalyptus oil	*Eucalyptus smithii*	Myrtaceae	Eucalypti aetheroleum	*Eucalyptusöl*

English	Botanical	Plant Family	Pharmacopeial	German
Eyebright herb	Euphrasia officinalis	Scrophulariaceae	Euphrasiae	Augentrostkraut
Fennel oil	Foeniculum vulgare	Apiaceae	Foeniculi aetheroleum	Fenchelöl
Fennel seed	Foeniculum vulgare	Apiaceae	Foeniculi fructus	Fenchel
Fenugreek seed	Trigonella foenum-graecum	Fabaceae	Foenugraeci semen	Bockshornsamen
Figs	Ficus carica	Moraceae	Caricae fructus	Feigen
Fir Needle oil	Abies alba	Pinaceae	Piceae aetheroleum	Fichtennadelöl
Fir Needle oil	Abies sachalinensis	Pinaceae	Piceae aetheroleum	Fichtennadelöl
Fir Needle oil	Abies sibirica	Pinaceae	Piceae aetheroleum	Fichtennadelöl
Fir Needle oil	Picea abies	Pinaceae	Piceae aetheroleum	Fichtennadelöl
Fir Needle oil	Picea excelsa	Pinaceae	Piceae aetheroleum	Fichtennadelöl
Fir shoots, fresh	Abies alba	Pinaceae	Piceae turiones recentes	Frische Fichtenspitzen
Flaxseed	Linum usitatissimum	Linaceae	Lini semen	Leinsamen
Frangula	Frangula alnus	Rhamnaceae	Frangulae cortex	Faulbaumrinde
Frangula	Rhamnus frangula	Rhamnaceae	Frangulae cortex	Faulbaumrinde
Fumitory	Fumaria officinalis	Fumariaceae	Fumariae herba	Erdrauchkraut
Galangal	Alpinia officinarium	Zingiberaceae	Galangae rhizoma	Galangtwurzelstock
Garlic	Allium sativum	Alliaceae	Allii sativi bulbus	Knoblauch
Gentian root	Gentiana lutea	Gentianaceae	Gentianae radix	Enzianwurzel
Ginger root	Zingiber officinale	Zingiberaceae	Zingiberis rhizoma	Ingwerwurzelstock
Ginkgo Biloba leaf	Ginkgo biloba	Ginkgoaceae	Ginkgo folium	Ginkgoblätter
Ginkgo Biloba leaf Extract	Ginkgo biloba	Ginkgoaceae	Ginkgo folium	Ginkgo biloba Blätter
Ginseng root	Panax ginseng	Araliaceae	Ginseng radix	Ginsengwurzel
Goat's Rue herb	Galega officinalis	Fabaceae	Galegae officinalis herba	Geißrautenkraut
Goldenrod	Solidago canadensis	Asteraceae	Solidago	Goldrute
Goldenrod	Solidago gigantea	Asteraceae	Solidago	Goldrute
Goldenrod	Solidago serotina	Asteraceae	Solidago	Goldrute
Goldenrod, European	Solidago virgaurea	Asteraceae	Solidago virgaureae herba	Echtes Goldrutenkraut
Guaiac wood	Guaiacum officinale	Zygophyllaceae	Guaiaci lignum	Guajakholz
Guaiac wood	Guaiacum sanctum	Zygophyllaceae	Guaiaci lignum	Guajakholz
Gumweed herb	Grindelia robusta	Asteraceae	Grindeliae herba	Grindeliakraut
Gumweed herb	Grindelia squarrosa	Asteraceae	Grindeliae herba	Grindeliakraut
Haronga bark and leaf	Harungana madagascariensis	Hypericaceae	Harunganae madagascariensis cortex et folium	Harongarinde

English	Botanical	Plant Family	Pharmacopeial	German
Hawthorn berry	*Crataegus laevigata*	Rosaceae	Crataegi fructus	*Weißdornfrüchte*
Hawthorn berry	*Crataegus monogyna*	Rosaceae	Crataegi fructus	*Weißdornfrüchte*
Hawthorn flower	*Crataegus laevigata*	Rosaceae	Crataegi flos	*Weißdornblätter*
Hawthorn flower	*Crataegus monogyna*	Rosaceae	Crataegi flos	*Weißdornblätter*
Hawthorn leaf	*Crataegus laevigata*	Rosaceae	Crataegi folium	*Weißdornblätter*
Hawthorn leaf	*Crataegus monogyna*	Rosaceae	Crataegi folium	*Weißdornblätter*
Hawthorn leaf with flower	*Crataegus laevigata*	Rosaceae	Crataegi folium cum flore	*Weißdornblätter mit Blüten*
Hawthorn leaf with flower	*Crataegus monogyna*	Rosaceae	Crataegi folium cum flore	*Weißdornblätter mit Blüten*
Hay flower	*Poa* spp.	Poaceae	Graminis flos	*Heublumen*
Heart's Ease herb	*Viola tricolor*	Violaceae	Violae tricoloris herba	*Stiefmütterchenkraut*
Heather flower	*Calluna vulgaris*	Ericaceae	Callunae vulgaris flos	*Heidekrautblüten*
Heather herb	*Calluna vulgaris*	Ericaceae	Callunae vulgaris herba	*Heidekraut*
Hempnettle herb	*Galeopsis ochroleuca*	Lamiaceae	Galeopsidis herba	*Hohlzahnkraut*
Hempnettle herb	*Galeopsis segetum*	Lamiaceae	Galeopsidis herba	*Hohlzahnkraut*
Henbane leaf	*Hyoscyamus niger*	Solanaceae	Hyoscyami folium	*Hyoscyamusblätter*
Hibiscus flower	*Hibiscus sabdariffa*	Malvaceae	Hibisci flos	*Hibiscusblüten*
Hollyhock flower	*Alcea rosea*	Malvaceae	Malvae arboreae flos	*Stockrosenblüten*
Hollyhock flower	*Althaea rosea*	Malvaceae	Malvae arboreae flos	*Stockrosenblüten*
Hops	*Humulus lupulus*	Moraceae	Lupuli strobulus	*Hopfenzapfen*
Horehound herb	*Marrubium vulgare*	Lamiaceae	Marrubii herba	*Andornkraut*
Horse Chestnut bark	*Aesculus hippocastanum*	Hippocastanaceae	Hippocastani cortex	*Roßkastanienrinde*
Horse Chestnut flower	*Aesculus hippocastanum*	Hippocastanaceae	Hippocastani flos	*Roßkastanienblüten*
Horse Chestnut leaf	*Aesculus hippocastanum*	Hippocastanaceae	Hippocastani folium	*Roßkastanienblätter*
Horse Chestnut seed	*Aesculus hippocastanum*	Hippocastanaceae	Hippocastani semen	*Roßkastiensamen*
Horseradish	*Armoracia rusticana*	Brassicaceae	Armoraciae rusticanae radix	*Meerrettich*
Horseradish	*Cochlearia armoracia*	Brassicaceae	Armoraciae rusticanae radix	*Meerrettich*
Horsetail herb	*Equisetum arvense*	Equisetaceae	Equiseti herba	*Schachtelhalmkraut*
Hound's Tongue herb	*Cynoglossum clandestinum*	Boraginaceae	Cynoglossi herba	*Hundszungenkraut*
Hound's Tongue herb	*Cynoglossum officinale*	Boraginaceae	Cynoglossi herba	*Hundszungenkraut*
Hyssop herb	*Hyssopus officinalis*	Lamiaceae	Hyssopi herba	*Ysopkraut*
Hyssop oil	*Hyssopus officinalis*	Lamiaceae	Hyssopi aetheroleum	*Ysopöl*

English	Botanical	Plant Family	Pharmacopeial	German
Iceland Moss	*Cetraria islandica*	Parmeliaceae	Lichen islandicus	*Isländisches Moos*
Indian Snakeroot	*Rauvolfia serpentina*	Apocynaceae	Rauwolfiae radix	*Rauwolfiawurzel*
Ivy leaf	*Hedera helix*	Araliaceae	Hederae helicis folium	*Efeublätter*
Jambolan bark	*Syzygium cumini*	Myrtaceae	Syzygii cumini cortex	*Syzygiumrinde*
Jambolan bark	*Syzygium jambolana*	Myrtaceae	Syzygii cumini cortex	*Syzygiumrinde*
Jambolan seed	*Syzygium cumini*	Myrtaceae	Syzygii cumini semen	*Syzygiumsamen*
Jambolan seed	*Syzygium jambolana*	Myrtaceae	Syzygii cumini semen	*Syzygiumsamen*
Java citronella oil	*Cymbopogon winterianus*	Poaceae	Cymbopoginis winteriani aetheroleum	*Cymbopogon-Arten*
Java tea	*Orthosiphon spicatus*	Lamiaceae	Orthosiphonis folium	*Orthosiphonblätter*
Java tea	*Orthosiphon stamineus*	Lamiaceae	Orthosiphonis folium	*Orthosiphonblätter*
Jimsonweed leaf	*Datura stramonium*	Solanaceae	Stramonii folium	*Stramoniumblätter*
Jimsonweed seed	*Datura stramonium*	Solanaceae	Stramonii semen	*Stramoniumsamen*
Johnny Jump-Up	*Viola tricolor*	Violaceae	Violae tricoloris	*Stiefmütterchenkraut*
Juniper berry	*Juniperus communis*	Cupressaceae	Juniperi fructus	*Wacholderbeeren*
Kava Kava	*Piper methysticum*	Piperaceae	Piperis methystici rhizoma	*Kava-Kava-Wurzelstock*
Kelp	*Laminaria hyperborea*	Laminariaceae	Laminariae stipites	*Laminariastiele*
Kelp	*Laminaria cloustonii*	Laminariaceae	Laminariae stipites	*Laminariastiele*
Kidney bean pods (without seeds)	*Phaseolus vulgaris*	Fabaceae	Phaseoli fructus sine semine	*Samenfreie Gartenbohnenhülsen*
Knotweed	*Polygonum aviculare*	Polygonaceae	Polygoni avicularis herba	*Vogelknöterichkraut*
Lady's Mantle	*Alchemilla vulgaris*	Rosaceae	Alchemillae herba	*Frauenmantelkraut*
Larch Turpentine	*Larix decidua*	Pinaceae	Terebinthina laricina	*Lärchenterpentin*
Lavender flower	*Lavandula angustifolia*	Lamiaceae	Lavandulae flos	*Lavendelblüten*
Lemon balm	*Melissa officinalis*	Lamiaceae	Melissae folium	*Melissenblätter*
Licorice root	*Glycyrrhiza glabra*	Fabaceae	Liquiritiae radix	*Süßholzwurzel*
Lily-of-the-valley herb	*Convallaria majalis*	Liliaceae	Convallariae herba	*Maiglöckchenkraut*
Linden charcoal	*Tilia cordata*	Tiliaceae	Tiliae carbo	*Lindenholzkohle*
Linden flower	*Tilia cordata*	Tiliaceae	Tiliae flos	*Lindenblüten*
Linden flower	*Tilia platyphyllos*	Tiliaceae	Tiliae flos	*Lindenblüten*
Linden leaf	*Tilia cordata*	Tiliaceae	Tiliae folium	*Lindenblätter*
Linden leaf	*Tilia platyphyllos*	Tiliaceae	Tiliae folium	*Lindenblätter*
Linden wood	*Tilia cordata*	Tiliaceae	Tiliae lignum	*Lindenholz*

English	Botanical	Plant Family	Pharmacopeial	German
Linden wood	Tilia platyphyllos	Tiliaceae	Tiliae lignum	Lindenholz
Liverwort herb	Hepatica nobilis	Ranunculaceae	Hepatici nobilis herba	Leberblümchenkraut
Loofa	Luffa aegyptiaca	Cucurbitaceae	Luffa aegyptiaca	Luffaschwamm
Lovage root	Levisticum officinale	Apiaceae	Levistici radix	Liebstöckelwurzel
Lungwort	Pulmonaria officinalis	Boraginaceae	Pulmonariae herba	Lungenkraut
Mace	Myristica fragrans	Myristicaceae	Myristica aril	Muskatnußbaum
Madder root	Rubia tinctorum	Rubiaceae	Rubiae tinctorum radix	Krappwurzel
Male fern herb	Dryopteris filix-mas	Aspleniaceae	Filicis maris herba	Wurmfarmkraut
Male fern leaf	Dryopteris filix-mas	Aspleniaceae	Filicis maris folium	Wurmfarmblätter
Male fern rhizome	Dryopteris filix-mas	Aspleniaceae	Filicis maris rhizoma	Wurmfarmwurzelstock
Mallow flower	Malva sylvestris	Malvaceae	Malvae flos	Malvenblüten
Mallow leaf	Malva sylvestris	Malvaceae	Malvae folium	Malvenblätter
Manna	Fraxinus ornus	Oleaceae	Manna	Manna
Marjoram herb	Majorana hortensis	Lamiaceae	Majoranae herba	Majoran
Marjoram herb	Origanum majorana	Lamiaceae	Majoranae herba	Majoran
Marjoram oil	Majorana hortensis	Lamiaceae	Majoranae aetheroleum	Majoranöl
Marjoram oil	Origanum majorana	Lamiaceae	Majoranae aetheroleum	Majoranöl
Marsh Tea	Ledum palustre	Lamiaceae	Ledi palustris herba	Sumpfporstkraut
Marshmallow leaf	Althaea officinalis	Malvaceae	Althaeae folium	Eibischblätter
Marshmallow root	Althaea officinalis	Malvaceae	Althaeae radix	Eibischwurzel
Maté	Ilex paraguariensis	Aquifoliaceae	Mate folium	Mateblätter
Mayapple resin	Podophyllum peltatum	Berberidiceae	Podophylli peltati resina	Podophyllumharz
Mayapple root	Podophyllum peltatum	Berberidiceae	Podophylli peltati rhizoma	Podophyllumwurzelstock
Meadow saffron	Colchicum autumnale	Liliaceae	Colchicum, Colchicum autumnale	Herbstzeitlose
Meadowsweet	Spiraea ulmaria	Rosaceae	Filipendula ulmaria	Mädesüß
Meadowsweet	Filipendula ulmaria	Rosaceae	Filipendula ulmaria	Mädesüß
Mentzelia	Mentzelia cordifolia	Loasaceae	Mentzeliae cordifoliae	Zweigspitzen, Stengel-und-Wurzel
Milk Thistle fruit	Silybum marianum	Asteraceae	Cardui mariae fructus	Mariendistelfrüchte
Milk Thistle herb	Silybum marianum	Asteraceae	Cardui mariae herba	Mariendistelkraut
Mint oil	Mentha arvensis	Lamiaceae	Menthae arvensis aetheroleum	Minzöl
Mistletoe berry	Viscum album	Viscaceae	Visci albi fructus	Mistelfrüchte

English	Botanical	Plant Family	Pharmacopeial	German
Mistletoe herb	*Viscum album*	Viscaceae	Visci albi herba	*Mistelkraut*
Mistletoe stem	*Viscum album*	Viscaceae	Visci albi stipitis	*Mistelstengel*
Monkshood herb	*Aconitum napellus*	Ranunculaceae	Aconiti herba	*Blauer Eisenhutkraut*
Monkshood root	*Aconitum napellus*	Ranunculaceae	Aconiti tuber	*Blauer Eisenhutwurzel*
Motherwort herb	*Leonurus cardiaca*	Lamiaceae	Leonuri cardiacae herba	*Herzgespannkraut*
Mountain Ash berry	*Sorbus aucuparia*	Rosaceae	Sorbi aucupariae fructus	*Ebereschenbeeren*
Mugwort herb	*Artemisia vulgaris*	Asteraceae	Artemisiae vulgaris herba	*Beifußkraut*
Mugwort root	*Artemisia vulgaris*	Asteraceae	Artemisiae vulgaris radix	*Beifußwurzel*
Muira Puama	*Ptychopetalum olacoides*	Olacaceae	Ptychopetali lignum	*Potenzholz*
Muira Puama	*Ptychopetalum unicatum*	Olacaceae	Ptychopetali lignum	*Potenzholz*
Mullein flower	*Verbascum densiflorum*	Scrophulariaceae	Verbasci flos	*Wollblumen*
Mullein flower	*Verbascum thapsus*	Scrophulariaceae	Verbasci flos	*Wollblumen*
Myrrh	*Commiphora molmol*	Burseraceae	Myrrha	*Myrrhe*
Nasturtium	*Tropaeolum majus*	Tropaeolaceae	Tropaeolum majus	*Kapuzinerkressenkraut*
Nettle herb	*Urtica dioica*	Urticaceae	Urticae herba	*Brennesselkraut*
Nettle herb	*Urtica urens*	Urticaceae	Urticae herba	*Brennesselkraut*
Nettle leaf	*Urtica dioica*	Urticaceae	Urticae folium	*Brennesselblätter*
Nettle leaf	*Urtica urens*	Urticaceae	Urticae folium	*Brennesselblätter*
Nettle root	*Urtica dioica*	Urticaceae	Urticae radix	*Brennesselwurzel*
Nettle root	*Urtica urens*	Urticaceae	Urticae radix	*Brennesselwurzel*
Niauli oil	*Melaleuca viridiflora*	Myrtaceae	Niauli aetheroleum	*Niauliöl*
Night-blooming Cereus flower	*Selenicereus grandiflorus*	Cactaceae	Selenicerei grandiflori flos	*Königin der Nacht*
Night-blooming Cereus herb	*Selenicereus grandiflorus*	Cactaceae	Selenicerei grandiflori herba	*Königin der Nacht*
Nutmeg	*Myristica fragrans*	Myristicaceae	Myristica fragrans	*Muskatnußbaum*
Nux Vomica	*Strychnos nux-vomica*	Loganiaceae	Strychni semen	*Brechnußsamen*
Oak bark	*Quercus robur*	Fagaceae	Quercus cortex	*Eichenrinde*
Oak bark	*Quercus petraea*	Fagaceae	Quercus cortex	*Eichenrinde*
Oat herb	*Avena sativa*	Poaceae	Avenae herba	*Haferkraut*
Oat straw	*Avena sativa*	Poaceae	Avenae stramentum	*Haferstroh*
Oats	*Avena sativa*	Poaceae	Avenae fructus	*Haferfrüchte*
Oleander leaf	*Nerium oleander*	Apocynaceae	Oleandri folium	*Oleanderblätter*
Olive leaf	*Olea europaea*	Oleaceae	Oleae folium	*Olivenblätter*
Olive oil	*Olea europaea*	Oleaceae	Olivae oleum	*Olivenöl*
Onion	*Allium cepa*	Alliaceae	Allii cepae bulbus	*Zwiebel*
Orange peel	*Citrus sinensis*	Rutaceae	Citri sinensis pericarpium	*Orangenschalen*

English	Botanical	Plant Family	Pharmacopeial	German
Oregano	*Origanum vulgare*	Lamiaceae	Origani vulgaris herba	*Dostenkraut*
Orris root	*Iris germanica*	Iridaceae	Iridis rhizoma	*Schwertlilienwurzelstock*
Orris root	*Iris pallida*	Iridaceae	Iridis rhizoma	*Schwertlilienwurzelstock*
Orris root	*Iris florentina* [*Iris germanica* var. *florentina*]	Iridaceae	Iridis rhizoma	*Schwertlilienwurzelstock*
Papain	*Carica papaya*	Caricaceae	Papainum crudum	*Papain*
Papaya leaf	*Carica papaya*	Caricaceae	Caricae papayae folium	*Baummelonenblätter*
Parsley herb and root	*Petroselinum crispum*	Apiaceae	Petroselini herba/radix	*Petersilienkraut/wurzel*
Paprika (Cayenne)	*Capsicum frutescens*	Solanaceae	Capsicum	*Paprika*
Paprika (Cayenne) species low in capsaicin	*Capsicum* spp.	Solanaceae	Capsicum	*capsaicinarme Paprika-Arten*
Parsley seed	*Petroselinum crispum*	Apiaceae	Petroselini fructus	*Petersilienfrüchte*
Pasque flower	*Pulsatilla pratensis*	Ranunculaceae	Pulsatillae herba	*Küchenschellenkraut*
Pasque flower	*Pulsatilla vulgaris*	Ranunculaceae	Pulsatillae herba	*Küchenschellenkraut*
Passionflower herb	*Passiflora incarnata*	Passifloraceae	Passiflorae herba	*Passionsblumenkraut*
Peony flower	*Paeonia mascula*	Paeoniaceae	Paeoniae flos	*Pfingstrosenblüten*
Peony flower	*Paeonia officinalis*	Paeoniaceae	Paeoniae flos	*Pfingstrosenblüten*
Peony root	*Paeonia mascula*	Paeoniaceae	Paeoniae radix	*Pfingstrosenwurzel*
Peony root	*Paeonia officinalis*	Paeoniaceae	Paeoniae radix	*Pfingstrosenwurzel*
Peppermint leaf	*Mentha x piperita*	Lamiaceae	Menthae piperitae folium	*Pfefferminzblätter*
Peppermint oil	*Mentha x piperita*	Lamiaceae	Menthae piperitae aetheroleum	*Pfefferminzöl*
Periwinkle	*Vinca minor*	Apocynaceae	Vincae minoris herba	*Immergrünkraut*
Peruvian Balsam	*Myroxylon balsamum*	Fabaceae	Balsamum peruvianum	*Perubalsam*
Petasites leaf	*Petasites* spp.	Asteraceae	Petasitidis folium	*Pestwurzblätter*
Petasites root	*Petasites hybridus*	Asteraceae	Petasitidis rhizoma	*Pestwurzwurzelstock*
Pheasant's Eye herb	*Adonis vernalis*	Ranunculaceae	Adonidis herba	*Adoniskraut*
Pimpinella herb	*Pimpinella major*	Apiaceae	Pimpinellae herba	*Bibernellkraut*
Pimpinella herb	*Pimpinella saxifraga*	Apiaceae	Pimpinellae herba	*Bibernellkraut*
Pimpinella root	*Pimpinella major*	Apiaceae	Pimpinellae radix	*Bibernellwurzel*
Pimpinella root	*Pimpinella saxifraga*	Apiaceae	Pimpinellae radix	*Bibernellwurzel*
Pine Needle oil	*Pinus mugo*	Pinaceae	Pini aetheroleum	*Kiefernnadelöl*
Pine Needle oil	*Pinus nigra*	Pinaceae	Pini aetheroleum	*Kiefernnadelöl*
Pine Needle oil	*Pinus pinaster*	Pinaceae	Pini aetheroleum	*Kiefernnadelöl*
Pine Needle oil	*Pinus sylvestris*	Pinaceae	Pini aetheroleum	*Kiefernnadelöl*

English	Botanical	Plant Family	Pharmacopeial	German
Pine Sprouts	*Pinus sylvestris*	Pinaceae	Pini turiones	*Kiefernsprossen*
Plantain	*Plantago lanceolata*	Plantaginaceae	Plantaginis lanceolatae herba	*Spitzwegerichkraut*
Poplar bud	*Populus* spp.	Salicaceae	Populi gemma	*Pappelknospen*
Potentilla	*Potentilla anserina*	Rosaceae	Potentillae anserinae herba	*Gänsefingerkraut*
Primrose flower	*Primula elatior*	Primulaceae	Primulae flos	*Schlüsselblumenblüten*
Primrose flower	*Primula veris*	Primulaceae	Primulae flos	*Schlüsselblumenblüten*
Primrose root	*Primula elatior*	Primulaceae	Primulae radix	*Primelwurzel*
Primrose root	*Primula veris*	Primulaceae	Primulae radix	*Primelwurzel*
Psyllium seed, Black	*Plantago afra*	Plantaginaceae	Psyllii semen	*Flohsamen*
Psyllium seed, Black	*Plantago arenaria*	Plantaginaceae	Psyllii semen	*Flohsamen*
Psyllium seed, Black	*Plantago indica*	Plantaginaceae	Psyllii semen	*Flohsamen*
Psyllium seed, Black	*Plantago psyllium*	Plantaginaceae	Psyllii semen	*Flohsamen*
Psyllium seed, Blonde	*Plantago isphagula*	Plantaginaceae	Plantaginis ovatae semen	*Indische Flohsamen*
Psyllium seed, Blonde	*Plantago ovata*	Plantaginaceae	Plantaginis ovatae semen	*Indische Flohsamen*
Psyllium seed husk, Blonde	*Plantago isphagula*	Plantaginaceae	Plantaginis ovatae testa	*Indische Flohsamenschalen*
Psyllium seed husk, Blonde	*Plantago ovata*	Plantaginaceae	Plantaginis ovatae testa	*Indische Flohsamenschalen*
Pulsatilla	*Pulsatilla pratensis*	Ranunculaceae	Pulsatillae herba	*Küchenschellenkraut*
Pulsatilla	*Pulsatilla vulgaris*	Ranunculaceae	Pulsatillae herba	*Küchenschellenkraut*
Pumpkin seed	*Cucurbita pepo*	Cucurbitaceae	Cucurbitae peponis semen	*Kürbissamen*
Purple Coneflower herb	*Echinacea purpurea*	Asteraceae	Echinaceae purpureae herba	*Purpursonnenhutkraut*
Purple Coneflower root	*Echinacea purpurea*	Asteraceae	Echinaceae purpureae radix	*Purpursonnenhutwurzel*
Radish	*Raphanus sativus*	Brassicaceae	Raphani sativi radix	*Rettich*
Raspberry leaf	*Rubus idaeus*	Rosaceae	Rubi idaei folium	*Himbeerblätter*
Rhatany root	*Krameria triandra*	Krameriaceae	Ratanhiae radix	*Ratanhiawurzel*
Rhododendron, Rusty-leaved	*Rhododendron ferrugineum*	Ericaceae	Rhododendri ferruginei folium	*Rostrote Alpenrosenblätter*
Rhubarb root	*Rheum officinale*	Polygonaceae	Rhei radix	*Rhabarber*
Rhubarb root	*Rheum palmatum*	Polygonaceae	Rhei radix	*Rhabarber*
Rose flower	*Rosa centifolia*	Rosaceae	Rosae flos	*Rosenblüten*
Rose flower	*Rosa gallica*	Rosaceae	Rosae flos	*Rosenblüten*
Rose hip	*Rosa* spp.	Rosaceae	Rosae pseudofructus	*Hagebuttenschalen*

English	Botanical	Plant Family	Pharmacopeial	German
Rose hip and seed	*Rosa* spp.	Rosaceae	Rosae pseudofructus cum fructibus	*Hagebutten*
Rose hip seed	*Rosa* spp.	Rosaceae	Rosae fructus	*Hagebuttenkerne*
Rosemary leaf	*Rosmarinus officinalis*	Lamiaceae	Rosmarini folium	*Rosmarinblätter*
Rue herb	*Ruta graveolens*	Rutaceae	Rutae herba	*Rautenkraut*
Rue leaf	*Ruta graveolens*	Rutaceae	Rutae folium	*Rautenblätter*
Rupturewort	*Herniaria glabra*	Caryophyllaceae	Herniariae	*Bruchkraut*
Rupturewort	*Herniaria hirsuta*	Caryophyllaceae	Herniariae	*Bruchkraut*
Saffron	*Crocus sativa*	Iridaceae	Croci stigma	*Safran*
Sage leaf	*Salvia officinalis*	Lamiaceae	Salviae folium	*Salbeiblätter*
Sandalwood, Red	*Pterocarpus santalinus*	Fabaceae	Santali lignum rubrum	*Rotes Sandelholz*
Sandalwood, White	*Santalum album*	Santalaceae	Santali albi lignum	*Weißes Sandelholz*
Sandy Everlasting	*Helichrysum arenarium*	Asteraceae	Helichrysi flos	*Ruhrkrautblüten*
Sanicle herb	*Sanicula europaea*	Apiaceae	Saniculae herba	*Sanikelkraut*
Sarsaparilla root	*Smilax aristolochiaefolii*	Smilacaceae	Sarsaparillae radix	*Sarsaparillewurzel*
Sarsaparilla root	*Smilax febrifuga*	Smilacaceae	Sarsaparillae radix	*Sarsaparillewurzel*
Sarsaparilla root	*Smilax regelii*	Smilacaceae	Sarsaparillae radix	*Sarsaparillewurzel*
Sarsaparilla root, German	*Carex arenaria*	Cyperaceae	Caricis rhizoma	*Sandriedgraswurzelstock*
Saw Palmetto berry	*Serenoa repens*	Arecaceae	Sabal fructus	*Sabalfrüchte*
Saw Palmetto berry	*Sabal serrulata*	Arecaceae	Sabal fructus	*Sabalfrüchte*
Scopolia root	*Scopolia carniolica*	Solanaceae	Scopolia rhizoma	*Glockenbilsenkraut Wurzelstock*
Scotch Broom flower	*Cytisus scoparius*	Fabaceae	Cytisi scoparii flos	*Besenginsterblüten*
Scotch Broom flower	*Sarothamnus scoparius*	Fabaceae	Cytisi scoparii flos	*Besenginsterblüten*
Scotch Broom herb	*Cytisus scoparius*	Fabaceae	Cytisi scoparii herba	*Besenginsterkraut*
Senecio herb	*Senecio nemorensis*	Asteraceae	Senecionis herba	*Fuchskreuzkraut*
Senega Snakeroot	*Polygala senega*	Polygalaceae	Polygalae radix	*Senegawurzel*
Senega Snakeroot	*Polygala* spp.	Polygalaceae	Polygalae radix	*Senegawurzel*
Senna leaf	*Cassia acutifolia*	Fabaceae	Sennae folium	*Sennesblätter*
Senna leaf	*Cassia angustifolia*	Fabaceae	Sennae folium	*Sennesblätter*
Senna leaf	*Cassia senna*	Fabaceae	Sennae folium	*Sennesblätter*
Senna leaf	*Senna alexandrina*	Fabaceae	Sennae folium	*Sennesblätter*
Senna pod	*Cassia acutifolia*	Fabaceae	Sennae fructus	*Alexandriner-Sennesfrüchte*
Senna pod	*Cassia angustifolia*	Fabaceae	Sennae fructus	*Tinnevelly-Sennesfrüchte*
Senna pod	*Cassia senna*	Fabaceae	Sennae fructus	*Alexandriner-Sennesfrüchte*

English	Botanical	Plant Family	Pharmacopeial	German
Senna pod	Senna alexandrina	Fabaceae	Sennae fructus	Sennesfrüchte
Shepherd's Purse	Capsella bursa pastoris	Brassicaceae	Bursae pastoris herba	Hirtentäschelkraut
Siberian Ginseng	Acanthopanax senticosus	Araliaceae	Eleutherococci radix	Eleutherococcus-senticosus-Wurzel
Siberian Ginseng	Eleutherococcus senticosus	Araliaceae	Eleutherococci radix	Eleutherococcus-senticosus-Wurzel
Silver Linden flower	Tilia argentea	Tiliaceae	Tiliae tomentosae flos	Silberlindenblüten
Silver Linden flower	Tilia tomentosa	Tiliaceae	Tiliae tomentosae flos	Silberlindenblüten
Silverweed	Potentilla anserina	Rosaceae	Potentillae anserinae herba	Gänsefingerkraut
Sloe berry	Prunus spinosa	Rosaceae	Pruni spinosae fructus	Schlehdornfrüchte
Snakeroot, Indian	Rauvolfia serpentina	Apocynaceae	Rauwolfiae radix	Rauwolfiawurzel
Snakeroot, Senega	Polygala senega	Polygalaceae	Polygalae radix	Senegawurzel
Snakeroot, Senega	Polygala spp.	Polygalaceae	Polygalae radix	Senegawurzel
Soapwort herb, Red	Saponaria officinalis	Caryophyllaceae	Saponariae rubrae herba	Seifenkraut
Soapwort root, Red	Saponaria officinalis	Caryophyllaceae	Saponariae rubrae radix	Rote Seifenwurzel
Soapwort root, White	Gypsophila paniculata	Caryophyllaceae	Gypsophilae radix	Wieße Seifenwurzel
Soapwort root, White	Gypsophila spp.	Caryophyllaceae	Gypsophilae radix	Wieße Seifenwurzel
Soy Lecithin	Glycine max	Fabaceae	Lecithin ex soja	Sojalecithin
Soy Phospholipid	Glycine max	Fabaceae	Phospholipide ex soja cum 73 - 79% (3-Sn Phosphatidyl) - cholin	Phosphalipide aus Sojabohnen
Speedwell	Veronica officinalis	Scrophulariaceae	Veronicae herba	Ehrenpreiskraut
Spinach leaf Spiny	Spinacia oleracea	Chenopodiaceae	Spinaciae folium	Spinatblätter
Restharrow root	Ononis spinosa	Fabaceae	Ononidis radix	Hauhechelwurzel
Sponge cucumber	Luffa aegyptiaca	Cucurbitaceae	Luffa aegyptiaca	Luffaschwamm
Sprouts, Pine	Pinus sylvestris	Pinaceae	Pini turiones	Kiefernsprossen
Squill	Urginea maritima	Liliaceae	Scillae bulbus	Meerzwiebel
St. John's Wort	Hypericum perforatum	Hypericaceae	Hyperici herba	Johanniskraut
Star Anise	Illicium verum	Illiciaceae	Anisi stellati	Sternanis
Stinging Nettle herb	Urtica dioica	Urticaceae	Urticae herba	Brennesselkraut
Stinging Nettle herb	Urtica urens	Urticaceae	Urticae herba	Brennesselkraut
Stinging Nettle leaf	Urtica dioica	Urticaceae	Urticae folium	Brennesselblätter
Stinging Nettle leaf	Urtica urens	Urticaceae	Urticae folium	Brennesselblätter
Stinging Nettle root	Urtica dioica	Urticaceae	Urticae radix	Brennesselwurzel

English	Botanical	Plant Family	Pharmacopeial	German
Stinging Nettle root	*Urtica urens*	Urticaceae	Urticae radix	*Brennesselwurzel*
Strawberry leaf	*Fragaria vesca*	Rosaceae	Fragariae folium	*Erdbeerblätter*
Strawberry leaf	*Fragaria viridis*	Rosaceae	Fragariae folium	*Erdbeerblätter*
Sundew	*Drosera intermedia*	Droseraceae	Droserae herba	*Sonnentaukraut*
Sundew	*Drosera longifolia*	Droseraceae	Droserae herba	*Sonnentaukraut*
Sundew	*Drosera ramentacea*	Droseraceae	Droserae herba	*Sonnentaukraut*
Sundew	*Drosera rotundifolia*	Droseraceae	Droserae herba	*Sonnentaukraut*
Sweet clover	*Melilotus altissimus*	Fabaceae	Meliloti herba	*Steinkleekraut*
Sweet clover	*Melilotus officinalis*	Fabaceae	Meliloti herba	*Steinkleekraut*
Sweet Violet root and herb	*Viola odorata*	Violaceae	Violae odoratae rhizoma and herba	*Märzveilchen/blüten*
Sweet Woodruff	*Galium odoratum*	Rubiaceae	Galii odorati herba	*Waldmeisterkraut*
Tansy flower	*Chrysanthemum vulgare*	Asteraceae	Chrysanthemi vulgaris flos	*Rainfarnblüten*
Tansy flower	*Tanacetum vulgare*	Asteraceae	Chrysanthemi vulgaris flos	*Rainfarnblüten*
Tansy herb	*Chrysanthemum vulgare*	Asteraceae	Chrysanthemi vulgaris herba	*Rainfarnkraut*
Tansy herb	*Tanacetum vulgare*	Asteraceae	Chrysanthemi vulgaris herba	*Rainfarnkraut*
Thyme	*Thymus vulgaris*	Lamiaceae	Thymi herba	*Thymiankraut*
Thyme	*Thymus zygis*	Lamiaceae	Thymi herba	*Thymiankraut*
Thyme, Wild	*Thymus serphyllum*	Lamiaceae	Serpylli herba	*Quendelkraut*
Tolu Balsam	*Myroxylon balsamum*	Fabaceae	Balsamum tolutanum	*Tolubalsam*
Tormentil root	*Potentilla erecta*	Rosaceae	Tormentillae rhizoma	*Tormentillwurzelstock*
Tormentil root	*Potentilla tormentilla*	Rosaceae	Tormentillae rhizoma	*Tormentillwurzelstock*
Turmeric root	*Curcuma aromatica*	Zingiberaceae	Curcumae longae rhizoma	*Curcumawurzelstock*
Turmeric root	*Curcuma domestica*	Zingiberaceae	Curcumae longae rhizoma	*Curcumawurzelstock*
Turmeric root	*Curcuma longa*	Zingiberaceae	Curcumae longae rhizoma	*Curcumawurzelstock*
Turmeric, Javanese	*Curcuma xanthorrhiza*	Zingiberaceae	Curcumae xanthorrhizae rhizoma	*Javanische Gelbwurzel*
Turpentine oil, Purified	*Pinus australis*	Pinaceae	Terebinthinae aetheroleum rectificatum	*Gereinigtes Terpentinöl*
Turpentine oil, Purified	*Pinus palustris*	Pinaceae	Terebinthinae aetheroleum rectificatum	*Gereinigtes Terpentinöl*
Turpentine oil, Purified	*Pinus pinaster*	Pinaceae	Terebinthinae aetheroleum rectificatum	*Gereinigtes Terpentinöl*
Turpentine oil, Purified	*Pinus* spp.	Pinaceae	Terebinthinae aetheroleum rectificatum	*Gereinigtes Terpentinöl*

English	Botanical	Plant Family	Pharmacopeial	German
Usnea	Usnea barbata	Usneaceae	Usnea	Bartflechten
Usnea	Usnea florida	Usneaceae	Usnea	Bartflechten
Usnea	Usnea hirta	Usneaceae	Usnea	Bartflechten
Usnea	Usnea plicata	Usneaceae	Usnea	Bartflechten
Usnea	Usnea spp.	Usneaceae	Usnea	Bartflechten
Uva Ursi leaf	Arctostaphylos uva-ursi	Ericaceae	Uvae ursi folium	Bärentraubenblätter
Uzara root	Xysmalobium undulatum	Asclepiadaceae	Uzarae radix	Uzarawurzel
Valerian root	Valeriana officinalis	Valerianaceae	Valerianae radix	Baldrianwurzel
Venetian Turpentine	Larix decidua	Pinaceae	Terebinthina veneta	Venezianischer Terpentin
Verbena herb	Verbena officinalis	Verbenaceae	Verbenae herba	Eisenkraut
Veronica herb	Veronica officinalis	Scrophulariaceae	Veronicae herba	Ehrenpreiskraut
Walnut hull	Juglans regia	Juglandaceae	Juglandis fructus cortex	Walnußfrüchtschalen
Walnut leaf	Juglans regia	Juglandaceae	Juglandis folium	Walnußblätter
Watercress	Nasturtium officinale	Brassicaceae	Nasturtii herba	Kapuzinerkressenkraut
West Indian Lemongrass	Cymbopogon citratus	Poaceae	Cymbopoginis citrati herba	Cymbopogon-Arten
West Indian Lemongrass oil	Cymbopogon citratus	Poaceae	Cymbopoginis citrati aetheroleum	Cymbopogon-Arten
White Dead Nettle flower	Lamium album	Lamiaceae	Lamii albi flos	Weiße Taubnesselblüten
White Dead Nettle herb	Lamium album	Lamiaceae	Lamii albi herba	Weißes Taubnesselkraut
White Mustard seed	Sinapis alba	Brassicaceae	Sinapis albae semen	Weiße Senfsamen
White Sandalwood	Santalum album	Santalaceae	Santali albi lignum	Weißes Sandelholz
White Soapwort root	Gypsophila paniculata	Caryophyllaceae	Gypsophilae radix	Wieße Seifenwurzel
White Soapwort root	Gypsophila spp.	Caryophyllaceae	Gypsophilae radix	Wieße Seifenwurzel
White Spruce oil	Abies alba	Pinaceae	Piceae aetheroleum	Ficthennadelöl
White Spruce oil	Abies sachalinensis	Pinaceae	Piceae aetheroleum	Ficthennadelöl
White Spruce oil	Abies sibirica	Pinaceae	Piceae aetheroleum	Ficthennadelöl
White Spruce oil	Picea abies	Pinaceae	Piceae aetheroleum	Ficthennadelöl
White Spruce oil	Picea excelsa	Pinaceae	Piceae aetheroleum	Fichtennadelöl
White Willow bark	Salix alba	Salicaceae	Salicis cortex	Weidenrinde
White Willow bark	Salix fragilis	Salicaceae	Salicis cortex	Weidenrinde
White Willow bark	Salix purpurea	Salicaceae	Salicis cortex	Weidenrinde

English	Botanical	Plant Family	Pharmacopeial	German
White Willow bark	*Salix* spp.	Salicaceae	Salicis cortex	*Weidenrinde*
Wild Oat herb	*Avena sativa*	Poaceae	Avenae herba	*Haferkraut*
Witch Hazel bark	*Hamamelis virginiana*	Hamamelidaceae	Hamamelidis cortex	*Hamamelisrinde*
Witch Hazel leaf	*Hamamelis virginiana*	Hamamelidaceae	Hamamelidis folium	*Hamamelisblätter*
Wood Sanicle	*Sanicula europaea*	Apiaceae	Saniculae herba	*Sanikelkraut*
Woody Nightshade	*Solanum dulcamara*	Solanaceae	Dulcamarae stipites	*Bittersüßstengel*
Wormwood	*Artemisia absinthium*	Asteraceae	Absinthii herba	*Wermutkraut*
Yarrow flower	*Achillea millefolium*	Asteraceae	Millefolii flos	*Schafgarbe*
Yarrow herb	*Achillea millefolium*	Asteraceae	Millefolii herba	*Schafgarbenkraut*
Yeast, Brewer's	*Candida utilis*	Cryptococcaeae	Faex medicinalis	*Medizinische Hefe*
Yeast, Brewer's	*Saccharomyces cerevisiae*	Saccharomycetaceae	Faex medicinalis	*Medizinische Hefe*
Brewer's Yeast/ Hansen CBS 5926	*Saccharomyces cerevisiae*	Saccharomycetaceae	Saccharomyces cerevisiae	*Trokenhefe aus Saccharomyces cerevisiae*
Yellow Jessamine	*Gelsemiums sempervirens*	Loganiaceae	Gelsemii rhizoma	*Gelsemiumwurzelstock*
Yohimbe bark	*Corynanthe yohimbi*	Rubiaceae	Yohimbehe cortex	*Yohimberinde*
Yohimbe bark	*Pausinystalia johimbe*	Rubiaceae	Yohimbehe cortex	*Yohimberinde*
Zedoary rhizome	*Curcuma zedoaria*	Zingiberaceae	Zedoariae rhizoma	*Zitwerwurzelstock*

By Botanical Name

Botanical	English	Plant Family	Pharmacopeial	German
Abies alba	Fir Needle oil	Pinaceae	Piceae aetheroleum	*Fichtennadelöl*
Abies alba	Fir shoots, fresh	Pinaceae	Piceae turiones recentes	*Frische Fichtenspitzen*
Abies alba	White Spruce oil	Pinaceae	Piceae aetheroleum	*Ficthennadelöl*
Abies sachalinensis	Fir Needle oil	Pinaceae	Piceae aetheroleum	*Fichtennadelöl*
Abies sachalinensis	White Spruce oil	Pinaceae	Piceae aetheroleum	*Ficthennadelöl*
Abies sibirica	Fir Needle oil	Pinaceae	Piceae aetheroleum	*Fichtennadelöl*
Abies sibirica	White Spruce oil	Pinaceae	Piceae aetheroleum	*Ficthennadelöl*
Acanthopanax senticosus	Eleuthero root	Araliaceae	Eleutherococci radix	*Eleutherococcus-senticosus-Wurzel*
Acanthopanax senticosus	Siberian Ginseng	Araliaceae	Eleutherococci radix	*Eleutherococcus-senticosus-Wurzel*

TAXONOMIC CROSS-REFERENCE, BOTANICAL — ANANAS COMOSUS

Botanical	English	Plant Family	Pharmacopeial	German
Achillea millefolium	Yarrow flower	Asteraceae	Millefolii flos	*Schafgarbe*
Achillea millefolium	Yarrow herb	Asteraceae	Millefolii herba	*Schafgarbenkraut*
Aconitum napellus	Aconite herb	Ranunculaceae	Aconiti herba	*Blauer Eisenhutkraut*
Aconitum napellus	Aconite tuber	Ranunculaceae	Aconiti tuber	*Blauer Eisenhutwurzel*
Aconitum napellus	Blue Monkshood herb	Ranunculaceae	Aconiti herba	*Blauer Eisenhutkraut*
Aconitum napellus	Blue Monkshood tuber	Ranunculaceae	Aconiti tuber	*Blauer Eisenhutwurzel*
Aconitum napellus	Monkshood herb	Ranunculaceae	Aconiti herba	*Blauer Eisenhutkraut*
Aconitum napellus	Monkshood root	Ranunculaceae	Aconiti tuber	*Blauer Eisenhutwurzel*
Adonis vernalis	Pheasant's Eye herb	Ranunculaceae	Adonidis herba	*Adoniskraut*
Aesculus hippocastanum	Horse Chestnut bark	Hippocastanaceae	Hippocastani cortex	*Roßkastanienrinde*
Aesculus hippocastanum	Horse Chestnut flower	Hippocastanaceae	Hippocastani flos	*Roßkastanienblüten*
Aesculus hippocastanum	Horse Chestnut leaf	Hippocastanaceae	Hippocastani folium	*Roßkastanienblätter*
Aesculus hippocastanum	Horse Chestnut seed	Hippocastanaceae	Hippocastani semen	*Roßkastiensamen*
Agathosma betulina	Buchu leaf	Rutaceae	Barosmae folium	*Buccoblätter*
Agrimonia eupatoria	Agrimony	Rosaceae	Agrimoniae herba	*Odermennigkraut*
Agrimonia eupatoria	Cocklebur	Rosaceae	Agrimoniae herba	*Odermennigkraut*
Agrimonia procera	Agrimony	Rosaceae	Agrimoniae herba	*Odermennigkraut*
Agrimonia procera	Cocklebur	Rosaceae	Agrimoniae herba	*Odermennigkraut*
Agropyron repens	Couch grass	Poaceae	Graminis rhizoma	*Queckenwurzelstock*
Alcea rosea	Hollyhock flower	Malvaceae	Malvae arboreae flos	*Stockrosenblüten*
Alchemilla alpina	Alpine Lady's Mantle herb	Rosaceae	Alchemillae alpinae herba	*Frauenmantelkraut*
Alchemilla vulgaris	Lady's Mantle	Rosaceae	Alchemillae herba	*Frauenmantelkraut*
Allium cepa	Onion	Alliaceae	Allii cepae bulbus	*Zwiebel*
Allium sativum	Garlic	Alliaceae	Allii sativi bulbus	*Knoblauch*
Aloe barbadensis	Aloe	Liliaceae	Aloe barbadensis	*Aloe*
Aloe barbadensis	Curaçao aloe	Liliaceae	Aloe barbadensis	*Curaçao-Aloe*
Aloe ferox	Aloe	Liliaceae	Aloe capensis	*Kap-Aloe*
Aloe ferox	Cape aloe	Liliaceae	Aloe capensis	*Kap-Aloe*
Aloe vera	Aloe	Liliaceae	Aloe barbadensis	*Aloe*
Aloe vera	Curaçao aloe	Liliaceae	Aloe barbadensis	*Curaçao-Aloe*
Alpinia officinarum	Galangal	Zingiberaceae	Galangae rhizoma	*Galangtwurzelstock*
Althaea officinalis	Marshmallow leaf	Malvaceae	Althaeae folium	*Eibischblätter*
Althaea officinalis	Marshmallow root	Malvaceae	Althaeae radix	*Eibischwurzel*
Althaea rosea	Hollyhock flower	Malvaceae	Malvae arboreae flos	*Stockrosenblüten*
Ammi daucoides	Bishop's Weed fruit	Apiaceae	Ammeos visnagae fructus	*Ammi-visnaga-Früchte*
Ammi visnaga	Bishop's Weed fruit	Apiaceae	Ammeos visnagae fructus	*Ammi-visnaga-Früchte*
Ananas comosus	Bromelain	Bromeliaceae	Bromelainum	*Ananas*

Botanical	English	Plant Family	Pharmacopeial	German
Anethum graveolens	Dill herb	Apiaceae	Anethi herba	Dillkraut
Anethum graveolens	Dill seed	Apiaceae	Anethi fructus	Dillfrüchte
Angelica archangelica	Angelica herb	Apiaceae	Angelicae herba	Angelikakraut
Angelica archangelica	Angelica root	Apiaceae	Angelicae radix	Angelikawurzel
Angelica archangelica	Angelica seed	Apiaceae	Angelicae fructus	Angelikafrüchte
Antennaria dioica	Cat's Ear flower	Asteraceae	Antennariae dioicae flos	Katzenpfötchenblüten
Antennaria dioica	Cat's Foot flower	Asteraceae	Antennariae dioicae flos	Katzenpfötchenblüten
Anthemis nobilis	Chamomile, Roman	Asteraceae	Chamomillae romanae flos	Römishe Kamillenblüten
Apium graveolens	Celery	Apiaceae	Apium graveolens	Sellerie
Apium graveolens	Celery herb	Apiaceae	Apii herba	Selleriekraut
Apium graveolens	Celery root	Apiaceae	Apii radix	Selleriewurzel
Apium graveolens	Celery seed	Apiaceae	Apii fructus	Selleriefrüchte
Arctium lappa	Burdock root	Asteraceae	Bardanae radix	Klettenwurzel
Arctium minus	Burdock root	Asteraceae	Bardanae radix	Klettenwurzel
Arctium tomentosum	Burdock root	Asteraceae	Bardanae radix	Klettenwurzel
Arctostaphylos uva-ursi	Uva Ursi leaf	Ericaeae	Uvae ursi folium	Bärentraubenblätter
Armoracia rusticana	Horseradish	Brassicaceae	Armoraciae rusticanae radix	Meerrettich
Arnica chamissonis	Arnica flower	Asteraceae	Arnicae flos	Arnikablüten
Arnica montana	Arnica flower	Asteraceae	Arnicae flos	Arnikablüten
Artemisia absinthium	Wormwood	Asteraceae	Absinthii herba	Wermutkraut
Artemisia vulgaris	Mugwort herb	Asteraceae	Artemisiae vulgaris herba	Beifußkraut
Artemisia vulgaris	Mugwort root	Asteraceae	Artemisiae vulgaris radix	Beifußwurzel
Ascophyllum nodosum	Bladderwrack	Fucaceae	Fucus	Tang
Asparagus officinalis	Asparagus herb	Liliaceae	Asparagi herba	Spargelkraut
Asparagus officinalis	Asparagus root	Liliaceae	Asparagi rhizoma	Spargelwurzelstock
Atropa belladonna	Belladonna leaf	Solanaceae	Belladonnae folium	Tollkirsche
Atropa belladonna	Belladonna root	Solanaceae	Belladonnae radix	Tollkirschewurzel
Atropa belladonna	Deadly Nightshade leaf	Solanaceae	Belladonnae folium	Tollkirsche
Atropa belladonna	Deadly Nightshade root	Solanaceae	Belladonnae radix	Tollkirschewurzel
Avena sativa	Oat herb	Poaceae	Avenae herba	Haferkraut
Avena sativa	Oat straw	Poaceae	Avenae stramentum	Haferstroh
Avena sativa	Oats	Poaceae	Avenae fructus	Haferfrüchte

Botanical	English	Plant Family	Pharmacopeial	German
Avena sativa	Wild Oat herb	Poaceae	Avenae herba	*Haferkraut*
Barosma betulina	Buchu leaf	Rutaceae	Barosmae folium	*Buccoblätter*
Berberis vulgaris	Barberry	Berberidaceae	Berberis vulgaris	*Berberitze*
Berberis vulgaris	Barberry	Berberidaceae	Berberidis fructus	*Berberitze*
Berberis vulgaris	Barberry bark	Berberidaceae	Berberidis cortex	*Berberitze*
Berberis vulgaris	Barberry root	Berberidaceae	Berberidis radix	*Berberitze*
Berberis vulgaris	Barberry root bark	Berberidaceae	Berberidis radicis cortex	*Berberitzenrinde*
Betula pendula	Birch leaf	Betulaceae	Betulae folium	*Birkenblätter*
Betula pubescens	Birch leaf	Betulaceae	Betulae folium	*Birkenblätter*
Borago officinalis	Borage flower	Boraginaceae	Boraginis flos	*Boretsch*
Borago officinalis	Borage herb	Boraginaceae	Boraginis herba	*Boretsch*
Bryonia alba	Bryonia root	Cucurbitaceae	Bryoniae radix	*Zaunrübenwurzel*
Bryonia cretica	Bryonia root	Cucurbitaceae	Bryoniae radix	*Zaunrübenwurzel*
Calendula officinalis	Calendula flower	Asteraceae	Calendulae flos	*Ringelblumenblüten*
Calendula officinalis	Calendula herb	Asteraceae	Calendulae herba	*Ringelblumenkraut*
Calluna vulgaris	Heather flower	Ericaceae	Callunae vulgaris flos	*Heidekrautblüten*
Calluna vulgaris	Heather herb	Ericaceae	Callunae vulgaris herba	*Heidekraut*
Candida utilis	Yeast, Brewer's	Cryptococcaeae	Faex medicinalis	*Medizinische Hefe*
Capsella bursa pastoris	Shepherd's Purse	Brassicaceae	Bursae pastoris herba	*Hirtentäschelkraut*
Capsicum frutescens	Cayenne (Paprika)	Solanaceae	Capsicum	*Paprika*
Capsicum frutescens	Paprika (Cayenne)	Solanaceae	Capsicum	*Paprika*
Capsicum spp.	Cayenne (Paprika) species low in capsaicin	Solanaceae	Capsicum	*capsaicinarme Paprika-Arten*
Capsicum spp.	Paprika (Cayenne) species low in capsaicin	Solanaceae	Capsicum	*capsaicinarme Paprika-Arten*
Carex arenaria	Sarsaparilla root, German	Cyperaceae	Caricis rhizoma	*Sandriedgraswurzelstock*
Carica papaya	Papain	Caricaceae	Papainum crudum	*Papain*
Carica papaya	Papaya leaf	Caricaceae	Caricae papayae folium	*Baummelonenblätter*
Carum carvi	Caraway oil	Apiaceae	Carvi aetheroleum	*Kümmelöl*
Carum carvi	Caraway seed	Apiaceae	Carvi fructus	*Kümmel*
Cassia acutifolia	Senna leaf	Fabaceae	Sennae folium	*Sennesblätter*
Cassia acutifolia	Senna pod	Fabaceae	Sennae fructus	*Alexandriner-Sennesfrüchte*
Cassia angustifolia	Senna leaf	Fabaceae	Sennae folium	*Sennesblätter*
Cassia angustifolia	Senna pod	Fabaceae	Sennae fructus	*Tinnevelly-Sennesfrüchte*
Cassia senna	Senna leaf	Fabaceae	Sennae folium	*Sennesblätter*
Cassia senna	Senna pod	Fabaceae	Sennae fructus	*Alexandriner-Sennesfrüchte*

Botanical	English	Plant Family	Pharmacopeial	German
Castanea sativa	Chestnut leaf	Fagaceae	Castaneae folium	Kastanienblätter
Castanea vesca	Chestnut leaf	Fagaceae	Castaneae folium	Kastanienblätter
Castanea vulgaris	Chestnut leaf	Fagaceae	Castaneae folium	Edelkastanienblätter
Centaurea cyanus	Cornflower	Asteraceae	Cyani flos	Kornblume
Centaurium minus	Centaury herb	Gentianaceae	Centaurii herba	Tausendgüldenkraut
Centaurium umbellatum	Centaury herb	Gentianaceae	Centaurii herba	Tausendgüldenkraut
Cetraria islandica	Iceland Moss	Parmeliaceae	Lichen islandicus	Isländisches Moos
Chamaemelum nobile	Chamomile, Roman	Asteraceae	Chamomillae romanae flos	Römische Kamillenblüten
Chamomilla recutita	Chamomile, German	Asteraceae	Matricariae flos	Kamilenblüten
Chelidonium majus	Celandine herb	Papaveraceae	Chelidonii herba	Schöllkraut
Chrysanthemum vulgare	Tansy flower	Asteraceae	Chrysanthemi vulgaris flos	Rainfarnblüten
Chrysanthemum vulgare	Tansy herb	Asteraceae	Chrysanthemi vulgaris herba	Rainfarnkraut
Cichorium intybus	Chicory	Asteraceae	Cichorium intybus	Wegwarte
Cimicifuga racemosa	Black Cohosh root	Ranunculaceae	Cimicifugae racemosae rhizoma	Cimicifugawurzelstock
Cinchona pubescens	Cinchona bark	Rubiaceae	Cinchonae cortex	Chinarinde
Cinchona succirubra	Cinchona bark	Rubiaceae	Cinchonae cortex	Chinarinde
Cinnamomum aromaticum	Cinnamon flower	Lauraceae	Cinnamomi flos	Zimtblüten
Cinnamomum aromaticum	Cinnamon bark, Chinese	Lauraceae	Cinnamomi cassiae cortex	Chinesischer Zimt
Cinnamomum camphora	Camphor	Lauraceae	Camphora	Campher
Cinnamomum cassia	Cinnamon flower	Lauraceae	Cinnamomi flos	Zimtblüten
Cinnamomum cassia	Cinnamon bark, Chinese	Lauraceae	Cinnamomi cassiae cortex	Chinesischer Zimt
Cinnamomum verum	Cinnamon	Lauraceae	Cinnamomi ceylanici cortex	Zimtrinde
Cinnamomum zeylanicum	Cinnamon	Lauraceae	Cinnamomi ceylanici cortex	Zimtrinde
Citrullus colocynthis	Colocynth	Cucurbitaceae	Colocynthidis fructus	Koloquinthen
Citrus aurantium	Bitter Orange flower	Rutaceae	Aurantii flos	Pomeranzenblüten
Citrus aurantium	Bitter Orange flower oil	Rutaceae	Aurantii flos aetheroleum	Pomeranzenblütenöl
Citrus aurantium	Bitter Orange peel	Rutaceae	Aurantii pericarpium	Pomeranzenschale
Citrus sinensis	Orange peel	Rutaceae	Citri sinensis pericarpium	Orangenschalen

Botanical	English	Plant Family	Pharmacopeial	German
Claviceps purpurea	Ergot	Clavicipitaceae	Secale cornutum	*Mutterkorn*
Cnicus benedictus	Blessed Thistle herb	Asteraceae	Cnici benedicti herba	*Benediktenkraut*
Cochlearia armoracia	Horseradish	Brassicaceae	Armoraciae rusticanae radix	*Meerrettich*
Coffea arabica	Coffee charcoal	Rubiaceae	Coffeae carbo	*Kaffeekohle*
Coffea canephora	Coffee charcoal	Rubiaceae	Coffeae carbo	*Kaffeekohle*
Coffea liberica	Coffee charcoal	Rubiaceae	Coffeae carbo	*Kaffeekohle*
Coffea spp.	Coffee charcoal	Rubiaceae	Coffeae carbo	*Kaffeekohle*
Cola nitida	Cola nut	Sterculiaceae	Colae semen	*Kolasamen*
Cola spp.	Cola nut	Sterculiaceae	Colae semen	*Kolasamen*
Colchicum autumnale	Autumn Crocus	Liliaceae	Colchicum, Colchicum autumnale	*Herbstzeitlose*
Colchicum autumnale	Meadow saffron	Liliaceae	Colchicum, Colchicum autumnale	*Herbstzeitlose*
Commiphora molmol	Myrrh	Burseraceae	Myrrha	*Myrrhe*
Convallaria majalis	Lily-of-the-valley herb	Liliaceae	Convallariae herba	*Maiglöckchenkraut*
Coriandrum sativum	Coriander	Apiaceae	Coriandri fructus	*Koriander*
Corynanthe yohimbi	Yohimbe bark	Rubiaceae	Yohimbehe cortex	*Yohimberinde*
Crataegus laevigata	Hawthorn berry	Rosaceae	Crataegi fructus	*Weißdornfrüchte*
Crataegus laevigata	Hawthorn flower	Rosaceae	Crataegi flos	*Weißdornblätter*
Crataegus laevigata	Hawthorn leaf	Rosaceae	Crataegi folium	*Weißdornblätter*
Crataegus laevigata	Hawthorn leaf with flower	Rosaceae	Crataegi folium cum flore	*Weißdornblätter mit Blüten*
Crataegus monogyna	Hawthorn berry	Rosaceae	Crataegi fructus	*Weißdornfrüchte*
Crataegus monogyna	Hawthorn flower	Rosaceae	Crataegi flos	*Weißdornblätter*
Crataegus monogyna	Hawthorn leaf	Rosaceae	Crataegi folium	*Weißdornblätter*
Crataegus monogyna	Hawthorn leaf with flower	Rosaceae	Crataegi folium cum flore	*Weißdornblätter mit Blüten*
Crocus sativa	Saffron	Iridaceae	Croci stigma	*Safran*
Cucurbita pepo	Pumpkin seed	Cucurbitaceae	Cucurbitae peponis semen	*Kürbissamen*
Curcuma aromatica	Turmeric root	Zingiberaceae	Curcumae longae rhizoma	*Curcumawurzelstock*
Curcuma domestica	Turmeric root	Zingiberaceae	Curcumae longae rhizoma	*Curcumawurzelstock*
Curcuma longa	Turmeric root	Zingiberaceae	Curcumae longae rhizoma	*Curcumawurzelstock*
Curcuma xanthorrhiza	Turmeric, Javanese	Zingiberaceae	Curcumae xanthorrhizae rhizoma	*Javanische Gelbwurzel*
Curcuma zedoaria	Zedoary rhizome	Zingiberaceae	Zedoariae rhizoma	*Zitwerwurzelstock*

Botanical	English	Plant Family	Pharmacopeial	German
Cymbopogon citratus	Citronella	Poaceae	Cymbopogon species	*Cymbopogon-Arten*
Cymbopogon citratus	West Indian Lemongrass	Poaceae	Cymbopoginis citrati herba	*Cymbopogon-Arten*
Cymbopogon citratus	West Indian Lemongrass oil	Poaceae	Cymbopoginis citrati aetheroleum	*Cymbopogon-Arten*
Cymbopogon nardus	Ceylon Citronella grass	Poaceae	Cymbopoginis nardi herba	*Cymbopogon-Arten*
Cymbopogon nardus	Citronella	Poaceae	Cymbopogon species	*Cymbopogon-Arten*
Cymbopogon spp.	Cymbopogon	Poaceae	Cymbopogon species	*Cymbopogon-Arten*
Cymbopogon winterianus	Citronella	Poaceae	Cymbopogon species	*Cymbopogon-Arten*
Cymbopogon winterianus	Java citronella oil	Poaceae	Cymbopoginis winteriani aetheroleum	*Cymbopogon-Arten*
Cynara scolymus	Artichoke leaf	Asteraceae	Cynarae folium	*Artischokenblätter*
Cynoglossum clandestinum	Hound's Tongue herb	Boraginaceae	Cynoglossi herba	*Hundszungenkraut*
Cynoglossum officinale	Hound's Tongue herb	Boraginaceae	Cynoglossi herba	*Hundszungenkraut*
Cytisus scoparius	Broom flower, Scotch	Fabaceae	Cytisi scoparius flos	*Besenginsterblüten*
Cytisus scoparius	Broom herb, Scotch	Fabaceae	Cytisi scoparius herba	*Besenginsterkraut*
Cytisus scoparius	Scotch Broom flower	Fabaceae	Cytisi scoparii flos	*Besenginsterblüten*
Cytisus scoparius	Scotch Broom herb	Fabaceae	Cytisi scoparii herba	*Besenginsterkraut*
Datura stramonium	Jimsonweed leaf	Solanaceae	Stramonii folium	*Stramoniumblätter*
Datura stramonium	Jimsonweed seed	Solanaceae	Stramonii semen	*Stramoniumsamen*
Delphinium consolida	Delphinium flower	Ranunculaceae	Delphinii flos	*Ritterspornblüten*
Drosera intermedia	Sundew	Droseraceae	Droserae herba	*Sonnentaukraut*
Drosera longifolia	Sundew	Droseraceae	Droserae herba	*Sonnentaukraut*
Drosera ramentacea	Sundew	Droseraceae	Droserae herba	*Sonnentaukraut*
Drosera rotundifolia	Sundew	Droseraceae	Droserae herba	*Sonnentaukraut*
Dryopteris filix-mas	Male fern herb	Aspleniaceae	Filicis maris herba	*Wurmfarnkraut*
Dryopteris filix-mas	Male fern leaf	Aspleniaceae	Filicis maris folium	*Wurmfarnblätter*
Dryopteris filix-mas	Male fern rhizome	Aspleniaceae	Filicis maris rhizoma	*Wurmfarnwurzelstock*
Echinacea angustifolia	Echinacea Angustifolia herb	Asteraceae	Echinaceae angustifoliae herba	*schmalblättriges Sonnenhutkraut*
Echinacea angustifolia	Echinacea Angustifolia root	Asteraceae	Echinaceae angustifoliae radix	*schmalblättriges Sonnenhutwurzel*
Echinacea pallida	Echinacea Pallida herb	Asteraceae	Echinaceae pallidae herba	*Blasses Kegelblumenkraut*
Echinacea pallida	Echinacea Pallida root	Asteraceae	Echinaceae pallidae radix	*Echinacea-pallida Wurzel*

Botanical	English	Plant Family	Pharmacopeial	German
Echinacea purpurea	Echinacea Purpurea herb	Asteraceae	Echinaceae purpureae herba	*Purpursonnenhutkraut*
Echinacea purpurea	Echinacea Purpurea root	Asteraceae	Echinaceae purpureae radix	*Purpursonnenhutwurzel*
Echinacea purpurea	Purple Coneflower herb	Asteraceae	Echinaceae purpureae herba	*Purpursonnenhutkraut*
Echinacea purpurea	Purple Coneflower root	Asteraceae	Echinaceae purpureae radix	*Purpursonnenhutwurzel*
Elettaria cardamomum	Cardamom	Zingiberaceae	Cardamomi fructus	*Kardamomen*
Eleutherococcus senticosus	Eleuthero root	Araliaceae	Eleutherococci radix	*Eleutherococcus-senticosus-Wurzel*
Eleutherococcus senticosus	Siberian Ginseng	Araliaceae	Eleutherococci radix	*Eleutherococcus-senticosus-Wurzel*
Ephedra shennungiana	Ephedra	Ephedraceae	Ephedrae herba	*Ephedrakraut*
Ephedra sinica	Ephedra	Ephedraceae	Ephedrae herba	*Ephedrakraut*
Equisetum arvense	Horsetail herb	Equisetaceae	Equiseti herba	*Schachtelhalmkraut*
Erythraea centaurium	Centaury herb	Gentianaceae	Centaurii herba	*Tausendgüldenkraut*
Eschscholzia californica	California Poppy	Papaveraceae	Eschscholziae	*Kalifornischer Goldmohn*
Eucalyptus fructicetorum	Eucalyptus oil	Myrtaceae	Eucalypti aetheroleum	*Eucalyptusöl*
Eucalyptus globulus	Eucalyptus leaf	Myrtaceae	Eucalypti folium	*Eucalyptusblätter*
Eucalyptus globulus	Eucalyptus oil	Myrtaceae	Eucalypti aetheroleum	*Eucalyptusöl*
Eucalyptus polybractea	Eucalyptus oil	Myrtaceae	Eucalypti aetheroleum	*Eucalyptusöl*
Eucalyptus smithii	Eucalyptus oil	Myrtaceae	Eucalypti aetheroleum	*Eucalyptusöl*
Eugenia caryophyllata	Cloves	Myrtaceae	Caryophylli flos	*Gewürznelken*
Euphrasia officinalis	Eyebright herb	Scrophulariaceae	Euphrasiae	*Augentrostkraut*
Ficus carica	Figs	Moraceae	Caricae fructus	*Feigen*
Filipendula ulmaria	Meadowsweet	Rosaceae	Filipendula ulmaria	*Mädesüß*
Foeniculum vulgare	Fennel oil	Apiaceae	Foeniculi aetheroleum	*Fenchelöl*
Foeniculum vulgare	Fennel seed	Apiaceae	Foeniculi fructus	*Fenchel*
Fragaria vesca	Strawberry leaf	Rosaceae	Fragariae folium	*Erdbeerblätter*
Fragaria viridis	Strawberry leaf	Rosaceae	Fragariae folium	*Erdbeerblätter*
Frangula alnus	Buckthorn bark	Rhamnaceae	Frangulae cortex	*Faulbaumrinde*
Frangula alnus	Frangula	Rhamnaceae	Frangulae cortex	*Faulbaumrinde*
Frangula purshiana	Cascara Sagrada bark	Rhamnaceae	Rhamni purshianae cortex	*Amerikanische Faulbaumrinde*
Fraxinus excelsior	Ash bark	Oleaceae	Fraxini cortex	*Esche*
Fraxinus excelsior	Ash leaf	Oleaceae	Fraxini folium	*Esche*
Fraxinus ornus	Manna	Oleaceae	Manna	*Manna*
Fucus vesiculosus	Bladderwrack	Fucaceae	Fucus	*Tang*

Botanical	English	Plant Family	Pharmacopeial	German
Fumaria officinalis	Fumitory	Fumariaceae	Fumariae herba	*Erdrauchkraut*
Galega officinalis	Goat's Rue herb	Fabaceae	Galegae officinalis herba	*Geißrautenkraut*
Galeopsis ochroleuca	Hempnettle herb	Lamiaceae	Galeopsidis herba	*Hohlzahnkraut*
Galeopsis segetum	Hempnettle herb	Lamiaceae	Galeopsidis herba	*Hohlzahnkraut*
Galium odoratum	Sweet Woodruff	Rubiaceae	Galii odorati herba	*Waldmeisterkraut*
Gelsemiums sempervirens	Yellow Jessamine	Loganiaceae	Gelsemii rhizoma	*Gelsemiumwurzelstock*
Gentiana lutea	Gentian root	Gentianaceae	Gentianae radix	*Enzianwurzel*
Ginkgo biloba	Ginkgo Biloba leaf	Ginkgoaceae	Ginkgo folium	*Ginkgoblätter*
Ginkgo biloba	Ginkgo Biloba leaf Extract	Ginkgoaceae	Ginkgo folium	*Ginkgo biloba Blätter*
Glycine max	Soy Lecithin	Fabaceae	Lecithin ex soja	*Sojalecithin*
Glycine max	Soy Phospholipid	Fabaceae	Phospholipide ex soja cum 73 - 79% (3-Sn Phosphatidyl) - cholin	*Phosphalipide aus Sojabohnen*
Glycyrrhiza glabra	Licorice root	Fabaceae	Liquiritiae radix	*Süßholzwurzel*
Grindelia robusta	Gumweed herb	Asteraceae	Grindeliae herba	*Grindeliakraut*
Grindelia squarrosa	Gumweed herb	Asteraceae	Grindeliae herba	*Grindeliakraut*
Guaiacum officinale	Guaiac wood	Zygophyllaceae	Guaiaci lignum	*Guajakholz*
Guaiacum sanctum	Guaiac wood	Zygophyllaceae	Guaiaci lignum	*Guajakholz*
Gypsophila paniculata	Soapwort root, White	Caryophyllaceae	Gypsophilae radix	*Wieße Seifenwurzel*
Gypsophila paniculata	White Soapwort root	Caryophyllaceae	Gypsophilae radix	*Wieße Seifenwurzel*
Gypsophila spp.	Soapwort root, White	Caryophyllaceae	Gypsophilae radix	*Wieße Seifenwurzel*
Gypsophila spp.	White Soapwort root	Caryophyllaceae	Gypsophilae radix	*Wieße Seifenwurzel*
Hamamelis virginiana	Witch Hazel bark	Hamamelidaceae	Hamamelidis cortex	*Hamamelisrinde*
Hamamelis virginiana	Witch Hazel leaf	Hamamelidaceae	Hamamelidis folium	*Hamamelisblätter*
Harpagophytum procumbens	Devil's Claw root	Pedaliaceae	Harpagophyti radix	*Südafrikanische Teufelskrallenwurzel*
Harungana madagascariensis	Haronga bark and leaf	Hypericaceae	Harunganae madagascariensis cortex et folium	*Harongarinde*
Hedera helix	Ivy leaf	Araliaceae	Hederae helicis folium	*Efeublätter*
Helichrysum arenarium	Sandy Everlasting	Asteraceae	Helichrysi flos	*Ruhrkrautblüten*
Hepatica nobilis	Liverwort herb	Ranunculaceae	Hepatici nobilis herba	*Leberblümchenkraut*
Herniaria glabra	Rupturewort	Caryophyllaceae	Herniariae	*Bruchkraut*
Herniaria hirsuta	Rupturewort	Caryophyllaceae	Herniariae	*Bruchkraut*

Botanical	English	Plant Family	Pharmacopeial	German
Hibiscus sabdariffa	Hibiscus flower	Malvaceae	Hibisci flos	*Hibiscusblüten*
Humulus lupulus	Hops	Moraceae	Lupuli strobulus	*Hopfenzapfen*
Hyoscyamus niger	Henbane leaf	Solanaceae	Hyoscyami folium	*Hyoscyamusblätter*
Hypericum perforatum	St. John's Wort	Hypericaceae	Hyperici herba	*Johanniskraut*
Hyssopus officinalis	Hyssop herb	Lamiaceae	Hyssopi herba	*Ysopkraut*
Hyssopus officinalis	Hyssop oil	Lamiaceae	Hyssopi aetheroleum	*Ysopöl*
Ilex paraguariensis	Maté	Aquifoliaceae	Mate folium	*Mateblätter*
Illicium verum	Star Anise	Illiciaceae	Anisi stellati	*Sternanis*
Inula helenium	Elecampane	Asteraceae	Helenii radix	*Alantwurzelstock*
Iris florentina [*Iris germanica* var. *florentina*]	Orris root	Iridaceae	Iridis rhizoma	*Schwertlilienwurzelstock*
Iris germanica	Orris root	Iridaceae	Iridis rhizoma	*Schwertlilienwurzelstock*
Iris pallida	Orris root	Iridaceae	Iridis rhizoma	*Schwertlilienwurzelstock*
Jambosa caryophyllus	Cloves	Myrtaceae	Caryophylli flos	*Gewürznelken*
Juglans regia	Walnut hull	Juglandaceae	Juglandis fructus cortex	*Walnußfrüchtschalen*
Juglans regia	Walnut leaf	Juglandaceae	Juglandis folium	*Walnußblätter*
Juniperus communis	Juniper berry	Cupressaceae	Juniperi fructus	*Wacholderbeeren*
Krameria triandra	Rhatany root	Krameriaceae	Ratanhiae radix	*Ratanhiawurzel*
Laminaria cloustonii	Kelp	Laminariaceae	Laminariae stipites	*Laminariastiele*
Laminaria hyperborea	Kelp	Laminariaceae	Laminariae stipites	*Laminariastiele*
Lamium album	White Dead Nettle flower	Lamiaceae	Lamii albi flos	*Weiße Taubnesselbüten*
Lamium album	White Dead Nettle herb	Lamiaceae	Lamii albi herba	*Weißes Taubnesselkraut*
Larix decidua	Larch Turpentine	Pinaceae	Terebinthina laricina	*Lärchenterpentin*
Larix decidua	Venetian Turpentine	Pinaceae	Terebinthina veneta	*Venezianischer Terpentin*
Lavandula angustifolia	Lavender flower	Lamiaceae	Lavandulae flos	*Lavendelblüten*
Ledum palustre	Marsh Tea	Lamiaceae	Ledi palustris herba	*Sumpfporstkraut*
Leonurus cardiaca	Motherwort herb	Lamiaceae	Leonuri cardiacae herba	*Herzgespannkraut*
Levisticum officinale	Lovage root	Apiaceae	Levistici radix	*Liebstöckelwurzel*
Linum usitatissimum	Flaxseed	Linaceae	Lini semen	*Leinsamen*
Luffa aegyptiaca	Loofa	Cucurbitaceae	Luffa aegyptiaca	*Luffaschwamm*
Luffa aegyptiaca	Sponge cucumber	Cucurbitaceae	Luffa aegyptiaca	*Luffaschwamm*
Lycopus europaeus	Bugleweed	Lamiaceae	Lycopi herba	*Wolfstrappkraut*
Lycopus virginicus	Bugleweed	Lamiaceae	Lycopi herba	*Wolfstrappkraut*

Botanical	English	Plant Family	Pharmacopeial	German
Majorana hortensis	Marjoram herb	Lamiaceae	Majoranae herba	Majoran
Majorana hortensis	Marjoram oil	Lamiaceae	Majoranae aetheroleum	Majoranöl
Malva sylvestris	Blue Mallow flower	Malvaceae	Malvae flos	Malvenblüten
Malva sylvestris	Mallow flower	Malvaceae	Malvae flos	Malvenblüten
Malva sylvestris	Mallow leaf	Malvaceae	Malvae folium	Malvenblätter
Marrubium vulgare	Horehound herb	Lamiaceae	Marrubii herba	Andornkraut
Marsdenia condurango	Condurango bark	Asclepiadaceae	Condurango cortex	Condurangorinde
Matricaria recutita	Chamomile, German	Asteraceae	Matricariae flos	Kamillenblüten
Melaleuca leucodendra	Cajeput oil	Myrtaceae	Cajuputi aetheroleum	Cajuputöl
Melaleuca viridiflora	Niauli oil	Myrtaceae	Niauli aetheroleum	Niauliöl
Melilotus altissimus	Sweet clover	Fabaceae	Meliloti herba	Steinkleekraut
Melilotus officinalis	Sweet clover	Fabaceae	Meliloti herba	Steinkleekraut
Melissa officinalis	Lemon balm	Lamiaceae	Melissae folium	Melissenblätter
Mentha arvensis	Mint oil	Lamiaceae	Menthae arvensis aetheroleum	Minzöl
Mentha x piperita	Peppermint leaf	Lamiaceae	Menthae piperitae folium	Pfefferminzblätter
Mentha x piperita	Peppermint oil	Lamiaceae	Menthae piperitae aetheroleum	Pfefferminzöl
Mentzelia cordifolia	Mentzelia	Loasaceae	Mentzeliae cordifoliae	Zweigspitzen, Stengel-und-Wurzel
Menyanthes trifoliata	Bogbean	Menyanthaceae	Menyanthis folium	Bitterkleeblätter
Myristica fragrans	Mace	Myristicaceae	Myristica aril	Muskatnußbaum
Myristica fragrans	Nutmeg	Myristicaceae	Myristica fragrans	Muskatnußbaum
Myroxylon balsamum	Peruvian Balsam	Fabaceae	Balsamum peruvianum	Perubalsam
Myroxylon balsamum	Tolu Balsam	Fabaceae	Balsamum tolutanum	Tolubalsam
Nasturtium officinale	Watercress	Brassicaceae	Nasturtii herba	Brunnenkressenkraut
Nerium oleander	Oleander leaf	Apocynaceae	Oleandri folium	Oleanderblätter
Ocimum basilicum	Basil herb	Lamiaceae	Basilici herba	Basilikumkraut
Ocimum basilicum	Basil oil	Lamiaceae	Basilici aetheroleum	Basilikumöl
Olea europaea	Olive leaf	Oleaceae	Oleae folium	Olivenblätter
Olea europaea	Olive oil	Oleaceae	Olivae oleum	Olivenöl
Ononis spinosa	Restharrow root	Fabaceae	Ononidis radix	Hauhechelwurzel
Origanum majorana	Marjoram herb	Lamiaceae	Majoranae herba	Majoran
Origanum majorana	Marjoram oil	Lamiaceae	Majoranae aetheroleum	Majoranöl
Origanum vulgare	Oregano	Lamiaceae	Origani vulgaris herba	Dostenkraut

Botanical	English	Plant Family	Pharmacopeial	German
Orthosiphon spicatus	Java tea	Lamiaceae	Orthosiphonis folium	*Orthosiphonblätter*
Orthosiphon stamineus	Java tea	Lamiaceae	Orthosiphonis folium	*Orthosiphonblätter*
Paeonia mascula	Peony flower	Paeoniaceae	Paeoniae flos	*Pfingstrosenblüten*
Paeonia mascula	Peony root	Paeoniaceae	Paeoniae radix	*Pfingstrosenwurzel*
Paeonia officinalis	Peony flower	Paeoniaceae	Paeoniae flos	*Pfingstrosenblüten*
Paeonia officinalis	Peony root	Paeoniaceae	Paeoniae radix	*Pfingstrosenwurzel*
Panax ginseng	Ginseng root	Araliaceae	Ginseng radix	*Ginsengwurzel*
Papaver rhoeas	Corn Poppy	Papaveraceae	Rhoeados flos	*Klatschmohnblüten*
Passiflora incarnata	Passionflower herb	Passifloraceae	Passiflorae herba	*Passionsblumenkraut*
Pausinystalia johimbe	Yohimbe bark	Rubiaceae	Yohimbehe cortex	*Yohimberinde*
Petasites hybridus	Petasites root	Asteraceae	Petasitidis rhizoma	*Pestwurzwurzelstock*
Petasites spp.	Petasites leaf	Asteraceae	Petasitidis folium	*Pestwurzblätter*
Petroselinum crispum	Parsley herb and root	Apiaceae	Petroselini herba/radix	*Petersilienkraut/wurzel*
Petroselinum crispum	Parsley seed	Apiaceae	Petroselini fructus	*Petersilienfrüchte*
Peumus boldus	Boldo leaf	Monimiaceae	Boldo folium	*Boldoblätter*
Phaseolus vulgaris	Kidney bean pods (without seeds)	Fabaceae	Phaseoli fructus sine semine	*Samenfreie Gartenbohnenhülsen*
Picea abies	Fir Needle oil	Pinaceae	Piceae aetheroleum	*Fichtennadelöl*
Picea abies	White Spruce oil	Pinaceae	Piceae aetheroleum	*Ficthennadelöl*
Picea excelsa	Fir Needle oil	Pinaceae	Piceae aetheroleum	*Fichtennadelöl*
Picea excelsa	White Spruce oil	Pinaceae	Piceae aetheroleum	*Fichtennadelöl*
Pimpinella anisum	Anise	Apiaceae	Anisi fructus	*Anis*
Pimpinella major	Pimpinella herb	Apiaceae	Pimpinellae herba	*Bibernellkraut*
Pimpinella major	Pimpinella root	Apiaceae	Pimpinellae radix	*Bibernellwurzel*
Pimpinella saxifraga	Pimpinella herb	Apiaceae	Pimpinellae herba	*Bibernellkraut*
Pimpinella saxifraga	Pimpinella root	Apiaceae	Pimpinellae radix	*Bibernellwurzel*
Pinus australis	Turpentine oil, Purified	Pinaceae	Terebinthinae aetheroleum rectificatum	*Gereinigtes Terpentinöl*
Pinus mugo	Pine Needle oil	Pinaceae	Pini aetheroleum	*Kiefernnadelöl*
Pinus nigra	Pine Needle oil	Pinaceae	Pini aetheroleum	*Kiefernnadelöl*
Pinus palustris	Turpentine oil, Purified	Pinaceae	Terebinthinae aetheroleum rectificatum	*Gereinigtes Terpentinöl*
Pinus pinaster	Pine Needle oil	Pinaceae	Pini aetheroleum	*Kiefernnadelöl*
Pinus pinaster	Turpentine oil, Purified	Pinaceae	Terebinthinae aetheroleum rectificatum	*Gereinigtes Terpentinöl*

Botanical	English	Plant Family	Pharmacopeial	German
Pinus spp.	Turpentine oil, Purified	Pinaceae	Terebinthinae aetheroleum rectificatum	*Gereinigtes Terpentinöl*
Pinus sylvestris	Pine Needle oil	Pinaceae	Pini aetheroleum	*Kiefernnadelöl*
Pinus sylvestris	Sprouts, Pine	Pinaceae	Pini turiones	*Kiefernsprossen*
Pinus sylvestris	Pine Sprouts	Pinaceae	Pini turiones	*Kiefernsprossen*
Piper methysticum	Kava Kava	Piperaceae	Piperis methystici rhizoma	*Kava-Kava-Wurzelstock*
Plantago afra	Psyllium seed, Black	Plantaginaceae	Psyllii semen	*Flohsamen*
Plantago arenaria	Psyllium seed, Black	Plantaginaceae	Psyllii semen	*Flohsamen*
Plantago indica	Psyllium seed, Black	Plantaginaceae	Psyllii semen	*Flohsamen*
Plantago psyllium	Psyllium seed, Black	Plantaginaceae	Psyllii semen	*Flohsamen*
Plantago isphagula	Psyllium seed, Blonde	Plantaginaceae	Plantaginis ovatae semen	*Indische Flohsamen*
Plantago isphagula	Psyllium seed husk, Blonde	Plantaginaceae	Plantaginis ovatae testa	*Indische Flohsamenschalen*
Plantago lanceolata	English plantain	Plantaginaceae	Plantaginis lanceolatae herba	*Spitzwegerichkraut*
Plantago lanceolata	Plantain	Plantaginaceae	Plantaginis lanceolatae herba	*Spitzwegerichkraut*
Plantago ovata	Psyllium seed, Blonde	Plantaginaceae	Plantaginis ovatae semen	*Indische Flohsamen*
Plantago ovata	Psyllium seed husk, Blonde	Plantaginaceae	Plantaginis ovatae testa	*Indische Flohsamenschalen*
Poa spp.	Hay flower	Poaceae	Graminis flos	*Heublumen*
Podophyllum peltatum	Mayapple resin	Berberidiceae	Podophylli peltati resina	*Podophyllumharz*
Podophyllum peltatum	Mayapple root	Berberidiceae	Podophylli peltati rhizoma	*Podophyllumwurzelstock*
Polygala senega	Senega Snakeroot	Polygalaceae	Polygalae radix	*Senegawurzel*
Polygala senega	Snakeroot, Senega	Polygalaceae	Polygalae radix	*Senegawurzel*
Polygala spp.	Senega Snakeroot	Polygalaceae	Polygalae radix	*Senegawurzel*
Polygala spp.	Snakeroot, Senega	Polygalaceae	Polygalae radix	*Senegawurzel*
Polygonum aviculare	Knotweed	Polygonaceae	Polygoni avicularis herba	*Vogelknöterichkraut*
Populus spp.	Aspen bark	Salicaceae	Populi cortex	*Pappelrinde*
Populus spp.	Aspen leaf	Salicaceae	Populi folium	*Pappelblätter*
Populus spp.	Poplar bud	Salicaceae	Populi gemma	*Pappelknospen*
Populus tremula	Aspen bark	Salicaceae	Populi cortex	*Pappelrinde*
Populus tremula	Aspen leaf	Salicaceae	Populi folium	*Pappelblätter*
Populus tremuloides	Aspen bark	Salicaceae	Populi cortex	*Pappelrinde*
Populus tremuloides	Aspen leaf	Salicaceae	Populi folium	*Pappelblätter*
Potentilla anserina	Potentilla	Rosaceae	Potentillae anserinae herba	*Gänsefingerkraut*
Potentilla anserina	Silverweed	Rosaceae	Potentillae anserinae herba	*Gänsefingerkraut*

Botanical	English	Plant Family	Pharmacopeial	German
Potentilla erecta	Tormentil root	Rosaceae	Tormentillae rhizoma	Tormentillwurzelstock
Potentilla tormentilla	Tormentil root	Rosaceae	Tormentillae rhizoma	Tormentillwurzelstock
Primula elatior	Primrose flower	Primulaceae	Primulae flos	Schlüsselblumenblüten
Primula elatior	Primrose root	Primulaceae	Primulae radix	Primelwurzel
Primula veris	Primrose flower	Primulaceae	Primulae flos	Schlüsselblumenblüten
Primula veris	Primrose root	Primulaceae	Primulae radix	Primelwurzel
Prunus spinosa	Blackthorn berry	Rosaceae	Pruni spinosae fructus	Schlehdornfrüchte
Prunus spinosa	Blackthorn flower	Rosaceae	Pruni spinosae flos	Schlehdornblüten
Prunus spinosa	Sloe berry	Rosaceae	Pruni spinosae fructus	Schlehdornfrüchte
Pterocarpus santalinus	Sandalwood, Red	Fabaceae	Santali lignum rubrum	Rotes Sandelholz
Ptychopetalum olacoides	Muira Puama	Olacaceae	Ptychopetali lignum	Potenzholz
Ptychopetalum unicatum	Muira Puama	Olacaceae	Ptychopetali lignum	Potenzholz
Pulmonaria officinalis	Lungwort	Boraginaceae	Pulmonariae herba	Lungenkraut
Pulsatilla pratensis	Pasque flower	Ranunculaceae	Pulsatillae herba	Küchenschellenkraut
Pulsatilla pratensis	Pulsatilla	Ranunculaceae	Pulsatillae herba	Küchenschellenkraut
Pulsatilla vulgaris	Pasque flower	Ranunculaceae	Pulsatillae herba	Küchenschellenkraut
Pulsatilla vulgaris	Pulsatilla	Ranunculaceae	Pulsatillae herba	Küchenschellenkraut
Quercus petraea	Oak bark	Fagaceae	Quercus cortex	Eichenrinde
Quercus robur	Oak bark	Fagaceae	Quercus cortex	Eichenrinde
Raphanus sativus	Radish	Brassicaceae	Raphani sativi radix	Rettich
Rauvolfia serpentina	Indian Snakeroot	Apocynaceae	Rauwolfiae radix	Rauwolfiawurzel
Rauvolfia serpentina	Snakeroot, Indian	Apocynaceae	Rauwolfiae radix	Rauwolfiawurzel
Rhamnus catharticus	Buckthorn berry	Rhamnaceae	Rhamni cathartici fructus	Kreuzdornbeeren
Rhamnus frangula	Buckthorn bark	Rhamnaceae	Frangulae cortex	Faulbaumrinde
Rhamnus frangula	Frangula	Rhamnaceae	Frangulae cortex	Faulbaumrinde
Rhamnus purshiana	Cascara Sagrada bark	Rhamnaceae	Rhamni purshianae cortex	Amerikanische Faulbaumrinde
Rheum officinale	Rhubarb root	Polygonaceae	Rhei radix	Rhabarber
Rheum palmatum	Rhubarb root	Polygonaceae	Rhei radix	Rhabarber
Rhododendron ferrugineum	Rhododendron, Rusty-leaved	Ericaceae	Rhododendri ferruginei folium	Rostrote Alpenrosenblätter
Rosa centifolia	Rose flower	Rosaceae	Rosae flos	Rosenblüten
Rosa gallica	Rose flower	Rosaceae	Rosae flos	Rosenblüten
Rosa spp.	Rose hip	Rosaceae	Rosae pseudofructus	Hagebuttenschalen

Botanical	English	Plant Family	Pharmacopeial	German
Rosa spp.	Rose hip and seed	Rosaceae	Rosae pseudofructus cum fructibus	*Hagebutten*
Rosa spp.	Rose hip seed	Rosaceae	Rosae fructus	*Hagebuttenkerne*
Rosmarinus officinalis	Rosemary leaf	Lamiaceae	Rosmarini folium	*Rosmarinblätter*
Rubia tinctorum	Madder root	Rubiaceae	Rubiae tinctorum radix	*Krappwurzel*
Rubus fruticosus	Blackberry leaf	Rosaceae	Rubi fruticosi folium	*Brombeerblätter*
Rubus fruticosus	Blackberry root	Rosaceae	Rubi fruticosi radix	*Brombeerwurzel*
Rubus idaeus	Raspberry leaf	Rosaceae	Rubi idaei folium	*Himbeerblätter*
Ruscus aculeatus	Butcher's Broom rhizome	Liliaceae	Rusci aculeati rhizoma	*Mäusedornwurzelstock*
Ruta graveolens	Rue herb	Rutaceae	Rutae herba	*Rautenkraut*
Ruta graveolens	Rue leaf	Rutaceae	Rutae folium	*Rautenblätter*
Sabal serrulata	Saw Palmetto berry	Arecaceae	Sabal fructus	*Sabalfrüchte*
Saccaromyces cerevisiae	Brewer's Yeast	Saccharomycetaceae	Saccharomyces cerevisiae	*Trokenhefe aus Saccharomyces cerevisiae*
Saccaromyces cerevisiae	Brewer's Yeast/Hansen CBS 5926	Saccharomycetaceae	Saccharomyces cerevisiae	*Trokenhefe aus Saccharomyces cerevisiae*
Saccaromyces cerevisiae	Yeast, Brewer's	Saccharomycetaceae	Faex medicinalis	*Medizinische Hefe*
Salix alba	White Willow bark	Salicaceae	Salicis cortex	*Weidenrinde*
Salix fragilis	White Willow bark	Salicaceae	Salicis cortex	*Weidenrinde*
Salix purpurea	White Willow bark	Salicaceae	Salicis cortex	*Weidenrinde*
Salix spp.	White Willow bark	Salicaceae	Salicis cortex	*Weidenrinde*
Salvia officinalis	Sage leaf	Lamiaceae	Salviae folium	*Salbeiblätter*
Sambucus nigra	Elder flower	Caprifoliaceae	Sambuci flos	*Holunderblüten*
Sanicula europaea	Sanicle herb	Apiaceae	Saniculae herba	*Sanikelkraut*
Sanicula europaea	Wood Sanicle	Apiaceae	Saniculae herba	*Sanikelkraut*
Santalum album	Sandalwood, White	Santalaceae	Santali albi lignum	*Weißes Sandelholz*
Santalum album	White Sandalwood	Santalaceae	Santali albi lignum	*Weißes Sandelholz*
Saponaria officinalis	Soapwort herb, Red	Caryophyllaceae	Saponariae rubrae herba	*Seifenkraut*
Saponaria officinalis	Soapwort root, Red	Caryophyllaceae	Saponariae rubrae radix	*Rote Seifenwurzel*
Sarothamnus scoparius	Broom flower, Scotch	Fabaceae	Cytisi scoparius flos	*Besenginsterblüten*
Sarothamnus scoparius	Broom herb, Scotch	Fabaceae	Cytisi scoparius herba	*Besenginsterkraut*
Sarothamnus scoparius	Scotch Broom flower	Fabaceae	Cytisi scoparii flos	*Besenginsterblüten*

Botanical	English	Plant Family	Pharmacopeial	German
Scopolia carniolica	Scopolia root	Solanaceae	Scopolia rhizoma	Glockenbilsenkraut Wurzelstock
Selenicereus grandiflorus	Night-blooming Cereus flower	Cactaceae	Selenicerei grandiflori flos	Königin der Nacht
Selenicereus grandiflorus	Night-blooming Cereus herb	Cactaceae	Selenicerei grandiflori herba	Königin der Nacht
Senecio nemorensis	Senecio herb	Asteraceae	Senecionis herba	Fuchskreuzkraut
Senna alexandrina	Senna leaf	Fabaceae	Sennae folium	Sennesblätter
Senna alexandrina	Senna pod	Fabaceae	Sennae fructus	Sennesfrüchte
Serenoa repens	Saw Palmetto berry	Arecaceae	Sabal fructus	Sabalfrüchte
Silybum marianum	Milk Thistle fruit	Asteraceae	Cardui mariae fructus	Mariendistelfrüchte
Silybum marianum	Milk Thistle herb	Asteraceae	Cardui mariae herba	Mariendistelkraut
Sinapis alba	White Mustard seed	Brassicaceae	Sinapis albae semen	Weiße Senfsamen
Smilax aristolochiaefolii	Sarsaparilla root	Smilacaceae	Sarsaparillae radix	Sarsaparillewurzel
Smilax febrifuga	Sarsaparilla root	Smilacaceae	Sarsaparillae radix	Sarsaparillewurzel
Smilax regelii	Sarsaparilla root	Smilacaceae	Sarsaparillae radix	Sarsaparillewurzel
Solanum dulcamara	Woody Nightshade	Solanaceae	Dulcamarae stipites	Bittersüßstengel
Solidago canadensis	Goldenrod	Asteraceae	Solidago	Goldrute
Solidago gigantea	Goldenrod	Asteraceae	Solidago	Goldrute
Solidago serotina	Goldenrod	Asteraceae	Solidago	Goldrute
Solidago virgaurea	Goldenrod, European	Asteraceae	Solidago virgaureae herba	Echtes Goldrutenkraut
Sorbus aucuparia	Mountain Ash berry	Rosaceae	Sorbi aucupariae fructus	Eberreschenbeeren
Spinacia oleracea	Spinach leaf Spiny	Chenopodiaceae	Spinaciae folium	Spinatblätter
Spiraea ulmaria	Meadowsweet	Rosaceae	Filipendula ulmaria	Mädesüß
Strychnos nux-vomica	Nux Vomica	Loganiaceae	Strychni semen	Brechnußsamen
Symphytum officinale	Comfrey herb	Boraginaceae	Symphyti herba	Beinwellkraut
Symphytum officinale	Comfrey leaf	Boraginaceae	Symphyti folium	Beinwellblätter
Symphytum officinale	Comfrey root	Boraginaceae	Symphyti radix	Beinwellwurzel
Syzygium aromaticum	Cloves	Myrtaceae	Caryophylli flos	Gewürznelken
Syzygium cumini	Jambolan bark	Myrtaceae	Syzygii cumini cortex	Syzygiumrinde
Syzygium cumini	Jambolan seed	Myrtaceae	Syzygii cumini semen	Syzygiumsamen
Syzygium jambolana	Jambolan bark	Myrtaceae	Syzygii cumini cortex	Syzygiumrinde
Syzygium jambolana	Jambolan seed	Myrtaceae	Syzygii cumini semen	Syzygiumsamen
Tanacetum vulgare	Tansy flower	Asteraceae	Chrysanthemi vulgaris flos	Rainfarnblüten

Botanical	English	Plant Family	Pharmacopeial	German
Tanacetum vulgare	Tansy herb	Asteraceae	Chrysanthemi vulgaris herba	*Rainfarnkraut*
Taraxacum officinale	Dandelion herb	Asteraceae	Taraxaci herba	*Löwenzahnkraut*
Taraxacum officinale	Dandelion root with herb	Asteraceae	Taraxaci radix cum herba	*Löwenzahn-wurzel-mit Kraut*
Theobroma cacao	Cocoa	Sterculiaceae	Cacao testes	*Kakaoschalen*
Theobroma cacao	Cocoa seed	Sterculiaceae	Cacao semen	*Kakaosamen*
Thymus serphyllum	Thyme, Wild	Lamiaceae	Serpylli herba	*Quendelkraut*
Thymus vulgaris	Thyme	Lamiaceae	Thymi herba	*Thymiankraut*
Thymus zygis	Thyme	Lamiaceae	Thymi herba	*Thymiankraut*
Tilia argentea	Silver Linden flower	Tiliaceae	Tiliae tomentosae flos	*Silberlindenblüten*
Tilia cordata	Linden charcoal	Tiliaceae	Tiliae carbo	*Lindenholzkohle*
Tilia cordata	Linden flower	Tiliaceae	Tiliae flos	*Lindenblüten*
Tilia cordata	Linden leaf	Tiliaceae	Tiliae folium	*Lindenblätter*
Tilia cordata	Linden wood	Tiliaceae	Tiliae lignum	*Lindenholz*
Tilia platyphyllos	Linden flower	Tiliaceae	Tiliae flos	*Lindenblüten*
Tilia platyphyllos	Linden leaf	Tiliaceae	Tiliae folium	*Lindenblätter*
Tilia platyphyllos	Linden wood	Tiliaceae	Tiliae lignum	*Lindenholz*
Tilia tomentosa	Silver Linden flower	Tiliaceae	Tiliae tomentosae flos	*Silberlindenblüten*
Trigonella foenum-graecum	Fenugreek seed	Fabaceae	Foenugraeci semen	*Bockshornsamen*
Tropaeolum majus	Nasturtium	Tropaeolaceae	Tropaeolum majus	*Kapuzinerkressen-kraut*
Turnera diffusa	Damiana herb	Turneraceae	Turnerae diffusae herba	*Damianakraut*
Turnera diffusa	Damiana leaf	Turneraceae	Turnerae diffusae folium	*Damianablätter*
Tussilago farfara	Coltsfoot flower	Asteraceae	Farfarae flos	*Huflattichblüten*
Tussilago farfara	Coltsfoot herb	Asteraceae	Farfarae herba	*Huflattichkraut*
Tussilago farfara	Coltsfoot leaf	Asteraceae	Farfarae folium	*Huflattichblätter*
Tussilago farfara	Coltsfoot root	Asteraceae	Farfarae radix	*Huflattichwurzel*
Urginea maritima	Squill	Liliaceae	Scillae bulbus	*Meerzwiebel*
Urtica dioica	Nettle herb	Urticaceae	Urticae herba	*Brennesselkraut*
Urtica dioica	Nettle leaf	Urticaceae	Urticae folium	*Brennesselblätter*
Urtica dioica	Nettle root	Urticaceae	Urticae radix	*Brennesselwurzel*
Urtica dioica	Stinging Nettle herb	Urticaceae	Urticae herba	*Brennesselkraut*
Urtica dioica	Stinging Nettle leaf	Urticaceae	Urticae folium	*Brennesselblätter*
Urtica dioica	Stinging Nettle root	Urticaceae	Urticae radix	*Brennesselwurzel*
Urtica urens	Nettle herb	Urticaceae	Urticae herba	*Brennesselkraut*
Urtica urens	Nettle leaf	Urticaceae	Urticae folium	*Brennesselblätter*
Urtica urens	Nettle root	Urticaceae	Urticae radix	*Brennesselwurzel*
Urtica urens	Stinging Nettle herb	Urticaceae	Urticae herba	*Brennesselkraut*

Botanical	English	Plant Family	Pharmacopeial	German
Urtica urens	Stinging Nettle leaf	Urticaceae	Urticae folium	*Brennesselblätter*
Urtica urens	Stinging Nettle root	Urticaceae	Urticae radix	*Brennesselwurzel*
Usnea barbata	Usnea	Usneaceae	Usnea	*Bartflechten*
Usnea florida	Usnea	Usneaceae	Usnea	*Bartflechten*
Usnea hirta	Usnea	Usneaceae	Usnea	*Bartflechten*
Usnea plicata	Usnea	Usneaceae	Usnea	*Bartflechten*
Usnea spp.	Usnea	Usneaceae	Usnea	*Bartflechten*
Vaccinium myrtillus	Bilberry fruit	Ericaceae	Myrtilli fructus	*Heidelbeeren*
Vaccinium myrtillus	Bilberry leaf	Ericaceae	Myrtilli folium	*Heidelbeerblätter*
Vaccinium myrtillus	Blueberry	Ericaceae	Myrtilli fructus	*Heidelbeeren*
Vaccinium myrtillus	Blueberry leaf	Ericaceae	Myrtilli folium	*Heidelbeerblätter*
Valeriana officinalis	Valerian root	Valerianaceae	Valerianae radix	*Baldrianwurzel*
Verbascum densiflorum	Mullein flower	Scrophulariaceae	Verbasci flos	*Wollblumen*
Verbascum thapsus	Mullein flower	Scrophulariaceae	Verbasci flos	*Wollblumen*
Verbena officinalis	Verbena herb	Verbenaceae	Verbenae herba	*Eisenkraut*
Veronica officinalis	Speedwell	Scrophulariaceae	Veronicae herba	*Ehrenpreiskraut*
Veronica officinalis	Veronica herb	Scrophulariaceae	Veronicae herba	*Ehrenpreiskraut*
Vinca minor	Periwinkle	Apocynaceae	Vincae minoris herba	*Immergrünkraut*
Viola odorata	Sweet Violet root and herb	Violaceae	Violae odoratae rhizoma and herba	*Märzveilchen/blüten*
Viola tricolor	Heart's Ease herb	Violaceae	Violae tricoloris herba	*Stiefmütterchenkraut*
Viola tricolor	Johnny Jump-Up	Violaceae	Violae tricoloris	*Stiefmütterchenkraut*
Viscum album	Mistletoe berry	Viscaceae	Visci albi fructus	*Mistelfrüchte*
Viscum album	Mistletoe herb	Viscaceae	Visci albi herba	*Mistelkraut*
Viscum album	Mistletoe stem	Viscaceae	Visci albi stipitis	*Mistelstengel*
Vitex agnus castus	Chaste Tree fruit	Verbenaceae	Agni casti fructus	*Keuschlammfrüchte*
Xysmalobium undulatum	Uzara root	Asclepiadaceae	Uzarae radix	*Uzarawurzel*
Zingiber officinale	Ginger root	Zingiberaceae	Zingiberis rhizoma	*Ingwerwurzelstock*

By Pharmacopeial Name

Pharmacopeial	English	Botanical	Plant Family	German
Absinthii herba	Wormwood	*Artemisia absinthium*	Asteraceae	*Wermutkraut*
Aconiti herba	Aconite herb	*Aconitum napellus*	Ranunculaceae	*Blauer Eisenhutkraut*
Aconiti herba	Blue Monkshood herb	*Aconitum napellus*	Ranunculaceae	*Blauer Eisenhutkraut*
Aconiti herba	Monkshood herb	*Aconitum napellus*	Ranunculaceae	*Blauer Eisenhutkraut*
Aconiti tuber	Aconite tuber	*Aconitum napellus*	Ranunculaceae	*Blauer Eisenhutwurzel*

Pharmacopeial	English	Botanical	Plant Family	German
Aconiti tuber	Blue Monkshood tuber	*Aconiti napellus*	Ranunculaceae	*Blauer Eisenhutwurzel*
Aconiti tuber	Monkshood root	*Aconiti napellus*	Ranunculaceae	*Blauer Eisenhutwurzel*
Adonidis herba	Pheasant's Eye herb	*Adonis vernalis*	Ranunculaceae	*Adoniskraut*
Agni casti fructus	Chaste Tree fruit	*Vitex agnus castus*	Verbenaceae	*Keuschlammfrüchte*
Agrimoniae herba	Agrimony	*Agrimonia eupatoria*	Rosaceae	*Odermennigkraut*
Agrimoniae herba	Cocklebur	*Agrimonia eupatoria*	Rosaceae	*Odermennigkraut*
Agrimoniae herba	Agrimony	*Agrimonia procera*	Rosaceae	*Odermennigkraut*
Agrimoniae herba	Cocklebur	*Agrimonia procera*	Rosaceae	*Odermennigkraut*
Alchemillae alpinae herba	Alpine Lady's Mantle herb	*Alchemilla alpina*	Rosaceae	*Frauenmantelkraut*
Alchemillae herba	Lady's Mantle	*Alchemilla vulgaris*	Rosaceae	*Frauenmantelkraut*
Allii cepae bulbus	Onion	*Allium cepa*	Alliaceae	*Zwiebel*
Allii sativi bulbus	Garlic	*Allium sativum*	Alliaceae	*Knoblauch*
Aloe barbadensis	Aloe	*Aloe barbadensis*	Liliaceae	*Aloe*
Aloe barbadensis	Curaçao aloe	*Aloe barbadensis*	Liliaceae	*Curaçao-Aloe*
Aloe barbadensis	Aloe	*Aloe vera*	Liliaceae	*Aloe*
Aloe barbadensis	Curaçao aloe	*Aloe vera*	Liliaceae	*Curaçao-Aloe*
Aloe capensis	Aloe	*Aloe ferox*	Liliaceae	*Kap-Aloe*
Aloe capensis	Cape aloe	*Aloe ferox*	Liliaceae	*Kap-Aloe*
Althaeae folium	Marshmallow leaf	*Althaea officinalis*	Malvaceae	*Eibischblätter*
Althaeae radix	Marshmallow root	*Althaea officinalis*	Malvaceae	*Eibischwurzel*
Ammeos visnagae fructus	Bishop's Weed fruit	*Ammi daucoides*	Apiaceae	*Ammi-visnaga-Früchte*
Ammeos visnagae fructus	Bishop's Weed fruit	*Ammi visnaga*	Apiaceae	*Ammi-visnaga-Früchte*
Anethi fructus	Dill seed	*Anethum graveolens*	Apiaceae	*Dillfrüchte*
Anethi herba	Dill herb	*Anethum graveolens*	Apiaceae	*Dillkraut*
Angelicae fructus	Angelica seed	*Angelica archangelica*	Apiaceae	*Angelikafrüchte*
Angelicae herba	Angelica herb	*Angelica archangelica*	Apiaceae	*Angelikakraut*
Angelicae radix	Angelica root	*Angelica archangelica*	Apiaceae	*Angelikawurzel*
Anisi fructus	Anise	*Pimpinella anisum*	Apiaceae	*Anis*
Anisi stellati	Star Anise	*Illicium verum*	Illiciaceae	*Sternanis*
Antennariae dioicae flos	Cat's Ear flower	*Antennaria dioica*	Asteraceae	*Katzenpfötchenblüten*
Antennariae dioicae flos	Cat's Foot flower	*Antennaria dioica*	Asteraceae	*Katzenpfötchenblüten*
Apii fructus	Celery seed	*Apium graveolens*	Apiaceae	*Selleriefrüchte*
Apii herba	Celery herb	*Apium graveolens*	Apiaceae	*Selleriekraut*
Apii radix	Celery root	*Apium graveolens*	Apiaceae	*Selleriewurzel*
Apium graveolens	Celery	*Apium graveolens*	Apiaceae	*Sellerie*
Armoraciae rusticanae radix	Horseradish	*Armoracia rusticana*	Brassicaceae	*Meerrettich*
Armoraciae rusticanae radix	Horseradish	*Cochlearia armoracia*	Brassicaceae	*Meerrettich*
Arnicae flos	Arnica flower	*Arnica chamissonis*	Asteraceae	*Arnikablüten*
Arnicae flos	Arnica flower	*Arnica montana*	Asteraceae	*Arnikablüten*

Pharmacopeial	English	Botanical	Plant Family	German
Artemisiae vulgaris herba	Mugwort herb	*Artemisia vulgaris*	Asteraceae	*Beifußkraut*
Artemisiae vulgaris radix	Mugwort root	*Artemisia vulgaris*	Asteraceae	*Beifußwurzel*
Asparagi herba	Asparagus herb	*Asparagus officinalis*	Liliaceae	*Spargelkraut*
Asparagi rhizoma	Asparagus root	*Asparagus officinalis*	Liliaceae	*Spargelwurzelstock*
Aurantii flos	Bitter Orange flower	*Citrus aurantium*	Rutaceae	*Pomeranzenblüten*
Aurantii flos aetheroleum	Bitter Orange flower oil	*Citrus aurantium*	Rutaceae	*Pomeranzenblütenöl*
Aurantii pericarpium	Bitter Orange peel	*Citrus aurantium*	Rutaceae	*Pomeranzenschale*
Avenae fructus	Oats	*Avena sativa*	Poaceae	*Haferfrüchte*
Avenae herba	Oat herb	*Avena sativa*	Poaceae	*Haferkraut*
Avenae herba	Wild Oat herb	*Avena sativa*	Poaceae	*Haferkraut*
Avenae stramentum	Oat straw	*Avena sativa*	Poaceae	*Haferstroh*
Balsamum peruvianum	Peruvian Balsam	*Myroxylon balsamum*	Fabaceae	*Perubalsam*
Balsamum tolutanum	Tolu Balsam	*Myroxylon balsamum*	Fabaceae	*Tolubalsam*
Bardanae radix	Burdock root	*Arctium lappa*	Asteraceae	*Klettenwurzel*
Bardanae radix	Burdock root	*Arctium minus*	Asteraceae	*Klettenwurzel*
Bardanae radix	Burdock root	*Arctium tomentosum*	Asteraceae	*Klettenwurzel*
Barosmae folium	Buchu leaf	*Agathosma betulina*	Rutaceae	*Buccoblätter*
Barosmae folium	Buchu leaf	*Barosma betulina*	Rutaceae	*Buccoblätter*
Basilici aetheroleum	Basil oil	*Ocimum basilicum*	Lamiaceae	*Basilikumöl*
Basilici herba	Basil herb	*Ocimum basilicum*	Lamiaceae	*Basilikumkraut*
Belladonnae folium	Belladonna leaf	*Atropa belladonna*	Solanaceae	*Tollkirsche*
Belladonnae folium	Deadly Nightshade leaf	*Atropa belladonna*	Solanaceae	*Tollkirsche*
Belladonnae radix	Belladonna root	*Atropa belladonna*	Solanaceae	*Tollkirschewurzel*
Belladonnae radix	Deadly Nightshade root	*Atropa belladonna*	Solanaceae	*Tollkirschewurzel*
Berberidis cortex	Barberry bark	*Berberis vulgaris*	Berberidaceae	*Berberitze*
Berberidis fructus	Barberry	*Berberis vulgaris*	Berberidaceae	*Berberitze*
Berberidis radicis cortex	Barberry root bark	*Berberis vulgaris*	Berberidaceae	*Berberitzenrinde*
Berberidis radix	Barberry root	*Berberis vulgaris*	Berberidaceae	*Berberitze*
Berberis vulgaris	Barberry	*Berberis vulgaris*	Berberidaceae	*Berberitze*
Betulae folium	Birch leaf	*Betula pendula*	Betulaceae	*Birkenblätter*
Betulae folium	Birch leaf	*Betula pubescens*	Betulaceae	*Birkenblätter*
Boldo folium	Boldo leaf	*Peumus boldus*	Monimiaceae	*Boldoblätter*
Boraginis flos	Borage flower	*Borago officinalis*	Boraginaceae	*Boretsch*
Boraginis herba	Borage herb	*Borago officinalis*	Boraginaceae	*Boretsch*

Pharmacopeial	English	Botanical	Plant Family	German
Bromelainum	Bromelain	*Ananas comosus*	Bromeliaceae	*Ananas*
Bryoniae radix	Bryonia root	*Bryonia alba*	Cucurbitaceae	*Zaunrübenwurzel*
Bryoniae radix	Bryonia root	*Bryonia cretica*	Cucurbitaceae	*Zaunrübenwurzel*
Bursae pastoris herba	Shepherd's Purse	*Capsella bursa pastoris*	Brassicaceae	*Hirtentäschelkraut*
Cacao semen	Cocoa seed	*Theobroma cacao*	Sterculiaceae	*Kakaosamen*
Cacao testes	Cocoa	*Theobroma cacao*	Sterculiaceae	*Kakaoschalen*
Cajuputi aetheroleum	Cajeput oil	*Melaleuca leucodendra*	Myrtaceae	*Cajuputöl*
Calendulae flos	Calendula flower	*Calendula officinalis*	Asteraceae	*Ringelblumenblüten*
Calendulae herba	Calendula herb	*Calendula officinalis*	Asteraceae	*Ringelblumenkraut*
Callunae vulgaris flos	Heather flower	*Calluna vulgaris*	Ericaceae	*Heidekrautblüten*
Callunae vulgaris herba	Heather herb	*Calluna vulgaris*	Ericaceae	*Heidekraut*
Camphora	Camphor	*Cinnamomum camphora*	Lauraceae	*Campher*
Capsicum	Cayenne (Paprika)	*Capsicum frutescens*	Solanaceae	*Paprika*
Capsicum	Paprika (Cayenne)	*Capsicum frutescens*	Solanaceae	*Paprika*
Capsicum	Cayenne (Paprika) species low in capsaicin	*Capsicum spp.*	Solanaceae	*capsaicinarme Paprika-Arten*
Capsicum	Paprika (Cayenne) species low in capsaicin	*Capsicum spp.*	Solanaceae	*capsaicinarme Paprika-Arten*
Cardamomi fructus	Cardamom	*Elettaria cardamomum*	Zingiberaceae	*Kardamomen*
Cardui mariae fructus	Milk Thistle fruit	*Silybum marianum*	Asteraceae	*Mariendistelfrüchte*
Cardui mariae herba	Milk Thistle herb	*Silybum marianum*	Asteraceae	*Mariendistelkraut*
Caricae fructus	Figs	*Ficus carica*	Moraceae	*Feigen*
Caricae papayae folium	Papaya leaf	*Carica papaya*	Caricaceae	*Baummelonenblätter*
Caricis rhizoma	Sarsaparilla root, German	*Carex arenaria*	Cyperaceae	*Sandriedgraswurzelstock*
Carvi aetheroleum	Caraway oil	*Carum carvi*	Apiaceae	*Kümmelöl*
Carvi fructus	Caraway seed	*Carum carvi*	Apiaceae	*Kümmel*
Caryophylli flos	Cloves	*Eugenia caryophyllata*	Myrtaceae	*Gewürznelken*
Caryophylli flos	Cloves	*Jambosa caryophyllus*	Myrtaceae	*Gewürznelken*
Caryophylli flos	Cloves	*Syzygium aromaticum*	Myrtaceae	*Gewürznelken*
Castaneae folium	Chestnut leaf	*Castanea sativa*	Fagaceae	*Kastanienblätter*
Castaneae folium	Chestnut leaf	*Castanea vesca*	Fagaceae	*Kastanienblätter*
Castaneae folium	Chestnut leaf	*Castanea vulgaris*	Fagaceae	*Edelkastanienblätter*
Centaurii herba	Centaury herb	*Centaurium minus*	Gentianaceae	*Tausendgüldenkraut*

Pharmacopeial	English	Botanical	Plant Family	German
Centaurii herba	Centaury herb	Centaurium umbellatum	Gentianaceae	Tausendgüldenkraut
Centaurii herba	Centaury herb	Erythraea centaurium	Gentianaceae	Tausendgüldenkraut
Chamomillae romanae flos	Chamomile, Roman	Anthemis nobilis	Asteraceae	Römische Kamillenblüten
Chamomillae romanae flos	Chamomile, Roman	Chamaemelum nobile	Asteraceae	Römische Kamillenblüten
Chelidonii herba	Celandine herb	Chelidonium majus	Papaveraceae	Schöllkraut
Chrysanthemi vulgaris flos	Tansy flower	Chrysanthemum vulgare	Asteraceae	Rainfarnblüten
Chrysanthemi vulgaris flos	Tansy flower	Tanacetum vulgare	Asteraceae	Rainfarnblüten
Chrysanthemi vulgaris herba	Tansy herb	Chrysanthemum vulgare	Asteraceae	Rainfarnkraut
Chrysanthemi vulgaris herba	Tansy herb	Tanacetum vulgare	Asteraceae	Rainfarnkraut
Cichorium intybus	Chicory	Cichorium intybus	Asteraceae	Wegwarte
Cimicifugae racemosae rhizoma	Black Cohosh root	Cimicifuga racemosa	Ranunculaceae	Cimicifugawurzelstock
Cinchonae cortex	Cinchona bark	Cinchona pubescens	Rubiaceae	Chinarinde
Cinchonae cortex	Cinchona bark	Cinchona succirubra	Rubiaceae	Chinarinde
Cinnamomi cassiae cortex	Cinnamon bark, Chinese	Cinnamomum aromaticum	Lauraceae	Chinesischer Zimt
Cinnamomi cassiae cortex	Cinnamon bark, Chinese	Cinnamomum cassia	Lauraceae	Chinesischer Zimt
Cinnamomi ceylanici cortex	Cinnamon	Cinnamomum verum	Lauraceae	Zimtrinde
Cinnamomi ceylanici cortex	Cinnamon	Cinnamomum zeylanicum	Lauraceae	Zimtrinde
Cinnamomi flos	Cinnamon flower	Cinnamomum aromaticum	Lauraceae	Zimtblüten
Cinnamomi flos	Cinnamon flower	Cinnamomum cassia	Lauraceae	Zimtblüten
Citri sinensis pericarpium	Orange peel	Citrus sinensis	Rutaceae	Orangenschalen
Cnici benedicti herba	Blessed Thistle herb	Cnicus benedictus	Asteraceae	Benediktenkraut
Coffeae carbo	Coffee charcoal	Coffea arabica	Rubiaceae	Kaffeekohle
Coffeae carbo	Coffee charcoal	Coffea canephora	Rubiaceae	Kaffeekohle
Coffeae carbo	Coffee charcoal	Coffea liberica	Rubiaceae	Kaffeekohle
Coffeae carbo	Coffee charcoal	Coffea spp.	Rubiaceae	Kaffeekohle
Colae semen	Cola nut	Cola nitida	Sterculiaceae	Kolasamen
Colae semen	Cola nut	Cola spp.	Sterculiaceae	Kolasamen
Colchicum, Colchicum autumnale	Autumn Crocus	Colchicum autumnale	Liliaceae	Herbstzeitlose
Colchicum, Colchicum autumnale	Meadow saffron	Colchicum autumnale	Liliaceae	Herbstzeitlose

Pharmacopeial	English	Botanical	Plant Family	German
Colocynthidis fructus	Colocynth	*Citrullus colocynthis*	Cucurbitaceae	*Koloquinthen*
Condurango cortex	Condurango bark	*Marsdenia condurango*	Asclepiadaceae	*Condurangorinde*
Convallariae herba	Lily-of-the-valley herb	*Convallaria majalis*	Liliaceae	*Maiglöckchenkraut*
Coriandri fructus	Coriander	*Coriandrum sativum*	Apiaceae	*Koriander*
Crataegi flos	Hawthorn flower	*Crataegus laevigata*	Rosaceae	*Weißdornblätter*
Crataegi flos	Hawthorn flower	*Crataegus monogyna*	Rosaceae	*Weißdornblätter*
Crataegi folium	Hawthorn leaf	*Crataegus laevigata*	Rosaceae	*Weißdornblätter*
Crataegi folium	Hawthorn leaf	*Crataegus monogyna*	Rosaceae	*Weißdornblätter*
Crataegi folium cum flore	Hawthorn leaf with flower	*Crataegus laevigata*	Rosaceae	*Weißdornblätter mit Blüten*
Crataegi folium cum flore	Hawthorn leaf with flower	*Crataegus monogyna*	Rosaceae	*Weißdornblätter mit Blüten*
Crataegi fructus	Hawthorn berry	*Crataegus laevigata*	Rosaceae	*Weißdornfrüchte*
Crataegi fructus	Hawthorn berry	*Crataegus monogyna*	Rosaceae	*Weißdornfrüchte*
Croci stigma	Saffron	*Crocus sativa*	Iridaceae	*Safran*
Cucurbitae peponis semen	Pumpkin seed	*Cucurbita pepo*	Cucurbitaceae	*Kürbissamen*
Curcumae longae rhizoma	Turmeric root	*Curcuma aromatica*	Zingiberaceae	*Curcumawurzelstock*
Curcumae longae rhizoma	Turmeric root	*Curcuma domestica*	Zingiberaceae	*Curcumawurzelstock*
Curcumae longae rhizoma	Turmeric root	*Curcuma longa*	Zingiberaceae	*Curcumawurzestock*
Curcumae xanthorrhizae rhizoma	Turmeric, Javanese	*Curcuma xanthorrhiza*	Zingiberaceae	*Javanische Gelbwurzel*
Cyani flos	Cornflower	*Centaurea cyanus*	Asteraceae	*Kornblume*
Cymbopoginis citrati aetheroleum	West Indian Lemongrass oil	*Cymbopogon citratus*	Poaceae	*Cymbopogon-Arten*
Cymbopoginis citrati herba	West Indian Lemongrass	*Cymbopogon citratus*	Poaceae	*Cymbopogon-Arten*
Cymbopoginis nardi herba	Ceylon Citronella grass	*Cymbopogon nardus*	Poaceae	*Cymbopogon-Arten*
Cymbopoginis winteriani aetheroleum	Java citronella oil	*Cymbopogon winterianus*	Poaceae	*Cymbopogon-Arten*
Cymbopogon species	Citronella	*Cymbopogon citratus*	Poaceae	*Cymbopogon-Arten*
Cymbopogon species	Citronella	*Cymbopogon nardus*	Poaceae	*Cymbopogon-Arten*
Cymbopogon species	Cymbopogon	*Cymbopogon spp.*	Poaceae	*Cymbopogon-Arten*
Cymbopogon species	Citronella	*Cymbopogon winterianus*	Poaceae	*Cymbopogon-Arten*
Cynarae folium	Artichoke leaf	*Cynara scolymus*	Asteraceae	*Artischokenblätter*
Cynoglossi herba	Hound's Tongue herb	*Cynoglossum clandestinum*	Boraginaceae	*Hundszungenkraut*

Pharmacopeial	English	Botanical	Plant Family	German
Cynoglossi herba	Hound's Tongue herb	Cynoglossum officinale	Boraginaceae	Hundszungenkraut
Cytisi scoparii flos	Scotch Broom flower	Cytisus scoparius	Fabaceae	Besenginsterblüten
Cytisi scoparii flos	Scotch Broom flower	Sarothamnus scoparius	Fabaceae	Besenginsterblüten
Cytisi scoparii herba	Scotch Broom herb	Cytisus scoparius	Fabaceae	Besenginsterkraut
Cytisi scoparius flos	Broom flower, Scotch	Cytisus scoparius	Fabaceae	Besenginsterblüten
Cytisi scoparius flos	Broom flower, Scotch	Sarothamnus scoparius	Fabaceae	Besenginsterblüten
Cytisi scoparius herba	Broom herb, Scotch	Cytisus scoparius	Fabaceae	Besenginsterkraut
Cytisi scoparius herba	Broom herb, Scotch	Sarothamnus scoparius	Fabaceae	Besenginsterkraut
Delphinii flos	Delphinium flower	Delphinium consolida	Ranunculaceae	Ritterspornblüten
Droserae herba	Sundew	Drosera intermedia	Droseraceae	Sonnentaukraut
Droserae herba	Sundew	Drosera longifolia	Droseraceae	Sonnentaukraut
Droserae herba	Sundew	Drosera ramentacea	Droseraceae	Sonnentaukraut
Droserae herba	Sundew	Drosera rotundifolia	Droseraceae	Sonnentaukraut
Dulcamarae stipites	Woody Nightshade	Solanum dulcamara	Solanaceae	Bittersüßstengel
Echinaceae angustifoliae herba	Echinacea Angustifolia herb	Echinacea angustifolia	Asteraceae	schmalblättriges Sonnenhutkraut
Echinaceae angustifoliae radix	Echinacea Angustifolia root	Echinacea angustifolia	Asteraceae	schmalblättriges Sonnenhutwurzel
Echinaceae pallidae herba	Echinacea Pallida herb	Echinacea pallida	Asteraceae	Blasses Kegelblumenkraut
Echinaceae pallidae radix	Echinacea Pallida root	Echinacea pallida	Asteraceae	Echinacea-pallida Wurzel
Echinaceae purpureae herba	Echinacea Purpurea herb	Echinacea purpurea	Asteraceae	Purpursonnenhut-kraut
Echinaceae purpureae herba	Purple Coneflower herb	Echinacea purpurea	Asteraceae	Purpursonnenhut-kraut
Echinaceae purpureae radix	Echinacea Purpurea root	Echinacea purpurea	Asteraceae	Purpursonnenhut-wurzel
Echinaceae purpureae radix	Purple Coneflower root	Echinacea purpurea	Asteraceae	Purpursonnenhut-wurzel
Eleutherococci radix	Eleuthero root	Acanthopanax senticosus	Araliaceae	Eleutherococcus-senticosus-Wurzel
Eleutherococci radix	Eleuthero root	Eleutherococcus senticosus	Araliaceae	Eleutherococcus-senticosus-Wurzel
Eleutherococci radix	Siberian Ginseng	Acanthopanax senticosus	Araliaceae	Eleutherococcus-senticosus-Wurzel
Eleutherococci radix	Siberian Ginseng	Eleutherococcus senticosus	Araliaceae	Eleutherococcus-senticosus-Wurzel
Ephedrae herba	Ephedra	Ephedra shennungiana	Ephedraceae	Ephedrakraut
Ephedrae herba	Ephedra	Ephedra sinica	Ephedraceae	Ephedrakraut
Equiseti herba	Horsetail herb	Equisetum arvense	Equisetaceae	Schachtelhalmkraut

Pharmacopeial	English	Botanical	Plant Family	German
Eschscholziae	California Poppy	Eschscholzia californica	Papaveraceae	Kalifornischer Goldmohn
Eucalypti aetheroleum	Eucalyptus oil	Eucalyptus fructicetorum	Myrtaceae	Eucalyptusöl
Eucalypti aetheroleum	Eucalyptus oil	Eucalyptus globulus	Myrtaceae	Eucalyptusöl
Eucalypti aetheroleum	Eucalyptus oil	Eucalyptus polybractea	Myrtaceae	Eucalyptusöl
Eucalypti aetheroleum	Eucalyptus oil	Eucalyptus smithii	Myrtaceae	Eucalyptusöl
Eucalypti folium	Eucalyptus leaf	Eucalyptus globulus	Myrtaceae	Eucalyptusblätter
Euphrasiae	Eyebright herb	Euphrasia officinalis	Scrophulariaceae	Augentrostkraut
Faex medicinalis	Yeast, Brewer's	Candida utilis	Cryptococcaeae	Medizinische Hefe
Faex medicinalis	Yeast, Brewer's	Saccharomyces cerevisiae	Saccharomycetaceae	Medizinische Hefe
Farfarae flos	Coltsfoot flower	Tussilago farfara	Asteraceae	Huflattichblüten
Farfarae folium	Coltsfoot leaf	Tussilago farfara	Asteraceae	Huflattichblätter
Farfarae herba	Coltsfoot herb	Tussilago farfara	Asteraceae	Huflattichkraut
Farfarae radix	Coltsfoot root	Tussilago farfara	Asteraceae	Huflattichwurzel
Filicis maris folium	Male fern leaf	Dryopteris filix-mas	Aspleniaceae	Wurmfarmblätter
Filicis maris herba	Male fern herb	Dryopteris filix-mas	Aspleniaceae	Wurmfarmkraut
Filicis maris rhizoma	Male fern rhizome	Dryopteris filix-mas	Aspleniaceae	Wurmfarmwurzelstock
Filipendula ulmaria	Meadowsweet	Filipendula ulmaria	Rosaceae	Mädesüß
Filipendula ulmaria	Meadowsweet	Spiraea ulmaria	Rosaceae	Mädesüß
Foeniculi aetheroleum	Fennel oil	Foeniculum vulgare	Apiaceae	Fenchelöl
Foeniculi fructus	Fennel seed	Foeniculum vulgare	Apiaceae	Fenchel
Foenugraeci semen	Fenugreek seed	Trigonella foenum-graecum	Fabaceae	Bockshornsamen
Fragariae folium	Strawberry leaf	Fragaria vesca	Rosaceae	Erdbeerblätter
Fragariae folium	Strawberry leaf	Fragaria viridis	Rosaceae	Erdbeerblätter
Frangulae cortex	Buckthorn bark	Frangula alnus	Rhamnaceae	Faulbaumrinde
Frangulae cortex	Frangula	Frangula alnus	Rhamnaceae	Faulbaumrinde
Frangulae cortex	Buckthorn bark	Rhamnus frangula	Rhamnaceae	Faulbaumrinde
Frangulae cortex	Frangula	Rhamnus frangula	Rhamnaceae	Faulbaumrinde
Fraxini cortex	Ash bark	Fraxinus excelsior	Oleaceae	Esche
Fraxini folium	Ash leaf	Fraxinus excelsior	Oleaceae	Esche
Fucus	Bladderwrack	Ascophyllum nodosum	Fucaceae	Tang
Fucus	Bladderwrack	Fucus vesiculosus	Fucaceae	Tang
Fumariae herba	Fumitory	Fumaria officinalis	Fumariaceae	Erdrauchkraut
Galangae rhizoma	Galangal	Alpinia officinarum	Zingiberaceae	Galangtwurzelstock

Pharmacopeial	English	Botanical	Plant Family	German
Galegae officinalis herba	Goat's Rue herb	Galega officinalis	Fabaceae	Geißrautenkraut
Galeopsidis herba	Hempnettle herb	Galeopsis ochroleuca	Lamiaceae	Hohlzahnkraut
Galeopsidis herba	Hempnettle herb	Galeopsis segetum	Lamiaceae	Hohlzahnkraut
Galii odorati herba	Sweet Woodruff	Galium odoratum	Rubiaceae	Waldmeisterkraut
Gelsemii rhizoma	Yellow Jessamine	Gelsemium sempervirens	Loganiaceae	Gelsemiumwurzelstock
Gentianae radix	Gentian root	Gentiana lutea	Gentianaceae	Enzianwurzel
Ginkgo folium	Ginkgo Biloba leaf	Ginkgo biloba	Ginkgoaceae	Ginkgoblätter
Ginkgo folium	Ginkgo Biloba leaf Extract	Ginkgo biloba	Ginkgoaceae	Ginkgo biloba Blätter
Ginseng radix	Ginseng root	Panax ginseng	Araliaceae	Ginsengwurzel
Graminis flos	Hay flower	Poa spp.	Poaceae	Heublumen
Graminis rhizoma	Couch grass	Agropyron repens	Poaceae	Queckenwurzelstock
Grindeliae herba	Gumweed herb	Grindelia robusta	Asteraceae	Grindeliakraut
Grindeliae herba	Gumweed herb	Grindelia squarrosa	Asteraceae	Grindeliakraut
Guaiaci lignum	Guaiac wood	Guaiacum officinale	Zygophyllaceae	Guajakholz
Guaiaci lignum	Guaiac wood	Guaiacum sanctum	Zygophyllaceae	Guajakholz
Gypsophilae radix	Soapwort root, White	Gypsophila paniculata	Caryophyllaceae	Wieße Seifenwurzel
Gypsophilae radix	Soapwort root, White	Gypsophila spp.	Caryophyllaceae	Wieße Seifenwurzel
Gypsophilae radix	White Soapwort root	Gypsophila paniculata	Caryophyllaceae	Wieße Seifenwurzel
Gypsophilae radix	White Soapwort root	Gypsophila spp.	Caryophyllaceae	Wieße Seifenwurzel
Hamamelidis cortex	Witch Hazel bark	Hamamelis virginiana	Hamamelidaceae	Hamamelisrinde
Hamamelidis folium	Witch Hazel leaf	Hamamelis virginiana	Hamamelidaceae	Hamamelisblätter
Harpagophyti radix	Devil's Claw root	Harpagophytum procumbens	Pedaliaceae	Südafrikanische Teufelskrallenwurzel
Harunganae madagascariensis cortex et folium	Haronga bark and leaf	Harungana madagascariensis	Hypericaceae	Harongarinde
Hederae helicis folium	Ivy leaf	Hedera helix	Araliaceae	Efeublätter
Helenii radix	Elecampane	Inula helenium	Asteraceae	Alantwurzelstock
Helichrysi flos	Sandy Everlasting	Helichrysum arenarium	Asteraceae	Ruhrkrautblüten
Hepatici nobilis herba	Liverwort herb	Hepatica nobilis	Ranunculaceae	Leberblümchenkraut
Herniariae	Rupturewort	Herniaria glabra	Caryophyllaceae	Bruchkraut
Herniariae	Rupturewort	Herniaria hirsuta	Caryophyllaceae	Bruchkraut
Hibisci flos	Hibiscus flower	Hibiscus sabdariffa	Malvaceae	Hibiscusblüten
Hippocastani cortex	Horse Chestnut bark	Aesculus hippocastanum	Hippocastanaceae	Roßkastanienrinde

Pharmacopeial	English	Botanical	Plant Family	German
Hippocastani flos	Horse Chestnut flower	Aesculus hippocastanum	Hippocastanaceae	Roßkastanienblüten
Hippocastani folium	Horse Chestnut leaf	Aesculus hippocastanum	Hippocastanaceae	Roßkastanienblätter
Hippocastani semen	Horse Chestnut seed	Aesculus hippocastanum	Hippocastanaceae	Roßkastiensamen
Hyoscyami folium	Henbane leaf	Hyoscyamus niger	Solanaceae	Hyoscyamusblätter
Hyperici herba	St. John's Wort	Hypericum perforatum	Hypericaceae	Johanniskraut
Hyssopi aetheroleum	Hyssop oil	Hyssopus officinalis	Lamiaceae	Ysopöl
Hyssopi herba	Hyssop herb	Hyssopus officinalis	Lamiaceae	Ysopkraut
Iridis rhizoma	Orris root	Iris florentina [Iris germanica var. florentina]	Iridaceae	Schwertlilienwurzelstock
Iridis rhizoma	Orris root	Iris germanica	Iridaceae	Schwertlilienwurzelstock
Iridis rhizoma	Orris root	Iris pallida	Iridaceae	Schwertlilienwurzelstock
Juglandis folium	Walnut leaf	Juglans regia	Juglandaceae	Walnußblätter
Juglandis fructus cortex	Walnut hull	Juglans regia	Juglandaceae	Walnußfrüchtschalen
Juniperi fructus	Juniper berry	Juniperus communis	Cupressaceae	Wacholderbeeren
Lamii albi flos	White Dead Nettle flower	Lamium album	Lamiaceae	Weiße Taubnesselbüten
Lamii albi herba	White Dead Nettle herb	Lamium album	Lamiaceae	Weißes Taubnesselkraut
Laminariae stipites	Kelp	Laminaria cloustonii	Laminariaceae	Laminariastiele
Laminariae stipites	Kelp	Laminaria hyperborea	Laminariaceae	Laminariastiele
Lavandulae flos	Lavender flower	Lavandula angustifolia	Lamiaceae	Lavendelblüten
Lecithin ex soja	Soy Lecithin	Glycine max	Fabaceae	Sojalecithin
Ledi palustris herba	Marsh Tea	Ledum palustre	Lamiaceae	Sumpfporstkraut
Leonuri cardiacae herba	Motherwort herb	Leonurus cardiaca	Lamiaceae	Herzgespannkraut
Levistici radix	Lovage root	Levisticum officinale	Apiaceae	Liebstöckelwurzel
Lichen islandicus	Iceland Moss	Cetraria islandica	Parmeliaceae	Isländisches Moos
Lini semen	Flaxseed	Linum usitatissimum	Linaceae	Leinsamen
Liquiritiae radix	Licorice root	Glycyrrhiza glabra	Fabaceae	Süßholzwurzel
Luffa aegyptiaca	Loofa	Luffa aegyptiaca	Cucurbitaceae	Luffaschwamm
Luffa aegyptiaca	Sponge cucumber	Luffa aegyptiaca	Cucurbitaceae	Luffaschwamm
Lupuli strobulus	Hops	Humulus lupulus	Moraceae	Hopfenzapfen
Lycopi herba	Bugleweed	Lycopus europaeus	Lamiaceae	Wolfstrappkraut
Lycopi herba	Bugleweed	Lycopus virginicus	Lamiaceae	Wolfstrappkraut
Majoranae aetheroleum	Marjoram oil	Majorana hortensis	Lamiaceae	Majoranöl

Pharmacopeial	English	Botanical	Plant Family	German
Majoranae aetheroleum	Marjoram oil	*Origanum majorana*	Lamiaceae	Majoranöl
Majoranae herba	Marjoram herb	*Majorana hortensis*	Lamiaceae	Majoran
Majoranae herba	Marjoram herb	*Origanum majorana*	Lamiaceae	Majoran
Malvae arboreae flos	Hollyhock flower	*Alcea rosea*	Malvaceae	Stockrosenblüten
Malvae arboreae flos	Hollyhock flower	*Althaea rosea*	Malvaceae	Stockrosenblüten
Malvae flos	Blue Mallow flower	*Malva sylvestris*	Malvaceae	Malvenblüten
Malvae flos	Mallow flower	*Malva sylvestris*	Malvaceae	Malvenblüten
Malvae folium	Mallow leaf	*Malva sylvestris*	Malvaceae	Malvenblätter
Manna	Manna	*Fraxinus ornus*	Oleaceae	Manna
Marrubii herba	Horehound herb	*Marrubium vulgare*	Lamiaceae	Andornkraut
Mate folium	Maté	*Ilex paraguariensis*	Aquifoliaceae	Mateblätter
Matricariae flos	Chamomile, German	*Chamomilla recutita*	Asteraceae	Kamilenblüten
Matricariae flos	Chamomile, German	*Matricaria recutita*	Asteraceae	Kamilenblüten
Meliloti herba	Sweet clover	*Melilotus altissimus*	Fabaceae	Steinkleekraut
Meliloti herba	Sweet clover	*Melilotus officinalis*	Fabaceae	Steinkleekraut
Melissae folium	Lemon balm	*Melissa officinalis*	Lamiaceae	Melissenblätter
Menthae arvensis aetheroleum	Mint oil	*Mentha arvensis*	Lamiaceae	Minzöl
Menthae piperitae aetheroleum	Peppermint oil	*Mentha x piperita*	Lamiaceae	Pfefferminzöl
Menthae piperitae folium	Peppermint leaf	*Mentha x piperita*	Lamiaceae	Pfefferminzblätter
Mentzeliae cordifoliae	Mentzelia	*Mentzelia cordifolia*	Loasaceae	Zweigspitzen, Stengel-und-Wurzel
Menyanthis folium	Bogbean	*Menyanthes trifoliata*	Menyanthaceae	Bitterkleeblätter
Millefolii flos	Yarrow flower	*Achillea millefolium*	Asteraceae	Schafgarbe
Millefolii herba	Yarrow herb	*Achillea millefolium*	Asteraceae	Schafgarbenkraut
Myristica aril	Mace	*Myristica fragrans*	Myristicaceae	Muskatnußbaum
Myristica fragrans	Nutmeg	*Myristica fragrans*	Myristicaceae	Muskatnußbaum
Myrrha	Myrrh	*Commiphora molmol*	Burseraceae	Myrrhe
Myrtilli folium	Bilberry leaf	*Vaccinium myrtillus*	Ericaceae	Heidelbeerblätter
Myrtilli folium	Blueberry leaf	*Vaccinium myrtillus*	Ericaceae	Heidelbeerblätter
Myrtilli fructus	Bilberry fruit	*Vaccinium myrtillus*	Ericaceae	Heidelbeeren
Myrtilli fructus	Blueberry	*Vaccinium myrtillus*	Ericaceae	Heidelbeeren
Nasturtii herba	Watercress	*Nasturtium officinale*	Brassicaceae	Brunnenkressenkraut
Niauli aetheroleum	Niauli oil	*Melaleuca viridiflora*	Myrtaceae	Niauliöl
Oleae folium	Olive leaf	*Olea europaea*	Oleaceae	Olivenblätter
Oleandri folium	Oleander leaf	*Nerium oleander*	Apocynaceae	Oleanderblätter
Olivae oleum	Olive oil	*Olea europaea*	Oleaceae	Olivenöl
Ononidis radix	Restharrow root	*Ononis spinosa*	Fabaceae	Hauhechelwurzel
Origani vulgaris herba	Oregano	*Origanum vulgare*	Lamiaceae	Dostenkraut

Pharmacopeial	English	Botanical	Plant Family	German
Orthosiphonis folium	Java tea	*Orthosiphon spicatus*	Lamiaceae	*Orthosiphonblätter*
Orthosiphonis folium	Java tea	*Orthosiphon stamineus*	Lamiaceae	*Orthosiphonblätter*
Paeoniae flos	Peony flower	*Paeonia mascula*	Paeoniaceae	*Pfingstrosenblüten*
Paeoniae flos	Peony flower	*Paeonia officinalis*	Paeoniaceae	*Pfingstrosenblüten*
Paeoniae radix	Peony root	*Paeonia mascula*	Paeoniaceae	*Pfingstrosenwurzel*
Paeoniae radix	Peony root	*Paeonia officinalis*	Paeoniaceae	*Pfingstrosenwurzel*
Papainum crudum	Papain	*Carica papaya*	Caricaceae	*Papain*
Passiflorae herba	Passionflower herb	*Passiflora incarnata*	Passifloraceae	*Passionsblumenkraut*
Petasitidis folium	Petasites leaf	*Petasites* spp.	Asteraceae	*Pestwurzblätter*
Petasitidis rhizoma	Petasites root	*Petasites hybridus*	Asteraceae	*Pestwurzwurzelstock*
Petroselini fructus	Parsley seed	*Petroselinum crispum*	Apiaceae	*Petersilienfrüchte*
Petroselini herba/radix	Parsley herb and root	*Petroselinum crispum*	Apiaceae	*Petersilienkraut/ wurzel*
Phaseoli fructus sine semine	Kidney bean pods (without seeds)	*Phaseolus vulgaris*	Fabaceae	*Samenfreie Gartenbohnenhülsen*
Phospholipide ex soja cum 73 - 79% (3-Sn Phosphatidyl) - cholin	Soy Phospholipid	*Glycine max*	Fabaceae	*Phosphalipide aus Sojabohnen*
Piceae aetheroleum	Fir Needle oil	*Abies alba*	Pinaceae	*Fichtennadelöl*
Piceae aetheroleum	Fir Needle oil	*Abies sachalinensis*	Pinaceae	*Fichtennadelöl*
Piceae aetheroleum	Fir Needle oil	*Abies sibirica*	Pinaceae	*Fichtennadelöl*
Piceae aetheroleum	Fir Needle oil	*Picea abies*	Pinaceae	*Fichtennadelöl*
Piceae aetheroleum	Fir Needle oil	*Picea excelsa*	Pinaceae	*Fichtennadelöl*
Piceae aetheroleum	White Spruce oil	*Abies alba*	Pinaceae	*Ficthennadelöl*
Piceae aetheroleum	White Spruce oil	*Abies sachalinensis*	Pinaceae	*Ficthennadelöl*
Piceae aetheroleum	White Spruce oil	*Abies sibirica*	Pinaceae	*Ficthennadelöl*
Piceae aetheroleum	White Spruce oil	*Picea abies*	Pinaceae	*Ficthennadelöl*
Piceae aetheroleum	White Spruce oil	*Picea excelsa*	Pinaceae	*Fichtennadelöl*
Piceae turiones recentes	Fir shoots, fresh	*Abies alba*	Pinaceae	*Frische Fichtenspitzen*
Pimpinellae herba	Pimpinella herb	*Pimpinella major*	Apiaceae	*Bibernellkraut*
Pimpinellae herba	Pimpinella herb	*Pimpinella saxifraga*	Apiaceae	*Bibernellkraut*
Pimpinellae radix	Pimpinella root	*Pimpinella major*	Apiaceae	*Bibernellwurzel*
Pimpinellae radix	Pimpinella root	*Pimpinella saxifraga*	Apiaceae	*Bibernellwurzel*
Pini aetheroleum	Pine Needle oil	*Pinus mugo*	Pinaceae	*Kiefernnadelöl*
Pini aetheroleum	Pine Needle oil	*Pinus nigra*	Pinaceae	*Kiefernnadelöl*
Pini aetheroleum	Pine Needle oil	*Pinus pinaster*	Pinaceae	*Kiefernnadelöl*
Pini aetheroleum	Pine Needle oil	*Pinus sylvestris*	Pinaceae	*Kiefernnadelöl*
Pini turiones	Pine Sprouts	*Pinus sylvestris*	Pinaceae	*Kiefernsprossen*
Pini turiones	Sprouts, Pine	*Pinus sylvestris*	Pinaceae	*Kiefernsprossen*
Piperis methystici rhizoma	Kava Kava	*Piper methysticum*	Piperaceae	*Kava-Kava-Wurzelstock*
Plantaginis lanceolatae herba	English plantain	*Plantago lanceolata*	Plantaginaceae	*Spitzwegerichkraut*

Pharmacopeial	English	Botanical	Plant Family	German
Plantaginis lanceolatae herba	Plantain	*Plantago lanceolata*	Plantaginaceae	*Spitzwegerichkraut*
Plantaginis ovatae semen	Psyllium seed, Blonde	*Plantago isphagula*	Plantaginaceae	*Indische Flohsamen*
Plantaginis ovatae semen	Psyllium seed, Blonde	*Plantago ovata*	Plantaginaceae	*Indische Flohsamen*
Plantaginis ovatae testa	Psyllium seed husk, Blonde	*Plantago isphagula*	Plantaginaceae	*Indische Flohsamenschalen*
Plantaginis ovatae testa	Psyllium seed husk, Blonde	*Plantago ovata*	Plantaginaceae	*Indische Flohsamenschalen*
Podophylli peltati resina	Mayapple resin	*Podophyllum peltatum*	Berberidiceae	*Podophyllumharz*
Podophylli peltati rhizoma	Mayapple root	*Podophyllum peltatum*	Berberidiceae	*Podophyllumwurzelstock*
Polygalae radix	Senega Snakeroot	*Polygala senega*	Polygalaceae	*Senegawurzel*
Polygalae radix	Senega Snakeroot	*Polygala* spp.	Polygalaceae	*Senegawurzel*
Polygalae radix	Snakeroot, Senega	*Polygala senega*	Polygalaceae	*Senegawurzel*
Polygalae radix	Snakeroot, Senega	*Polygala* spp.	Polygalaceae	*Senegawurzel*
Polygoni avicularis herba	Knotweed	*Polygonum aviculare*	Polygonaceae	*Vogelknöterichkraut*
Populi cortex	Aspen bark	*Populus* spp.	Salicaceae	*Pappelrinde*
Populi cortex	Aspen bark	*Populus tremula*	Salicaceae	*Pappelrinde*
Populi cortex	Aspen bark	*Populus tremuloides*	Salicaceae	*Pappelrinde*
Populi folium	Aspen leaf	*Populus* spp.	Salicaceae	*Pappelblätter*
Populi folium	Aspen leaf	*Populus tremuloides*	Salicaceae	*Pappelblätter*
Populi folium	Aspen leaf	*Populus tremula*	Salicaceae	*Pappelblätter*
Populi gemma	Poplar bud	*Populus* spp.	Salicaceae	*Pappelknospen*
Potentillae anserinae herba	Potentilla	*Potentilla anserina*	Rosaceae	*Gänsefingerkraut*
Potentillae anserinae herba	Silverweed	*Potentilla anserina*	Rosaceae	*Gänsefingerkraut*
Primulae flos	Primrose flower	*Primula elatior*	Primulaceae	*Schlüsselblumenblüten*
Primulae flos	Primrose flower	*Primula veris*	Primulaceae	*Schlüsselblumenblüten*
Primulae radix	Primrose root	*Primula elatior*	Primulaceae	*Primelwurzel*
Primulae radix	Primrose root	*Primula veris*	Primulaceae	*Primelwurzel*
Pruni spinosae flos	Blackthorn flower	*Prunus spinosa*	Rosaceae	*Schlehdornblüten*
Pruni spinosae fructus	Blackthorn berry	*Prunus spinosa*	Rosaceae	*Schlehdornfrüchte*
Pruni spinosae fructus	Sloe berry	*Prunus spinosa*	Rosaceae	*Schlehdornfrüchte*
Psyllii semen	Psyllium seed, Black	*Plantago afra*	Plantaginaceae	*Flohsamen*
Psyllii semen	Psyllium seed, Black	*Plantago arenaria*	Plantaginaceae	*Flohsamen*
Psyllii semen	Psyllium seed, Black	*Plantago indica*	Plantaginaceae	*Flohsamen*
Psyllii semen	Psyllium seed, Black	*Plantago psyllium*	Plantaginaceae	*Flohsamen*

Pharmacopeial	English	Botanical	Plant Family	German
Ptychopetali lignum	Muira Puama	*Ptychopetalum olacoides*	Olacaceae	*Potenzholz*
Ptychopetali lignum	Muira Puama	*Ptychopetalum unicatum*	Olacaceae	*Potenzholz*
Pulmonariae herba	Lungwort	*Pulmonaria officinalis*	Boraginaceae	*Lungenkraut*
Pulsatillae herba	Pasque flower	*Pulsatilla pratensis*	Ranunculaceae	*Küchenschellenkraut*
Pulsatillae herba	Pasque flower	*Pulsatilla vulgaris*	Ranunculaceae	*Küchenschellenkraut*
Pulsatillae herba	Pulsatilla	*Pulsatilla pratensis*	Ranunculaceae	*Küchenschellenkraut*
Pulsatillae herba	Pulsatilla	*Pulsatilla vulgaris*	Ranunculaceae	*Küchenschellenkraut*
Quercus cortex	Oak bark	*Quercus petraea*	Fagaceae	*Eichenrinde*
Quercus cortex	Oak bark	*Quercus robur*	Fagaceae	*Eichenrinde*
Raphani sativi radix	Radish	*Raphanus sativus*	Brassicaceae	*Rettich*
Ratanhiae radix	Rhatany root	*Krameria triandra*	Krameriaceae	*Ratanhiawurzel*
Rauwolfiae radix	Indian Snakeroot	*Rauvolfia serpentina*	Apocynaceae	*Rauwolfiawurzel*
Rauwolfiae radix	Snakeroot, Indian	*Rauvolfia serpentina*	Apocynaceae	*Rauwolfiawurzel*
Rhamni cathartici fructus	Buckthorn berry	*Rhamnus catharticus*	Rhamnaceae	*Kreuzdonnbeeren*
Rhamni purshianae cortex	Cascara Sagrada bark	*Frangula purshiana*	Rhamnaceae	*Amerikanische Faulbaumrinde*
Rhamni purshianae cortex	Cascara Sagrada bark	*Rhamnus purshiana*	Rhamnaceae	*Amerikanische Faulbaumrinde*
Rhei radix	Rhubarb root	*Rheum officinale*	Polygonaceae	*Rhabarber*
Rhei radix	Rhubarb root	*Rheum palmatum*	Polygonaceae	*Rhabarber*
Rhododendri ferruginei folium	Rhododendron, Rusty-leaved	*Rhododendron ferrugineum*	Ericaceae	*Rostrote Alpenrosenblätter*
Rhoeados flos	Corn Poppy	*Papaver rhoeas*	Papaveraceae	*Klatschmohnblüten*
Rosae flos	Rose flower	*Rosa centifolia*	Rosaceae	*Rosenblüten*
Rosae flos	Rose flower	*Rosa gallica*	Rosaceae	*Rosenblüten*
Rosae fructus	Rose hip seed	*Rosa* spp.	Rosaceae	*Hagebuttenkerne*
Rosae pseudofructus	Rose hip	*Rosa* spp.	Rosaceae	*Hagebuttenschalen*
Rosae pseudofructus cum fructibus	Rose hip and seed	*Rosa* spp.	Rosaceae	*Hagebutten*
Rosmarini folium	Rosemary leaf	*Rosmarinus officinalis*	Lamiaceae	*Rosmarinblätter*
Rubi fruticosi folium	Blackberry leaf	*Rubus fruticosus*	Rosaceae	*Brombeerblätter*
Rubi fruticosi radix	Blackberry root	*Rubus fruticosus*	Rosaceae	*Brombeerwurzel*
Rubi idaei folium	Raspberry leaf	*Rubus idaeus*	Rosaceae	*Himbeerblätter*
Rubiae tinctorum radix	Madder root	*Rubia tinctorum*	Rubiaceae	*Krappwurzel*
Rusci aculeati rhizoma	Butcher's Broom rhizome	*Ruscus aculeatus*	Liliaceae	*Mäusedornwurzelstock*
Rutae folium	Rue leaf	*Ruta graveolens*	Rutaceae	*Rautenblätter*
Rutae herba	Rue herb	*Ruta graveolens*	Rutaceae	*Rautenkraut*
Sabal fructus	Saw Palmetto berry	*Sabal serrulata*	Arecaceae	*Sabalfrüchte*

Pharmacopeial	English	Botanical	Plant Family	German
Sabal fructus	Saw Palmetto berry	*Serenoa repens*	Arecaceae	*Sabalfrüchte*
Saccharomyces cerevisiae	Brewer's Yeast	*Saccaromyces cerevisiae*	Saccharomycetaceae	*Medizinische Hefe*
Saccharomyces cerevisiae	Brewer's Yeast/ Hansen CBS 5926	*Saccaromyces cerevisiae*	Saccharomycetaceae	*Trokenhefe aus Saccharomyces cerevisiae*
Salicis cortex	White Willow bark	*Salix alba*	Salicaceae	*Weidenrinde*
Salicis cortex	White Willow bark	*Salix fragilis*	Salicaceae	*Weidenrinde*
Salicis cortex	White Willow bark	*Salix purpurea*	Salicaceae	*Weidenrinde*
Salicis cortex	White Willow bark	*Salix* spp.	Salicaceae	*Weidenrinde*
Salviae folium	Sage leaf	*Salvia officinalis*	Lamiaceae	*Salbeiblätter*
Sambuci flos	Elder flower	*Sambucus nigra*	Caprifoliaceae	*Holunderblüten*
Saniculae herba	Sanicle herb	*Sanicula europaea*	Apiaceae	*Sanikelkraut*
Saniculae herba	Wood Sanicle	*Sanicula europaea*	Apiaceae	*Sanikelkraut*
Santali albi lignum	Sandalwood, White	*Santalum album*	Santalaceae	*Weißes Sandelholz*
Santali albi lignum	White Sandalwood	*Santalum album*	Santalaceae	*Weißes Sandelholz*
Santali lignum rubrum	Sandalwood, Red	*Pterocarpus santalinus*	Fabaceae	*Rotes Sandelholz*
Saponariae rubrae herba	Soapwort herb, Red	*Saponaria officinalis*	Caryophyllaceae	*Seifenkraut*
Saponariae rubrae radix	Soapwort root, Red	*Saponaria officinalis*	Caryophyllaceae	*Rote Seifenwurzel*
Sarsaparillae radix	Sarsaparilla root	*Smilax aristolochiaefolii*	Smilacaceae	*Sarsaparillewurzel*
Sarsaparillae radix	Sarsaparilla root	*Smilax febrifuga*	Smilacaceae	*Sarsaparillewurzel*
Sarsaparillae radix	Sarsaparilla root	*Smilax regelii*	Smilacaceae	*Sarsaparillewurzel*
Scillae bulbus	Squill	*Urginea maritima*	Liliaceae	*Meerzwiebel*
Scopolia rhizoma	Scopolia root	*Scopolia carniolica*	Solanaceae	*Glockenbilsenkraut Wurzelstock*
Secale cornutum	Ergot	*Claviceps purpurea*	Clavicipitaceae	*Mutterkorn*
Selenicerei grandiflori flos	Night-blooming Cereus flower	*Selenicereus grandiflorus*	Cactaceae	*Königin der Nacht*
Selenicerei grandiflori herba	Night-blooming Cereus herb	*Selenicereus grandiflorus*	Cactaceae	*Königin der Nacht*
Senecionis herba	Senecio herb	*Senecio nemorensis*	Asteraceae	*Fuchskreuzkraut*
Sennae folium	Senna leaf	*Cassia acutifolia*	Fabaceae	*Sennesblätter*
Sennae folium	Senna leaf	*Cassia angustifolia*	Fabaceae	*Sennesblätter*
Sennae folium	Senna leaf	*Cassia senna*	Fabaceae	*Sennesblätter*
Sennae folium	Senna leaf	*Senna alexandrina*	Fabaceae	*Sennesblätter*
Sennae fructus	Senna pod	*Cassia acutifolia*	Fabaceae	*Alexandriner-Sennesfrüchte*
Sennae fructus	Senna pod	*Cassia angustifolia*	Fabaceae	*Tinnevelly-Sennesfrüchte*
Sennae fructus	Senna pod	*Cassia senna*	Fabaceae	*Alexandriner-Sennesfrüchte*
Sennae fructus	Senna pod	*Senna alexandrina*	Fabaceae	*Sennesfrüchte*
Serpylli herba	Thyme, Wild	*Thymus serphyllum*	Lamiaceae	*Quendelkraut*

Pharmacopeial	English	Botanical	Plant Family	German
Sinapis albae semen	White Mustard seed	*Sinapis alba*	Brassicaceae	*Weiße Senfsamen*
Solidago	Goldenrod	*Solidago canadensis*	Asteraceae	*Goldrute*
Solidago	Goldenrod	*Solidago gigantea*	Asteraceae	*Goldrute*
Solidago	Goldenrod	*Solidago serotina*	Asteraceae	*Goldrute*
Solidago virgaureae herba	Goldenrod, European	*Solidago virgaurea*	Asteraceae	*Echtes Goldrutenkraut*
Sorbi aucupariae fructus	Mountain Ash berry	*Sorbus aucuparia*	Rosaceae	*Ebereschenbeeren*
Spinaciae folium	Spinach leaf Spiny	*Spinacia oleracea*	Chenopodiaceae	*Spinatblätter*
Stramonii folium	Jimsonweed leaf	*Datura stramonium*	Solanaceae	*Stramoniumblätter*
Stramonii semen	Jimsonweed seed	*Datura stramonium*	Solanaceae	*Stramoniumsamen*
Strychni semen	Nux Vomica	*Strychnos nux-vomica*	Loganiaceae	*Brechnußsamen*
Symphyti folium	Comfrey leaf	*Symphytum officinale*	Boraginaceae	*Beinwellblätter*
Symphyti herba	Comfrey herb	*Symphytum officinale*	Boraginaceae	*Beinwellkraut*
Symphyti radix	Comfrey root	*Symphytum officinale*	Boraginaceae	*Beinwellwurzel*
Syzygii cumini cortex	Jambolan bark	*Syzygium cumini*	Myrtaceae	*Syzygiumrinde*
Syzygii cumini cortex	Jambolan bark	*Syzygium jambolana*	Myrtaceae	*Syzygiumrinde*
Syzygii cumini semen	Jambolan seed	*Syzygium cumini*	Myrtaceae	*Syzygiumsamen*
Syzygii cumini semen	Jambolan seed	*Syzygium jambolana*	Myrtaceae	*Syzygiumsamen*
Taraxaci herba	Dandelion herb	*Taraxacum officinale*	Asteraceae	*Löwenzahnkraut*
Taraxaci radix cum herba	Dandelion root with herb	*Taraxacum officinale*	Asteraceae	*Löwenzahn-wurzel-mit Kraut*
Terebinthina laricina	Larch Turpentine	*Larix decidua*	Pinaceae	*Lärchenterpentin*
Terebinthina veneta	Venetian Turpentine	*Larix decidua*	Pinaceae	*Venezianischer Terpentin*
Terebinthinae aetheroleum rectificatum	Turpentine oil, Purified	*Pinus australis*	Pinaceae	*Gereinigtes Terpentinöl*
Terebinthinae aetheroleum rectificatum	Turpentine oil, Purified	*Pinus palustris*	Pinaceae	*Gereinigtes Terpentinöl*
Terebinthinae aetheroleum rectificatum	Turpentine oil, Purified	*Pinus pinaster*	Pinaceae	*Gereinigtes Terpentinöl*
Terebinthinae aetheroleum rectificatum	Turpentine oil, Purified	*Pinus* spp.	Pinaceae	*Gereinigtes Terpentinöl*
Thymi herba	Thyme	*Thymus vulgaris*	Lamiaceae	*Thymiankraut*
Thymi herba	Thyme	*Thymus zygis*	Lamiaceae	*Thymiankraut*
Tiliae carbo	Linden charcoal	*Tilia cordata*	Tiliaceae	*Lindenholzkohle*

Pharmacopeial	English	Botanical	Plant Family	German
Tiliae flos	Linden flower	*Tilia cordata*	Tiliaceae	*Lindenblüten*
Tiliae flos	Linden flower	*Tilia platyphyllos*	Tiliaceae	*Lindenblüten*
Tiliae folium	Linden leaf	*Tilia cordata*	Tiliaceae	*Lindenblätter*
Tiliae folium	Linden leaf	*Tilia platyphyllos*	Tiliaceae	*Lindenblätter*
Tiliae lignum	Linden wood	*Tilia cordata*	Tiliaceae	*Lindenholz*
Tiliae lignum	Linden wood	*Tilia platyphyllos*	Tiliaceae	*Lindenholz*
Tiliae tomentosae flos	Silver Linden flower	*Tilia argentea*	Tiliaceae	*Silberlindenblüten*
Tiliae tomentosae flos	Silver Linden flower	*Tilia tomentosa*	Tiliaceae	*Silberlindenblüten*
Tormentillae rhizoma	Tormentil root	*Potentilla erecta*	Rosaceae	*Tormentillwurzelstock*
Tormentillae rhizoma	Tormentil root	*Potentilla tormentilla*	Rosaceae	*Tormentillwurzelstock*
Tropaeolum majus	Nasturtium	*Tropaeolum majus*	Tropaeolaceae	*Kapuzinerkressenkraut*
Turnerae diffusae folium	Damiana leaf	*Turnera diffusa*	Turneraceae	*Damianablätter*
Turnerae diffusae herba	Damiana herb	*Turnera diffusa*	Turneraceae	*Damianakraut*
Urticae folium	Nettle leaf	*Urtica dioica*	Urticaceae	*Brennesselblätter*
Urticae folium	Nettle leaf	*Urtica urens*	Urticaceae	*Brennesselblätter*
Urticae folium	Stinging Nettle leaf	*Urtica dioica*	Urticaceae	*Brennesselblätter*
Urticae folium	Stinging Nettle leaf	*Urtica urens*	Urticaceae	*Brennesselblätter*
Urticae herba	Nettle herb	*Urtica dioica*	Urticaceae	*Brennesselkraut*
Urticae herba	Nettle herb	*Urtica urens*	Urticaceae	*Brennesselkraut*
Urticae herba	Stinging Nettle herb	*Urtica dioica*	Urticaceae	*Brennesselkraut*
Urticae herba	Stinging Nettle herb	*Urtica urens*	Urticaceae	*Brennesselkraut*
Urticae radix	Nettle root	*Urtica dioica*	Urticaceae	*Brennesselwurzel*
Urticae radix	Nettle root	*Urtica urens*	Urticaceae	*Brennesselwurzel*
Urticae radix	Stinging Nettle root	*Urtica dioica*	Urticaceae	*Brennesselwurzel*
Urticae radix	Stinging Nettle root	*Urtica urens*	Urticaceae	*Brennesselwurzel*
Usnea	Usnea	*Usnea barbata*	Usneaceae	*Bartflechten*
Usnea	Usnea	*Usnea florida*	Usneaceae	*Bartflechten*
Usnea	Usnea	*Usnea hirta*	Usneaceae	*Bartflechten*
Usnea	Usnea	*Usnea plicata*	Usneaceae	*Bartflechten*
Usnea	Usnea	*Usnea* spp.	Usneaceae	*Bartflechten*
Uvae ursi folium	Uva Ursi leaf	*Arctostaphylos uva-ursi*	Ericaeae	*Bärentraubenblätter*
Uzarae radix	Uzara root	*Xysmalobium undulatum*	Asclepiadaceae	*Uzarawurzel*
Valerianae radix	Valerian root	*Valeriana officinalis*	Valerianaceae	*Baldrianwurzel*
Verbasci flos	Mullein flower	*Verbascum densiflorum*	Scrophulariaceae	*Wollblumen*

Pharmacopeial	English	Botanical	Plant Family	German
Verbasci flos	Mullein flower	*Verbascum thapsus*	Scrophulariaceae	*Wollblumen*
Verbenae herba	Verbena herb	*Verbena officinalis*	Verbenaceae	*Eisenkraut*
Veronicae herba	Speedwell	*Veronica officinalis*	Scrophulariaceae	*Ehrenpreiskraut*
Veronicae herba	Veronica herb	*Veronica officinalis*	Scrophulariaceae	*Ehrenpreiskraut*
Vincae minoris herba	Periwinkle	*Vinca minor*	Apocynaceae	*Immergrünkraut*
Violae odoratae rhizoma and herba	Sweet Violet root and herb	*Viola odorata*	Violaceae	*Märzveilchen/blüten*
Violae tricoloris	Johnny Jump-Up	*Viola tricolor*	Violaceae	*Stiefmütterchenkraut*
Violae tricoloris herba	Heart's Ease herb	*Viola tricolor*	Violaceae	*Stiefmütterchenkraut*
Visci albi fructus	Mistletoe berry	*Viscum album*	Viscaceae	*Mistelfrüchte*
Visci albi herba	Mistletoe herb	*Viscum album*	Viscaceae	*Mistelkraut*
Visci albi stipitis	Mistletoe stem	*Viscum album*	Viscaceae	*Mistelstengel*
Yohimbehe cortex	Yohimbe bark	*Corynanthe yohimbi*	Rubiaceae	*Yohimberinde*
Yohimbehe cortex	Yohimbe bark	*Pausinystalia johimbe*	Rubiaceae	*Yohimberinde*
Zedoariae rhizoma	Zedoary rhizome	*Curcuma zedoaria*	Zingiberaceae	*Zitwerwurzelstock*
Zingiberis rhizoma	Ginger root	*Zingiber officinale*	Zingiberaceae	*Ingwerwurzelstock*

Part Five

European Regulatory Literature

18. Excerpts from the *German Pharmacopoeia*
    Hawthorn fluidextract   553
    Hawthorn leaf with flower   555
    Horse Chestnut seed   557
    Horse Chestnut seed standardized extract   560
    Lemon Balm   561
    Milk Thistle fruit   563

19. Excerpts from the *European Pharmacopoeia*
    Extracts   567
    Powders   569
    Tinctures   570
    Witch Hazel leaf   571
    German Chamomile flower   573
    Senna leaf   575
    Alexandrian Senna Pods   577
    Tinnevelly Senna Pods   579
    Valerian root   581

20. European Economic Community (EEC)
    Standards for Quality of Herbal Remedies   583

Chapter 18

Excerpts from the German Pharmacopoeia

The *German Pharmacopoeia* (*Deutsches Arzneibuch*, usually referred to as *DAB*) contains monographs on the quality and standards of numerous herbal drugs, medicinal plant preparations, and natural substances (e.g., essential oils) sold in Germany. As is customary in pharmacopeial monographs, they do not list the approved medicinal uses of the herb, but instead contain the standards for assuring the proper identity and purity of the herbal drug. This section contains six monographs as examples of the level of quality control measures required for manufacturers of phytomedicines in Germany. Included are monographs taken from *DAB 10*; Hawthorn fluidextract (Crataegi extractum fluidum), Hawthorn leaf with flower (Crataegi folium cum flore), Horse Chestnut seed (Hippocastani semen), Standardized Horse Chestnut seed extract (Hippocastani semen extractum siccum normatum), Lemon Balm (Melissae folium), and Milk Thistle fruit (Cardui mariae fructus). Four of these monographs have been revised in the most recent edition, *DAB 1997*, as noted.

Hawthorn fluidextract
Crataegi extractum fluidum
DAB 10

Hawthorn fluidextract contains 0.25 - 0.50 percent flavonoids calculated as hyperoside ($C_{21}H_{20}O_{12}$; MW 464.4); the content must be declared. The content determined should not differ more than +10 percent from the content declared.

Preparation
Hawthorn fluidextract is prepared from comminuted hawthorn leaf with flower and ethanol 70 percent (v/v) in accordance with a process for fluidextracts described in the **Extracts** monograph, preferably by percolation. The fluidextract thus obtained is stored for 5 days at a temperature between 2 and 8° C and then filtered. Subsequently, the content of flavonoids, calculated as hyperoside, is determined.

Properties
Greenish-brown, clear liquid with weak, characteristic odor.

Test for Identity
The test is performed by means of thin-layer chromatography (V.6.20.2) using a layer of silica gel GR.
Test solution:
Use the fluidextract undiluted as the test solution.
Reference solution:
Dissolve 1 mg chlorogenic acid *RN* and 2.5 mg hyperoside *RN* and rutoside *R* respectively in 10 ml methanol *R*.

Apply separately to the plate 10 µl of each solution in the form of bands (20 mm times 3 mm). Chromatography is carried out with a mixture of 10 parts by volume anhydrous formic acid R, 10 parts by volume water, 30 parts by volume ethyl methyl ketone R, and 50 parts by volume ethyl acetate R over a distance of 15 cm. After drying at 100 - 105° C, spray the still warm plate with approximately 10 ml of a 1 percent solution (m/V) of diphenylboryl oxethylamine R in methanol R (for a 200 mm by 200 mm plate) and then with approximately 10 ml of a 5 percent solution (v/v) of macrogol 400 R in methanol R. Carry out the evaluation after approximately 30 minutes under ultraviolet light at 365 nm. The chromatogram of the reference solution shows in the lower third the yellow-brown fluorescent rutoside area, approximately in the middle the light-blue fluorescent chlorogenic acid area and slightly above the middle the intensive yellow-brown fluorescent hyperoside area. Corresponding areas are seen in the chromatogram of the reference solution; additionally, a greenish fluorescent area is visible above the hyperoside area (vitexin-2"-rhamnoside) and above the hyperoside area another greenish fluorescent area (vitexin). In the upper third, 1 or 2 blue fluorescent areas appear. Further, weaker areas can be found in the chromatogram of the test solution.

Test for Purity
Content of ethanol (V.5.3.1)
50 - 65 percent (v/v).
Methanol, isopropyl alcohol (V.5.3.2)
The fluidextract has to comply with the test fixed in the extract monograph for fluidextracts.

Assay
In a 100 ml round bottomed flask, reduced to dryness 1.5 g fluidextract at a temperature of no more than 40° C applying reduce pressure. Mix the residue with 2 ml of a 0.5 percent solution (m/V) of methenamine R, 20 ml acetone R, and 2 ml hydrochloric acid 25 percent R and heat to boiling under reflux for 30 minutes. Filter the hot mixture through a small quantity of cotton wool into a 100 ml volumetric flask; heat to boiling under reflux the extract residue and the cotton in a round-bottomed flask twice for 10 minutes with 20 ml acetone R each; filter the hot solutions through cotton into the volumetric flask.

After cooling down to room temperature, dilute with acetone R to make 100 ml. Add 20 ml water to 20 ml of the solution in a separating funnel, and shake out once with 15 ml and 3 times with 10 ml ethyl acetate R in each case. Combine the shaken out quantities of ethyl acetate solution in a separating funnel, and wash 2 times using 50 ml water each time, then decant immediately after into a 50 ml volumetric flask and dilute to 50 ml with ethyl acetate R by rinsing filter. Add 1 ml aluminium chloride reagent RN to 10 ml of this solution, and dilute to 25 ml with 5 percent methanolic acetic acid RN (test solution).

At the same time, dilute 10 ml of the solution only with methanolic acetic acid 5 percent RN to 25 ml (compensation liquid). After 30 minutes, measure the absorption (V.6.19) of the test solution at 425 nm against the compensation liquid.

The calculation of the content of flavonoids in percent, calculated as hyperoside, is based on a specific absorption A 1 percent 1 cm = 500.

Storage
Keep tightly closed and protected from light.

Labeling
The content of flavonoids in percent, calculated as hyperoside, has to be indicated on the container.

Hawthorn leaf with flower
Crataegi folium cum flore
DAB 10*

Hawthorn leaf with flower consists of dried approximately 7 cm long flowering twig tops of *Crataegus monogyna* Jaquin emend. Lindman or *C. laevigata* (Poiret) de Candolle (synonym: *C. oxyacantha* L. p. p. et duct.) and more seldomly of other European *Crataegus* species such as *C. pentagyna* Waldstein et Kitaibel ex Willdenow, *C. nigra* Waldstein et Kitaibel, and *C. azarolus* L. It contains at least 0.7 percent flavonoids, calculated as hyperoside ($C_{21}H_{20}O_{12}$; MW 464.4).

Description
The drug has a weak, peculiar odor and a slightly sweet to slightly bitter somewhat astringent taste. The drug consists of the dark-brown, woody, from approximately 1 to a maximum 2.5 mm thick stalk pieces bearing alternate petiolated deciduous leaves with small, often fallen, leaflets, and, on their ends, numerous false-umbelliform white flowers. The leaves are more or less pronouncedly lobed and slightly to barely serrate on the margin. In the case of *C. laevigata* they are dull 3-, 5-, or 7-lobed with short incisions reaching at maximum the middle of each half-blade; *C. monogyna* has 3 - 5 sharp lobes and deep incisions reaching near the midrib. The upper surface of the leaf is dark-green to brownish green, the lower surface light gray-green with noticeable narrow net-venation and slightly protuberant main veins. The leaves of *C. laevigata*, *C. monogyna* and *C. pentagyna* are glabrous to pubescent; those of *C. azarolus* are hairy.

The flowers have a brownish-green receptacle with 5 triangular calyx tips, 5 free yellowish-white to brownish, rounded to broadly ovate, short ungulated petals, and numerous stamens. The ovary attached to the receptacle bears 1 - 5 long styles and contains as much loculi with one fertile ovule in each.

Crataegus monogyna has 1, *C. laevigata* 2 - 3, *C. azarolus* 2 or 3 but sometimes only 1, *C. nigra* and *C. pentagyna* 5, in rare cases 4, styles and loculi.

Microscopic Characteristics
The lower surface of the deciduous leaf has numerous large anomocytic stomata (V.4.3). Epidermis cells are rounded-polygonal, partially with slightly wavy cuticular striation. The epidermis of the upper surface of the leaf consists of irregular-polygonal cells with clearly wavy striated cuticle and only sparse anomocytic stomata (V.4.3). The mesophyll is bifacial with mostly 2 layers of very narrow palisades.

Veins are accompanied by crystal cells containing single crystals, more seldomly clusters of calcium oxalate. Small, approximately 10 - 20 µm large calcium oxalate clusters, more seldomly single crystals are further to be found in numerous mesophyll cells. Covering hairs are unicellular, more or less coarse- to thick-walled with wide lumen, almost straight to more or less curved to twisted, blunt or pointed and pitted on the base. On the leaves of *C. monogyna*, *C. laevigata* and *C. pentagyna* there are very sparse hairs on the leaf surface. Calyx and receptacle have the same structure as the deciduous leaves but with only few stomata. The inner part of the receptacle bears numerous covering hairs.

The epidermis of the petals consists on both sides of coarse-walled, rounded polygonal, strongly papillous cells with clearly wavy striated cuticle. Its mesophyll contains, in particular on the petal base and near the vascular bundles, small clusters and more seldomly single crystals of calcium oxalate. Style and filaments have thin-walled elongated slightly papillous epidermis cells with striated cuticle. The endothelium has regular bow-shaped thickenings.

Pollen grains are up to 44 nm large, rounded, triangular to elliptic, with smooth exine and 3 germinal pores.

The stalk is covered with a multilayered dark red-brown cork. The phelloderm consists of collenchymatic cells with thick bright walls. The consecutive bark parenchyma bears changing quantities of calcium oxalate clusters or single crystals which are partially arranged in short longitudinal rows. Outside of the phloem, there are small bundles of narrow-lumen lignified sclerenchyma fibers accompanied by crystal cell rows. The xylem, made up of numerous collateral vascular bundles, forms on the thicker parts of the stalk a more or less closed wood ring interrupted only by 1 - 3-lined medullary rays and consisting of numerous narrow-lumen spiral, reticulate, and border-pitted tracheae and tracheids, pitted wood parenchyma, and single narrow sclerenchyma fibers. This ring encloses a large medulla made of rounded, coarse-walled, pitted and partly lignified cells, sometimes containing single clusters or single crystals of calcium oxalate.

Test for Identity

The test is carried out by means of thin-layer chromatography (V.6.20.2) using a layer of silica gel GR.

Test solution:
Shake 1 g pulverized drug (710) for 5 minutes with 10 ml methanol R on a water-bath at 65° C. Use the cooled filtrated solution as the test solution.

Reference solution:
Dissolve 1 mg each of chlorogenic acid RN and caffeic acid R and 2.5 mg each hyperoside R and rutoside R in 10 ml methanol R.

Apply separately to the plate 30 μl test solution and 10 μl reference solution in the form of bands (20 mm times 3 mm). Chromatography is carried out with a mixture of 10 parts by volume water, 10 parts by volume anhydrous formic acid R, 30 parts by volume ethyl methyl ketone R, and 50 parts by volume ethyl acetate R over a distance of 15 cm. After drying at 100 - 105° C, spray the still warm plate with approximately 10 ml of a 1 percent solution (m/V) of diphenylboryl oxyethylamine R in methanol R (for a 200 mm times 200 mm plate) and then with approximately 10 ml of a 5 percent solution (v/v) of macrogol 400 R in methanol R. Carry out the evaluation after approximately 30 minutes under ultraviolet light at 365 nm. The lowest area of the reference solution and the test solution to be seen is the medium-strong, yellow-brown fluorescent rutoside area. In upward direction, both chromatograms show the light-blue fluorescent area of chlorogenic acid and the intense yellow-brown to orange fluorescent hyperoside area. Directly above this area, a fluorescent area of the same color is to be found for the test solution. A light-blue fluorescent area is situated near the solvent front. Further, weaker areas are to be found in the chromatogram of the test solution.

Test for Purity
Foreign matter (V.4.2)
Not more than 2 percent. Flowers of other genera are not permitted. Flowers of *Sorbus* species can be identified by their ovary with respectively two ovules in each loculus. Flowers of *Prunus* L. can be identified by the ovary standing free in the center of the receptacle and consisting of only one carpel and by its small bud scales (short shoot) at the base of the pedicel.

Loss on drying (V.6.22)
Not more than 10 percent determined with 1 g pulverized drug (355) by drying for 2 hours in a desiccator at 100 - 105° C.

Ash (V.3.2.16)
Not more than 9 percent, determined with 1.00 g pulverized drug.

Assay

In a 100 ml round bottomed flask, mix 0.600 g pulverized drug (250) with 1 ml of a 0.5 percent solution (w/v) of methenamine R, 20 ml acetone R and 2 ml hydrochloric acid 25 percent R and heat to boiling under reflux for 30 minutes. Filter the hot mixture through a small quantity of cotton wool into a 100 ml volumetric flask; heat to boiling under reflux the drug residue and the cotton in a round-bottomed flask twice for 10 minutes with 20 ml acetone R in each; filter the hot solutions through cotton into a volumetric flask.

After cooling to room temperature, dilute with acetone R to 100 ml. In a separating funnel, add 20 ml water to 20 ml of the solution and extract by shaking out once with 15 ml and 3 times with 10 ml ethyl acetate R. Wash the ethyl acetate extractions combined in a separating funnel twice with 50 ml water respectively, then decant into a 540 ml volumetric flask and dilute to 50 ml with ethyl acetate R.

To 10 ml of this solution add 1 ml aluminum chloride reagent RN and dilute to 25 ml with methanolic acetic acid 5 percent RN.

At the same time, dilute 10 ml of the solution only with methanolic acetic acid 5 percent RN to 25 ml (compensation liquid). After 30 minutes, measure the absorption (V.6.19) of the test solution at 425 nm against the compensation liquid.

The calculation of the content of flavonoids in percent, calculated as hyperoside, is based on a specific absorption A 1 percent 1 cm = 500.

Storage
Keep tightly closed and protected from light.

*[This monograph is superseded by a new monograph in DAB 1997.]

Horse Chestnut seed
Hippocastani semen
DAB 10*

Horse chestnut seed comprises the dry seeds of *Aesculus hippocastanum* L. The drug contains at least 3 percent triterpene glycosides, calculated as anhydrous aescin ($C_{54}H_{84}O_{23}$; MW = 1101) and related to the dry drug.

Properties
The drug has no odor. It demonstrates the macroscopic and microscopic features described below under "Test for Identity," sections A and B.

Test for Identity
A. The seeds are round to oval, approximately 2 - 4 cm in diameter, somewhat flattened, surrounded by a dark brown skin, shiny only when fresh, and have a large, roundish light brown spot or scar (hilum). The entire area beneath the skin is occupied by the very large embryo with large, slightly yellow cotyledons.

B. Carry out investigation under the microscope using chloral hydrate solution R or water. The epidermis of the seed skin is made up of polygonal, brown-walled cells extending radially along the cross section of the seed, shaped somewhat in palisade fashion. Beneath these, many layers of sclerenchymatic cells are found with thick, coarsely stippled, yellowish to brownish cell walls and, directly adjoining, a colorless parenchyma rich in intercellular spaces consisting of a few layers of coarse-walled, only unclearly stippled cells, and a small number of annular and spiral vessels. The tissue of the cotyledons consists of colorless, thin-walled cells tightly filled with starch and fat. It is not possible to demonstrate the presence of oil droplets until after dissolving the starch in a chloral hydrate preparation or by coloring them red with Sudan-III-Glycerol RN.

To test for the starch, first make an aqueous preparation. Typical aesculus starch consists of individual pear- or kidney-shaped grains approximately 15 - 25 µm in size, in rare cases up to approximately 30 µm, and vary from having a number of rounded corners up to being irregularly roundish to oval, often with wart-like excrescences; a large number of small, roundish individual grains approximately 5 - 10 µm in size, and a few groups of 2 - 4 joined grains arranged in rows, which, according to the number of grains involved, may be up to approximately 35 µm or even in some cases up to 45 µm long. A large number of the starch grains display a biradiate to multiradiate intranuclear space, being only monoradiate in rare cases.

Pulverize the drug (355). The powder is yellowish-gray. Carry out investigation under the microscope using water or chloral hydrate solution R. As an aqueous preparation, the powder reveals the following features: a very large number of typical starch grains and, in the chloral hydrate preparation, a very large number of fat droplets differing in size, freely suspended, and in the thin-walled, colorless tissue of the cotyledons: the yellowish-brown fragments of the seed skin with thick-walled, stippled sclerenchymal cells; coarse-walled, unclearly stippled, colorless parenchymal cells as well as sporadic annular and spiral vessels from the inner layers of the seed skin.

C. Carry out the investigation with thin-layer chromatography (V.6.20.2) using a layer of GF 254 R silica gel.

Test solution:
Heat 1 g pulverized drug (500) for 15 minutes using 10 ml 70 percent ethanol RN in a reflux system, and filter after cooling. Use this filtrate as a test solution.

Reference solution:
Dissolve 10 mg aescin R in 1 ml 70 percent ethanol RN.

Apply 20 µl test solution and 10 µl reference solution in the form of bands (20 mm times 3 mm) separately to the silica gel plate. Carry out chromatography over a test length of 12 cm using the upper phase of a mixture of 10 parts 98 percent acetic acid R by volume, 40 parts water by volume, and 50 parts 1-butanol R by volume. After complete removal of the mobile phase by drying at 100 - 105° C, the fluorescence-reducing zones are characterized in ultraviolet light at 254 nm. Following this, spray the plate with approximately 10 ml anisaldehyde reagent R (for a plate measuring 200 mm times 200 mm), and heat to 100 - 105° C for 5 - 10 minutes under observation. The fluorescence-reducing zone of the aescin (escin) is recognizable in ultraviolet light at 254 nm in the chromatograph of the reference solution; another fluorescence-reducing zone which is just as clear can be seen at approximately the same level in the chomatograph of the test solution. After spraying, the blue/violet-colored zone of the aescin is recognizable in daylight both in the chromatograph of the test solution and in the chromatograph of the reference solution. In addition, a series of narrower and weaker brown to brownish-red colored zones are visible above the chromatograph of the test solution; a brown/gray-colored zone is prominent in the lower region; a brown-colored zone is situated somewhat below this.

Test for Purity
Foreign matter (V.4.2)
The drug must meet the requirements of the test.
Loss on drying (V.6.22)
Maximum 10 percent, with 1 g powdered drug (355), determined through desiccation in a drying cabinet at 100 - 105° C for 2 hours.
Ash (V.3.2.16)
Maximum 4 percent.

Assay
Add 100 ml of a 65 percent solution (v/v) of methanol R to 1 g powdered drug (500) in a 250 ml flask. Weigh the flask with its contents within an accuracy of 0.1 g. After this, heat for 30 minutes in a reflux system at boiling point in a water bath. After cooling, complement to the original mass with the 65 percent solution (v/v) of methanol R, and filter the mixture. In a 100 ml round-bottomed flask, reduce 30.0 ml of the filtrate to dryness at a pressure between 1.5 and 2.5 kPa. Dissolve the residue in 20 ml 0.1N hydrochloric acid, transfer to a 250 ml separating funnel, and subsequently rinse out the flask 2 times using 5 ml 0.1N hydrochloric acid each time. Add 20 ml 1-propanol R and 50 ml chloroform R to the combined hydrochlorous solutions, and shake thoroughly for 2 minutes. After separation of the lower phase, add the lower phase of a shaken out mixture consisting of 30 ml 0.1N hydrochloric acid, 20 ml 1-propanol R and 50 ml chloroform R to the upper phase remaining in the separation funnel and shake thoroughly for 2 minutes. Reduce the combined shaken out mixtures (lower phase) to dryness at a pressure between 1.5 and 2.5 kPa in a round-bottomed flask.

Wash the residue 2 times using 10 ml peroxide-free ether R each time, filter the ether phase and subsequently wash the filter with 210 ml peroxide-free ether R. Reject the filtrates. After removal of the remaining ether, add 10 ml anhydrous acetic acid R to the residue 3 times; filter the solutions through the previously used, now dried, filter into a 50 ml volumetric flask. Subsequently wash the round-bottomed flask and the filter with a little anhydrous acetic acid R. Filter the wash liquid into the volumetric flask, and dilute the combined filtrates to 50 ml with anhydrous acetic acid R.

Dilute 5 ml of the solution with iron (III)-chloride/acetic acid reagent RN to 25 ml in a 25 ml volumetric flask, heat in a water bath at 60° C for 25 minutes, swishing the mixture round in the flask a number of times while doing so, and cool to room temperature under running cold water. Prepare a compensation liquid from 5 ml anhydrous acetic acid R and iron (III) chloride/acetic acid reagent RN under the same conditions.

Measure the absorption (V.6.19) of the solution at 540 nm using the compensation liquid as reference. Take a specific absorption of A 1 percent/1 cm = 60 as a basis for calculation of the content in percent of triterpene glycosides, calculated as anhydrous aescin and related to the dry drug.

Storage
Store protected from light.

*[This monograph is superseded by a new monograph in DAB 1997.]

Horse Chestnut seed standardized extract

Hippocastani semen extractum siccum normatum
DAB 10*

Standardized horse chestnut seed extract contains at least 16 and at most 20 percent triterpene glycosides, calculated as anhydrous aescin and related to the dry extract.

Preparation
Standardized horse chestnut seed extract is prepared in accordance with a process for dry extracts described in the monograph entitled Extracts from chopped horse chestnut seed and ethanol/water mixtures or methanol/water mixtures (ethanol or methanol content approximately 40 - 60 v/v percent).

Properties
A yellowish to yellow-brown, powdery or pulverizable mass with a weak, characteristic odor; soluble in water and 50 percent ethanol, practically insoluble in ether or chloroform.

Test for Identity
A. Dissolve 10 mg extract in 10 ml anhydrous acetic acid R. An intense yellow-green color is produced on the addition of iron (III) chloride/acetic acid reagent RN.
B. Carry out this test by thin layer chromatography (V.6.20.2) using a layer of GF 254 R silica gel.

Test solution:
Dissolve 0.25 g extract in 10 ml 50 percent ethanol RN.

Reference solution:
Dissolve 10 mg aescin R in 1 ml 70 percent ethanol RN.

Apply 20 µl test solution and 10 µl reference solution in the form of bands (20 mm times 3 mm) separately to the silica gel plate. Carry out chromatography with the upper phase of a mixture of 10 parts 98 percent acetic acid R by volume, 40 parts water by volume, and 50 parts 1-butanol R by volume over a test length of 12 cm. After complete removal of the mobile phase by drying at 100 - 105° C, evaluate the chromatographs in ultraviolet light at 254 nm. The fluorescence-reducing zone of the aescin is recognizable in ultraviolet light at 254 nm in the chromatograph of the reference solution; a number of other fluorescence-reducing zones are present in the chromatograph of the test solution beside a fluorescence-reducing zone at the same level as the aescin zone in the chromatograph of the reference solution in the upper half. After this, spray the plate with approximately 10 ml anisaldehyde reagent R (for a 200 mm x 200 mm plate) and heat at 100 - 105° C under observation for 5 - 10 minutes. The intense blue/violet-colored zone of the aescin is recognizable in daylight in the chromatograph of the reference solution. A blue-violet zone of approximately equal intensity is found at the same level in the chromatograph of the test solution; here, a series of narrower and weaker brown to brownish-red colored zones are visible in the upper half, as well as wider, greenish gray to brown/gray-colored zones in the lower third.

Test for Purity
Loss on drying
Maximum 5 percent. Testing is carried out as described for dry extracts in the monograph entitled **Extracts**.
Ash (V.3.2.16)
Maximum 5 percent, determined with 1 g pulverized extract.
[Purity test for methanol residue added DAB 1997 monograph.]

Assay
Dissolve 0.250 g of the extract in a flask

with 20 ml 0.1N hydrochloric acid, and transfer to a 250 ml separating funnel; subsequently rinse out the flask 2 times using 5 ml 0.1N hydrochloric acid each time. Add 20 ml 1-propanol R and 50 ml chloroform R to the combined hydrochlorous solutions, and shake thoroughly for 2 minutes. After separation of the lower phase, add the lower phase of a shaken out mixture consisting of 30 ml 0.1N hydrochloric acid, 20 ml 1-propanol R and 50 ml chloroform R to the upper phase remaining in the separation funnel, and shake thoroughly for 2 minutes. Reduce the combined shaken out mixtures (lower phase) to dryness at a pressure between 1.5 and 2.5 kPa in a flask.

Wash the residue 2 times using 10 ml peroxide-free ether R each time, filter the ether phase and subsequently wash the filter with 10 ml peroxide-free ether R. Reject the filtrates. After removal of the remaining ether, add 10 ml anhydrous acetic acid R to the residue 3 times; filter the solutions through the previously used, now dried, filter into a 50 ml volumetric flask. Subsequently wash the round-bottomed flask and the filter with a little anhydrous acetic acid R, filter the wash liquid into the volumetric flask, and dilute the combined filtrates to 100 ml with anhydrous acetic acid R.

Dilute 5 ml of the solution with iron (III) chloride/acetic acid reagent RN to 25 ml in a 25 ml volumetric flask, heat in a water bath at 60° C for 25 minutes, swirling the mixture round in the flask a number of times while doing so, and cool to room temperature under flowing cold water.

Dissolve 25 mg aescin RN to 50 ml in anhydrous acetic acid R. Treat 5 ml of this solution with iron (III) chloride/acetic acid reagent RN under the same conditions as the test solution (reference solution).

Treat 5 ml anhydrous acetic acid R with iron (III) chloride/acetic acid reagent RN under the same conditions as the test solution (compensation liquid).

Measure the absorption (V.6.19) of the test solution and the reference solution at 540 nm using the compensation liquid as reference. In order to calculate the content in percent of triterpene glycosides, calculated as anhydrous aescin and related to the dry drug, use the following formula:

$$\frac{200 \cdot A1 \cdot m2 \cdot (100 - b)}{A2 \cdot m1 \cdot (100 - a)}$$

where

$A1$	=	absorption of the test solution
$A2$	=	absorption of the reference solution
$m1$	=	initial weight of the extract in g
$m2$	=	initial weight of the aescin RN in g
a	=	loss on drying of the extract in percent
b	=	loss on drying of the aescin RN in percent

Storage
Store tightly sealed and protect from light.

*[This monograph is superseded by a new monograph in DAB 1997.]

Lemon Balm
Melissae folium
DAB 10

Lemon Balm consists of the dried foliage of *Melissa officinalis* L. It contains volatile oil with citral.

Description
The crude plant material has an aromatic and slightly spicy, lemony aroma and taste. The blades of the more or less long-stalked leaves can be up to about 8 cm long and

up to some 4 cm wide; they are in the shape of a flattened egg, truncated at the base, or even heart-shaped. The leaf blade is thick and somewhat crumpled; the upper surface is dark green, the under surface lighter green. The edge of the leaf is irregularly notched or serrated. The upper surface exhibits a small number of hairs; hairs may also be visible on the strongly protruding veins on the under surface.

Microscopic characteristics: The epidermis cells of both surfaces have sinuous side walls; both sides of the leaf carry small 1-2-celled, conical or triangular tooth-shaped hairs with a smooth to finely verrucose cuticle. There are also multicellular, solid-walled, long articulated hairs with a pointed end cell and finely threadlike verrucose cuticle. Here and there are observed small glandular hairs with a 1 - 3-celled stalk and a 1 - 2-celled head; glandular hairs of type B (V.4.N3). Stomata of the diacytic type (V.4.3.) are found mainly on the leaf undersurface.

Powdered crude drug material: The powder is green. It contains leaf fragments with sinuous epidermis cells, diacytic stomata (V.4.3), and numerous cone-shaped or triangular tooth-shaped hairs; a few solid-walled, 3-5-celled glandular hairs with verrucose or streaked cuticle or their fragments; small glandular hairs with 1 - 3-celled stalks and usually single-celled heads; glandular hairs of type B (V.4.N3). Calcium oxalate crystals are absent.

Test for Identity

The testing is performed by thin-layer chromatography (V.6.20.2) on a layer of silica gel G R.

Test solution:
Shake out 0.30 g freshly pulverized crude plant material (355) with 5 ml dichloromethane R for 2 - 3 minutes and filter off about 2 g anhydrous sodium sulfate R. Flush out the flask and the filter with 2 ml dichloromethane R. Combine the filtrates and evaporate gently to dryness. Take up the residue in 0.2 ml ethyl acetate R.

Reference solution:
Dissolve 5 µl citral R and 4 mg guaiazulene R in 10 ml toluene R.

Apply 20 µl test solution and 10 µl reference solution to the plate in separate strips (20 times 3 mm), and chromatograph with a mixture of 10 parts by volume of ethyl acetate R and 90 parts by volume of hexane R, developing twice with the same solvent system over a migration distance of 10 cm. After evaporation of the solvent system at room temperature, two green-gray zones are visible a little way above the start, which fluoresce deep red in ultraviolet light at 365 nm (chlorophyll). A yellow zone is visible under the solvent front.

Spray the plate with approximately 10 ml of anisaldehyde reagent R (for a 200 mm times 200 mm plate), heat to 100 - 105° C for 10 minutes under continuous observation, and evaluate in daylight. Citral appears as a pale gray-violet zone more or less in the middle of the chromatograms of the reference and test solutions. Slightly above this citral zone in the chromatogram of the test solution there may be a pink zone (= caryophyllene epoxide). In the upper third of the chromatogram of the test solution a pale gray-violet zone (= citronellal) is visible just below the orange-brown zone of guaiazulene in the reference chromatogram. The violet main zone in the chromatogram of the test solution (caryophyllene and other hydrocarbons) is situated close to the solvent front, just above the guaiazulene zone. Other, mostly pale gray-violet or reddish, zones will be present in the lower half of the chromatogram of the test solution (= citronellal, granules, etc.).

Test for Purity

Foreign matter (V.4.2)
Maximum 3 percent.
Loss on drying (V.6.22)
Maximum 12 percent; determined by dry-

ing 1 g pulverized crude plant material (355) in a drying cabinet for 2 hours at 100 - 105° C.

Ash (V.3.2.16)
Maximum 12 percent; determined on 1 g pulverized crude plant material.

Storage
Store protected from light.

Milk Thistle fruit
Cardui mariae fructus
DAB 10*

Milk thistle fruit consists of the ripe liberated fruit of *Silybum marianum* Gaertner (syn. *Carduus marianus* L.). The drug contains no less than 1 percent silymarin, calculated as silybin ($C_{25}H_{22}O_{10}$, MW=482.4), and related to the dried drug. [Minimum content silymarin = 1.5 percent in *DAB* 1997.]

Properties
The drug is practically free of odor, the fruit husks are bitter, and the seeds have an oily taste. The drug manifests the macroscopic and microscopic features described below in Sections A and B under Test for Identity.

Test for Identity
A. The obliquely ovate to elongate, somewhat flattened fruit (achenes) which are approximately 6 - 7 mm long, approximately 3 mm wide and approximately 1.5 mm thick, possess an extruding, cartilaginous, shining, yellowish edge on their top side and a navel at their base. The husks are shiny brown-black or clouded gray/brown, striated with dark or white gray, and surround the straight embryo with two thick, flattened cotyledons containing fatty oil and aleuronic granules.

B. Carry out the assay under the microscope, whereby chloral hydrate solution *R* is used. The epidermis of the pericarp consists of almost colorless cells elongated in palisade form with markedly thickened external walls arranged to face the surface of the fruit vertically and in which part of the lumen continues, thus protruding outward in a slotted fashion. In plain view at high magnification, the cells only reveal a slot-shaped lumen. They are equipped with thickening supports that in plain view appear as nodular thickenings of the cell wall. The subepidermal layer of the pericarp consists of non-ligneous, thin-walled parenchymal cells and is structured in the form of a pigment layer. Colorless cells and cell groups alternate with pigment cells, whose number is variable, whereby the frequently patterned appearance of the pericarp is formed. Following this, we find the pericarpal tissue consisting of punctuated parenchymal cells stretched longitudinally to the fruit and approximately eight layers of cells thick. The innermost layer of the pericarp may be collapsed, and contains large "cigar-shaped" or monoclinous calcium oxalate prisms. The epidermis of the seed husk is made up of large, yellow cells stretched in palisade form. These cells possess a narrow lumen, that widens only towards the ends of the cells, and the cell walls possess a markedly protruding layer formation. The subepidermal membranes are equipped with closely adjacent, pronounced thickening supports ("retiform cells"). These are followed by an adjacent single layer of cells with coarse, somewhat "swollen" walls and lipophilic cellular content (residual endosperm). The seed embryo consists of fragile-walled cells containing a large number of crystal clusters and oil drops in addition to small encapsulated granules (druses).

Subject the drug to pulverization (355). The powder is brown/yellow. Carry out the assay under the microscope, using chloral hydrate solution R. The powder shows the following features: fragments of the colorless, palisade-shaped epidermis cells of the pericarp up to approximately 75 µm long and approximately 8 µm wide, with attached pigment layer, which turns a red color in chloral hydrate preparation; in plain view, gray fragments with the slot-shaped lumen liberated by the thick wall strengthening, or the cell wall nodes formed by the thickening supports; fragments of the pigment layer in plain view, running red in the chloral hydrate preparation, pigment cells alternating with colorless parenchymal cells; markedly punctuated, colorless cells with translucently appearing pigment cells in plain view; "cigar-shaped" or monoclinous fragments of the yellow, seed husk with very narrow lumens arranged in palisade form and approximately 150 µm long, very markedly punctuated in plain view; weak yellowish colored fragments from the "retiform cell layer" as well as fragments of the seed embryo consisting of fragile-walled cells with small encapsulated granules (druses) and lipophilic substances.

C. Carry out the assay with the aid of thin-layer chromatography (V.6.20.2), using a thin layer of silica gel G R.

Test solution:
In a reflux system, heat 1 g pulverized drug (500) for 5 minutes with 10 ml methanol R in a hot water bath at 70° C. Filter the solution after cooling, carefully reduce to dryness, and absorb in 1 ml of methanol R.

Reference solution:
Dissolve 1 mg caffeic acid in 10 ml methanol R.

On the silica gel plate, apply separately 30 µl test solution and 10 µl reference solution in the form of strips (20 mm times 3 mm). Carry out chromatography using a mixture of 8.5 parts by volume anhydrous formic acid R, 16.5 parts by volume acetone R and 75 parts by volume chloroform R, developing each chromatograph two times using the same mobile phase over a column of 10 cm. After drying at 100 - 105° C, spray the plate while still warm with approximately 10 ml of a 1 percent solution (m/V) of diphenylboryl oxyethylamine R in methanol R (for a 200 mm times 200 mm plate), followed by approximately 10 ml of a 5 percent solution (v/v) of Macrogol 400 R in methanol R. Perform the evaluation after approximately 30 minutes in UV light at a wavelength of 365 nm. Approximately in its middle, the chromatograph of the reference solution shows the bright blue fluorescent zone of caffeic acid. The chromatograph of the reference solution shows, at the level of the caffeic acid zone, the yellow-green fluorescent zone of silybin, above the silybin zone a number of weaker fluorescent zones and below this up to the initial strip further clearly fluorescent zones (silydianin, silychristin, taxifolin, and others). The taxifolin shows a brown-yellow fluorescence.

Test for Purity
State of decomposition
The drug should have neither a rancid odor nor a rancid taste.
Foreign matter (V.4.2)
The drug must meet the requirements of the assay.
Loss on drying (V.6.22)
Maximum 8 percent, determined with 1 g pulverized drug (500) by drying for two hours in a drying cabinet at a temperature

of 100 - 105° C.

Ash (V.3.2.16)
Maximum 8 percent.

Assay

Extract 5 g pulverized drug (500) for 4 hours with petroleum ether R1 and after drying in air for 5 hours with methanol R in a Soxhlet type extraction unit. Reduce the methanolic extract by drying to approximately 25 - 230 ml at a pressure between 1.5 and 2.5 kPa, filter the solution into a 50 ml volumetric flask, and dilute with methanol R to 50 ml under continuous washing of the filter. In a 10 ml volumetric flask, add 2 ml dinitrophenylhydrazine sulfuric acid reagent R into 1 ml test solution, and after tightly sealing the volumetric flask, heat for 50 minutes at 50° C. After cooling, dilute with methanolic potassium hydroxide solution R to give a final volume of 10 ml, and mix thoroughly. After 120 seconds, calculating from the time of the point of filling, dilute 1 ml of the solution in a centrifuging glass with 20 ml methanol R, and centrifuge. Pour the clear overstanding, colored solution into a 50 ml volumetric flask, distribute the residue in 20 ml methanol R, and centrifuge once more. Pour the clear overstanding solution into the volumetric flask and finally dilute with methanol R to make 50 ml.

Measure the absorption (V.6.19) of the solution at a wavelength of 490 nm using as reference a compensatory liquid which has been prepared with 1 ml methanol R instead of the test solution.

Take a specific absorption of A 1 percent/1 cm = 585 as a basis for calculation of the content in percent silymarin, calculated as silybin and related to the dry drug.

Storage

Store protected from light.

*[This monograph is superseded by a new monograph in DAB 1997.]

Chapter 19

Excerpts from the European Pharmacopoeia

The *European Pharmacopoeia* monographs represent quality and identity standards and test methods for many herbal drugs sold in Europe. Monographs are produced by a joint effort of scientists and health professionals from many countries in Western Europe.

The first three monographs define and explain formulation methods for leading dosage forms: Extracts (extracta), Powders (pulveres), and Tinctures (tincturae). The following six monographs are included: Witch Hazel leaf (Hamamelidis Folium), German Chamomile flower (Matricariae Flos), Senna leaf (Sennae Folium), Alexandrian Senna pods (Sennae Fructus Acutifoliae), Tinnevelly Senna pods (Sennae Fructus Angustifoliae), and Valerian root (Valerianae Radix). These monographs contain pharmaceutical quality parameters and methods, with specific methods to determine identity, and descriptions of tests and assay methods to determine purity, with the types of reagents and related chemicals required.

Extracts
Extracta

Extracts

Extracts are concentrated preparations of liquid, dry or intermediate consistency, usually obtained from dried vegetable or animal matter. For some preparations, the matter to be extracted may undergo a preliminary treatment, for example, inactivation of enzymes, grinding, or defatting.

Extracts are prepared by maceration, percolation or other suitable, justified methods using ethanol or another suitable solvent. After extraction, unwanted matter is removed, if necessary.

Production by percolation

If necessary, reduce the drug to pieces of suitable size. Mix thoroughly with a portion of the prescribed extraction solvent and allow to stand for an appropriate time. Transfer to a percolator and allow the percolate to flow slowly, making sure that the drug is always covered with the remaining extraction solvent. The drug residue may be pressed out and the expressed fluid combined with the percolate.

Production by maceration

Unless otherwise prescribed, reduce the drug to pieces of suitable size, mix thoroughly with the prescribed extraction solvent and allow to stand in a closed container for an appropriate time. The drug residue is separated from the extraction solvent, and, if necessary, pressed out. In the latter case, the two liquids obtained are combined.

Concentration to the intended consistency is carried out using suitable methods, generally under reduced pressure and a temperature at which deterioration of the constituents is at a minimum. The residual solvents in the extract do not exceed the prescribed limits.

Standardized extracts are adjusted to the defined content of constituents using suitable inert materials or using another extract of the vegetable or animal matter used for the preparation.

Liquid Extracts

Liquid extracts are fluid preparations of which, in general, one part is equivalent to one part of the original dried drug (m/m or v/m). These preparations are adjusted, if necessary, so that they satisfy the requirements for content of solvent concentration for constituents or for dry residue.

Liquid extracts may be prepared by the methods described above using only ethanol of suitable concentration or water or by dissolving a soft or dry extract in the same solvents and, if necessary, filtering; whatever their method of preparation, the extracts obtained have a comparable composition. A slight sediment may form on standing, as long as the composition is not changed significantly.

Liquid extracts may contain suitable antimicrobial preservatives.

Tests
Relative density (V.6.4)
The liquid extract complies with the limits prescribed.
Ethanol content (V.5.3.1)
For alcoholic extracts, carry out the determination of ethanol content. The ethanol content complies with that prescribed.
Methanol and 2-propanol (V.5.3.2)
For alcoholic extracts, not more than 0.05 percent v/v of methanol or 2-propanol, unless otherwise prescribed.
Dry residue
In a flat-bottomed dish about 50 mm in diameter and about 30 mm in height, introduce rapidly 2 g or 2 ml of the extract to be examined. Evaporate to dryness on a water-bath and dry in an oven at 100 - 105° C for 3 hours. Allow to cool in a desiccator over diphosphorous pentoxide R and weigh. Calculate the result as a percentage mass in mass (m/m) or mass in volume (m/v).

Storage
Store in a well-closed container, protected from light.

Labeling
The label on the container states: the vegetable or animal matter used; where applicable, that fresh vegetable or animal matter was used; the name and concentration of the solvent used for the preparation; where applicable, the concentration of ethanol in the final extract; the content of active principle and/or the ratio of starting material to final liquid extract; and the name and concentration of any added antimicrobial preservative.

Soft Extracts
Soft extracts are preparations of consistency intermediate between liquid and dry extracts. They are obtained by partial evaporation of the solvent used for preparation. Only ethanol of suitable concentration or water is used. Soft extracts generally have a dry residue of not less than 70 percent (m/m). They may contain suitable antimicrobial preservatives.

Tests
Dry residue
In a flat-bottomed dish about 50 mm in diameter and about 30 mm in height, weigh rapidly 2 g of the extract to be examined. Heat to dryness on a water-bath and dry in an oven at 100 - 105° C for 3 hours. Allow to cool in a desiccator over diphosphorous pentoxide R and weight. Calculate the result as a percentage mass in mass (m/m).

Storage
Store in a well-closed container, protected from light.

Labeling
The label on the container states: the vegetable or animal matter used; where

applicable, that fresh vegetable or animal matter was used; the content of active principle and/or the ratio of starting material to final liquid extract; the name and concentration of any added antimicrobial preservative.

Dry Extracts

Dry extracts are solid preparations obtained by evaporation of the solvent used for their production. Dry extracts generally have a dry residue of not less than 95 percent (m/m). Suitable inert materials may be added.

Standardized dry extracts are adjusted to the defined content of constituents, using suitable inert materials or a dry extract of the vegetable or animal matter used for the preparation.

Where applicable, the monograph on a dry extract prescribes a limit test for the solvent used for extraction.

Tests
Loss on drying
In a flat-bottomed dish about 50 mm in diameter and about 30 mm in height, weight rapidly 0.50 g of the extract to be examined, finely powdered. Dry in an oven at 100 - 105° C for 3 hours. Allow to cool in a desiccator over diphosphorous pentoxide R and weigh. Calculate the result as a percentage mass in mass (m/m).

Storage
Store in an airtight container, protected from light.

Labeling
The label on the container states: the vegetable or animal matter used; where applicable, that fresh vegetable or animal matter was used; the content of active principle and/or the ratio of starting material to final liquid extract; the name and concentration of any added antimicrobial preservative.

Powders
Pulveres

Powders
Powders are preparations consisting of solid, loose, dry particles of varying degrees of fineness. They contain one or more active ingredients, with or without auxiliary substances and, if necessary, authorized coloring matters and flavoring substances.

Several categories of powders may be distinguished, such as:

Powders for oral administration; powders for the preparation of liquids for oral use; powders for parenteral use; powders for topical use.

When justified and authorized, the requirements of this monograph do not necessarily apply to powders for veterinary use.

Tests
Fineness
If prescribed, the fineness of a powder is determined by the sieve test (V.5.5.1) and another appropriate method.

Uniformity of content (V.5.2.2)
Unless otherwise prescribed or justified and authorized, single-dose powders with a content of active ingredient less than 2 mg or less than 2 percent of the total mass comply with the test for uniformity of content of single-dose preparations. If the preparation has more than one active ingredient, the requirement applies only to those ingredients that correspond to the above conditions. The test is not required for multivitamin and trace-element preparations. If the test for uniformity of

content is prescribed for all the active ingredients, the test for uniformity of mass is not required.

Uniformity of mass (V.5.2.1)
Single-dose powders comply with the test for uniformity of mass of single-dose preparations.

Storage
Store in an airtight container.

Powders for Oral Administration
Powders for oral administration are generally administered in or with water or another suitable liquid. They may also be swallowed directly. They are presented as single-dose or multidose powders.

Multidose powders require the provision of a measuring device capable of delivering the quantity prescribed. Each dose of a single-dose powder is enclosed in an individual container, for example a sachet, a paper packet or a vial.

Effervescent powders
Effervescent powders are presented as single-dose or multidose powders and generally contain acid substances and carbonates or hydrogen carbonates that react rapidly in the presence of water to release carbon dioxide. They are intended to be dissolved or dispersed in water before administration.

Powders for Topical Use
Powders for topical use are presented as single-dose powders or multidose powders. They are free from grittiness. Powders specifically intended for use on large open wounds or on severely injured skin must be sterile. Powders required to be sterile must comply with the test for sterility.

Tests
Sterility (V.2.1.1)
If the label states that the preparation is sterile, it complies with the test for sterility.

Labeling
The label states that preparation is for external use and, where necessary, that the preparation is sterile.

Requirements additional to those prescribed in this monograph may be imposed by the national authority in respect of preparations not specifically provided for in the Pharmacopoeia.

Tinctures
Tincturae

Tinctures
Tinctures are liquid preparations usually obtained from dried vegetable or animal matter.

For some preparations, the matter to be extracted must undergo a preliminary treatment, for example, inactivation of enzymes, grinding or defatting.

Tinctures are prepared by maceration, percolation or other suitable, justified methods, using ethanol of suitable concentration. Tinctures may also be obtained by dissolving or diluting extracts in ethanol of suitable concentration.

Tinctures are usually obtained either using 1 part of drug and 10 parts of extraction solvent or 1 part of drug and 5 parts of extraction solvent. Tinctures are usually clear. A slight sediment may form on standing as long as the composition is not changed significantly.

Production by percolation
If necessary, reduce the drug to pieces of suitable size. Mix thoroughly with a portion of solvent and allow to stand for an appropriate time. Transfer to a percolator and allow the percolate to flow slowly, making sure that the drug is always cov-

ered with the remaining extraction solvent. The drug residue may be pressed out and the expressed fluid combined with the percolate.

Production by maceration
Unless otherwise prescribed, reduce the drug to pieces of suitable size, mix thoroughly with the prescribed extraction solvent and allow to stand in a closed container for an appropriate time. The drug residue is separated from the extraction solvent and, if necessary, pressed out. In the latter case, the two liquids obtained are combined.

Production from extracts
The tincture is prepared by dissolving or diluting an extract, using ethanol of appropriate concentration. The content of solvent and constituents or, where applicable, the content of solvent and of dry residue correspond to that of tinctures obtained by maceration or percolation.

Adjustment of the constituents
When the content of constituents must be adjusted, such adjustment may be carried out, if necessary, either by adding the extraction solvent of suitable concentration or by adding another tincture of the vegetable or animal matter used for the preparation.

Tests
Relative density (V.6.4)
The tincture complies with the limits prescribed.

Ethanol content (V.5.3.1)
The ethanol content complies with that prescribed.

Methanol and 2-propanol (V.5.3.2)
Not more than 0.05 percent v/v of methanol or 2-propanol, unless otherwise prescribed.

Dry residue
In a flat-bottomed dish about 50 mm in diameter and about 30 mm in height, introduce rapidly 2 g or 2 ml of the tincture. Evaporate to dryness on a water-bath and dry in an oven at 100 - 105° C for 3 hours. Allow to cool in a desiccator over diphosphorous pentoxide R and weigh. Calculate the result as a percentage mass in mass (m/m) or mass in volume (m/v).

Storage
Store in an airtight container, protected from light.

Labeling
The label on the container states: the vegetable or animal matter used; where applicable, that fresh vegetable or animal matter was used; the concentration of ethanol used for the preparation; the concentration of ethanol in the final tincture; the content of active principle and/or the ratio of starting material to extraction fluid and of starting material to final tincture.

Hamamelis (Witch Hazel) Leaf
Hamamelidis Folium

Hamamelis leaf consists of the dried leaf of *Hamamelis virginiana* L [Fam. Hamamelidaceae]. It contains not less than 7 percent of tannins, calculated with reference to the dried drug.

Characteristics
The lamina is 5 - 12 cm long and 3 - 8 cm wide and is broadly ovate to obovate; the base is oblique and asymmetric and the apex is acute or, rarely, obtuse.

Hamamelis leaf has the macroscopic and microscopic characteristics described under identification tests A and B.

Identification

A. The leaf is green or greenish-brown, often broken, crumpled, and compressed into more or less compact masses. The margins of the lamina are roughly crenate or dentate. The venation is pinnate and prominent on the abaxial surface. Usually, four to six pairs of secondary veins are attached to the main vein, leaving at an acute angle and curving gently to the marginal points where there are fine veins, often at right angles to the secondary veins.

B. Reduce to a powder (355). The powder is brownish-green. Examine under a microscope using chloral hydrate solution R. The powder shows the following diagnostic characteristics: fragments of adaxial epidermis with wavy anticlinal walls; abaxial epidermis with stomata, some of them paracytic (V.4.3), other atypical; star-shaped covering trichomes, either entire or broken, composed of four to twelve unicellular branches which are united by their bases, elongated, conical and curved, up to 250 µm long, thick-walled and with a clearly visible lumen, with contents often brown-colored; fibers are lignified and thick-walled, isolated or in groups, and they are accompanied by a sheath of prismatic calcium oxalate crystals; small cylindrical parenchymatous cells of palisade; irregularly shaped cells of spongy mesophyll; sclereids, frequently enlarged at one or both ends, 150 - 180 µm long, whole or fragmented; fragments of annular or spiral vessels; isolated prisms of calcium oxalate. Examine by thin-layer chromatography (V.6.20.2), using silica gel G R as the coating substance.

Test solution:
To 1 g of the powdered drug (355) add 10 ml of alcohol (60 percent v/v), shake for 15 minutes and filter.

Reference solution:
A. Dissolve 30 mg of tannic acid R in 5 ml of alcohol (60 percent v/v).

B. Dissolve 5 mg of gallic acid R in 5 ml of alcohol (60 percent v/v).

Apply separately to the plate as bands 10 l of each solution. Develop over a path of 10 cm using a mixture of 10 volumes water, 10 volumes of anhydrous formic acid R and 80 volumes of ethyl formate R. Dry the plate at 100 - 105° C for 10 minutes and allow to cool. Spray with ferric chloride solution R2 until bluish-gray zones (phenolic compounds) appear. The chromatogram obtained with the test solution shows in its lower third a principal zone similar in position to the principal zone in the chromatogram obtained with reference solution (A) and, in its upper part, a narrow zone similar in position to the principal zone in the chromatogram obtained with reference solution (B). The chromatogram obtained with the test solution shows in addition several slightly colored zones in the central part.

Tests

Foreign matter (V.4.2)
Not more than 7 percent of stem and not more than 2 percent of other foreign matter, determine on 50 g.

Loss on drying (V.6.22)
Not more than 10 percent, determined on 2 g of powdered drug (355) by drying in an oven at 100 - 105° C for 4 hours.

Total ash (V.3.2.16)
Not more than 7 percent.

Ash insoluble in hydrochloric acid (V.4.1)
Not more than 2 percent.

Assay

Carry out all the extraction and dilution operations protected, as far as possible, from light. Use carbon dioxide-free water R for all operations.

To 0.750 g of the powdered drug (180) in a conical flask add 150 ml of water. Heat to boiling and maintain in a water-bath for 30 minutes. Cool in running water, transfer the mixture to a volumetric flask and dilute to 250 ml with water. Allow the solids to settle and filter the liquid through a filter paper 12 cm in diameter. Discard the first 50 ml of the filtrate.

Total polyphenols
Dilute 5 ml of the filtrate to 25 ml with water. Mix 5 ml of this solution with 2 ml of phosphotungstic acid solution R and dilute to 50 ml with sodium carbonate solution R. Exactly 3 minutes after addition of the last reagent, measure the absorbance (V.6.19) at 715 nm (A1) using water as the compensation liquid.

Polyphenols not adsorbed by hide powder
To 20 ml of the filtrate add 0.20 g of hide powder CRS and shake vigorously for 60 minutes. Filter. Dilute 5 ml of the filtrate to 25 ml with water. Mix 5 ml of this solution with 2 ml of phosphotungstic acid solution R and dilute to 50 ml with sodium carbonate solution R. Exactly 3 minutes after addition of the last reagent measure the absorbance at 715 nm (A2), using water as the compensation liquid.

Standard
Dissolve 50 mg of pyrogallol R in water and dilute to 100 ml with the same solvent. Dilute 5 ml of the solution to 100 ml with water. Mix 5 ml of this solution with 2 ml of phosphotungstic acid solution R, mix and dilute to 50 ml with sodium carbonate solution R. Exactly 3 minutes after addition of the last reagent and within 15 minutes after dissolution of the pyrogallol, measure the absorbance at 715 nm (A3), using water as the compensation liquid.

Calculate the percentage content of tannins from the expression:

$$\frac{13.12 \, (A_1 - A_2)}{A_3 \times m}$$

m = mass of substance to be examined in grams.

Storage
Store in a well-closed container, protected from light.

VII.1.1. Reagents
Chloral hydrate.
Complies with the requirements prescribed in the monograph on Chlorali Hydras.
   Chloral hydrate solution.
   A solution of 80 g in 20 ml of water.

Matricaria (German Chamomile) Flower
Matricariae Flos

Matricaria flower consists of the dried flower heads of *Matricaria recutita* L. (*Chamomilla recutita* (L.) Rauschert) [Fam. Asteraceae]. It contains not less than 0.4 percent v/m of blue essential oil.

Characteristics
Matricaria flower has a characteristically pleasant and aromatic odor.

The capitula, when spread out, consist of an involucre made up of many bracts arranged in one to three rows; an elongated-conical receptacle, occasionally hemispherical (young capitula); twelve to twenty marginal ligulate florets with a white ligule; several dozen yellow central tubular florets.

Matricaria flower has the macroscopic and microscopic characters described under identification tests A and B.

Identification
A. The bracts of the involucre are obovate to lanceolate, with a brownish-gray scarious margin. The receptacle is essentially conical and hollow, without

paleae. The base of the corolla of ligulate florets consists of a light yellow to brownish-yellow tube extending to an elongated-oval, white ligule. The corolla of tubular florets is yellow and broadens at the apex, where it splits into five teeth; its base is yellowish-brown to brown.

B. Separate the capitulum into its different parts. Examine under a microscope, using chloral hydrate solution R. The outer epidermis (abaxial) of the involucral bracts shows a scarious margin with a single layer of radially elongated cells and a central part made up of chlorophyll tissue covered with elongated epidermal cells with sinuous lateral walls, stomata and secretory trichomes. Surrounding the vascular bundles are numerous elongated, pitted sclereids with a fairly large lumen. In surface view, the corolla of ligulate florets and tubular florets show isodiametric or elongated cells with a more or less wavy wall and a few glandular trichomes. The outer part of the epidermis of the ligulate florets consists of papillary cells with cuticular striations radiating from their tips. In the mesophyll, very small clusters of calcium oxalate are sometimes seen. Four main veins run lengthwise through the entire mesophyll, sometimes accompanied by one or two other veins, which are shorter and run parallel to the main veins. The two main median veins both split into two near the tip and, with the lateral veins, anastomose two by two, forming three arcs at the three terminal teeth of the ligule. The ovaries, oval to spherical, of both kinds of florets, have at their base a sclerous ring consisting of a single row of cells. The epidermis of the ovary is made up of elongated cells with sinuous walls between which are inserted secretory trichomes. The ovaries contain numerous very small clusters of calcium oxalate. In the tubular florets the lower part of each stamen filament is surrounded by thick-walled cells. The epidermal cells of the ends of the two stigmata are very papillose. The pollen grains have a diameter of about 30 µm and are rounded and triangular, with three germinal pores and a spiny exine. Examine by thin-layer chromatography (V.6.20.2) using silica gel GF 254 R as the coating substance.

Test solution

In a porcelain mortar, coarsely pound 1 g of the drug, transfer to a chromatography column 15 cm long and 1.5 cm in internal diameter and tap lightly with a glass rod. Rinse the mortar and the pestle with two quantities, each of 10 ml, of methylene chloride R and pour the rinsings into the column. Collect the percolate in a flask with a long, narrow neck and remove the solvent by evaporation on a water-bath. Dissolve the residue in 0.5 ml of toluene R.

Reference solution

Dissolve 10 mg of borneol R, 20 mg of bornyl acetate R and 4 mg of guaiazulene R in toluene R and dilute to 10 ml with the same solvent. Apply separately to the plate as bands 20 mm by 3 mm 10 l of each solution. Develop over a path of 10 cm using chloroform R. Allow the plate to dry in air and examine in ultraviolet light at 254 nm. The chromatogram obtained with the test solution shows a number of quenching zones. The largest zone (en-yne-dicycloether) is situated at the same level as the zone due to bornyl acetate in the chromatogram obtained with the reference solution; a further zone is seen near the starting-point (matricin). Spray the plate with anisaldehyde solution R, using 10 ml for a plate 200 mm square, and examine in daylight while heating to 100 - 105° C for 5 - 10 minutes. The chromatogram obtained with the reference solution shows: in the lower third, a brownish-yellow zone (borneol) that becomes violet-gray after a few hours; in the middle a yellowish-brown to gray zone (bornyl acetate); and in the upper third a deep red zone with a blue edge (guaiazulene).

The chromatogram obtained with the test solution shows: a blue zone (matricin) near the starting-point; several violet-red zones (one of which is due to bisabolol) with Rf values between those of borneol and bornyl acetate; a brownish zone (en-yne-dicycloether) with an Rf value similar to that of bornyl acetate; red zones (terpenes) with Rf values similar to that of guaiazulene; other zones appear in the middle and lower parts of the chromatogram. Place 0.1 ml of the test solution used in identification test C in a test tube, add 2.5 ml of a solution prepared by dissolving 0.25 g of dimethylaminobenzaldehyde R in a mixture of 5 ml of phosphoric acid R, 45 ml of acetic acid R and 45 ml of water. Heat for 2 minutes in a water-bath and allow to cool. Add 5 ml of light petroleum R and shake. The aqueous layer has a distinct greenish-blue to blue color.

Tests
Broken drug
Not more than 25 percent passes through a no. 710 sieve.
Foreign matter (V.4.2)
Complies with the test for foreign matter.
Total ash (V.3.2.16)
Not more than 13 percent.

Assay
Carry out the determination of essential oils in vegetable drugs (V.4.5.8). Use 30 g of whole drug, a 100 ml flask, 300 ml of water as the distillation liquid and 0.50 ml of xylene R in the graduated tube. Distill at a rate of 3 - 4 ml per minute for 4 hours.

Storage
Store in a well-closed container, protected from light.

VII.1.1. Reagents
Chloral hydrate.
Complies with the requirements prescribed in the monograph on Chlorali Hydras.
Chloral hydrate solution.
A solution of 80 g in 20 ml of water.

Senna Leaf
Sennae Folium

Senna leaf consists of the dried leaflets of *Cassia senna* L. (syn. *C. acutifolia* Delile) [Fam. Fabaceae], known as Alexandrian or Khartoum senna, of *C. angustifolia* Vahl [Fam. Fabaceae], known as Tinnevelly senna, or a mixture of the two species. It contains not less than 2.5 percent of hydroxyanthracene glycosides, calculated as sennoside B ($C_{42}H_{38}O_{20}$; MW=863) with reference to the dried drug.

Characteristics
Senna leaf has a slight characteristic odor and has macroscopic and microscopic characteristics described under identification tests A and B.

Identification
A. *C. senna* occurs as grayish-green to brownish-green, thick, fragile leaflets, lanceolate, mucronate, asymmetrical at the base, usually 15 - 40 mm long and 5 - 15 mm wide, the maximum width being at a point slightly below the center; the lamina is slightly undulant with both surfaces covered with fine short trichomes. Pinnate venation is visible mainly on the lower surface, with lat-

eral veins leaving the midrib at an angle of about 60 and anastomosing to form a ridge near the margin.

Stomatal index (V.4.3) 10-12.5-15

B. *C. angustifolia* occurs as yellowish-green to brownish-green leaflets, elongated and lanceolate, slightly asymmetrical at the base, usually 20 - 50 mm long and 7 - 20 mm wide at the center. Both surfaces are smooth with a very small number of short trichomes and are frequently marked with transverse or oblique lines.

Stomatal index (V.4.3) 14-17.5-20

C. Reduce to a powder (355). The powder is light green to greenish-yellow. Examine under a microscope using chloral hydrate solution R. The powder shows the following diagnostic characteristics: polygonal epidermal cells showing paracytic stomata (V.4.3); unicellular trichomes, conical in shape, with warted walls, isolated or attached to fragments of epidermis; fragments of vascular bundles with a crystal sheath of prismatic crystals of calcium oxalate; cluster crystals isolated or in fragments of parenchyma.

Examine by thin-layer chromatography (V.6.20.2), using silica gel G R as the coating substance.

Test solution

To 0.5 of the powdered drug (180) add 5 ml of a mixture of equal volumes of alcohol R and water and heat to boiling. Centrifuge and use the supernatant liquid.

Reference solution

Dissolve 10 mg of senna extract CRS in 1 ml of a mixture of equal volumes of alcohol R and water (a slight residue remains).

Apply separately to the plate as bands 20 mm by 2 mm 10 l of each solution. Develop over a path of 10 cm using a mixture of 1 volume of glacial acetic acid R, 30 volumes of water, 40 volumes of ethyl acetate R and 40 volumes of propanol R. Allow the plate to dry in air, spray with a 20 percent v/v solution of nitric acid R and heat at 120° C for 10 minutes. Allow to cool and spray with a 5 percent m/v solution of potassium hydroxide R in alcohol (50 percent v/v) until the zones appear. The principal zones in the chromatogram obtained with the test solution are similar in position (sennosides B, A, D, and C in the order of increasing Rf values up to the central part), color and size to the principal zones in the chromatogram obtained with the reference solution. Between the zones corresponding to the sennosides D and C a red zone corresponding to rhein-8-glucoside may be visible. Place about 25 mg of the powdered drug (180) in a conical flask and add 50 ml of water and 2 ml of hydrochloric acid R. Heat in a water-bath for 15 minutes, cool and shake with 40 ml of ether R. Separate the ether, dry over anhydrous sodium sulfate R, evaporate 5 ml to dryness and to the cooled residue add 5 ml of dilute ammonia R 1. A yellow or orange color develops. Heat in a water-bath for 2 minutes. A reddish-violet color develops.

Tests

Foreign matter (V.4.2)

Not more than 3 percent of foreign organs and not more than 1 percent of foreign elements.

Loss on drying (V.6.22)

Not more than 12 percent, determined on 1 g of the powdered drug (355) by drying in an oven at 100 - 105° C for 2 hours.

Total ash (V.3.2.16)

Not more than 12 percent.

Ash insoluble in hydrochloric acid (V.4.1)

Not more than 2.5 percent.

Assay

Carry out the assay protected from bright light. Place 0.150 g of the powdered dry (180) in a 100 ml flask. Add 30 ml of water, mix, weigh, and place in a water-bath. Heat under a reflux condenser for 15 minutes. Allow to cool, weigh, and adjust to the original mass with water. Centrifuge and transfer 20 ml of the supernatant liquid to a 150 ml separating funnel. Add 0.1 ml of dilute hydrochloric acid R and shake with three quantities, each of 15 ml, of chloroform R. Allow to separate and discard the chloroform layer. Add 0.10 g of sodium bicarbonate R and shake for 3 minutes. Centrifuge and transfer 10 ml of the supernatant liquid to a 100 ml round-bottomed flask with a ground-glass neck. Add 20 ml of ferric chloride solution R1 and mix. Heat for 20 minutes under a reflux condenser in a water-bath with the water level above that of the liquid in the flask; add 1 ml of hydrochloric acid R and heat for a further 20 minutes, with frequent shaking, to dissolve the precipitate. Cool, transfer the mixture to a separating funnel and shake with three quantities each of 25 ml of ether R previously used to rinse the flask. Combine the ether layers and wash with two quantities, each of 15 ml, of water. Transfer the three layers to a volumetric flask and dilute to 100 ml with ether R. Evaporate 10 ml carefully to dryness and dissolve the residue in 10 ml of a 0.5 percent m/v solution of magnesium acetate R in methanol R. Measure the absorbance (V.6.19) at 515 nm, using methanol R as the compensation liquid.

Calculate the percentage content of sennoside B from the expression

$$\frac{A \times 1.25}{m}$$

i.e., taking specific absorbance to 240.
A = absorbance at 515 nm.
m = mass of the substance to be examined in grams.

Storage
Store protected from light and moisture.

VII.1.1. Reagents
Chloral hydrate.
Complies with the requirements prescribed in the monograph on Chlorali Hydras.
    Chloral hydrate solution.
    A solution of 80 g in 20 ml of water.

Alexandrian Senna Pods
Sennae Fructus Acutifoliae

Alexandrian senna pod consists of the dried fruit of *Cassia senna* L. (syn. *C. acutifolia* Delile) [Fam. Fabaceae]. They contain not less than 3.4 percent of hydroxyanthracene glycosides, calculated as sennoside B ($C_{42}H_{38}O_{20}$, MW=863) with reference to the dried drug.

Characteristics
Alexandrian senna pods have a slight odor. They have the macroscopic and microscopic characteristics described under identification tests A and B.

Identification
A. Alexandrian senna pods occur as flattened reniform pods, green to greenish-brown with brown patches at the positions corresponding to the seeds, usually 40 - 50 mm long and at least 20 mm wide. At one end is a stylar point and at the other a short stalk. The pods contain six or seven flattened and obovate seeds, green to pale brown, with a continuous network of prominent ridges on the testa.
B. Reduce to a powder (355). The powder is brown. Examine under a microscope using chloral hydrate solution R. The powder shows the following diagnostic

characteristics: epicarp with polygonal cells and a small number of conical warty trichomes and occasional anomocytic or paracytic stomata (V.4.3); fibers in two crossed layers accompanied by a crystal sheath of calcium oxalate prisms; characteristic palisade cells in the seed and stratified cells in the endosperm; clusters and prisms of calcium oxalate.

Examine by thin-layer chromatography (V.6.20.2), using silica gel G R as the coating substance.

Test solution
To 0.5 g of the powdered drug (180) add 5 ml of a mixture of equal volumes of alcohol R and water and heat to boiling. Centrifuge and use the supernatant liquid.

Reference solution
Dissolve 10 mg of senna extract CRS in 1 ml of a mixture of equal volumes of alcohol R and water (a slight residue remains).

Apply separately to the plate as bands 20 mm by 2 mm 10 l of each solution. Develop over a path of 10 cm using a mixture of 1 volume of glacial acetic acid R, 30 volumes of water, 40 volumes of ethyl acetate R and 40 volumes of propanol R. Allow the plate to dry in air, spray with a 20 percent v/v solution of nitric acid R and heat at 120° C for 10 minutes. Allow to cool and spray with a 5 percent m/v solution of potassium hydroxide R in alcohol (50 percent v/v) until the zones appear. The principal zones in the chromatogram obtained with the test solution are similar in position (sennosides B, A, D, and C in the order of increasing Rf value up to the central part), color and size to the principal zones in the chromatogram obtained with the reference solution. Between the zones corresponding to sennosides D and C a red zone corresponding to rhein-8-glucoside may be visible. The zones corresponding to sennosides D and C are faint in the chromatogram obtained with the test solution. Place about 25 mg of the powdered drug (180) in a conical flask and add 50 ml of water and 2 ml of hydrochloric acid R. Heat in a water-bath for 15 minutes, cool and shake with 40 ml of ether R. Separate the ether, dry over anhydrous sodium sulfate R, evaporate 5 ml to dryness and to the cooled residue add 5 ml of dilute ammonia R1. A yellow orange color develops. Heat in a water-bath for 2 minutes. A reddish-violet color develops.

Tests
Foreign matter (V.4.2)
Not more than 1 percent.
Loss on drying (V.6.22)
Not more than 12 percent, determined on 1 g of the powdered drug (355) by drying in an oven at 100 - 105° C for 2 hours.
Total ash (V.3.2.16)
Not more than 9 percent.
Ash insoluble in hydrochloric acid (V.4.1)
Not more than 2 percent.

Assay
Carry out the assay protected from bright light. Place 0.150 g of the powdered drug (180) in a 100 ml flask. Add 30 ml of water, mix, weigh, and place in a water-bath. Heat under a reflux condenser for 15 minutes. Allow to cool, weigh, and adjust to the original mass with water. Centrifuge and transfer 20 ml of the supernatant liquid to a 150 ml separating funnel. Add 0.10 g of sodium bicarbonate R and shake for 3 minutes. Centrifuge and transfer 10 ml of the supernatant liquid to a 100 ml round-bottomed flask with a ground-glass neck. Add 20 ml of ferric chloride solution R1 and mix. Heat for 20 minutes under a reflux condenser in a water-bath with the water level above that of the liquid in the flask; add 1 ml of hydrochloric acid R and heat for a further 20 minutes, with frequent shaking, to dissolve the precipitate. Cool, transfer the mixture to a separating funnel and shake with three quantities, each of 25 ml, of ether R previously used to rinse the flask. Combine the ether layers and wash with two quantities, each of 15 ml, of water. Transfer the three layers to a

volumetric flask and dilute to 100 ml with ether R. Evaporate 10 ml carefully to dryness and dissolve the residue in 10 ml of a 0.5 percent m/v solution of magnesium acetate R in methanol R. Measure the absorbance (V.6.19) at 515 nm, using methanol R as the compensation liquid.

Calculate the percentage content of sennoside B from the expression

$$\frac{A \times 1.25}{m}$$

i.e., taking specific absorbance to 240.
A = absorbance at 515 nm.
m = mass of the substance to be examined in grams.

Storage
Store protected from light and moisture.

VII.1.1. Reagents
Chloral hydrate.
 Complies with the requirements prescribed in the monograph on Chlorali Hydras.
 Chloral hydrate solution.
 A solution of 80 g in 20 ml of water.

Tinnevelly Senna Pods
Sennae Fructus Angustifoliae

Tinnevelly senna pod consists of the dried fruit of *Cassia angustifolia* Vahl [Fam. Fabaceae]. They contain not less than 2.2 percent of hydroxyanthracene glycosides, calculated as sennoside B ($C_{42}H_{38}O_{20}$, MW=863) with reference to the dried drug.

Characteristics
Tinnevelly senna pods have a slight odor. They have the macroscopic and microscopic characteristics described under identification tests A and B.

Identification
A. Alexandrian senna pods occur as flattened reniform pods, green to greenish-brown with brown patches at the positions corresponding to the seeds, usually 35 - 60 mm long and 14 - 18 mm wide. At one end is a stylar point and at the other a short stalk. The pods contain five to eight flattened and obovate seeds, green to pale brown, with incomplete, wavy, transverse ridges on the testa.
B. Reduce to a powder (355). The powder is brown. Examine under a microscope using chloral hydrate solution R. The powder shows the following diagnostic characteristics: epicarp with polygonal cells and a small number of conical warty trichomes and occasional anomocytic or paracytic stomata (V.4.3); fibers in two crossed layers accompanied by a crystal sheath of calcium oxalate prisms; characteristic palisade cells in the seed and stratified cells in the endosperm; clusters and prisms of calcium oxalate.
 Examine by thin-layer chromatography (V.6.20.2), using silica gel G R as the coating substance.

Test solution
To 0.5 g of the powdered drug (180) add 5 ml of a mixture of equal volumes of alcohol R and water and heat to boiling. Centrifuge and use the supernatant liquid.

Reference solution
Dissolve 10 mg of senna extract CRS in 1 ml of a mixture of equal volumes of alcohol R and water (a slight residue remains).
 Apply separately to the plate as band 20 mm by 2 mm 10 l of each solution. Develop over a path of 10 cm using a mix-

ture of 1 volume of glacial acetic acid R, 30 volumes of water, 40 volumes of ethyl acetate R and 40 volumes of propanol R. Allow the plate to dry in air, spray with a 20 percent v/v solution of nitric acid R and heat at 120° C for 10 minutes. Allow to cool and spray with a 5 percent m/v solution of potassium hydroxide R in alcohol (50 percent v/v) until the zones appear. The principal zones in the chromatogram obtained with the test solution are similar in position (sennosides B, A, D, and C in the order of increasing Rf value up to the central part), color and size to the principal zones in the chromatogram obtained with the reference solution. Between the zones corresponding to sennosides D and C a red zone corresponding to rhein-8-glucoside may be visible. The zones corresponding to sennosides D and C are faint in the chromatogram obtained with the test solution. Place about 25 mg of the powdered drug (180) in a conical flask and add 50 ml of water and 2 ml of hydrochloric acid R. Heat in a water-bath for 15 minutes, cool and shake with 40 ml of ether R. Separate the ether, dry over anhydrous sodium sulfate R, evaporate 5 ml to dryness and to the cooled residue add 5 ml of dilute ammonia R1. A yellow orange color develops. Heat on a water-bath for 2 minutes. A reddish-violet color develops.

Tests

Foreign matter (V.4.2)
Not more than 1 percent.
Loss on drying (V.6.22)
Not more than 12 percent, determined on 1 g of the powdered drug (355) by drying in an oven at 100 - 105° C for 2 hours.
Total ash (V.3.2.16)
Not more than 9 percent.
Ash insoluble in hydrochloric acid (V.4.1)
Not more than 2 percent.

Assay

Carry out the assay protected from bright light. Place 0.150 g of the powdered drug (180) in a 100 ml flask. Add 30 ml of water, mix, weigh, and place in a water-bath. Heat under a reflux condenser for 15 minutes. Allow to cool, weigh, and adjust to the original mass with water. Centrifuge and transfer 20 ml of the supernatant liquid to a 150 ml separating funnel. Add 0.10 g of sodium bicarbonate R and shake for 3 minutes. Centrifuge and transfer 10 ml of the supernatant liquid to a 100 ml round-bottomed flask with a ground-glass neck. Add 20 ml of ferric chloride solution R1 and mix. Heat for 20 minutes under a reflux condenser in a water-bath with the water level above that of the liquid in the flask; add 1 ml of hydrochloric acid R and heat for a further 20 minutes, with frequent shaking to dissolve the precipitate. Cool, transfer the mixture to a separating funnel and shake with three quantities, each of 25 ml, of ether R previously used to rinse the flask. Combine the ether layers and wash with two quantities, each of 15 ml, of water. Transfer the three layers to a volumetric flask and dilute to 100 ml with ether R. Evaporate 10 ml carefully to dryness and dissolve the residue in 10 ml of a 0.5 percent m/v solution of magnesium acetate R in methanol R. Measure the absorbance (V.6.19) at 515 nm, using methanol R as the compensation liquid.

Calculate the percentage content of sennoside B from the expression

$$\frac{A \times 1.25}{m}$$

i.e., taking specific absorbance to 240.

A = absorbance at 515 nm.
m = mass of the substance to be examined in grams.

Storage

Store protected from light and moisture.

VII.1.1. Reagents

Chloral hydrate.
Complies with the requirements prescribed in the monograph on Chlorali Hydras.

Chloral hydrate solution.
A solution of 80 g in 20 ml of water.

Valerian root
Valerianae Radix

Valerian root consists of the subterranean organs of *Valeriana officinalis* L. s.l. [Fam. Valerianaceae], including the rhizome, roots and stolons, carefully dried at a temperature below 40° C. It contains not less than 0.5 percent v/m of essential oil.

Description

Valerian root has a characteristic and penetrating odor, resembling that of valeric acid and camphor; the taste is somewhat sweet at first, then spicy and slightly bitter.

The rhizome is yellowish-gray to pale grayish-brown, obconical to cylindrical, up to 50 mm long and 30 mm in diameter; the base is elongated or compressed, covered by and merging with numerous roots. The apex usually exhibits a cup-shaped scar from the aerial parts; stem-bases are rarely present. In longitudinal section, the pith exhibits a central cavity traversed by septa. The roots are numerous, almost cylindrical, of the same color as the rhizome, 1 - 3mm in diameter and sometimes more than 100 mm long. A few filiform fragile secondary roots are present. The fracture is short. The stolons are pale yellowish-gray, showing prominent nodes separated by longitudinally striated internodes, each 20 - 50 mm long, with a fibrous fracture.

Examined under a microscope, the transverse section of the root shows small, suberised, epidermal cells, some with root hair; the exodermis consists of one or occasionally two layers of suberised cells often containing droplets of essential oil. The outer cortex comprises two to four layers of resin-containing cells with thin or collenchymatous, sometimes suberised walls. The inner cortex is composed of numerous layers of polygonal to rounded cells filled with starch. The starch granules are simple to compound; the simple granules are rounded, 5 - 15 µm in diameter, sometimes showing a cleft or stellate hilum; the compound granules, with two to six components, are up to 20 µm in diameter. The endodermis consists of a single layer of suberised, tangentially elongated cells. The pericycle is continuous and starch-filled; parenchyma surrounds the phloem zone; the cambium is frequently indistinct; the vascular bundles form an interrupted ring surrounding the starch-filled cells. The rhizome in transverse section has a different anatomy from the root. Its structure is complicated by the presence of numerous vascular bundles coming from the roots and stolons. The epidermis and exodermis are partly replaced by poorly developed periderm. The central pith is wide and has cavities of various sizes, the larger ones being separated by plates of partially sclerified tissue.

The powder is light brown and is characterized by numerous fragments of parenchyma with rounded or elongated cells and containing starch granules as described above; cells containing light-brown resin; rectangular sclereids with pitted walls, 5 - 15 µm thick; xylem, isolated or in non-compact bundles, 10 - 50 µm in diameter; some absorbing root hairs and cork fragments are also present.

Identification

To 0.2 g of freshly powdered drug add 5 ml of methylene chloride R, allow to stand for 5 minutes, shaking several times, and filter. Rinse the filter with 2 ml of methylene chloride R. Collect the filtrate and washings in a test-tube and heat in a water-bath for the minimum time necessary to remove the solvent. Dissolve the residue in 0.2 ml of methanol R (solution a). To 0.2 ml of solution (a) add 3 ml of a mixture of equal volumes of glacial acetic acid R and hydrochloric acid R1 and shake several times. The solution becomes blue within 15 minutes.

Tests

Chromatography
Examine by thin-layer chromatography (V.6.20.2), using silica gel G R as the coating substance.

Test solution
Use solution (a) prepared for the identification test.

Reference solution
Dissolve 2 mg of aminoazobenzene R and 2 mg of Sudan red G R in methanol R and dilute to 10 µl with the same solvent. Apply separately to the plate as bands 20 mm by 3 mm 10 µl of each solution. Develop twice over a path of 10 cm using a mixture of 30 volumes of ethyl acetate R and 70 volumes of hexane R. Spray with anisaldehyde solution R using 10 ml for a plate 200 mm square and examine while heating at 100 - 105° C for 5 - 10 minutes. The chromatogram obtained with the test solution shows: in the middle, at an Rf between those of the pink zone (Sudan red G) and the orange zone (aminoazobenzene) in the chromatogram obtained with the reference solution, a deep-violet zone (valerenic acid) and sometimes above this zone a grayish-brown zone (valtrate and isovaltrate); a faint violet zone (acetoxyvalerenic acid) with an Rf value lower than that of the zone due to aminoazobenze; gray zones situated between the zone due to valerenic acid and the starting point; in the upper part, a number of violet zones of variable intensity; any violet zone immediately above the starting point is at most very faint.

Extractable matter
To 2 g of the powdered drug (25) add a mixture of 8 g of water and 12 g of alcohol R and allow to macerate for 2 hours, shaking frequently. Filter, evaporate 5 g of the filtrate to dryness on a water-bath and dry at 100 - 105° C. The residue weighs not less than 75 mg (15 percent).

Sulfated ash (V.3.2.14)
Not more than 15 percent, determined on 1 g of powdered drug.

Ash insoluble in hydrochloric acid (V.4.1)
Not more than 7 percent.

Assay

Carry out the determination of essential oil in vegetable drugs (V.4.5.8). Use 215 g of freshly powdered drug (500), a 1000 ml flask, 300 ml of water as distillation liquid and 0.50 ml of xylene R in the graduated tube. Distill at a rate of 3 - 4 ml per minute for 4 hours.

Storage

Store in a well-closed container, protected from light.

VII.1.1 Reagents

Aminoazobenzene. – $C_{12}H_{11}N_3$ (Mr 197.2) Color Index No. 11000. Azobenzene-4-amine.

Brownish-yellow needles with a bluish tinge, slightly soluble in water, freely soluble in alcohol, chloroform, and ether. mp: about 128° C.

Chapter 20

European Economic Community (EEC) Standards for Quality of Herbal Remedies

This section includes guidelines for detailed qualitative and quantitative labeling standards, description of the method of preparation, quality control of vegetable drug preparations and other control tests that must be conducted during the manufacturing process.

The following quote is taken from a directive published by the EEC in reference to defining quality standards for herbal drugs sold in the EEC:

> Note for guidance concerning the application of Part 1 of the Annex to Directive 75/318/EEC, as amended. The special problems of herbal remedies and the differences between medicinal products containing chemically defined active ingredients are described in this note for guidance.
>
> Consistent quality for products of vegetable origin can only be assured if the starting materials are defined in a rigorous and detailed manner, including the specific botanical identification of the plant material used. It is also important to know the geographical source and the conditions under which the vegetable drug is obtained in order to ensure material of consistent quality.
>
> Reference substances used in the control of all stages of the manufacturing process should be clearly defined.

A. Qualitative and Quantitative Labeling Standards

(1) In the case of a vegetable drug *either*
    (a) the quantity of the vegetable drug must be stated *or*
    (b) the quantity of a vegetable drug may be given as a range corresponding to a defined quantity of constituents with known therapeutic activity.

Example:
(a) Active ingredient

Name	Quantity
Sennae folium dry 60% ethanolic extract (8:1)	125 mg
or	
Sennae folium dry 60% ethanolic extract	125 mg equivalent to 1000 mg Sennae folium

or

(b) Active ingredient

Name	Quantity
Sennae folium dry 60% extract (8:1)	100 - 130 mg, corresponding to 25 mg of hydroxyanthracene glycosides, calculated as sennoside B

Other ingredients Name	Quantity
Dextrin	20 - 50 mg

B. Description of the Method of Preparation

The manufacturing process, within the meaning of this section, is the preparation of the finished product from the starting materials. The description should include details of any comminution or size reduction step, and details of any process, such as fumigation, etc., used to reduce the levels of microbial contamination, together with the controls exercised over the process. If vegetable drug preparations are the starting material, the manufacture of the vegetable drug preparations and their controls do not belong under this section but under section C.

C. Quality Control of Vegetable Drug Preparations

If the herbal remedy contains not the vegetable drug itself but a preparation, the monograph on the drug must be followed by a description and validation of the manufacturing process for the vegetable drug preparation.

For each vegetable drug preparation, a monograph must be submitted. This must be established on the basis of recent scientific data and must give particulars of the characteristics, identification tests, and purity tests. This has to be done, e.g., by appropriate chromatographic methods. If deemed necessary by the results of the analysis of the starting material, tests on microbiological quality, residues of pesticides, fumigation agents, radioactivity, solvents, and toxic metals have to be carried out. Quantitative determination (assay) of characteristic constituents is required. The test methods must be described in detail.

If preparations from vegetable drugs with constituents with known therapeutic activity are standardized (i.e., adjusted to a certain level of constituents with known therapeutic activity) it must be stated how such standardization is achieved. If another ingredient is used for this purpose, it is necessary to specify as a range the quantity that can be added.

D. Control Test Carried Out at an Intermediate Stage of the Manufacturing Process of the Finished Product

Details of all control tests, with details of test procedures and limits applied at any intermediate stages of the manufacturing processes, are required, especially if these tests cannot be done on the finished product.

PART SIX

APPENDIX

Abbreviations and Symbols	587
Weights and Measures	591
German *Federal Gazette* (*Bundesanzeiger*) Numbers and Publication Dates of Commission E Monographs	593
List of European Scientific Cooperative on Phytotherapy (ESCOP) Monographs	613
List of World Health Organization (WHO) Monographs	615
General Glossary	617
General References	641
General Index	643
Addendum – Contraindications of Unapproved Herbs	681
Errata	685

ABBREVIATIONS AND SYMBOLS

ASK — *Bearbeitungsnummern des Bundesinstituts für Arzneimittel und Medizinprodukte*, working numbers of the Federal Institute for Drug Agents and Medicinal Products for individual chemical reagents

B. Anz. — *Bundesanzeiger* (German *Federal Gazette*), edited by the Minister of Justice

BfArM — German Federal Institute of Drugs and Medical Devices (formerly BGA)

BGA — German Federal Health Agency (now BfArM)

C — Celsius, Centigrade

ca — circa, approximately

cm, cm^2 — centimeter(s), square centimeter(s)

DAB 6 — *Deutsches Arzneibuch* (*German Pharmacopoeia*), Sixth edition 1926

DAB 7 — *Deutsches Arzneibuch* (*German Pharmacopoeia*), Seventh edition 1968

DAB 8 — *Deutsches Arzneibuch* (*German Pharmacopoeia*), Eighth edition 1978; First Supplement 1980; Second Supplement 1983

DAB 9 — *Deutsches Arzneibuch* (*German Pharmacopoeia*), Ninth edition 1986; First Supplement 1989; Second Supplement 1990

DAB 10 — *Deutsches Arzneibuch* (*German Pharmacopoeia*), Tenth edition 1991; First Supplement 1992; Second Supplement 1993

DAC — *Deutscher Arzneimittel-Codex* (*German Drug Formulary*)

D.C. — de Candolle (botanical authority)

emend. — *emendavit*, as corrected (in botanical name)

Erg. B. 6 — *Ergänzungsbuch zum Deutschen Arzneibuch* (*Supplement Volume to the German Pharmacopoeia*), Sixth edition 1926. Reprinted 1953

Fam. — plant family

FIP — Federacion Internacionale Pharmaceutique (International Pharmaceutical Federation)

FIP unit — measurement of calorie content in bread units issued by the Federacion Internacionale Pharmaceutique

g — gram

GPU — guinea pig units, ad hoc measure used for fixed combination of pheasant's eye fluidextract, lily-of-the-valley powdered extract, squill powdered extract, and oleander leaf powdered extract

HPLC — High performance liquid chromatography

kPa — kiloPascals

L. — Linnaeus (botanical authority)

l — liter

LD^{50} — Lethal-dosage-50, dose causing death in 50% of test animals

LD^{100} — Lethal-dosage-100, dose causing death in 100% of test animals

m/m — mass in mass measurement

m/v — mass in volume measurement

mcg — microgram

mg — milligram

mg/kg — milligrams drug per kilogram body weight

ml — milliliter

mm — millimeters

m — meters

MAO — monoamine oxidase

MMR — Molar Mass

MW — molecular weight

N — normal (solution)

nm — nanometers

Nutt. — Nuttall (botanical authority)

NYHA — New York Heart Association

ÖAB — Österreichisches Arzneibuch (Austrian Pharmacopoeia), 2 volumes, 1981; First Supplement 1983

PA — pyrrolizidine alkaloid

Ph. Helv. VI — *Pharmacopoea Helvetica* (*Swiss Pharmacopeia*), sixth edition

p.p. — *pro parte*, in part (in botanical name)

R — reagent

R*f* — radiative frequency (in HPLC)

RN — normalized reagent

s.l. — *sensu lato*, in a broad sense (in botanical name)

spp. — species

syn. — synonym

var. — *varietas*, variety (variety of plant within species)

v/v — volume in volume measurement

v/w — volume in weight measurement

UV — ultraviolet

WHO — World Health Organization

μ — microns

μg — microgram

μl — microliter

μm — micrometer

α — alpha

ß — beta

γ — gamma

Weights and Measures

Metric Weight

kg (kilo)	one kilogram	= 1000 grams
cg	one centigram	= 0.01 gram
mg	one milligram	= 0.001 grams
µg (mcg)	one microgram	= 0.0001 gram

Avoirdupois Weight

pounds	ounces	drachma	grains
1	16	256	7000
	1	16	437.5
		1	27.34375

Apothecaries Weight

pounds	ounces	drachma	scruples	grains
1	12	96	288	5760
	1	8	24	480
		1	3	60
			1	24

1 grain	= .065 mg
1 grain	= 0.097 minims
1 minim	= 1 drop
60 drops	= 1 fluid dram

Comparison of United States, British Imperial, and Metric Systems of Liquid Measures

1 U.S. minim	= 1.04 Imperial minims
1 U.S. gallon	= 0.8237 Imperial gallon
1 U.S. pint	= 0.8237 Imperial pint
1 Imperial gallon	= 1.2009 U.S. gallons
1 Imperial pint	= 1.2009 U.S. pints
1 Imperial fluid ounce	= 437.5 grains
1 U.S. gallon	= 128 fluid ounces = 61440 minims = 3.785 liters
8 pints or 6.66 Imp. pints	= 8.3283 lbs. avoirdupois at 60° F
1 Imperial gallon	=160 fluid ounces = 76800 minims = 4.5460 liters
8 Imperial pints or 9.6072 U.S. pints	= 10 lbs. avoirdupois at 60° F

Metric to English Length

mm	millimeter	= 0.04 inches (in)
cm	centimeter	= 0.39 in
dm	decimeter	= 3.93 in
m	meter	= 39.3 in

English to Metric Length

1 inch (in) = 25.4 millimeters (mm) = 2.54 cm
1 foot (ft) = 304.8 mm = 30.48 cm = 0.3048 m

German Federal Gazette (Bundesanzeiger) Numbers and Publication Dates of Commission E Monographs

This table lists by English name all the monographs published by the Commission. The original monographs were published by their pharmacopeial name in the *Bundesanzeiger*, the German equivalent of the United States *Federal Register*. This list includes the specific volume of the *Bundesanzeiger*, the date of publication, and the date of any revisions.

English Name	Pharmacopeial Name	Issue Number	Date
Agrimony	Agrimoniae herba	B. Anz. No. 50	Mar. 13, 1986
Agrimony	Agrimoniae herba *Rev.*	B. Anz. No. 50	Mar. 13, 1990
Aloe	Aloe	B. Anz. No. 133	July 21, 1993
Alpine Lady's Mantle herb	Alchemillae alpinae herba	B. Anz. No. 162	Aug. 29, 1992
Angelica root	Angelicae radix	B. Anz. No. 101	June 1, 1990
Angelica seed and herb	Angelicae fructus/-herba	B. Anz. No. 101	June 1, 1990
Anise seed	Anisi fructus	B. Anz. No. 122	July 6, 1988
Arnica flower	Arnicae flos	B. Anz. No. 228	Dec. 5, 1984
Artichoke leaf	Cynarae folium	B. Anz. No. 122	July 6, 1988
Artichoke leaf	Cynarae folium *Rev.*	B. Anz. No. 164	Sep. 1, 1990
Ash bark and leaf	Fraxinus excelsior	B. Anz. No. 22a	Feb. 1, 1990
Asparagus herb	Asparagi herba	B. Anz. No. 127	July 12, 1991
Asparagus root	Asparagus rhizoma	B. Anz. No. 127	July 12, 1991
Aspen bark and leaf	Populi cortex/-folium	B. Anz. No. 162	Aug. 29, 1992
Autumn Crocus	Colchicum autumnale	B. Anz. No. 173	Sep. 18, 1986
Barberry	Berberis vulgaris	B. Anz. No. 43	Mar. 2, 1989
Basil herb	Basilici herba	B. Anz. No. 54	Mar. 18, 1992
Basil oil	Basilici aetheroleum	B. Anz. No. 54	Mar. 18, 1992
Belladonna	Atropa belladonna	B. Anz. No. 223	Nov. 30, 1985
Bilberry fruit	Myrtilli fructus	B. Anz. No. 76	Apr. 23, 1987
Bilberry fruit	Myrtilli fructus *Rev.*	B. Anz. No. 50	Mar. 13, 1990

English Name	Pharmacopeial Name	Issue Number	Date
Bilberry leaf	Myrtilli folium	*B. Anz.* No. 76	Apr. 23, 1987
Birch leaf	Betulae folium	*B. Anz.* No. 50	Mar. 13, 1986
Bishop's Weed fruit	Ammeos visnagae fructus	*B. Anz.* No. 71	Apr. 15, 1994
Bitter Orange flower	Aurantii flos	*B. Anz.* No. 128	July 14, 1993
Bitter Orange peel	Aurantii pericarpium	*B. Anz.* No. 193a	Oct. 15, 1987
Bitter Orange peel	Aurantii pericarpium *Rev.*	*B. Anz.* No. 50	Mar. 13, 1990
Black Cohosh root	Cimicifugae racemosae rhizoma	*B. Anz.* No. 43	Mar. 2, 1989
Blackberry leaf	Rubi fruticosi folium	*B. Anz.* No. 22a	Feb. 1, 1990
Blackberry root	Rubi fruticosi radix	*B. Anz.* No. 22a	Feb. 1, 1990
Blackthorn berry	Pruni spinosae fructus	*B. Anz.* No. 101	June 1, 1990
Blackthorn flower	Pruni spinosae flos	*B. Anz.* No. 101	June 1, 1990
Bladderwrack	Fucus	*B. Anz.* No. 101	June 1, 1990
Blessed Thistle herb	Cnici benedicti herba	*B. Anz.* No. 193a	Oct. 15, 1987
Bogbean leaf	Menyanthis folium	*B. Anz.* No. 22a	Feb. 1, 1990
Boldo leaf	Boldo folium	*B. Anz.* No. 76	Apr. 23, 1987
Boldo leaf	Boldo folium *Rev.*	*B. Anz.* No. 164	Sep. 1, 1990
Borage	Borago	*B. Anz.* No. 127	July 12, 1991
Brewer's Yeast	Saccharomyces cerevisiae	*B. Anz.* No. 71	Apr. 15, 1994
Bromelain	Bromelainum	*B. Anz.* No. 48	Mar. 10, 1994
Bryony root	Bryoniae radix	*B. Anz.* No. 122	July 6, 1988
Buchu leaf	Barosmae folium	*B. Anz.* No. 22a	Feb. 1, 1990
Buckthorn bark	Frangulae cortex	*B. Anz.* No. 133	July 21, 1993
Buckthorn berry	Rhamni cathartici fructus	*B. Anz.* No. 221	Nov. 25, 1993
Bugleweed	Lycopi herba	*B. Anz.* No. 22a	Feb. 1, 1990
Burdock root	Bardanae radix	*B. Anz.* No. 22a	Feb. 1, 1990
Butcher's Broom	Rusci aculeati rhizoma	*B. Anz.* No. 127	July 12, 1991
Cajeput oil	Cajeputi aetheroleum	*B. Anz.* No. 128	July 14, 1993
Calendula flower	Calendulae flos	*B. Anz.* No. 50	Mar. 13, 1986
Calendula herb	Calendulae herba	*B. Anz.* No. 128	July 14, 1993
California Poppy	Eschscholzia californica	*B. Anz.* No. 178	Sep. 21, 1991
Camphor	Camphora	*B. Anz.* No. 228	Dec. 5, 1984
Camphor	Camphora *Rev.*	*B. Anz.* No. 50	Mar. 13, 1990
Caraway oil	Carvi aetheroleum	*B. Anz.* No. 22a	Feb. 1, 1990
Caraway seed	Carvi fructus	*B. Anz.* No. 22a	Feb. 1, 1990
Cardamom seed	Cardamomi fructus	*B. Anz.* No. 223	Nov. 30, 1985
Cardamom seed	Cardamomi fructus *Rev.*	*B. Anz.* No. 50	Mar. 13, 1990
Cardamom seed	Cardamomi fructus *Rev.*	*B. Anz.* No. 164	Sep. 1, 1990

English Name	Pharmacopeial Name	Issue Number	Date
Cascara Sagrada bark	Rhamni purshianae cortex	B. Anz. No. 133	July 21, 1993
Cat's Foot flower	Antennariae dioicae flos	B. Anz. No. 162	Aug. 29, 1992
Celandine herb	Chelidonii herba	B. Anz. No. 90	May 15, 1985
Celery	Apium graveolens	B. Anz. No. 127	July 12, 1991
Centaury herb	Centaurii herba	B. Anz. No. 122	July 6, 1988
Centaury herb	Centaurii herba Rev.	B. Anz. No. 50	Mar. 13, 1990
Chamomile flower, German	Matricariae flos	B. Anz. No. 228	Dec. 5, 1984
Chamomile flower, German	Matricariae flos Rev.	B. Anz. No. 50	Mar. 13, 1990
Chamomile flower, Roman	Chamomillae romanae flos	B. Anz. No. 221	Nov. 25, 1993
Chaste Tree fruit	Agni casti fructus	B. Anz. No. 90	May 15, 1985
Chaste Tree fruit	Agni casti fructus Repl.	B. Anz. No. 226	Dec. 2, 1992
Chestnut leaf	Castaneae folium	B. Anz. No. 76	Apr. 23, 1987
Chicory	Cichorium intybus	B. Anz. No. 76	Apr. 23, 1987
Chicory	Cichorium intybus Rev.	B. Anz. No. 164	Sep. 1, 1990
Cinchona bark	Cinchonae cortex	B. Anz. No. 22a	Feb. 1, 1990
Cinnamon bark	Cinnamomi ceylanici cortex	B. Anz. No. 22a	Feb. 1, 1990
Cinnamon bark, Chinese	Cinnamomi cassiae cortex	B. Anz. No. 22a	Feb. 1, 1990
Cinnamon flower	Cinnamomi flos	B. Anz. No. 49	Mar. 11, 1992
Cloves	Caryophylli flos	B. Anz. No. 223	Nov. 30, 1985
Cocoa	Cacao testes	B. Anz. No. 40	Feb. 27, 1991
Cocoa seed	Cacao semen	B. Anz. No. 40	Feb. 27, 1991
Coffee Charcoal	Coffeae carbo	B. Anz. No. 85	May 5, 1988
Cola nut	Colae semen	B. Anz. No. 127	July 12, 1991
Colocynth	Colocynthidis fructus	B. Anz. No. 164	Sep. 1, 1990
Coltsfoot flower/herb/root	Farfarae flos/-herba/-radix	B. Anz. No. 138	July 27, 1990
Coltsfoot leaf	Farfarae folium	B. Anz. No. 138	July 27, 1990
Comfrey herb and leaf	Symphyti herba/-folium	B. Anz. No. 138	July 27, 1990
Comfrey root	Symphyti radix	B. Anz. No. 138	July 27, 1990
Condurango bark	Condurango cortex	B. Anz. No. 193a	Oct. 15, 1987
Condurango bark	Condurango cortex Rev.	B. Anz. No. 50	Mar. 13, 1990
Coriander seed	Coriandri fructus	B. Anz. No. 173	Sep. 18, 1986
Corn Poppy	Rhoeados flos	B. Anz. No. 85	May 5, 1988
Cornflower	Centaurea cyanus	B. Anz. No. 43	Mar. 2, 1989

English Name	Pharmacopeial Name	Issue Number	Date
Couch Grass	Graminis rhizoma	*B. Anz.* No. 22a	Feb. 1, 1990
Damiana leaf and herb	Turnera diffusa	*B. Anz.* No. 43	Mar. 2, 1989
Dandelion herb	Taraxaci herba	*B. Anz.* No. 162	Aug. 29, 1992
Dandelion root with herb	Taraxaci radix cum herba	*B. Anz.* No. 228	Dec. 5, 1984
Dandelion root with herb	Taraxaci radix cum herba *Rev.*	*B. Anz.* No. 164	Sep. 1, 1990
Delphinium flower	Delphinii flos	*B. Anz.* No. 80	Apr. 27, 1989
Devil's Claw root	Harpagophyti radix	*B. Anz.* No. 43	Mar. 2, 1989
Devil's Claw root	Harpagophyti radix *Rev.*	*B. Anz.* No. 164	Sep. 1, 1990
Dill seed	Anethi fructus	*B. Anz.* No. 193a	Oct. 15, 1987
Dill seed	Anethi fructus *Rev.*	*B. Anz.* No. 50	Mar. 13, 1990
Dill weed	Anethi herba	*B. Anz.* No. 193a	Oct. 15, 1987
Echinacea Angustifolia herb and root/ Pallida herb	Echinaceae angustifoliae herba et radix / pallidae herba	*B. Anz.* No. 162	Aug. 29, 1992
Echinacea Pallida root	Echinaceae pallidae radix	*B. Anz.* No. 162	Aug. 29, 1992
Echinacea Purpurea herb	Echinaceae purpureae herba	*B. Anz.* No. 43	Mar. 2, 1989
Echinacea Purpurea root	Echinaceae purpureae radix	*B. Anz.* No. 162	Aug. 29, 1992
Elder flower	Sambuci flos	*B. Anz.* No. 50	Mar. 13, 1986
Elecampane root	Helenii radix	*B. Anz.* No. 85	May 5, 1988
Eleuthero (Siberian Ginseng) root	Eleutherococci radix	*B. Anz.* No. 11	Jan. 17, 1991
Ephedra	Ephedrae herba	*B. Anz.* No. 11	Jan. 17, 1991
Ergot	Secale cornutum	*B. Anz.* No. 173	Sep. 18, 1986
Eucalyptus leaf	Eucalypti folium	*B. Anz.* No. 177a	Sep. 24, 1986
Eucalyptus leaf	Eucalypti folium *Rev.*	*B. Anz.* No. 50	Mar. 13, 1990
Eucalyptus oil	Eucalypti aetheroleum	*B. Anz.* No. 177a	Sep. 24, 1986
Eucalyptus oil	Eucalypti aetheroleum *Rev.*	*B. Anz.* No. 50	Mar. 13, 1990
Eyebright	Euphrasia officinalis	*B. Anz.* No. 162	Aug. 29, 1992
Fennel oil	Foeniculi aetheroleum	*B. Anz.* No. 74	Apr. 19, 1991
Fennel seed	Foeniculi fructus	*B. Anz.* No. 74	Apr. 19, 1991
Fenugreek seed	Foenugraeci semen	*B. Anz.* No. 22a	Feb. 1, 1990
Figs	Caricae fructus	*B. Anz.* No. 101	June 1, 1990
Fir Needle oil	Piceae aetheroleum	*B. Anz.* No. 154	Aug. 21, 1985
Fir Needle oil	Piceae aetheroleum *Rev.*	*B. Anz.* No. 50	Mar. 13, 1990
Fir Shoots, Fresh	Piceae turiones recentes	*B. Anz.* No. 193a	Oct. 15, 1987
Flaxseed	Lini semen	*B. Anz.* No. 228	May 12, 1984

English Name	Pharmacopeial Name	Issue Number	Date
Fumitory	Fumariae herba	B. Anz. No. 173	Sep. 18, 1986
Galangal	Galangae rhizoma	B. Anz. No. 173	Sep. 18, 1986
Galangal	Galangae rhizoma *Rev.*	B. Anz. No. 50	Mar. 13, 1990
Garlic	Allii sativi bulbus	B. Anz. No. 122	July 6, 1988
Gentian root	Gentianae radix	B. Anz. No. 223	Nov. 30, 1985
Gentian root	Gentianae radix *Rev.*	B. Anz. No. 50	Mar. 13, 1990
Ginger root	Zingiberis rhizoma	B. Anz. No. 85	May 5, 1988
Ginger root	Zingiberis rhizoma *Rev.*	B. Anz. No. 50	Mar. 13, 1990
Ginger root	Zingiberis rhizoma *Rev.*	B. Anz. No. 164	Sep. 1, 1990
Ginkgo Biloba Leaf Extract	Ginkgo folium	B. Anz. No. 133	July 19, 1994
Ginkgo Biloba leaf	Ginkgo folium	B. Anz. No. 133	July 19, 1994
Ginseng root	Ginseng radix	B. Anz. No. 11	Jan. 17, 1991
Goat's Rue herb	Galegae officinalis herba	B. Anz. No. 180	Sep. 24, 1993
Goldenrod	Solidago	B. Anz. No. 193a	Oct. 15, 1987
Goldenrod	Solidago *Rev.*	B. Anz. No. 50	Mar. 13, 1990
Guaiac Wood	Guajaci lignum	B. Anz. No. 76	Apr. 23, 1987
Gumweed herb	Grindeliae herba	B. Anz. No. 11	Jan. 17, 1991
Haronga bark and leaf	Harunganae madagascariensis cortex et folium	B. Anz. No. 50	Mar. 13, 1990
Hawthorn berry	Crataegi fructus	B. Anz. No. 133	July 19, 1994
Hawthorn flower	Crataegi flos	B. Anz. No. 133	July 19, 1994
Hawthorn leaf	Crataegi folium	B. Anz. No. 133	July 19, 1994
Hawthorn leaf with flower	Crataegi folium cum flore	B. Anz. No. 133	July 19, 1994
Hay flower	Graminis flos	B. Anz. No. 85	May 5, 1988
Heart's Ease herb	Violae tricoloris herba	B. Anz. No. 50	Mar. 13, 1986
Heather herb and flower	Callunae vulgaris	B. Anz. No. 101	June 1, 1990
Hempnettle herb	Galeopsidis herba	B. Anz. No. 76	Apr. 23, 1987
Henbane leaf	Hyoscyami folium	B. Anz. No. 85	May 5, 1988
Hibiscus	Hibisci flos	B. Anz. No. 22a	Feb. 1, 1990
Hollyhock flower	Malvae arboraeae flos	B. Anz. No. 43	Mar. 2, 1989
Hops	Lupuli strobulus	B. Anz. No. 228	Dec. 5, 1984
Hops	Lupuli strobulus *Rev.*	B. Anz. No. 50	Mar. 13, 1990
Horehound herb	Marrubii herba	B. Anz. No. 22a	Feb. 1, 1990
Horse Chestnut bark and flower	Hippocastani cortex/-flos	B. Anz. No. 221	Nov. 25, 1993
Horse Chestnut leaf	Hippocastani folium	B. Anz. No. 128	July 14, 1993

English Name	Pharmacopeial Name	Issue Number	Date
Horse Chestnut seed	Hippocastani semen	*B. Anz.* No. 71	Apr. 15, 1994
Horseradish	Armoraciae rusticanae radix	*B. Anz.* No. 85	May 5, 1988
Horsetail herb	Equiseti herba	*B. Anz.* No. 173	Sep. 18, 1986
Hound's Tongue herb	Cynoglossi herba	*B. Anz.* No. 43	Mar. 2, 1989
Hyssop	Hyssopus officinalis	*B. Anz.* No. 162	Aug. 29, 1992
Iceland Moss	Lichen islandicus	*B. Anz.* No. 43	Mar. 2, 1989
Indian Snakeroot	Rauwolfiae radix	*B. Anz.* No. 173	Sep. 18, 1986
Ivy leaf	Hederae helicis folium	*B. Anz.* No. 122	July 6, 1988
Jambolan bark	Syzygii cumini cortex	*B. Anz.* No. 76	Apr. 23, 1987
Jambolan seed	Syzygii cumini semen	*B. Anz.* No. 76	Apr. 23, 1987
Java Tea	Orthosiphonis folium	*B. Anz.* No. 50	Mar. 13, 1986
Java Tea	Orthosiphonis folium *Rev.*	*B. Anz.* No. 50	Mar. 13, 1990
Jimsonweed leaf and seed	Stramonii folium/-semen	*B. Anz.* No. 22a	Feb. 1, 1990
Juniper berry	Juniperi fructus	*B. Anz.* No. 228	Dec. 5, 1984
Kava Kava	Piperis methystici rhizoma	*B. Anz.* No. 101	June 1, 1990
Kelp	Laminariae stipites	*B. Anz.* No. 128	July 14, 1993
Kidney Bean pods (without seeds)	Phaseoli fructus sine semine	*B. Anz.* No. 50	Mar. 13, 1986
Kidney Bean pods (without seeds)	Phaseoli fructus sine semine *Rev.*	*B. Anz.* No. 50	Mar. 13, 1990
Knotweed herb	Polygoni avicularis herba	*B. Anz.* No. 76	Apr. 23, 1987
Knotweed herb	Polygoni avicularis herba *Rev.*	*B. Anz.* No. 50	Mar. 13, 1990
Lady's Mantle	Alchemillae herba	*B. Anz.* No. 173	Sep. 18, 1986
Larch Turpentine	Terebinthina Laricina	*B. Anz.* No. 228	Dec. 5, 1984
Larch Turpentine	Terebinthina Laricina *Rev.*	*B. Anz.* No. 50	Mar. 13, 1990
Lavender flower	Lavandulae flos	*B. Anz.* No. 228	Dec. 5, 1984
Lavender flower	Lavandulae flos *Rev.*	*B. Anz.* No. 50	Mar. 13, 1990
Lemon Balm	Melissae folium	*B. Anz.* No. 228	Dec. 5, 1984
Lemon Balm	Melissae folium *Rev.*	*B. Anz.* No. 50	Mar. 13, 1990
Lemongrass	Cymbopogon species	*B. Anz.* No. 22a	Feb. 1, 1990
Licorice root	Liquiritiae radix	*B. Anz.* No. 90	May 15, 1985
Licorice root	Liquiritiae radix *Rev.*	*B. Anz.* No. 50	Mar. 13, 1990
Licorice root	Liquiritiae radix *Rev.*	*B. Anz.* No. 74	Apr. 19, 1991
Licorice root	Liquiritiae radix *Rev.*	*B. Anz.* No. 178	Sep. 21, 1991
Lily-of-the-valley herb	Convallariae herba	*B. Anz.* No. 76	Apr. 23, 1987
Lily-of-the-valley herb	Convallariae herba *Rev.*	*B. Anz.* No. 22a	Feb. 1, 1990
Linden Charcoal	Tiliae carbo	*B. Anz.* No. 164	Sep. 1, 1990

English Name	Pharmacopeial Name	Issue Number	Date
Linden flower	Tiliae flos	B. Anz. No. 164	Sep. 1, 1990
Linden flower, Silver	Tiliae tomentosae flos	B. Anz. No. 164	Sep. 1, 1990
Linden leaf	Tiliae folium	B. Anz. No. 164	Sep. 1, 1990
Linden wood	Tiliae lignum	B. Anz. No. 164	Sep. 1, 1990
Liverwort herb	Hepatici nobilis herba	B. Anz. No. 128	July 14, 1993
Loofa	Luffa aegyptiaca	B. Anz. No. 180	Sep. 24, 1993
Lovage root	Levistici radix	B. Anz. No. 101	June 1, 1990
Lungwort	Pulmonariae herba	B. Anz. No. 193a	Oct. 15, 1987
Madder root	Rubiae tinctorum radix	B. Anz. No. 162	Aug. 29, 1992
Male Fern	Filicis maris folium/herba/rhizoma	B. Anz. No. 180	Sep. 24, 1993
Mallow flower	Malvae flos	B. Anz. No. 43	Mar. 2, 1989
Mallow leaf	Malvae folium	B. Anz. No. 43	Mar. 2, 1989
Manna	Manna	B. Anz. No. 22a	Feb. 1, 1990
Marjoram	Origanum majorana	B. Anz. No. 226	Dec. 2, 1992
Marsh Tea	Ledi palustris herba	B. Anz. No. 177a	Sep. 24, 1986
Marshmallow leaf	Althaeae folium	B. Anz. No. 43	Mar. 2, 1989
Marshmallow root	Althaeae radix	B. Anz. No. 43	Mar. 2, 1989
Maté leaf	Mate folium	B. Anz. No. 85	May 5, 1988
Mayapple root and resin	Podophylli peltati rhizoma/resina	B. Anz. No. 50	Mar. 13, 1986
Meadowsweet	Filipendula ulmaria	B. Anz. No. 43	Mar. 2, 1989
Mentzelia	Mentzelia cordifolia	B. Anz. No. 180	Sep. 24, 1993
Milk Thistle fruit	Cardui mariae fructus	B. Anz. No. 50	Mar. 13, 1986
Milk Thistle herb	Cardui mariae herba	B. Anz. No. 49	Mar. 11, 1992
Mint oil	Menthae arvensis aetheroleum	B. Anz. No. 177a	Sep. 24, 1986
Mint oil	Menthae arvensis aetheroleum *Rev.*	B. Anz. No. 50	Mar. 13, 1990
Mint oil	Menthae arvensis aetheroleum *Rev.*	B. Anz. No. 164	Sep. 1, 1990
Mint oil	Menthae arvensis aetheroleum *Rev.*	B. Anz. No. 128	July 14, 1993
Mistletoe berry	Visci albi fructus	B. Anz. No. 128	July 14, 1993
Mistletoe herb	Visci albi herba	B. Anz. No. 228	Dec. 5, 1984
Mistletoe stem	Visci albi stipites	B. Anz. No. 119	June 29, 1994
Monkshood	Aconitum napellus	B. Anz. No. 193a	Oct. 15, 1987
Motherwort herb	Leonuri cardiacae herba	B. Anz. No. 50	Mar. 13, 1986
Mountain Ash berry	Sorbi aucupariae fructus	B. Anz. No. 122	July 6, 1988

English Name	Pharmacopeial Name	Issue Number	Date
Mugwort herb and root	Artemisia vulgaris herba et radix	B. Anz. No. 122	July 6, 1988
Muira Puama	Ptychopetali lignum	B. Anz. No. 193a	Oct. 15, 1987
Mullein flower	Verbasci flos	B. Anz. No. 22a	Feb. 1, 1990
Myrrh	Myrrha	B. Anz. No. 193a	Oct. 15, 1987
Nasturtium	Tropaeolum majus	B. Anz. No. 162	Aug. 29, 1992
Niauli oil	Niauli aetheroleum	B. Anz. No. 162	Aug. 29, 1992
Night-blooming Cereus	Selenicereus grandiflorus	B. Anz. No. 22a	Feb. 1, 1990
Nutmeg	Myristica fragans	B. Anz. No. 173	Sep. 18, 1986
Nux Vomica	Strychni semen	B. Anz. No. 173	Sep. 18, 1986
Oak bark	Quercus cortex	B. Anz. No. 22a	Feb. 1, 1990
Oat herb	Avenae herba	B. Anz. No. 193a	Oct. 15, 1987
Oat Straw	Avenae stramentum	B. Anz. No. 193a	Oct. 15, 1987
Oats	Avenae fructus	B. Anz. No. 85	May 5, 1988
Oleander leaf	Oleandri folium	B. Anz. No. 122	July 6, 1988
Oleander leaf	Oleandri folium *Rev.*	B. Anz. No. 43	Mar. 2, 1989
Oleander leaf	Oleandri folium *Rev.*	B. Anz. No. 22a	Feb. 1, 1990
Olive leaf	Oleae folium	B. Anz. No. 11	Jan. 17, 1991
Olive oil	Olivae oleum	B. Anz. No. 178	Sep. 21, 1991
Onion	Allii cepae bulbus	B. Anz. No. 50	Mar. 13, 1986
Orange peel	Citri sinensis pericarpium	B. Anz. No. 22a	Feb. 1, 1990
Oregano	Origani vulgaris herba	B. Anz. No. 122	July 6, 1988
Orris root	Iridis rhizoma	B. Anz. No. 221	Nov. 25, 1993
Papain	Papainum crudum	B. Anz. No. 160	Aug. 25, 1994
Papaya leaf	Caricae papayae folium	B. Anz. No. 193a	Oct. 15, 1987
Paprika (Cayenne)	Capsicum	B. Anz. No. 22a	Feb. 1, 1990
Paprika (Cayenne) species low in Capsaicin	Capsicum	B. Anz. No. 80	Apr. 27, 1989
Parsley herb/root	Petroselini herba/radix	B. Anz. No. 43	Mar. 2, 1989
Parsley seed	Petroselini fructus	B. Anz. No. 43	Mar. 2, 1989
Pasque flower	Pulsatillae herba	B. Anz. No. 223	Nov. 30, 1985
Passionflower herb	Passiflorae herba	B. Anz. No. 223	Nov. 30, 1985
Passionflower herb	Passiflorae herba *Rev.*	B. Anz. No. 50	Mar. 13, 1990
Peony flower and root	Paeonia flos/radix	B. Anz. No. 85	May 5, 1988
Peppermint leaf	Menthae piperitae folium	B. Anz. No. 223	Nov. 30, 1985
Peppermint leaf	Menthae piperitae folium *Rev.*	B. Anz. No. 50	Mar. 13, 1990
Peppermint leaf	Menthae piperitae folium *Rev.*	B. Anz. No. 164	Sep. 1, 1990

English Name	Pharmacopeial Name	Issue Number	Date
Peppermint oil	Menthae piperitae aetheroleum	B. Anz. No. 50	Mar. 13, 1986
Peppermint oil	Menthae piperitae aetheroleum *Rev.*	B. Anz. No. 50	Mar. 13, 1990
Peppermint oil	Menthae piperitae aetheroleum *Rev.*	B. Anz. No. 164	Sep. 1, 1990
Peppermint oil	Menthae piperitae aetheroleum *Rev.*	B. Anz. No. 128	July 14, 1993
Periwinkle	Vincae minoris herba	B. Anz. No. 173	Sep. 18, 1986
Peruvian Balsam	Balsamum peruvianum	B. Anz. No. 173	Sep. 18, 1986
Petasites leaf	Petasitidis hybridus/-folium	B. Anz. No. 138	July 27, 1990
Petasites root	Petasitidis rhizoma	B. Anz. No. 138	July 27, 1990
Pheasant's Eye herb	Adonidis herba	B. Anz. No. 85	May 5, 1988
Pheasant's Eye herb	Adonidis herba *Rev.*	B. Anz. No. 22a	Feb. 1, 1990
Pimpinella herb	Pimpinellae herba	B. Anz. No. 101	June 1, 1990
Pimpinella root	Pimpinellae radix	B. Anz. No. 101	June 1, 1990
Pine Needle oil	Pini aetheroleum	B. Anz. No. 154	Aug. 21, 1985
Pine Needle oil	Pini aetheroleum *Rev.*	B. Anz. No. 50	Mar. 13, 1990
Pine Sprouts	Pini turiones	B. Anz. No. 173	Sep. 18, 1986
Pine Sprouts	Pini turiones *Rev.*	B. Anz. No. 50	Mar. 13, 1990
Plantain	Plantaginis lanceolatae herba	B. Anz. No. 223	Nov. 30, 1985
Pollen	Pollen	B. Anz. No. 11	Jan. 17, 1991
Poplar bark and leaf	Populi cortex/-folium	B. Anz. No. 162	Aug. 29, 1992
Poplar bud	Populi gemma	B. Anz. No. 22a	Feb. 1, 1990
Potentilla	Potentillae anserinae herba	B. Anz. No. 223	Nov. 30, 1985
Potentilla	Potentillae anserinae herba *Rev.*	B. Anz. No. 50	Mar. 13, 1990
Primrose flower	Primulae flos	B. Anz. No. 122	July 6, 1988
Primrose flower	Primulae flos *Rev.*	B. Anz. No. 50	Mar. 13, 1990
Primrose root	Primulae radix	B. Anz. No. 122	July 6, 1988
Primrose root	Primulae radix *Rev.*	B. Anz. No. 50	Mar. 13, 1990
Psyllium seed husk, Blonde	Plantaginis ovatae testa	B. Anz. No. 22a	Feb. 1, 1990
Psyllium seed husk, Blonde	Plantaginis ovatae testa *Rev.*	B. Anz. No. 74	Apr. 19, 1991
Psyllium seed, Black	Psyllii semen	B. Anz. No. 223	Nov. 30, 1985
Psyllium seed, Black	Psyllii semen *Rev.*	B. Anz. No. 50	Mar. 13, 1990

English Name	Pharmacopeial Name	Issue Number	Date
Psyllium seed, Blonde	Plantaginis ovatae semen	B. Anz. No. 22a	Feb. 1, 1990
Psyllium seed, Blonde	Plantaginis ovatae semen Rev.	B. Anz. No. 74	Apr. 19, 1991
Pumpkin seed	Curcurbitae peponis semen	B. Anz. No. 223	Nov. 30, 1985
Pumpkin seed	Curcurbitae peponis semen Rev.	B. Anz. No. 11	Jan. 17, 1991
Radish	Raphani sativi radix	B. Anz. No. 177a	Sep. 24, 1986
Raspberry leaf	Rubi idaei folium	B. Anz. No. 193a	Oct. 15, 1987
Rhatany root	Ratanhiae radix	B. Anz. No. 43	Mar. 2, 1989
Rhododendron, Rusty-leaved	Rhododendri ferruginei folium	B. Anz. No. 164	Sep. 1, 1990
Rhubarb root	Rhei radix	B. Anz. No. 133	July 21, 1993
Rose flower	Rosae flos	B. Anz. No. 164	Sep. 1, 1990
Rose Hip	Rosae pseudofructus	B. Anz. No. 164	Sep. 1, 1990
Rose Hip and seed	Rosae pseudofructus cum fructibus	B. Anz. No. 164	Sep. 1, 1990
Rose Hip seed	Rosae fructus	B. Anz. No. 164	Sep. 1, 1990
Rosemary leaf	Rosmarini folium	B. Anz. No. 223	Nov. 30, 1985
Rosemary leaf	Rosmarini folium Rev.	B. Anz. No. 221	Nov. 28, 1986
Rosemary leaf	Rosmarini folium Rev.	B. Anz. No. 50	Mar. 13, 1990
Rue	Ruta folium/herba	B. Anz. No. 43	Mar. 2, 1989
Rupturewort	Herniariae herba	B. Anz. No. 173	Sep. 18, 1986
Saffron	Croci stigma	B. Anz. No. 76	Apr. 23, 1987
Sage leaf	Salviae folium	B. Anz. No. 90	May 15, 1985
Sage leaf	Salviae folium Rev.	B. Anz. No. 50	Mar. 13, 1990
Sandalwood, Red	Santali lignum rubrum	B. Anz. No. 193a	Oct. 15, 1987
Sandalwood, White	Santali lignum albi	B. Anz. No. 43	Mar. 2, 1989
Sandy Everlasting	Helichrysi flos	B. Anz. No. 122	July 6, 1988
Sandy Everlasting	Helichrysi flos Rev.	B. Anz. No. 164	Sep. 1, 1990
Sanicle herb	Saniculae herba	B. Anz. No. 177a	Sep. 24, 1986
Sanicle herb	Saniculae herba Rev.	B. Anz. No. 50	Mar. 13, 1990
Sarsaparilla root	Sarsaparillae radix	B. Anz. No. 164	Sep. 1, 1990
Sarsaparilla, German	Caricis rhizoma	B. Anz. No. 101	June 1, 1990
Saw Palmetto berry	Sabal fructus	B. Anz. No. 43	Mar. 2, 1989
Saw Palmetto berry	Sabal fructus Rev.	B. Anz. No. 22a	Feb. 1, 1990
Saw Palmetto berry	Sabal fructus Rev.	B. Anz. No. 11	Jan. 17, 1991
Scopolia root	Scopoliae rhizoma	B. Anz. No. 177a	Sep. 24, 1986
Scotch Broom flower	Cytisi scoparii flos	B. Anz. No. 11	Jan. 17, 1991

English Name	Pharmacopeial Name	Issue Number	Date
Scotch Broom herb	Cytisi scoparii herba	B. Anz. No. 11	Jan. 17, 1991
Senecio herb	Senecionis herba	B. Anz. No. 138	July 27, 1990
Senega Snakeroot	Polygalae radix	B. Anz. No. 50	Mar. 13, 1986
Senega Snakeroot	Polygalae radix *Rev.*	B. Anz. No. 50	Mar. 13, 1990
Senna leaf	Sennae folium	B. Anz. No. 133	July 21, 1993
Senna pod	Sennae fructus	B. Anz. No. 133	July 21, 1993
Shepherd's Purse	Bursae pastoris herba	B. Anz. No. 173	Sep. 18, 1986
Shepherd's Purse	Bursae pastoris herba *Rev.*	B. Anz. No. 50	Mar. 13, 1990
Soapwort herb, Red	Saponariae herba	B. Anz. No. 80	Apr. 27, 1989
Soapwort root, Red	Saponariae rubrae radix	B. Anz. No. 80	Apr. 27, 1989
Soapwort root, White	Gypsophilae radix	B. Anz. No. 101	June 1, 1990
Soy Lecithin	Lecithinum ex soja	B. Anz. No. 85	May 5, 1988
Soy Phospholipid	Lecithinum ex soja Phospholipide 73-79% (3-sn Phosphatidyl)-cholin	B. Anz. No. 133	July 19, 1994
Spinach leaf	Spinaciae folium	B. Anz. No. 85	May 5, 1988
Spiny Restharrow root	Ononidis radix	B. Anz. No. 76	Apr. 23, 1987
Spiny Restharrow root	Ononidis radix *Rev.*	B. Anz. No. 50	Mar. 13, 1990
Squill	Scillae bulbus	B. Anz. No. 154	Aug. 21, 1985
Squill	Scillae bulbus *Rev.*	B. Anz. No. 43	Mar. 2, 1989
St. John's Wort	Hyperici herba	B. Anz. No. 228	Dec. 5, 1984
St. John's Wort	Hyperici herba *Rev.*	B. Anz. No. 43	Mar. 13, 1989
Star Anise seed	Anisi stellati fructus	B. Anz. No. 122	July 6, 1988
Stinging Nettle herb and leaf	Urticae herba/-folium	B. Anz. No. 76	Apr. 23, 1987
Stinging Nettle root	Urticae radix	B. Anz. No. 173	Sep. 18, 1986
Stinging Nettle root	Urticae radix *Rev.*	B. Anz. No. 43	Mar. 2, 1989
Stinging Nettle root	Urticae radix *Rev.*	B. Anz. No. 50	Mar. 13, 1990
Stinging Nettle root	Urticae radix *Rev.*	B. Anz. No. 11	Jan. 17, 1991
Strawberry leaf	Fragariae folium	B. Anz. No. 22a	Feb. 1, 1990
Sundew	Droserae herba	B. Anz. No. 228	May 12, 1984
Sweet Clover	Meliloti herba	B. Anz. No. 50	Mar. 13, 1986
Sweet Clover	Meliloti herba *Rev.*	B. Anz. No. 50	Mar. 13, 1990
Sweet Violet root and herb	Violae odoratae rhizoma et herba	B. Anz. No. 111	June 17, 1994
Sweet Violet flower	Violae odoratae flos	B. Anz. No. 111	June 17, 1994
Sweet Woodruff herb	Galii odorati herba	B. Anz. No. 193a	Oct. 15, 1987
Tansy	Chrysanthemi vulgaris	B. Anz. No. 122	July 6, 1988
Thyme	Thymi herba	B. Anz. No. 228	Dec. 5, 1984

English Name	Pharmacopeial Name	Issue Number	Date
Thyme	Thymi herba *Rev.*	*B. Anz.* No. 50	Mar. 13, 1990
Thyme	Thymi herba *Rev.*	*B. Anz.* No. 226	Dec. 2, 1992
Thyme, Wild	Serpylli herba	*B. Anz.* No. 193a	Oct. 15, 1987
Thyme, Wild	Serpylli herba *Rev.*	*B. Anz.* No. 50	Mar. 13, 1990
Tolu Balsam	Balsamum tolutanum	*B. Anz.* No. 173	Sep. 18, 1986
Tormentil root	Tormentillae rhizoma	*B. Anz.* No. 85	May 5, 1988
Tormentil root	Tormentillae rhizoma *Rev.*	*B. Anz.* No. 50	Mar. 13, 1990
Turmeric root	Curcumae longae rhizoma	*B. Anz.* No. 223	Nov. 30, 1985
Turmeric root	Curcumae longae rhizoma *Rev.*	*B. Anz.* No. 164	Sep. 1, 1990
Turmeric root, Javanese	Curcumae xanthorrhizae rhizoma	*B. Anz.* No. 122	July 6, 1988
Turmeric root, Javanese	Curcumae xanthorrhizae rhizoma *Rev.*	*B. Anz.* No. 164	Sep. 1, 1990
Turpentine oil, Purified	Terebinthinae aetheroleum rectificatum	*B. Anz.* No. 90	May 15, 1985
Turpentine oil, Purified	Terebinthinae aetheroleum rectificatum *Rev.*	*B. Anz.* No. 50	Mar. 13, 1990
Usnea	Usnea species	*B. Anz.* No. 80	Apr. 27, 1989
Uva Ursi leaf	Uvae ursi folium	*B. Anz.* No. 109	June 15, 1994
Uzara root	Uzarae radix	*B. Anz.* No. 164	Sep. 1, 1990
Valerian root	Valerianae radix	*B. Anz.* No. 90	May 15, 1985
Valerian root	Valerianae radix *Rev.*	*B. Anz.* No. 50	Mar. 13, 1990
Verbena herb	Verbenae herba	*B. Anz.* No. 22a	Feb. 1, 1990
Veronica herb	Veronicae herba	*B. Anz.* No. 43	June 1, 1990
Walnut hull	Juglandis fructus cortex	*B. Anz.* No. 101	June 1, 1990
Walnut leaf	Juglandis folium	*B. Anz.* No. 101	June 1, 1990
Watercress	Nasturtii herba	*B. Anz.* No. 22a	Feb. 1, 1990
White Dead Nettle flower	Lamii albi flos	*B. Anz.* No. 76	Apr. 23, 1987
White Dead Nettle herb	Lamii albi herba	*B. Anz.* No. 128	July 14, 1993
White Mustard seed	Sinapis albae semen	*B. Anz.* No. 22a	Feb. 1, 1990
White Willow bark	Salicis cortex	*B. Anz.* No. 228	May 12, 1984
Witch Hazel leaf and bark	Hamamelidis folium et cortex	*B. Anz.* No. 154	Aug. 21, 1985
Witch Hazel leaf and bark	Hamamelidis folium et cortex *Rev.*	*B. Anz.* No. 50	Mar. 13, 1990
Woody Nightshade stem	Dulcamarae stipites	*B. Anz.* No. 101	June 1, 1990
Wormwood	Absinthii herba	*B. Anz.* No. 228	Dec. 5, 1984

English Name	Pharmacopeial Name	Issue Number	Date
Yarrow	Achillea millefolia	*B. Anz.* No. 22a	Feb. 1, 1990
Yeast, Brewer's	Faex medicinalis	*B. Anz.* No. 85	May 5, 1988
Yeast, Brewer's/ Hansen CBS 5926	Saccharomyces cerevisiae	*B. Anz.* No. 71	April 15, 1984
Yellow Jessamine root	Gelsemii rhizoma	*B. Anz.* No. 178	Sep. 21, 1991
Yohimbe bark	Yohimbehe cortex	*B. Anz.* No. 193a	Oct. 15, 1987
Yohimbe bark	Yohimbehe cortex *Rev.*	*B. Anz.* No. 22a	Feb. 1, 1990
Zedoary rhizome	Zedoariae rhizoma	*B. Anz.* No. 122	July 6, 1988

English Name	Fixed Combinations	Issue Number	Date
Angelica root, Gentian root, Bitter orange peel	Angelicae radix, Gentianae radix, Aurantii pericarpium	*B. Anz.* No. 234	Dec. 18, 1991
Angelica root, Gentian root, Caraway seed Belladonna leaf with homeopathic preparations	Angelicae radix, Gentianae radix, Carvi fructus, Belladonnae folium with homeopathic preparations	*B. Anz.* No. 49	Mar. 11, 1992
Angelica root, Gentian root, Fennel seed	Angelicae radix, Gentianae radix, Foeniculi fructus	*B. Anz.* No. 40	Feb. 27, 1991
Angelica root, Gentian root, Wormwood herb	Angelicae radix, Gentianae radix, Absinthii herba	*B. Anz.* No. 49	Mar. 11, 1992
Angelica root, Gentian root, Wormwood, Peppermint oil	Angelicae radix, Gentianae radix, Absinthii herba, Menthae piperitae aetheroleum	*B. Anz.* No. 234	Dec. 18, 1991
Anise oil and Iceland moss	Anisi aetheroleum et Lichen islandicus	*B. Anz.* No. 67	Apr. 4, 1992
Anise oil, Fennel oil, Licorice root, Thyme herb	Anisi aetheroleum, Foeniculi aetheroleum, Liquiritiae radix, Thymi herba	*B. Anz.* No. 149	Aug. 13, 1991
Anise oil, Primrose root, Thyme herb	Anisi aetheroleum, Primulae radix, Thymi herba	*B. Anz.* No. 67	Apr. 4, 1992

English Name	Fixed Combinations	Issue Number	Date
Anise seed, Fennel seed, Caraway seed	Anisi fructus, Foeniculi fructus, Carvi fructus	B. Anz. No. 67	Apr. 4, 1992
Anise seed, Fennel seed, Ivy leaf, Licorice root	Anisi fructus, Foeniculi fructus, Hederae helicis folium, Liquiritiae radix	B. Anz. No. 234	Dec. 18, 1991
Anise seed, Linden flower, Thyme herb	Anisi fructus, Tiliae flos, Thymi herba	B. Anz. No. 149	Aug. 13, 1991
Anise seed, Marshmallow root, Eucalyptus oil, Licorice root	Anisi fructus, Althaeae radix, Eucalypti aetheroleum, Liquiritiae radix	B. Anz. No. 67	Apr. 4, 1992
Anise seed, Marshmallow root, Iceland moss, Licorice root	Anisi fructus, Althaeae radix, Lichen islandicus, Liquiritiae radix	B. Anz. No. 67	Apr. 4, 1992
Anise seed, Marshmallow root, Primrose root, Sundew herb	Anisi fructus, Althaeae radix, Primulae radix, Droserae herba	B. Anz. No. 67	Apr. 4, 1992
Belladonna leaf with chemically defined substances	Belladonnae folium (with chemically defined compounds)	B. Anz. No. 180	Sep. 24, 1993
Belladonna leaf with other drugs	Belladonnae folium (with other drugs)	B. Anz. No. 180	Sep. 24, 1993
Birch leaf, Goldenrod, and Java tea	Betulae folium, Solidaginis herba, Orthosiphonis folium	B. Anz. No. 180	Sep. 24, 1993
Camphor, Eucalyptus oil, Purified Larch Turpentine	Camphora, Eucalypti aetheroleum, Terebinthinae, aetheroleum rectificatum	B. Anz. No. 162	Aug. 29, 1992
Caraway oil and Fennel oil	Carvi aetheroleum et Foeniculi aetheroleum	B. Anz. No. 234	Dec. 18, 1991
Caraway oil, Fennel oil, Chamomile flower	Carvi aetheroleum, Foeniculi aetheroleum, Matricariae flos	B. Anz. No. 149	Aug. 13, 1991
Caraway seed, Fennel seed, Chamomile flower	Carvi fructus, Foeniculi fructus, Matricariae flos	B. Anz. No. 234	Dec. 18, 1991

English Name	Fixed Combinations	Issue Number	Date
Dandelion root with herb, Celandine herb, Artichoke leaf	Taraxaci radix cum herba, Chelidonii herba, Cynarae folium	B. Anz. No. 149	Aug. 13, 1991
Dandelion root with herb, Cendine herb, Wormwood herb	Taraxaci radix cum herba, Chelidonii herba, Absinthii herba	B. Anz. No. 221	Nov. 25, 1993
Dandelion root with herb, Peppermint leaf, Artichoke leaf	Taraxaci radix cum herba, Menthae piperitae folium, Cynarae folium	B. Anz. No. 149	Aug. 13, 1991
Eucalyptus oil and Pine oil	Eucalypti aetheroleum et Pini aetheroleum	B. Anz. No. 128	July 14, 1993
Eucalyptus oil, Primrose root, Thyme herb	Eucalypti aetheroleum, Primulae radix, Thymi herba	B. Anz. No. 67	Apr. 4, 1992
Fennel oil, Anise oil, Caraway oil	Foeniculi aetheroleum, Anisi aetheroleum, Carvi aetheroleum	B. Anz. No. 67	Apr. 4, 1992
Ginger root, Gentian root, Wormwood herb	Zingiberis rhizoma, Gentianae radix, Absinthii herba	B. Anz. No. 67	Apr. 4, 1992
Gumweed herb, Primrose root, Thyme herb	Grindeliae herba, Primulae radix, Thymi herba	B. Anz. No. 67	Apr. 4, 1992
Ivy leaf, Licorice root, Thyme	Hederae helicis folium, Liquiritiae radix, Thymi herba	B. Anz. No. 85	May 8, 1991
Licorice root and Chamomile flower	Liquiritiae radix et Matricariae flos	B. Anz. No. 128	July 14, 1993
Licorice root, Peppermint leaf, Chamomile flower	Liquiritiae radix, Menthae piperitae folium, Matricariae flos	B. Anz. No. 128	July 14, 1993
Licorice root, Primrose root, Marshmallow root, Anise seed	Liquiritiae radix, Primulae radix, Althaeae radix, Anisi fructus	B. Anz. No. 49	Mar. 11, 1992
Lily-of-the-valley herb and Squill	Convallariae herba et Scillae bulbus	B. Anz. No. 128	July 14, 1993
Marshmallow root, Fennel seed, Iceland moss, Thyme herb	Althaeae radix, Foeniculi fructus, Lichen islandicus, Thymi herba	B. Anz. No. 234	Dec. 18, 1991

English Name	Fixed Combinations	Issue Number	Date
Marshmallow root, Licorice root, Primrose root, Thyme oil	Althaeae radix, Liquiritiae radix, Primulae radix, Thymi aetheroleum	B. Anz. No. 67	Apr. 4, 1992
Milk Thistle fruit, Peppermint leaf, Wormwood	Cardui mariae fructus, Menthae piperitae folium, Absinthii herba	B. Anz. No. 149	Aug. 13, 1991
Passionflower herb, Valerian root, Lemon Balm leaf	Passiflorae herba, Valerianae radix, Melissae folium	B. Anz. No. 234	Dec. 18, 1991
Peppermint herb and Caraway seed	Menthae piperitae folium et Carvi fructus	B. Anz. No. 234	Dec. 18, 1991
Peppermint herb, Fennel seed, Chamomile flower	Menthae piperitae folium, Foeniculi fructus, Matricariae flos	B. Anz. No. 95	May 25, 1991
Peppermint leaf and Fennel seed	Menthae piperitae folium et Foeniculi fructus	B. Anz. No. 234	Dec. 18, 1991
Peppermint leaf, Caraway seed, Chamomile flower	Menthae piperitae folium, Carvi fructus, Matricariae flos	B. Anz. No. 149	Aug. 13, 1991
Peppermint leaf, Caraway seed, Chamomile flower, Bitter Orange peel	Menthae piperitae folium, Carvi fructus, Matricariae flos, Aurantii pericarpium	B. Anz. No. 149	Aug. 13, 1991
Peppermint leaf, Caraway seed, Fennel seed	Menthae piperitae folium, Carvi fructus, Foeniculi fructus	B. Anz. No. 149	Aug. 13, 1991
Peppermint leaf, Caraway seed, Fennel seed, Chamomile flower	Menthae piperitae folium, Carvi fructus, Foeniculi fructus, Matricariae flos	B. Anz. No. 149	Aug. 13, 1991
Peppermint leaf, Chamomile flower, Caraway seed	Menthae piperitae folium, Matricariae flos, Carvi fructus	B. Anz. No. 49	Mar. 11, 1992
Peppermint oil, Caraway oil	Menthae piperitae aetheroleum, Carvi aetheroleum	B. Anz. No. 149	Aug. 13, 1991
Peppermint oil, Caraway oil, Chamomile flower	Menthae piperitae aetheroleum, Carvi aetheroleum, Matricariae flos	B. Anz. No. 149	Aug. 13, 1991

English Name	Fixed Combinations	Issue Number	Date
Peppermint oil, Caraway oil, Fennel oil	Menthae piperitae aetheroleum, Carvi aetheroleum, Foeniculi aetheroleum	B. Anz. No. 149	Aug. 13, 1991
Peppermint oil, Caraway oil, Fennel oil, Chamomile flower	Menthae piperitae aetheroleum, Carvi aetheroleum, Foeniculi aetheroleum, Matricariae flos	B. Anz. No. 149	Aug. 13, 1991
Peppermint oil, Fennel oil	Menthae piperitae aetheroleum, Foeniculi aetheroleum	B. Anz. No. 149	Aug. 13, 1991
Peppermint oil, Fennel oil, Chamomile flower	Menthae piperitae aetheroleum, Foeniculi aetheroleum, Matricariae flos	B. Anz. No. 234	Dec. 18, 1991
Pheasant's Eye fluidextract, Lily-of-the-valley herb, Squill, Oleander dry extract	Adonidis herba, extr., Convallariae herba, Scillae bulbus, Oleandri sec. extr.	B. Anz. No. 180	Sep. 24, 1993
Pheasant's Eye herb and Lily-of-the-valley herb	Adonidis herba et Convallariae herba	B. Anz. No. 128	July 14, 1993
Pheasant's Eye herb, Lily-of-the-valley, Squill bulb, Oleander leaf with Bishop's weed fruit	Adonidis herba, Convallariae herba, Scillae bulbus, Oleandri folium cum Ammeos visnagae fructus	B. Anz. No. 160	Aug. 25, 1994
Pheasant's Eye herb, Lily-of-the-valley, Squill bulb, Oleander leaf with Bishop's weed fruit	Adonidis herba, Convallariae herba, Scillae bulbus, Oleandri folium with Ammeos visnagae fructus	B. Anz. No. 142	July 30, 1994
Pheasant's Eye herb, Lily-of-the-valley, Squill bulb, Oleander leaf with chem. def. drugs	Adonidis herba, Convallariae herba, Scillae bulbus, Oleandri folium (with chem. def. drugs)	B. Anz. No. 128	July 14, 1993

English Name	Fixed Combinations	Issue Number	Date
Pheasant's Eye herb, Lily-of-the-valley, Squill bulb, Oleander leaf with homeopathic preparations	Adonidis herba, Convallariae herba, Scillae bulbus, Oleandri folium (with homeopathic preparations)	B. Anz. No. 128	July 14, 1993
Pheasant's Eye herb, Lily-of-the-valley, Squill, Oleander leaf with herbs that don't contain cardiac glycosides	Adonidis herba, Convallariae herba, Scillae bulbus, Oleandri folium (with herbs that don't contain cardiac glycosides)	B. Anz. No. 128	July 14, 1993
Primrose root and Thyme	Primulae radix et Thymi herba	B. Anz. No. 149	Aug. 13, 1991
Primrose root, Marshmallow root, Anise seed	Primulae radix, Althaeae radix, Anisi fructus	B. Anz. No. 40	Feb. 27, 1991
Primrose root, Sundew, Thyme	Primulae radix, Droserae herba, Thymi herba	B. Anz. No. 149	Aug. 13, 1991
Senna leaf and Psyllium husk	Sennae folium et Plantaginis ovatae testa	B. Anz. No. 221	Nov. 25, 1993
Senna leaf, Peppermint oil, Caraway oil	Sennae folium, Menthae piperitae aetheroleum, Carvi aetheroleum	B. Anz. No. 49	Mar. 11, 1992
Star Anise seed and Thyme	Anisi stellati fructus et Thymi herba	B. Anz. No. 67	Apr. 4, 1992
Sundew and Thyme	Droserae herba et Thymi herba	B. Anz. No. 149	Aug. 13, 1991
Thyme and White Soapwort root	Thymi herba et Gyposophilae radix	B. Anz. No. 67	Apr. 4, 1992
Turmeric root and Celandine herb	Curcumae longae rhizoma et Chelidonii herba	B. Anz. No. 85	May 8, 1991
Javanese Turmeric root, Celandine herb, Wormwood, Caraway seed and Fennel seed	Curcumae xanthorrhizae rhizoma, Chelidonii herba, Absinthii herba, Carvi fructus et Foeniculi fructus	B. Anz. No. 234	Dec. 18, 1991
Turmeric root, Javanese, Peppermint leaf, Wormwood herb	Curcumae xanthorrhizae rhizoma, Menthae piperitae folium, Absinthii herba	B. Anz. No. 67	Apr. 4, 1992

English Name	Fixed Combinations	Issue Number	Date
Uva Ursi leaf, Goldenrod herb, Java tea	Uvae ursi folium, Solidaginis herba, Orthosiphonis folium	B. Anz. No. 49	Mar. 11, 1992
Valerian root and Hops	Valerianae radix et Lupuli strobulus	B. Anz. No. 162	Aug. 29, 1992
Valerian root, Hops, and Lemon Balm	Valerianae radix, Lupuli strobulus et Melissae folium	B. Anz. No. 67	Apr. 4, 1992
Valerian root, Hops and Passionflower herb	Valerianae radix, Lupuli strobulus, et Passiflorae herba		

List of European Scientific Cooperative on Phytotherapy (ESCOP) Monographs

The European Scientific Cooperative on Phytotherapy (ESCOP) was formed in 1990 as an organization of scientists with expertise in various aspects of phytomedicine. In an effort to help harmonize therapeutic data on herbal drug products sold in the European Union, ESCOP has published 50 monographs on medicinal plants used in western Europe, although, unlike those of the Commission E, ESCOP monographs are not official on a regulatory level. ESCOP monographs cover therapeutic aspects of the herbal drug; there are no data on quality control measures for determining identity or assaying purity. Such information is usually found in the respective pharmacopeias of European countries. Except for Feverfew, all herbal drugs reviewed by ESCOP also have been evaluated by Commission E. They are published in fascicules (volumes) of ten herbs.

Common Name	Pharmacopeial Name	Latin Binomial
Fascicule 1		
Marshmallow root	Altheae radix	*Althaea officinalis*
Birch leaf	Betulae folium	*Betula spp.*
Boldo leaf	Boldo folium	*Peumus boldus*
Calendula flower	Calendula Flos	*Calendula officinalis*
Fennel Seed	Foeniculi Fructus	*Foeniculum vulgare*
St. John's Wort	Hyperici Herba	*Hypericum perforatum*
Linseed	Lini Semen	*Linum usitatissimum*
Java Tea	Orthosiphonis Folium	*Orthosiphon spicatus*
Thyme herb	Thymi Herba	*Thymus vulgaris*
Ginger root	Zingiberis Rhizoma	*Zingiber officinale*
Fascicule 2		
Devil's Claw root	Harpagophyti Radix	*Harpagophytum procumbens*
Lemon Balm leaf	Melissa Folium	*Melissa officinalis*
Ispaghula (Psyllium seed)	Plantaginis Ovatae Semen	*Plantago psyllium*
Ispaghula (Psyllium husk)	Plantaginis Ovatae Testa	*Plantago psyllium*
Sage leaf	Salviae Folium	*Salvia officinalis*
Goldenrod herb	Solidaginis virgaureae herba	*Solidago virgaurea*
Feverfew leaf and herb	Tanaceti Parthenii Herba/Folium	*Tanacetum parthenium*

Common Name	Pharmacopeial Name	Latin Binomial
Dandelion leaf	Taraxaci Folium	*Taraxacum officinale*
Dandelion root	Taraxaci Radix	*Taraxacum officinale*
Nettle root	Urticae Radix	*Urtica dioica*

Fascicule 3

Common Name	Pharmacopeial Name	Latin Binomial
Garlic	Allii sativi bulbus	*Allium sativum*
Anise seed	Anisi fructu	*Pimpinella anisum*
Caraway seed	Carvi fructus	*Carum carvi*
Juniper berry	Juniperi fructus	*Juniperus communis*
Iceland Moss	Lichen islandicu	*Cetraria islandica*
Peppermint oil	Menthae piperitae aetholeum	*Mentha x piperita*
Peppermint leaf	Menthae piperitae folium	*Mentha x piperita*
Senega snake root	Polygalae radix	*Polygala senega*
Cowslip root	Primulae radix	*Primula veris*
Rosemary leaf with flower	Rosmarini folium cum flore	*Rosmarinus officinalis*

Fascicule 4

Common Name	Pharmacopeial Name	Latin Binomial
Wormwood	Absinthii herba	*Artemisia absinthium*
Arnica flower	Arnicae flos	*Arnica montana*
Gentian root	Gentianae radix	*Gentiana lutea*
Hops flower	Lupuli flos	*Humulus lupulus*
Melilot	Meliloti herba	*Melilotus officinalis*
Passionflower herb	Passiflorae herba	*Passiflora spp.*
Blackcurrant leaf	Ribis nigri folium	*Ribes nigrum*
Willow bark	Salicis cortex	*Salix spp.*
Nettle leaf/herb	Urticae folium/herba	*Urtica dioica*
Valerian root	Valeriana radix	*Valeriana officinalis*

Fascicule 5

Common Name	Pharmacopeial Name	Latin Binomial
Cape Aloes	Aloe capensis	*Aloe ferox*
Buckthorn bark (Frangula)	Frangulae cortex	*Rhamnus frangula*
Witch hazel leaf	Hamamelis folium	*Hamamelis virginiana*
Rest-harrow root	Ononidis radix	*Ononis spinosa*
Psyllium seed	Psylli semen	*Plantago psyllium*
Cascara sagrada bark	Rhamni purshiani cortex	*Rhamnus purshianus*
Senna leaf	Sennae folium	*Cassia senna*
Alexandrian Senna pods	Sennae fructus acutifoliae	*Cassia senna*
Tinnevelly Senna pods	Sennae fructus angustifoliae	*Cassia senna*
Uva-ursi leaf	Uvae ursi folium	*Arctostaphylos uva-ursi*

List of World Health Organization (WHO) Monographs

In 1991 the World Health Organization (WHO) published "Guidelines for the Assessment of Herbal Medicines," a document that established guidelines designed to assist regulatory bodies in evaluation of the quality, safety and efficacy of herbal medicines. WHO established a criterion that historical and traditional use of an herb should be considered as part of the evaluation process in determining the safety and efficacy, when combined with modern scientific data. WHO also called for the development of monographs on important medicinal herbs. In 1998 WHO is expected to publish the first 28 herbal monographs covering 41 species of medicinal plants. WHO monographs include sections covering criteria for the determination of the proper botanical identity and purity of the herbal drug, as well as sections on the chemistry, pharmacology, toxicology and clinical pharmacology of the herb. Herbs also evaluated by Commission E are marked with an asterisk (*).

Common Name	Latin Name/Monograph Title
*Aloe vera	*Aloe vera* (gel)
*Aloe vera	*Aloe vera* (juice)
Astragalus	*Astragalus membranaceus*
Astragalus	*Astragalus mongholicus*
Bupleurum	*Bupleurum falcatum*
Bupleurum	*Bupleurum falcatum* var. *scorzonerifolium*
*Cassia	*Cinnamomum cassia*
*Chamomile	*Chamomilla recutita*
*Cinnamon	*Cinnamomum verum*
*Echinacea	*Echinacea angustifolia* var. *angustifolia*
*Echinacea	*Echinacea angustifolia* var. *strigosa*
*Echinacea	*Echinacea pallida*
*Echinacea, purple coneflower	*Echinacea purpurea*

Common Name	Latin Name/Monograph Title
*Ephedra, ma huang	*Ephedra sinica*
*Garlic	*Allium sativum*
*Ginger	*Zingiber officinale*
*Ginkgo	*Ginkgo biloba*
*Ginseng, Asian	*Panax ginseng*
Goldthread	*Coptis chinensis*
Goldthread	*Coptis deltoides*
Goldthread	*Coptis japonica*
Gotu kola	*Centella asiatica*
*Indian snakeroot	*Rauvolfia serpentina*
Java brucea	*Brucea javanica*
*Licorice	*Glycyrrhiza glabra*
*Licorice	*Glycyrrhiza uralensis*
*Onion	*Allium cepa*
*Peony	*Paeonia lactiflora*
Platycodon	*Platycodon grandiflorum*
*Psyllium	*Plantago afra*
*Psyllium	*Plantago indica*
*Psyllium	*Plantago ovata*
*Psyllium	*Plantago asiatica*
*Rhubarb	*Rheum officinale*
*Rhubarb	*Rheum palmatum*
*Senna leaf	*Cassia senna* (leaf)
*Senna pod	*Cassia senna* (fruit)
*Thyme	*Thymus vulgaris*
*Thyme	*Thymus zygis*
*Turmeric	*Curcuma longa*
*Valerian	*Valeriana officinalis*

GENERAL GLOSSARY
of Anatomical, Botanical, Medical, Pharmaceutical, and Physiological Terms

abortifacient — a drug or chemical agent that induces abortion

absorption — uptake of a substance into the body or a tissue through skin or mucous membrane

accommodation disturbance — disturbance in the ability of the eye to focus

acetylcholinesterase — nuerotransmitter enzyme that hydrolyzes acetylcholine, affecting functioning of the parasympathetic nervous system

acetylcholinesterase inhibitor — agent that counteracts hydrolysis of acetylcholine to acetate and choline

acid — a solution having a pH of less than seven

acinus — small sac-like dilatation

acne — a chronic skin disorder due to inflammation of hair follicles and sebaceous glands (secretion glands in the skin)

actino- — in botany, rayed, starlike

active transport — movement of particles across cell membranes requiring the expenditure of energy

acute — an illness or symptom of sudden onset, which generally has a short duration

addiction — habitual dependence on a substance

Addison's disease — characterized by the chronic destruction of the adrenal cortex, which leads to an increased loss of sodium and water in the urine, muscle weakness and low blood pressure. The bronze color of the skin is due to the increased production of the skin pigment, melanin.

additive — the substance being added to another to obtain the desired product (e.g., food colors and food processing).

adenoma — an ordinarily benign growth of epithelial tissue in which the tumor cells form glands or gland-like structures that tend to exhibit glandular function

adjuvant — a substance added to a drug that affects the action of the active ingredient in a predictable way

adnexitis — inflammation of organ appendages, typically referring to the fallopian tube

adrenoceptors — sites on nerve cells or fibers which react to epinephrine or norepinephrine

adsorbent — a solid substance which binds other substances to its surface but does not interact chemically with them

adsorption — the property of a solid substance to attract and hold other molecules to its surface

aegyptiacus — in botany, of Egypt

aglycone — non-carbohydrate portion of a glycoside

agranulocytosis — condition characterized by a marked decrease in the number of white blood cells called granulocytes

AIDS — acquired immunodeficiency syndrome, a syndrome of the immune system caused by the HIV virus which weakens the immune system by destroying T4 helper/inducer lymphocytes

akathisia — condition of motor restlessness that can range from a sense of inner disquiet to inability to sleep, seen in toxic reaction to neuroleptic and antipsychotic medication

albuminuria — presence of albumin in the urine

alcoholic solution — in the case of herb preparations, mixture of water and ethanol used to dissolve an herb or its constituents

-alis — in botany, pertaining to, e.g. digitalis, pertaining to a finger

alkaline — a solution having a pH greater than seven

allergic keratitis — inflammation of the cornea due to allergic response

allergy — hypersensitivity caused by exposure to a particular antigen (allergen), resulting in an increased reactivity to that antigen on subsequent exposure, sometimes with harmful immunologic consequences

alopecia — loss of hair

alpinus — in botany, of high mountains

alterative — a term used in botanical medicine referring to a substance that restores health gradually, similar to a tonic

alveolar — pertaining to a small hollow space, as in the lung, e.g. pulmonary alveolus

amantadine (amantadine hydrochloride) — antiviral agent used to prevent or treat influenza; also used to treat Parkinson's disease

amarum — bitter vegetable drug

ammi — in botany, from an umbelliferous plant

analeptic — central nervous system stimulant

analgesic — agent which relieves pain without causing loss of consciousness

anancastic — pertaining to any form of repetitious stereotyped behavior that causes anxiety if prevented

anaphylactic — intense allergic reaction to a foreign substance

anaphylactic shock — life-threatening allergic response characterized by decreased blood pressure and impaired respiration

ancyclostoma — parasitic hookworm in the human duodenum

anemia — low amounts of red blood cells with clinical symptoms such as shortness of breath, lethargy and heart palpitations

anemo- — in botany, pertaining to wind

anesthesia — loss of sensation caused by neurological dysfunction or a pharmacological depression of nerve function

anesthetic — agent causing loss of sensation by neurological dysfunction or a pharmacological depression of nerve function

aneurysm — localized enlargement of an artery

angina — severe, restricting pain, usually referring to the pectoris

angina pectoris — severe chest pain

angioedema — recurring attacks of transient, subcutaneous edema, often due to an allergic reaction

angioneuropathy — any neuropathy affecting primarily blood vessels as angiospasm, angioparalysis, or vasomotor paralysis

angioneurosis — vasomotor (causing dilation or constriction of the blood vessels) nervous disease for which there is no detectable damage to nerve tissue

angusti- — in botany, narrow

anhydrous — water deficient

aniso- — in botany, uneven, unequal

anorectic — agent that decreases appetite

anterior — in the front or forward part of the organ or toward the head of the body

anthelmintic — agent that expels or destroys intestinal worms

antiandrogenic — substance capable of preventing full expression of the biological effects of androgenic hormones on responsive tissues, either by producing an antagonistic effect, as in the case of estrogen, or by competing for receptor sites on the cell surface

antiarrhythmic — combating an irregular heart beat

antibacterial — destroying or inhibiting the growth of bacteria

antibody — immunoglobulin molecule evoked as a response to an antigen which then interacts with the antigen

anti-chemotactic — preventing the movement of cells or organisms in response to chemicals

anticholinergic — antagonistic to the cholinergic nerve fibers

anticoagulant — preventing clotting

antiedamatous — preventing swelling

antiemetic — preventing vomiting

anti-exudative — preventing oozing

antifungal — destroying or combating fungi

antigonadotropic — agent preventing growth or function of the testes or ovary

antihistamine — drugs, used to treat allergy symptoms, which block the action of histamine

antiinflammatory — reducing inflammation by acting on body mechanisms, without directly acting on the cause of inflammation, e.g., glucocorticoids, aspirin

antimicrobial — tending to destroy microbes, hinder their multiplication or growth

antimuscarinic — inhibiting the toxic effect of muscarine or muscarine-like substances

antimycotic — fungicidal

antiparasitic — destructive to parasites

antiphlogistic — preventing inflammation

antiseptic — inhibiting growth of infectious organisms

antisialagogue — counteracts formation of saliva

antispasmodic — preventing spasms

antithyrotropic — inhibiting thyroid hormones

antitussive — cough suppressant

anuria — inability to urinate

-anus — in botany, belonging to, e.g., *virginianus*, of Virginia

anxiety — apprehension of danger, or dread, accompanied by nervous restlessness, tension, increased heart rate, and shortness of breath unrelated to a clearly identifiable stimulus

aortic stenosis — narrowing of the aortic valve of the heart

aphrodisiac — substance increasing or arousing sexual desire

aplasia — absence of tissue or defective organ development

aplastic anemia — anemia caused by failure of red blood cells to regenerate

apnea — cessation of breathing

apoplexy — sudden neurologic impairment due to a cerebrovascular disorder, e.g., cerebral stroke

aqueous extract — water extract

argyro- — in botany, silvery

-arium — in botany, place where something is done, e.g., herbarium, collection of dried plants

armoracia — in botany, designation for horseradish

aroma corrigent — substance that reduces, neutralizes or enhances an odor

aromatic bitter — bitter used as a flavoring due to its volatile oils

arrhythmia — any deviation from the normal rhythm of the heart

arrythmogenic — causing a change in the normal rhythm of the heart

arteriosclerosis — arterial hardening

arthralgia — joint pain

arthritis — joint inflammation

arthrosis — joint disease

arthrosis deformans — noninfectious degeneration of a joint characterized by pain, cracking, and loss of bone

ascarid — large, heavy-bodied roundworms parasitic in the human intestine

-ascens — in botany, process of becoming, e.g., *violascens*, becoming violet

ascites — accumulation of serous fluid in the abdominal cavity

aspiration — inhalation, or removal of fluids or gases from a cavity using suction

asthenia — diminishing strength and energy

astringent — agent causing contraction, especially after topical application

ataxia — failed muscular coordination, irregular muscular action

ataxic — relating to or suffering from ataxia

atelectasis — incomplete lung expansion or lung collapse and airlessness

atherosclerosis — common form of arteriosclerosis with deposits of yellow plaques containing cholesterol, lipids, and lipophages within the intima and inner media of arteries

-aticus — in botany, place of growth, e.g., *aquaticus*, growing in water

atony — lack of muscle tone of the supportive musculature of the bladder sphincter, resulting in incontinence

atopic — genetically predisposed toward developing immediate hypersensitivity reactions to common environmental allergens

atopic allergy — genetically determined state of hypersensitivity to environmental allergens

atropine-like effect — anticholinergic effect, resulting in tachycardia, mydriasis, constipation, retention of urine, limited perspiration attributable to the blockade of acetylcholine at muscarinic type cholinergic receptors in the nervous system

-atus — in botany, likeness of possession, rostratus, having a beak

Auerbach's myenteric plexus — network of nerves in the muscular layer of the wall of the digestive tract

autoimmune disease — immune response directed against tissues within one's own body

autumnalis — in botany, of the fall season

axon — an extended process of a neuron that conducts impulses traveling away from the cell body

bacteriostatic — preventing multiplication of bacteria

balneological treatment — treatment by immersing part of the body in a bath

balneotherapy — healing bath

barbadensis — in botany, from Barbados, e.g., *Aloe barbadensis*

bathmotropic — a response to stimulants which influences nervous and muscular irritability; negatively bathmotropic—lessening nervous or muscular irritability; positively bathmotropic—increasing nervous or muscular irritability

biliary dyskinesia — inability to secrete bile

biliary excretion (of drug) — removal of the drug metabolites formed in the body through bile, usually important for compounds with higher molecular weights (greater than 500)

bilirubinuria — presence of bilirubin (yellow-red pigment of bile) in urine

-bilis — in botany, ability or capacity, *sensibilis*, capable of sensitivity

binding to plasma protein — attachment of a compound, usually pharmaceutically active, to proteins in the blood, an important consideration when two or more drugs are simultaneously administered and displace each other

bitter — a bitter-tasting infusion or tonic that affects digestion or appetite by stimulating the increasing output of saliva and gastric juices; gentian and hops are among the plants used for this purpose

bitter principle — alkaloid

bitter principles — constituents possessing a bitter taste

bitterness value — inverse of the dilution at which a compound imparts a perceptible, bitter taste (e.g., a bitterness value of 50,000 means a part of the compound in 50,000 parts of water still tastes bitter)

bladder and kidney congestion — accumulation of fluid in the tissues resulting from congestive heart failure

blennorrhea — excess discharge from mucous surfaces, such as the urethra or vagina; term used in the past for gonorrhea

blood purification — the process by which an agent or organ enhances the body's normal function of removing impurities from the blood stream

blood viscosity — fluid flexibility of the blood

borealis — in botany, northern

brachialgia — arm pain

brachy- — in botany, short

bradycardia — slow heart rate

brevi- — in botany, short

brightening agent — filler

bronchitis — inflammation of the mucous membrane of the bronchial tubes, frequently accompanied by cough, hypersecretion of mucus, and expectoration of sputum

broncholytic — agent that reduces viscosity of bronchial secretions

bronchospasmolytic — reducing spasms of the bronchial tubes

bronchospasm — sudden involuntary contraction of the smooth muscles surrounding the bronchial tubes

bruise — injury producing a hematoma or diffuse extravasation of blood without breaking the skin

buccal — pertaining to, located near, the cheek

bud — immature vegetative or floral shoot, often covered by scales

-bundus — in botany, fullness, abundance, floribundus, full of flowers

bunion — localized swelling at the first metatarsophalangeal joint (between the instep and the toes) due to an inflamed bursa (fluid-filled sac)

bursitis — inflammation of bursa or fluid-filled sacs which normally function to reduce friction

cachexia — weight loss due to chronic disease or prolonged emotional stress

calyx — external leafy portion of flower consisting of sepals

cancer — refers to the various types of malignant neoplasms which contain cells growing out of control and invading adjacent tissues, which can metastasize to distant tissues

candidiasis — infection with *Candida*, especially *Candida albicans*, usually resulting from debilitation (AIDS, prolonged administration of antibiotics)

canker sore — a small, painful ulcer that occurs on the inside of the cheek, lip or underside of the tongue

carbon clearance test — method of measuring the activity of the immune system

carcinogenicity — tendency to cause cancer

carcinoma — malignant growth of epithelial cells tending to infiltrate the surrounding tissue and giving rise to metastasis

cardiac — pertaining to the heart, also, pertaining to the stomach area adjacent to the esophagus

cardiac asthma — sudden intensification of impaired breathing associated with heart disease such as left ventricular failure; cardiasthma

cardiac dysrhythmia — any irregularity of heart beat

cardiac glycoside — compound consisting of a plant steroid with one or more sugars that exerts an effect on the contraction and conduction of the heart muscle

cardiac neurasthenia — general fatigue originating from dysfunction of the heart

cardiac neurosis — heart irregularity of psychogenic origin

cardiomegaly — enlargement of the heart

carminative — agent relieving flatulence or gas

carpo- — in botany, pertaining to fruit

caryo- — in botany, nutlike

cataplasm — poultice

catarrh — mucous membrane inflammation

celery-carrot-mugwort syndrome — skin photosensitivity caused by massive consumption of vegetables containing psoralens, chemicals which can cause toxic effects when exposed to sunlight

cepa — in botany, Latin name for onion

cephalalgia — headache

cephalic — pertaining to the head

cervical syndrome — syndrome involving neck pain

cheilitis — inflammation affecting the lips

chloralized — anesthetized using chloral hydrate

cholagogue — agent that stimulates bile flow from the gallbladder into the duodenum

cholangitis — bile duct inflammation

cholecystitis — gallbladder inflammation

cholecystokinetic — increasing secretion of the gastrointestinal hormone cholecystokinin, which promotes emptying of the gallbladder

cholelithiasis — presence of gallstones in the gallbladder or bile duct

choleretic — agent stimulating the liver to increase bile production

cholestasis — cessation or suppression of bile flow

cholestatic liver disorder — an arrest in the flow of bile from the liver

choline absorption — intake of choline in free form or as lecithin (phosphatidylcholine), acetate (acetylcholine) from the vitamin B complex, or cytidine diphosphate

chologenic — producing bile

chondrosis — formation of cartilaginous tissue; term used in the past for a cartilaginous tumor

chronic illness — illness extending over a long period of time

chronotropic — affecting time or rate, especially heart rate

chryso- — in botany, golden

cicatricial keloid — nodular, firm, movable, nonencapsulated mass of scar tissue, tender and frequently painful

ciliary activity — activity of the eyelashes or any hairlike processes (cilia)

cinnamomeus — in botany, light reddish-brown

cirrhosis — disease of liver characterized by loss of normal microscopic lobular structure

claudication (intermittent) — condition caused by interruptions of blood supply to the muscles, characterized by limping and pain chiefly in the calf muscles

cleansing the blood — see blood purification

climacteric — period of transition from fertility to menopause

clonic — form of movement marked by contractions and relaxations of a muscle, occurring in rapid succession

coelo- — in botany, pertaining to a hollow

colitis ulcerosa (ulcerative colitis) — ulceration of the colon and rectum, usually chrinic, characterized by rectal bleeding, abdominal pain and diarrhea

collagen — primary protein within white fibers of connective tissue, cartilage, and bone

collagenosis — a disease affecting collagen

collateral circulation — blood flow through a side branch of a blood vessel

comminuted — crushed, pulverized

Composite — in botany, annual or perennial herb of the family Asteraceae (aka Compositae), with watery or milky sap, often with fleshy roots, simple leaves, flower corolla with five petals

condyloma — viral warts of the anal-genital region

congestive — pertaining to accumulation of blood or fluid within a vessel or organ

conjunctiva — mucous membrane covering the posterior surface of the eyelids and the anterior surface of the eyeball

constipation — infrequent or incomplete bowel movements

convulsant poison — a substance causing violent spasms of the face, trunk, and/or extremities

cornea — transparent structure forming the anterior part of the eye

coronary infarction — sudden lack of blood supply to the heart that results an area of dead cardiac tissue

coronary/myocardial perfusion — flow of blood to the heart and/or blood vessels surrounding the heart

cor pulmonale — hypertrophy of the right ventricle of the heart resulting from excessive pressure in the pulmonary artery

corpus luteum — yellow endocrine body formed in the ovary that secretes estrogen

corrigent — modifying or correcting

cortex — in botany, bark

corticosteroid — steroid hormone produced by the adrenal cortex

Crohn's disease — chronic inflammatory disease of the gastrointestinal tract

cross reaction — reaction between an antibody and antigen, separate from the reaction which initially evoked formation of the antibody

crypto- — in botany, hidden

cteno- — in botany, pertaining to a term

curare-like effect — paralysis of skeletal muscle

cuti-visceral reflex — reaction of the digestive, respiratory, urogenital, or endocrine system to sensation on the skin

cyath- — in botany, cuplike

cystitis — inflammation of the urinary bladder

cytoplasmic — pertaining to the contents of a cell outside the nucleus

cytostatic — characterized by the slowing of movement and accumulation of blood cells

dasy- — in botany, shaggy, hairy

decoction — liquid prepared by boiling plant material in water for a period of time

decubitus ulcer — bed sore

demulcent — an agent which soothes and relieves irritation, especially of the mucous membranes

dermatitis — inflammatory skin condition

diabetes insipidus — excessive production of urine, usually due to insufficient production of antidiuretic hormone

diabetes mellitus — a disease with increased blood glucose levels due to lack or ineffectiveness of insulin

diaphoretic — sudorific, an agent promoting sweating

diarrhea — excessive discharge of contents of bowel

diastole — relaxation phase of the heart beat

diathesis — constitutional state of increased susceptibility to disease

disorders of kidney secretions — insufficient kidney flow

diuresis — excretion of urine

diuretic — agent increasing urine output

dopamine — a neurohormone; precursor to norepinephrine which acts as a stimulant to the nervous system

dosage — amount of therapeutic substance

dose — amount of a therapeutic substance to be taken during a specified time period

dragée — pill or capsule with a sugar coating

dromotropic — affecting conductivity of nerve fibers

dropsy — edema, abnormal accumulation of water in the body, usually associated with weak heart performance

duodenum — first portion of the small intestine — between the pylorus and jejunum

dyscrasia — abnormal or pathological imbalance due to excessive material in the blood

dyskinesia — a condition characterized by spasmodic, uncoordinated, or other abnormal movements; i.e., those which result from a reaction to phenothiazines

dysmenorrhea — difficult or painful menstruation

dyspepsia — indigestion

dysplasia — abnormal development of tissue

dyspnea — difficult breathing

dystonia — impaired muscle tonus

dystrophic nervous disturbance — progressive changes that may result from defective nutrition of nervous tissue

dysuria — painful urination

ecchymosis — small, flat hemorrhagic spots on the skin or mucous membranes

eclampsia — convulsions, unrelated to other cerebral conditions, in pregnant or puerperal women (women who have just given birth)

ectopic — located outside normal position, e.g., location of fetus in pregnancy

eczema — inflammatory skin condition

edema — abnormal accumulation of fluids within tissues

edematous dermatitis — skin irritation marked by an accumulation of watery fluid

ejaculatio praecox — premature ejaculation during sexual intercourse

electrolyte — substance in solution that conducts an electrical current

-ellus — in botany, diminutive, e.g., echinellus, minutely spiny

embolism — obstruction of a vessel by an abnormal body, usually a detached blood clot

embrocation — liniment; external application of a liniment

embryotoxic — poisonous to the developing embryo

emetic — substance causing vomiting

empyema — pus located in a body cavity

emulsion — system containing two unmixable liquids in which one is dispersed in the form of small globules throughout the other

endangiitis obliterans — inflammation of the inner blood vessel membrane leading to vessel occlusion

endogenous depression — depressive mental state not resulting from life events

endplate — termination, referring to a motor nerve fiber that enervates to a skeletal muscle fiber

-ensis — in botany, origin, country, or place of growth; e.g., texensis, found in Texas

enteral — referring to the inside of the intestinal tract

enteral absorption — absorption by means of the intestine

enteritis regionalis — localized inflammation of the intestine

enuresis nocturna — bed-wetting

epicondylitis — infection or inflammation of a projection from a long bone near the extremity

epidermis — superficial epithelial layers of the skin

epigastric — relating to the area immediately above the stomach

epilemma — interstitial sheath-like connective tissue in a peripheral nerve that separates the individual nerve fibers

epilepsy — chronic brain disorder associated with some seizures and, typically, alteration of consciousness

epileptiform convulsion — violent spasms; similar to those of epilepsy

erythema nodosum — acute inflammation of skin with red nodules

erythro- — in botany, reddish

-escens — in botany, process of becoming; e.g., florescens, blooming

essential oil — volatile terpene derivatives responsible for the odor or taste of a plant

-estris — in botany, place of growth; *e.g.*, campestris, growing in the field

estrogen receptor site binding — site on the surface of a cell receiving estrogen from circulation

estrogen-like — exerting biological effects similar to the effect of estrogen

exanthem — rash, symptomatic of viral or bacterial diseases

exocrine pancreas insufficiency — inability of the pancreas to secrete enzymes into the gastrointestinal tract for the digestion of proteins and fat

expectorant — promoting mucous secretion of the bronchi or facilitating its expulsion

extrapyramidal — referring to brain structures other than those needed for motor activities

extrasystole — an ectopic or asynchronous beat from any source in the heart

exudative diathesis — a constitutional or inborn predisposition to loss of fluids

familial Mediterranean fever — transient, recurrent attacks of fever with or without abdominal or joint pain, found usually among persons of Armenian or Sephardic (Jewish) descent

fatty liver — accumulation of triglycerides in the liver

febrifuge — antipyretic, agent fighting fever

febrile — having to do with a fever

fenestrated — anatomical, window-like opening

fermentative dyspepsia, fermentative digestive disturbances — impaired digestion associated with fermented foods

fibrinolytic activity — clot removal

fili- — in botany, threadlike

first-degree burn — burn involving only the epidermis and causing irritation and edema without blisters

fistula — an abnormal passageway, allowing movement between organs

flatulence — abnormal amount of gas in the stomach and intestines

flavor corrigent — agent accenting the flavors of components in a mixture

flower — reproductive structure of flowering plants with or without protective envelopes, the calyx and corolla

fluidextract — concentrated hydroalcoholic extract in which 1 ml is equivalent to 1 g of the original botanical

fluor albus — see leukorrhea

flux — profuse discharge from a body cavity

Foehn Illness — syndrome including sleep and mood disturbances accompanying strong warm winds in the Alps

folium — in botany, leaf

frostbite — damage to local tissue from exposure to extreme cold

fruit — matured ovary of flowering plants, with or without accessory parts

fruticosus — in botany, bushy

fungistatic — inhibiting the growth of fungi

furunculosis — localized skin infection

galactogogue — stimulating secretion of milk

galenical preparations — preparations of botanical drugs

gallstone — a gallbladder or bileduct concretion composed of cholesterol, occasionally mixed with calcium

ganglions — nerve cell bodies grouped in the peripheral nervous system

gargle — fluid used therapeutically as a throat wash

gastroenteritis — gastrointestinal tract inflammation; characterized by abdominal pain, nausea, diarrhea, vomiting; which may be caused by bacteria, parasites or a virus

gingivitis — inflammation of the fibrous tissues that surround the teeth

gland-stimulating remedy — expectorant

glaucoma — eye disease with increased ocular pressure

glaucoma, narrow-angle — form of glaucoma in which contact of the iris with the peripheral cornea prevents normal drainage of aqueous humor

glosso- — in botany, tongue-like

glucocorticoid — any steroid-like compound capable of significantly influencing intermediary metabolism, such as promotion of deposition of glycogen in the liver, and of exerting a useful antiinflammatory effect

glucosuria — glucose in the urine

glycine — the simplest amino acid which is a contituent of normal protein and an inhibitory transmitter; used as a dietary supplement

glycogenolytic — breaking down glycogen to glucose

glycoside — a molecule which upon hydrolysis produces at least one simple sugar and non-sugar component

goiter — chronic thyroid gland enlargement, not due to cancerous growth

gout — a disease characterized by an increased blood uric acid level and sudden onset of episodes of acute arthritis

grandi- — in botany, large

granulation — pink, fleshy overgrowth of capillaries and collagen within a wound

granulatory — encouraging granulation

granulocyte — a mature white blood cell with cytoplasm containing granules

hallucination — perception of objects or events that are not actually present

hallux valgus — twisting of the big toe toward the outer side of the foot

helminthiasis — diseased state due to intestinal parasites such as nematodes, cestodes, trematodes, and acanthocephalans

hematoma — localized blood clot within an organ or tissue

hematuria — blood in the urine

hemodialysis — process of separating water and small soluble substances from the blood

hemolysis — breaking down of red blood cells

hemolytic icterus — jaundice due to hemolysis

hemorrhage — profuse blood flow

hemorrhagic nephritis — acute glomerulonephritis accompanied by hematuria (blood in the urine)

hemorrhoids — varicose disorder causing painful swellings at the anus; piles

hemostatic — stopping blood flow; antihemorrhagic agent

hepatitis — liver inflammation, typically due to a virus or toxic substance

hepatotoxic — poisonous to the liver

herpes simplex — infection, often recurrent, caused by herpes virus type 1 and 2 and typically found on the the lip or genetalia

hetero- — in botany, different

hippocampus — brain structure that forms the edge of the cortical mantle of the cerebral hemisphere

HIV — abbreviation for human immunodeficiency virus

holo- — in botany, entire

homeopathic — a product containing infinitesimal doses of a drug that would, in normal doses, produce symptoms of the disease that it is intended to treat

homo- — in botany, like, same

HPLC — high performance liquid chromatography

human immunodeficiency virus (HIV) — a retrovirus associated with onset of advanced immunodeficiency syndrome (AIDS)

hybrid — an individual (plant or animal) whose parents are different varieties of the same species or belong to different but closely allied species

hydrops (dropsy) — an excessive accumulation of clear, watery fluid in any of the tissues or cavities of the body; edema, ascites, anasarca

hypercalcemia — excess calcium in the blood

hypercholesterolemia — excess cholesterol in the blood

hypercrinia — excessive secretion of mucus

hyperemia — condition of increased blood accumulation in a portion of the body, due to inflammation, obstruction to blood flow, or local relaxation of arterioles

hyperemic — causing increased blood accumulation in a portion of the body; relating to hyperemia

hyperhidrosis — excessive sweating

hypertension — high blood pressure

hyperthyroidism — an abnormal condition of the thyroid gland resulting in excessive secretion of thyroid hormones characterized by an increased metabolism and weight loss

hypertonia — excessive concentration of salts in the blood; condition of having a greater osmotic pressure than a reference solution (blood or interstitial fluid), having a fluid in which cells shrink

hypertrophy — increase in the size of an organ due to enlargement of its cells; frequently with a corresponding increase in functional capacity

hypokalemia — abnormally low blood potassium

hypothermia — abnormally low body temperature

hypothrombinemia — abnormally low amounts of thrombin circulating in the blood, resulting in an increased tendency to bleed

hypothyroidism — diminished production of thyroid hormone, leading to low metabolic rate, tendency to gain weight, and somnolence

hypotonia — lessened tension; arterial relaxation

hypotonic-asthenic dyskinesia — condition characterized by weakened voluntary movements

hypoxic tolerance — ability to function despite below-normal availability of oxygen to tissue

ichthyosis — skin disease with extreme scaling

icterus — jaundice

ileus — bowel obstruction

in vitro — in an artificial environment, such as the test tube

in vivo — in a living animal

-ineus — in botany, color or material, stramineus, straw-colored

inotropic — affecting force of muscle contraction

intermittent claudication — symptom characterized by pain during walking

intestinal flora — bacteria living in the large intestine

intraperitoneal — in the peritoneal cavity underlying the abdomen, often referring to the location of experimental injections

involutional — reducing an enlarged organ to normal size

irrigation therapy — washing out a cavity or wound with a fluid; irrigation of the kidney parenchyma and the urinary tract by addition of increased amounts of liquid, usually a mild herbal teas with aquaretic or diuretic properties

ischialgia — hip pain

ischuria — retention or suppression of urine

iso- — in botany, equal

itch — irritating sensation of the skin that arouses the urge to scratch; pruritis

jaundice — increased blood plasma level of bile pigments causing yellowish staining of the integument, sclera, deeper tissues, and excreta

kali — pertaining to potassium

kaliuretic — substance increasing elimination of potassium into the urine

keloid — a nodular, firm, movable, nonencapsulated, often linear mass of scar tissue, tender and frequently painful, consisting of wide, irregularly distributed bands of collagen, usually occurring after trauma, surgery, a burn, or severe acne, more common among people of African orgin

kidney gravel — small concretions formed in the kidney

kyphosis — spinal deformity characterized by extensive flexion

lactation — production of milk; period after giving birth during which milk is secreted in the breasts

laevi- — in botany, smooth

lamina — in botany, blade

lanci- — in botany, spear-shaped

lani- — in botany, woolly

latex — milky emulsion or suspension formed by some seed plants; contains suspended particles of natural rubber or related compounds

lati- — in botany, broad

laxative — mild cathartic; agent having the property of loosening the bowels

leaf — a photosynthetic and transpiring organ, usually developed from leaf primordium in the bud; an expanded, usually green, organ borne on the stem of a plant

lepido- — in botany, scaly

lepto- — in botany, slender

leuco-, leuko- — in botany, white

leukopenia — low white blood cell count

leukoplakia — thickened, white patch on mucous membrane of the mouth, in some cases precancerous

leukorrhea — discharge from the vagina of a white or yellowish viscous fluid with pus and mucus cells

leukosis — abnormal proliferation of any of the tissues that produce white blood cells

lignum — in botany, wood

ligulate flowers — strap-shaped, as in the case of the flattened corolla in the ray florets of composites

limbic system — brain structures, including hippocampus, dentate gyrus, and amygdala

liniment — ointment

lipid — fat-soluble substances derived from animal or vegetable cells by nonpolar solvents (e.g. ether); the term can include the following types of materials: fatty acids, glycerides, phospholipids, alcohols and waxes

lipid peroxidation — the introduction of a great number of oxygen molecules into unsaturated fatty acids

lipid-lowering — reducing levels of serum lipids in the circulation, usually refers to serum cholesterol

lipolytic — breaking down fat

lipophilic — agent that dissolves fats, e.g., alcohol

loop diuretic — fast-acting, highly effective agents increasing excretion of urine by acting on the loop of Henle in the kidney

lumbago — pain in the mid- and lower back

lumen — space in the interior of a tubular structure

luteinizing hormone — anterior pituitary hormone stimulating estrogen production by the ovary; promoting formation of progesterone by the corpus luteum in women and stimulating testosterone release in men

luteus — in botany, deep yellow

maceration — herb preparation softened by soaking

macro- — in botany, giant

manager disease — obesity and/or congestive heart failure associated with sedentary lifestyle and high emotional stress

MAO inhibitor — monoamine oxidase inhibitor

mastodynia — breast pain

medulla — in botany, pith

megacolon — massive dilation of the colon

melano- — in botany, black, very dark

Ménière's disease — affliction of the middle ear characterized by vertigo, nausea, vomiting, tinnitus, and progressive deafness

menopause — permanent cessation of menstruation

menorrhagia — abnormally heavy menstrual period

mesenchyma — cells developing into the synovial membrane of a joint

mesenchymal — refers to connective tissue, blood, and lymphatics that originate from embryonic mesoderm

metabolite — any product (foodstuff, intermediate, waste product) of metabolism

meteorism — tympania; swelling of the abdomen from gas in the intestinal or peritoneal cavity

methemoglobinuria — excretion of methemoglobin, a transformation product of hemoglobin, into urine

metrorrhagia — any irregular, acyclic bleeding from the uterus between periods

micro- — in botany, small, little

micturition — urination

migraine — a symptom complex occurring periodically and characterized by pain in the head, dizziness, nausea, vomiting, photophobia, and visual disturbance

milk scall — seborrhea of the scalp in infants; cradle cap

mineralocorticoid — one of the steroids of the adrenal cortex that influences salt (sodium, potassium) metabolism

mitosis — cell division

monoamine oxidase (MAO) — enzyme catalyzing the removal of an amine group from a variety of substrates, including norepinephrine and dopamine

montanus — in botany, of the mountains

motility — capacity for spontaneous movement, frequently in reference to the intestine

mucilage — preparation consisting of a solution in water of the viscous principles of plants; used as a soothing application to mucous membranes

mucolytic — agent breaking down or dissolving mucus

mucosa — mucous tissue layer lining tubular structures (nasal passages, ear canal, etc.)

mucous — containing or producing mucus

mucus — the clear secretion of the muous membrane

multiple sclerosis — demyelinating disorder of the central nervous system, causing patches of sclerosis (plaques) in the brain and spinal cord, manifested by loss of normal neurological functions, e.g., muscle weakness, loss of vision, and mood alterations

muscarine-like effect — having an effect similar to a muscarinic, cholinergic compound; e.g., causing vasodilation, salivation, bronchoconstriction, and gastrointestinal stimulation

muscarinergic cholinoceptors — parasympathetic receptors

musculotropic — affecting, attracted to, or acting upon muscle tissue

mutagenicity — production of genetic alterations

myalgia — diffuse muscle pain

mydriasis — dilation of the pupil

myocardium — heart muscle

myodegenenation — muscular degeneration

myogelosis — a localized hardened mass found in muscle tissue

myoglobinuria — excretion of the muscle's oxygen-transport protein, myoglobin, in the urine

myopathy — any disease or abnormal condition of the muscular tissues

myxedema — a condition arising from diminished thyroid function, characterized by hard swelling of subcutaneous tissue, hair loss, lower temperature, muscle debility, hoarseness and the slow return of a muscle to neutral position after a tendon jerk

native dry extract — an extract, typically hydroalcoholic, of plant material from which the solvent has evaporated to leave a solid residue

natriuretic — agent causing sodium to be excreted into the urine

nausea — symptoms resulting from an inclination to vomit

ne- — in botany, not, free from

necrosis — death of one or more cells, or of a portion of a tissue or organ

neonate — newborn

nephritis — kidney inflammation

nephro- — in botany, kidney-shaped

nephrolithiasis — presence of kidney stones or gravel

nephrosclerosis — hardening of the kidney from overgrowth and contraction of the interstitial connective tissue

nervous bladder — tendency to urinate in response to emotion stress

neuralgia/neuralgic ailment — pain of severe throbbing or stabbing nature along a nerve

neurasthenia — ill-defined condition, accompanying or following depression, characterized by vague fatigue believed to be brought about by psychological factors

neuritis — nerve inflammation

neuroleptic — a therapeutic agent which produces a state of altered awareness and tranquilization

neurotoxic — poisonous to the nerves

neurovegetative (neurovisceral) — referring to the innervation of the internal organs by the autonomic nervous system

nicotine-like effects — producing an effect which stimulates (small doses) and then depresses (large doses) autonomic nervous function

noradrenaline, norepinephrine — a catecholamine hormone secreted from the adrenal medulla and post-ganglionic adrenergic fibers in response to hypotension or emotional stress

NYHA guidelines — New York Heart Association guidelines specifying degrees of heart failure:

>stage I — no effect on physical performance
>
>stage II — performance of patient under major stress is decreased
>
>stage III — performance affected even during normal activity but not during rest
>
>stage IV — symptoms during rest, no physical stress is possible, patient must remain in bed

ochro- — in botany, yellowish

odonto- — in botany, toothlike

-oideus — in botany, resembling; *e.g*, helianthoides, resembling the genus *Helianthus*

ointment — semisolid preparation usually containing medicinal substances and intended for external therapeutic application

oral — by mouth or of the mouth

organ neurosis — dysfunction for which there is no apparent organic cause

ortho- — in botany, straight

orthostatic circulatory disturbance — changes in circulation upon assuming an upright position

osteochondritis — inflammation of a bone and its cartilage

-osus — in botany, abundance; e.g., foliosus, full of leaves

oxy- — in botany, sharp

oxytocin — a peptide hormone from the pituitary that stimulates lactation; used to induce labor, manage postpartum hemorrhage, and reduce painful breast engorgement

oxyurid — pin worm

pachy- — in botany, thick

PAF antagonist — platelet activating factor inhibitor. PAF activates platelets to secrete serotonin and other mediators to cause smooth-muscle contraction and vascular permeability, involved in asthma; a PAF antagonist counters these effects

pancreatitis — inflammation of the pancreas

papaverine-like — mildly analgesic, powerfully antispasmodic

paracrine — hormonal response from cell to cell near a secretory site

parametritis — inflammation of the tissues adjacent to the uterus

parasympathetic nervous system — portion of the autonomic nervous system that is generally associated with increasing digestion and intestinal muscle activity; decreasing blood circulation and respiration

parasympatholytic — agent, such as atropine, that annuls or antagonizes the effects of the parasympathetic nervous system

parasympathomimetic — drugs or chemicals having an action resembling that caused by stimulation of the parasympathetic nervous system, e.g., acetylcholine

parenteral administration — administration by means other than the digestive tract, such as intravenous, subcutaneous, intramuscular, or intramedullary injection

paresthesia — abnormal sensation, such as burning or prickling

parvi- — in botany, small

pericarditis sicca — fibrinous inflammation of the external surface of the heart and its surrounding membrane without the accumulation of fluid

periodontitis — inflammation of the area around a tooth

periostitis — inflammation of the thick fibrous membrane surrounding a bone

peristalsis — movement characterized by alternate circular contraction and relaxation of the intestine or other tubular structure which propels the contents onward

peritoneum — serous sac lining the abdominal cavity and covering most of the organs inside it

phaeo- — in botany, dark

phagocytosis — process of ingestion and digestion by cells of solid substances such as other cells, bacteria, dead tissue, and foreign particles

phanero- — in botany, easily seen

pharmacokinetics — the study of the absorption, distribution, metabolism and excretion of drugs and other substances in living organisms

pharyngeal — related to the upper expanded portion of the digestive tube, between the esophagus below and the mouth and nasal cavities above and in front

pheochromocytoma — encapsulated tumor of the adrenal gland secreting epinephrine and norepinephrine

phlebectasia — dilation of the veins

phlebitis — inflammation of a vein

phospholipid — a phosphorus-containing lipid; an important constituent of cell membranes

photosensitization — process of increasing sensitivity to sunlight

picro- — in botany, bitter

podo- — in botany, of a foot

polydipsia — chronic excessive thirst

portal circulation — circulation in which the outflow from one organ goes directly to a second organ, most commonly used to refer to the venous circulation of the intestine which goes to the liver

poultice — soft mass prepared by moistening botanicals or other absorbent substances with oil or water, usually applied hot to the skin

proctitis — inflammation of the mucous membranes of the rectum

prodrug — a drug whose actions result from its conversion by metabolic processes within the body

prolactin — an anterior pituitary peptide hormone that initiates and maintains lactation

prostaglandin — any of a class of physiologically active substances present in many tissues, with effects such as vasodilation, vasoconstriction, stimulation of the smooth muscles of the bronchus or intestine, uterine stimulation; also involved in pain, inflammation, fever, allergic diarrhea, and dysmennorhea

prostatectomy — removal of the prostate gland

prothrombin — protein needed for clotting of the blood

pruritis ani — anal itching

pruritus — itching

pseudomelanosis coli — changes in the pigmentation of the colon

psoriasis — inherited condition characterized by the eruption of reddish, scaled papules on the skin of the elbows, knees, scalp, and trunk

psychoanaleptic drugs — central nervous system stimulants that reverse depression

psychogenic — of a psychological origin

ptycho- — in botany, pertaining to grooves or folds

pulmonary edema — accumulation of fluid in the lung

pungent principles — essential oils imparting odor

purpura — bleeding into the tissues directly beneath skin or mucous membranes

pustule — small elevation of the skin containing pus

pyelonephritis — inflammation of the renal pelvis

pylorospasm — abnormal contraction of the lower sphincter of the stomach

pyretic — fever-inducing agent

pyro- — in botany, fiery

pyrrho- — in botany, fire red, ruby red

rachis — in botany, axis

radiculitis — disorders of the roots of the nerves

radix — in botany, root

rami- — in botany, pertaining to branches

ramus — in botany, branch

ranunculus dermatitis — type of dermatitis resulting from contact of skin with plants of the genus Ranunculus

Raynaud's disease — neurovascular disorder characterized by local vascular contractions resulting in attacks of decreased blood flow to the extremities upon exposure to cold

rectification — purification, usually through repeated steam distillations

resin — amorphous brittle substance consisting of the hardened secretion of a various plants, typically derived from the oxidation of terpenes

retina — receptive field of the eye

retinal edema — accumulation of fluid in the retina

rhagades — chaps, cracks, or fissures

rheological — deformative flow of materials, usually blood

rheumatism — general term applied to conditions of pain, or inability to articulate, various elements of the musculoskeletal system

rhinitis — inflammation of the nasal mucous membrane

rhizome — in botany, underground stem

rhodo- — in botany, rose-colored

rickets — vitamin-D deficiency characterized by abnormal calcification of bone tissues

roborant — strengthening agent, tonic

Roemheld's syndrome — gastro-cardiac syndrome

root — an absorbing and anchoring organ of the plant, usually developed from the radicle and growing downward

roseus — in botany, rosy

rubefacient — reddening agent, usually in reference to a counter-irritant

saluretic — substance increasing elimination of salts into the urine

sapro- — in botany, rotten

sativus — in botany, cultivated

scabies — skin eruption due to a mite

scar tissue — fibrous tissue replacing normal tissues destroyed by injury or disease

schisto- — in botany, split, cleft

sciatica — pain in the lower back and hip radiating down the back of the thigh into the leg, often due to herniated lumbar disk

seborrhea, seborrheic skin disease — skin inflammation characterized by dry or moist, greasy, yellow crusts or scales

secretagogue — agent promoting secretion

secretolytic — agent breaking down secretions

secretomotory — stimulating secretion

sedative — calming, quieting; drug that quiets nervous excitement

seed — mature ovule of seed plants

semper- — in botany, always

sequalae — consequences, subsequent events

sexual neurasthenia — psychogenic inhibition of sexual performance

sitz bath — immersion bath

soporific — sleep-inducing agent

spasm — involuntary contraction of one or more muscle groups

spondylarthritis — intervertebral arthritis

spondylitis — inflammation of one or more vertebrae

static edema — fluid accumulation in condition of confinement

status lymphaticus — thymicolymphaticus, old term for a syndrome of supposed enlargement of the thymus and lymph nodes in infants and young children, formerly believed to be associated with unexplained sudden death

stem — a supporting and conducting organ usually developed initially from the epicotyl and growing upward

steno- — in botany, narrow

stenocardia — angina pectoris

stenosis (esophageal, GI tract) — narrowing

stipule — in botany, a leaf-like appendage located singly (usually) in pairs at the base of the stem (petiole) of a leaf

stolon — stem

stomachic — agent that improves appetite and digeston

stomach-strengthening remedy — stomachic

stomatitis — inflammation of the mucous membrane of the mouth

strobile — in botany, a conelike inflorescence, as in hops

strongyloid — nematode parasite

struma — goiter, any enlargement of a tissue

subsidence — sinking or settling in bone, as in the case of prosthetic component of an artificial joint

sunburn — reddening of the skin, with or without blistering, caused by exposure to ultraviolet light

sympathetic nervous system — portion of the autonomic nervous system that is generally associated with "flight or fight" reactions by increasing blood circulation and respiration and decreasing digestion

sympathomimetic effect — mimicking the action of the sympathetic nervous system

synergistic — having the property that the total combined effect of two or more factors exceeds the sum of their individual effects

syrup — a liquid preparation of medicinal substances in a concentrated aqueous solution of sucrose

systole — contraction of the heart

T4 — thyroxine, thyroid hormone also prepared synthetically, for treatment of hypothyroidism and myxedema

tachycardia — excessively rapid heart rate

tachyphylaxis — progressive decrease in response following repetitive administration of a pharmacologically or physiologically active substance

tea — an infusion made by pouring boiling water over plant material and allowing to steep for a period of time

tendovaginitis — inflammation of a tendon and its sheath

tenesmus — painful spasm of the anal sphincter accompanied by an urgent desire to evacuate the bowel or bladder, involuntary straining, and the passage of little fecal matter or urine

tenui- — in botany, slender

teratogenic — causing abnormal embryonic growth processes

teratogenicity — property of an agent that causes physical defects in the developing embryo

testa — in botany, seed coat

thermolabile — altered or destroyed by heat

thiazide — a class of diuretics that increase the excretion of sodium and chloride and accompanying volume of water

thrombasthenia — platelet defect with impaired ability to form blood clots

thrombocyte — platelet

thrombocytopenia — condition of abnormally small number of platelets circulating in the blood, characterized by inability to properly clot blood and easy bruising

thrombophlebitis — venous inflammation with formation of clots

thrombosis — formation of blood clots causing vascular obstruction

thyrotoxicosis — state produced by excessive thyroid hormone

tincture — an alcohol or water-alcohol solution, usually referring to a preparation from herbal materials

tinnitus — ringing or roaring in the ear

T-lymphocyte — long-lived white blood cell responsible for cell-mediated immunity

tonic — remedy utilized to restore strength and vigor; typically taken for an extended period of time

tonic for the kidneys — diuretic

toniclonic — a muscle spasm which is both tonic, occurring over an extended period of time, and clonic, marked by contractions and relaxations of the muscle occurring in rapid succession

topical application — administration to the skin

tracheobronchitis — inflammation of the mucous membrane of the trachea and bronchi

trigeminal neuralgia — pain in the trigeminus, chief sensory nerve of the face and the motor nerve enabling chewing

tuberculosis — a specific disease caused by *Mycobacterium tuberculosis*, which may affect almost any tissue or organ of the body, most commonly the lungs

ulcer — lesion on the skin or mucous membrane

ulcus cruris — indolent leg ulcer, ulcer of the diaphragm

uremia — condition characterized by excessive urea and other nitrogen compounds in the blood due to renal insufficiency

uric acid diathesis — inherited tendency to gout

urinary calculi — concretions in the urethra

urticaria — hives, vascular reaction of upper layers of skin marked by wheals

-utus — in botany, possessing; e.g., cornutus, having horns

varicosis — unnatural and permanent distention of the veins

vascular dementia — mental incapacity due to inadequate blood flow to the brain

vasodilator — agent causing widening of the lumen (interior space) of blood vessels

vasomotor cephalalgia — migraine headache

vasomotor dysfunction — disorder involving blood vessel constriction

vasoneurosis — vascular abnormality without discernible physiological cause

vegetative dystonia — abnormal tissue tonicity resulting from autonomic nervous system dysfunction

vegetative nervous system — portion of the nervous system associated with involuntary functions; autonomic nervous system

venectasia — phlebectasia, dilation of the veins

venous tone — firmness of tension of vascular walls

ventricular tachycardia — excessively rapid heart beat due to uncontrolled ectopic focus in the ventricle

vermifuge — agent used to treat worm infestation

vernalis — in botany, of the spring

vertigo — dizziness

vesicle — small sac

villi — small processes protruding from absorptive or secretory surfaces

virens — in botany, green

virustatic — inhibiting viral action

viti- — in botany, pertaining to a vine

volatile oil — easily evaporated terpene derivatives found in plants which impart taste and aroma

vomit — to eject matter from the stomach through the mouth

vulgaris — in botany, common

whooping cough — cough characterized by spasm of the larynx; pertussis

xantho- — in botany, yellow

xylo- — in botany, woody

zygo- — in botany, joined

GENERAL REFERENCES

Arky, R. 1996. *Physicians' Desk Reference*, 50th ed. Montvale, New Jersey: Medical Economics.

Arnaudov, G. 1964. *Terminologia Medica Polyglotta: Medical Terminology in Six Languages*. Sofia, Bulgaria: Medicina et Physcultura.

Betteridge, H.T. 1971. *New Cassell's German Dictionary*. New York: Funk & Wagnalls.

Bradley, P. R. 1992. *British Herbal Compendium: A Handbook of Scientific Information on Widely Used Plant Drugs*. Vol. I. Bournemouth: British Herbal Medicine Association.

Bruneton, J. 1995. *Pharmacognosy, Phytochemistry, Medicinal Plants*. New York: Lavoisier Publishing.

Evans, W. C. 1992. *Trease and Evans' Pharmacognosy*. London: Balliere Tindall.

Fincher, J. H. 1986. *Dictionary of Pharmacy*. Columbia: University of South Carolina.

Foster, S. (ed.) 1992. *Herbs of Commerce*. Austin, Texas: American Herbal Products Association.

Hocking, G. M. 1997. *A Dictionary of Natural Products*. Medford, New Jersey: Plexus Publishing.

Hocking, G. M. 1955. *A Dictionary of Terms in Pharmacognosy and Economic Botany*. Springfield, Illinois: Charles C. Thomas.

Isselbacher, K., E. Braunwald, J. Wilson, J. Martin, A. Fauci, D. Kasper. 1994. *Harrison's Principles of Internal Medicine*. 13th ed. New York: McGraw-Hill.

Kartesz, J. T. 1994. *A Synonymized Checklist of the Vascular Flora of the United States, Canada, and Greenland*. 2nd ed. Portland: Timber Press.

Leung, A. Y. and S. Foster. 1996. *Encyclopedia of Natural Products Used in Foods, Drugs and Cosmetics*. New York: Wiley-Interscience.

Mutschler, E., H. Derendorf, M. Schafer-Korting, K. Elrod, K. Estes. 1995. *Drug Actions: Basic Principles and Therapeutic Aspects*. Stuttgart: MedPharm Scientific Publishers.

Newall, C. A., L. A. Anderson, J. D. Phillipson. 1996. *Herbal Medicines: A Guide for Health-care Professionals*. London: The Pharmaceutical Press.

Radford, A. 1986. *Fundamentals of Plant Systematics*. New York: Harper & Row.

Robbera, J., M. Speedie, V. Tyler. 1996. *Pharmacognosy and Pharmacobiotechnology*. Baltimore: Williams & Witkins.

Salisbury, F., C. Ross. 1992. *Plant Physiology*. Belmont, California: Wadsworth.

Schilcher, H. 1997. *Phytotherapy in Paediatrics: Handbook for Physicians and Pharmacists*. Stuttgart: Medpharm Scientific Publishers.

Stearn, W. T. 1966. *Botanical Latin: History, Grammar, Syntax, Terminology and Vocabulary*. New York: Hafner Publishing Co.

Stedman, T. 1982. *Stedman's Illustrated Medical Dictionary*. 24th ed. Baltimore: Williams & Wilkins.

Trease, G. E. and W. C. Evans. 1966. *A Textbook of Pharmacognosy*. 9th ed. London: Bailliere, Tindal and Cassell.

Wichtl, M., N. G. Bisset (eds.) 1994. *Herbal Drugs and Phytopharmaceuticals: A Handbook for Practice on a Scientific Basis*. Stuttgart: MedPharm Scientific Publishers.

Wren, R. C., E. M. Williamson, F. J. Evans. 1988. *Potter's New Cyclopaedia of Botanical Drugs and Preparations*. Saffron Walden: C. W. Daniels Co. Ltd.

GENERAL INDEX

This General Index is compiled from the material in this book, including the Introduction, Monographs, Therapeutic Indexes, Chemical and Taxonomic Indexes, Glossary and other indexes. For quick reference, the page numbers of monographs are printed in bold type after the common names, Latin names, pharmacopeial names and German names of the herbs upon which the monographs are based. Other than the pages of the monographs themselves, detailed information from the sample monographs from the *German Pharmacopoeia* and *European Pharmacopoeia* are not included. Due to the fact that the Unapproved Component Characteristics section (Chapter 6) contains monographs listing combinations with many herbs — such combinations not being approved by Commission E — and because there are so many of these relatively minor combinations, the editors have decided that these herbs are too numerous and inconsequential to include in this index. German and Latin names are italicized.

Abdominal Pain of Unknown Origin, 80, 96, 104, 195, 205, 207, 297, 298, 433, 435
Abies
    alba, **130-131**, 505, 515-516, 544
    sachalinensis, **130**, 505, 515-516, 544
    sibirica, **130**, 505, 515-516, 544
Abortifacient, 35, 48, 353, 354, 371, 471, 473, 617
Abortion, 36, 45, 317, 349, 362, 370, 379, 451, 453, 617
Absinthii herba, **232**, 518, 533, 604, 605, 607, 608, 610, 614
Absinthin, 233, 490
Absorbent, 113, 459, 462
Acanthopanax senticosus, **61**, 124, 504, 513, 516, 539
Accommodation Disturbance, Ocular, 444, 445
Acetylcholinesterase Inhibitor, 158, 460, 462, 617
Achillea millefolium, **233**, 516, 517, 543
Acne, 25, 234, 236, 419, 422, 617
Aconite
    herb, 499, 517, 533
    tuber, 499, 517, 533
Aconiti
    herba, **351**, 499, 500, 509, 517, 533, 534
    tuber, **351**, 499, 500, 509, 517, 533, 534
Aconitine, 351, 490
Aconitum napellus, *Aconitum napellus*, **351**, 500, 509, 517, 533, 599
Adonidis herba, **183**, 510, 517, 534, 601, 609-610

Adonis vernalis, **183**, 510, 517, 534,
Adoniskraut, **183**, 510, 517, 534,
aescin (escin), 64, 148-149
Aesculus hippocastanum, **148**, 337, 393, 506, 517, 541, 542, **557-559**
Agathosma betulina, **317**, 501, 517, 535
Aglycones, 47, 80, 95-96, 100, 104, 143, 195, 204-207, 489, 490
Agni casti fructus, **108**, 502, 533, 534, 595
Agnuside, 490
Agranulocytosis, 86, 444, 445, 618
Agrimonia
    eupatoria, **79**, 499, 503, 517, 534
    procera, **79**, 499, 503, 517, 534
Agrimoniae herba, **79**, 499, 503, 517, 534, 593
Agrimony, 73, **79**, 425, 428, 431, 464, 494, 497, 499, 517, 534, 593
Agropyron repens, **118**, 503, 517, 541
AIDS, 45, 122, 328, 392, 420, 434, 435, 444, 452, 460, 472, 618, 622, 629
Alantolactone, 35, 329, 490, 491
Alantwurzelstock, 328, 504, 525, 541
Albumin, 59, 132, 212, 491, 618
Albuminuria, 46, 81, 96, 98, 105, 195, 205, 207, 243, 297, 298, 347, 444, 445, 452, 453, 618
Alcea rosea, **336**, 506, 517, 543
Alchemilla
    alpina, **307**, 499, 517, 534
    vulgaris, **158**, 507, 517, 534

Alchemillae
	alpinae herba, **307**, 499, 517, 534, 593
	herba, **158**, 499, 507, 517, 534, 598
Alexandriner-Sennesfrüchte, **206**, 512, 519, 547
Alkaloids, xii, 35-36, 49, 57, 87, 93, 105-106, 109-110, 114-116, 125, 146, 152-153, 172, 175, 180, 183, 202, 203, 232, 310, 316, 324, 326, 329, 338, 340, 351, 355, 365, 373, 376, 383, 389, 476, 479, 487-488, 491
Allantoin, 115, 116, 491
Allergic Reactions/Allergies, 16, 45-46, 84, 92, 109, 119, 123, 178, 189, 235, 251, 253-254, 256, 264, 266, 321, 392, 413, 433-435, 452-453, 618, 621
	Mucosa Reactions, 35, 110, 445, 452-453
		Allergy/Hypersensitivity, 434, 435
			Gastrointestinal Tract, 82, 250-253, 255-259, 275, 294, 444-445, 451
		Respiratory Tract, 82, 129, 246, 250-253, 255-259, 275-276, 281, 283-285, 288-290, 294, 415, 444-445
	Skin Reactions, 35, 85, 109-110, 144, 156, 159, 179, 182, 188, 251, 253, 256, 309, 323, 375, 390, 444, 451, 453-454
		and migraine, 35
Alliaceae, 134, 176, 505, 509, 517, 534
Allii
	cepae bulbus, **176**, 509, 517, 534, 600
	sativi bulbus, **134**, 505, 517, 534, 597, 614
Alliin, 134, 177, 491
Allium
	cepa, **176**, 509, 517, 534, 616
	sativum, **134**, 505, 517, 534, 614, 616
Aloe, *Aloe*, 12, 47, 49, 499, 501, 503, 517, 534
	barbadensis, *barbadensis*, 80, 499, 503, 517, 534, 621
	capensis, 80, 499, 501, 517, 534, 614
	ferox, 80, 499, 501, 517, 534, 614
	vera, 80, 499, 503, 517, 534, 615
Aloe-emodin, 47, 80, 96-97, 104, 195, 204-207, 489, 491
Aloin, 80-81, 489, 491
Alopecia, 86, 443, 446, 618
Alpine Lady's Mantle herb, 36, 76, **307**, 499, 517, 534, 593
Alpinia officinarium, 505, 517, 540
Altesherz, 63
Althaea
	officinalis, **166-167**, 506, 508, 517, 534, 542, 613
	rosea, **336**, 506, 517, 543

Althaeae
	folium, **166**, 508, 517, 534, 599, 606, 608, 610
	radix, **167**, 508, 517, 534, 599, 606-608, 610
Alveolitis, 35, 341, 452-453
Amarogentin, 135, 491
American Botanical Council, 38
American Herbal Pharmacopoeia — AHP, 16
American Herbal Products Association, 41
Amerikanische Faulbaumrinde, **104**, 501-502, 523, 529, 546
Amines, biogenic, 491
Ammeos visnagae fructus, 312, 500, 517, 534, 594, 609
Ammi daucoides, **312**, 500, 517, 534
Ammi visnaga, **312-313**, 397, 500, 517, 534
Ammi-visnaga-Früchte, **312**, 500, 517, 534
Anabsin, 233, 491
Anabsinthin, 233, 491
Anal fissures, 53, 165, 191-192, 337, 364, 394, 406, 419-420, 422
Analeptic, Respiratory, 260, 461-462
Analgesic, 84, 121, 230, 309, 360, 400-401, 460, 462, 472-473, 618, 634
Ananas, 501, 517, 536
	comosus, **94**, 501, 517, 536
Anaphylactic shock, 320-321, 452-453, 618
Andornkraut, **148**, 506, 526, 543
Andromeda derivatives, 367, 491
Anesthesia/Anesthestic, Topical, 420, 422, 460, 462
Anethi
	fructus, **121**, 504, 518, 534, 596
	herba, **327**, 504, 518, 534, 596
Anethole, 53, 82, 128-129, 250-254, 256-259, 275, 294, 433, 489, 491
Anethum graveolens, **121**, **327**, 504, 518, 534
Angelica, *Angelica*
	archangelica, **81**, **308**, 499, 518, 534
	herb, 26, 35, 39, 50, 73, 76, 245, 247-248, **308**, 387, 400, 422-423, 425, 427, 431, 435, 438, 447-448, 456, 463-466, 468, 492-494, 499, 518, 534, 593, 605
	root, 26, 39, 50, 73, 75-76, **81-82**, 245-249, 308, 387, 397-398, 400, 422-423, 425-427, 431, 435, 437-438, 440-442, 445-449, 463-466, 468, 492-494, 499, 518, 534, 593, 605
	seed, 35, 39, 50, 73, 75-76, 81, 245, **308**, 397, 422-423, 425-427, 431, 440-442, 445-446, 448-449, 456, 463-466, 468, 492-494, 499, 518, 534, 593, 605
		and herb, 35

Angelicae
  fructus, **308**, 499, 518, 534, 593, 605
  herba, **308**, 499, 518, 534, 605
  radix, **81**, 499, 518, 534, 593, 605
Angelikafrüchte, **308**, 499, 518, 534
Angelikakraut, **308**, 499, 518, 534
Angelikawurzel, **81**, 499, 518, 534
Angina, 172, 312, 334, 354, 365, 380, 404, 406, 415, 443, 446, 619, 638
Anis, **82**, 499, 527, 534
Anise
  oil, 45, 74-76, 82-83, 215, 237-238, **250-253**, **258**, 387, 401, 423-426, 435-442, 445-446, 448-449, 462-463, 466, 468, 477, 493, 499, 525, 527, 534, 605-607, 614
  seed, **82**, **253-259**
Anisi
  fructus, **82**, 215, 499, 525, 527, 534, 593, 603, 605-607, 610, 614
    stellati fructus, **215**, 513, 525, 534, 603, 610
Ano-genital Irritation, 419, 422
Antennaria dioica, **319**, 502, 518, 534
Antennariae dioicae flos, **319**, 502, 518, 534, 595
Anthemis nobilis, **320-321**, 502, 518, 537
Anthocyanins, 88, 188, 214, 488, 491
Anthranoids, 80, 95, 97, 104, 195-196, 204-207, 491
Antiandrogenic, 201, 459, 462, 619
Anti-anxiety, 157, 460, 462
Antiarrhythmic, 81, 96, 98, 208, 297, 299, 357, 471, 473, 475, 477, 479, 619
Antibacterial, 83, 107, 111-112, 134, 141, 171, 174, 177, 182, 187-188, 198-199, 220, 225, 234, 250-255, 257-259, 261-262, 268, 270-271, 276-277, 286-290, 294, 296, 300-301, 313, 348, 392, 460, 462, 477, 488, 619
Antichemotactic, 460, 462
Anticholinergic, 87-88, 146, 202, 232, 404, 407, 460, 462, 475-476, 619, 621
Anticonvulsant, 460, 462
Antidepressant, 25, 68, 215, 460, 462
Anti-edematous, 219, 461-462
Antiemetic, 69, 136, 460, 462, 619
Anti-exudative, 148, 201, 309, 459, 463, 471, 473, 619
Antiflatulent, 160, 460, 463
Antifungal, 112, 460, 463, 619
Antigonadotropic, 99, 459, 463, 619
Antihemorrhagic, 471, 473, 629
Antihypertensive, 357, 459, 463

Anti-infectious, 363, 392, 472-473
Antiinflammatory, 25, 57, 100, 115-116, 215, 222, 231, 239, 316, 349, 375, 379, 463, 472, 473, 488, 619, 628
Anti-irritant, 461, 463, 467
Antimicrobial, 102-103, 118, 129, 150, 152, 194, 220, 224-225, 232, 237, 310, 387, 460, 463, 472-473, 489, 568-569, 619
Antiparasitic, 182, 460, 463, 619
Antiperspirant, 459, 463
Antiphlogistic, 57, 84, 86, 100, 107, 121, 134, 140, 230, 232, 260, 273-274, 303, 309, 460, 463, 473, 619
Antipyretic, 230, 357, 460, 463, 472-473, 627
Antiseptic, 49, 84, 112, 130-131, 159, 182, 185-186, 224, 260, 267, 328, 460, 463, 620
Antispasmodic, xxi, 82-83, 94, 102-103, 106-107, 112, 121, 127-129, 133-134, 136, 140, 153, 155, 157, 162, 164, 180, 182-183, 197, 216, 234, 260, 266, 273-274, 276, 286, 294, 298, 303, 307, 339, 342, 348, 354, 357-358, 370-371, 396, 460, 463-464, 472-473, 620, 634
Antithyrotropic, 99, 459, 464, 620
Antitussive, 126, 218, 257, 295, 300, 349, 406, 461, 464, 472-473, 620
Antiviral, 112, 460, 464, 489, 618
Anuria, 362, 452-453, 620
Anwendungsgebiete, 44
Anxiety, xxi, 26, 33, 36, 125, 147, 152, 156, 215, 319, 353, 355, 383, 394, 397-399, 401, 406, 413, 416, 420, 422, 434-435, 452-453, 618, 620
Apiaceae, 44, 81-82, 102, 117, 121, 128-129, 163, 179, 184, 200, 308, 312, 320, 327, 362, 366, 499, 500, 501, 502, 503, 504, 505, 508, 510, 512, 516, 517, 518, 519, 521, 523, 525, 527, 530, 534, 536, 538, 540, 542, 544, 547
Apigenin, 60, 70, 107, 491
Apigenin-7-glucoside, 107, 491
Apii
  fructus, **320**, 502, 518, 534
  herba, **320**, 502, 518, 534
  radix, **320**, 502, 518, 534
Apiol, 35, 362-363, 491
Apium graveolens, *Apium graveolens*, **320**, 502, 518, 534, 595
Aplastic Anemia, 86, 444, 446, 620
Apocynaceae, 152, 356, 364, 490, 507, 509-510, 513, 526, 529, 533, 543, 546, 550
Apotheke, 22
Appendicitis, 80, 96-97, 104, 195, 205, 207, 297-298, 433, 435

Appetite, Loss of, 120, 351, 420, 422, 476
aquaresis, 58
aquaretic, 19, 45
Aquifoliaceae, 168, 508, 525, 543
Araliaceae, 124, 138, 153, 504, 505, 507, 513, 516, 523, 524, 527, 539, 541
Arbor vitae tips (*Thuja occidentalis*), 26
Arbutin, 35, 49, 225, 303, 348, 367, 484, 488, 491
Arctium
    lappa, **318**, 501, 518, 535
    minus, **318**, 501, 518, 535
    tomentosum, **318**, 501, 518, 535
Arctostaphylos uva-ursi, 515, 518, 549, 614
Arecaceae, 201, 512, 530, 531, 546, 547
Armoracia rusticana, **150**, 506, 518, 534
Armoraciae rusticanae radix, **150**, 506, 518, 521, 534, 598
Arnica, *Arnica*
    chamissonis, **83**, 499, 518, 534
        flower, 73, **83-84**, 238, 242, 374, 390, 393, 396, 401, 405, 411, 423, 425-431, 435, 447, 450, 462-463, 491-499, 518, 534, 593, 614
    montana, **83**, 403, 499, 518, 534, 614
Arnicae flos, **83**, 499, 518, 534, 593, 614
Arnikablüten, **83**, 499, 518, 534
Arrhythmia, Stabilizes, 471, 473
Arrhythmogenic, 357, 471, 473
Artabsin, 233, 490-491
Artemisia, *Artemisia*
    absinthium, **232**, 516, 518, 533, 614
    vulgaris, *vulgaris*, 43, **352**, 509, 518, 535, 600
Artemisiae vulgaris
    herba, 43, **352**, 509, 518, 535
    radix, 43, **352**, 509, 518, 535
Arterial Occlusive Disease, 137, 419, 422
Arthritis, 144, 239-240, 242, 308, 311, 316-318, 335, 337, 347, 351-352, 359, 364, 368-369, 371, 373, 375, 378, 381, 421-422, 620, 628, 637
Arthrosis, 239-240, 337, 421-422, 620
Artichoke, 25
    leaf, 50, 73, 75, **84**, **264-266**, 425-427, 435-439, 465, 469, 491-493, 497, 499, 522, 538, 593, 607
Artischokenblätter, **84**, 499, 522, 538
Artubiin, 491
Asarone, 491
Ascaridol, 94, 491
Asclepiadaceae, 117, 226, 490, 503, 515, 526, 533, 538, 549
Ascophyllum nodosum, **315**, 500, 518, 540

Ascorbic acid, 233, 491
Ash, 36
    bark, 76, 165, **308-309**, 386, 473, 499, 509, 523, 531, 540, 548, 593
    leaf, 36-37, 76-77, **308-309**, 386, 473, 499, 509, 523, 531, 540, 548, 593, 599
Asparagi
    herba, **309**, 499, 518, 535, 593
    rhizoma, **85**, 499, 518, 535, 593
Asparagus, *Asparagus*
    herb, 40, 45, 58, 73, 76, **309**, 412, 428, 429, 432, 440, 446, 453, 466, 473, 499, 518, 535, 593
    officinalis, **85**, 309, 499, 518, 535
    root, 45, 58, 73, 76, **85**, 412, 428, 429, 432, 440, 442, 446, 453, 466, 473, 499, 518, 535, 593
Aspen
    bark, 52, 77, **385-386**, 430, 453, 499, 528, 545, 593
    leaf, 77, **385-386**, 430, 453, 499, 528, 545, 593
Aspleniaceae, **346-347**, 508, 522, 540
Asteraceae, 44, 83-84, 92, 100, 107, 109, 114, 118-119, 121, 123, 139-140, 169, 183, 199, 232-233, 318-319, 321, 324-325, 327-328, 350, 352, 365, 376, 379, 391-392, 490, 499-505, 508-512, 514, 516-526, 531-541, 543-544, 547-548, 573, 624
Asthma, 312, 324, 340, 359, 371, 380, 390, 406, 421, 422, 434, 435
    Bronchial, 267, 390, 399, 415, 421
Astragalin, 83, 491
Astragalus, 12
Astringent, 79, 88, 91-92, 113, 154, 158, 174, 176, 187, 189, 194, 197-198, 228, 231-232, 234, 323, 341, 345, 348, 369, 372, 459, 464, 489, 555, 620
Atherosclerosis, 177, 419, 422
Atropa belladonna, 43, **87**, 403, 405, 500, 504, 518, 535, 593
Atropine, 17, 87, 293, 400, 488, 491, 635
Aucubin, 186, 491
Aufgüsse, 59
Augentrostkraut, **329**, 505, 523, 540
Aurantii
    flos, **313**, 500, 520, 535, 594
    flos aetheroleum, **313**, 500, 520, 535, 608
    pericarpium, **89**, 500, 520, 535, 594, 605, 608
Austrian Pharmacopoeia, 59
Autoimmune Diseases, 122, 328, 392, 434-435
Autumn Crocus, 73, **86**, 427, 441, 445-450, 462-463, 467, 483, 492, 499, 521, 537, 593

Avena sativa, **176**, **355-356**, 509, 516, 518, 535
Avenae
    fructus, **356**, 509, 518, 519, 535, 600
    herba, **355**, 509, 516, 518, 519, 535, 600
    stramentum, **176**, 509, 518, 535, 600
BAH, 31
Baldrianwurzel, **226**, 515, 533, 549
balneology, 53
Balsamum
    peruvianum, **182**, 510, 526, 535, 601
    tolutanum, **220**, 514, 526, 535, 604
Barberry, 76, **309-310**, 454, 455, 456, 491, 500, 519, 535, 593
    bark, **309-310**, 375, 454, 491, 500, 519, 535
    root bark, **309-310**, 375, 454, 500, 519, 535
Bardanae radix, 43, **318**, 501, 518, 535, 594
Bärentraubenblätter, **224**, 515, 518, 549
Barosma betulina, **317**, 501, 519, 535
Barosmae folium, **317**, 501, 517, 519, 535, 594
Bartflechten, **224**, 515, 533, 549
Basil
    herb, 35, 58, 76, 77, **310-311**, 387, 473, 493, 500, 526, 535, 593
    leaf, 58
    oil, 52, 77, 311, **387-388**, 473, 493, 500, 526, 535, 593
Basilici
    aetheroleum, **387**, 500, 526, 535, 593
    herba, **310**, 500, 526, 535, 593
Basilikumkraut, **310**, 500, 526, 535
Basilikumöl, **387**, 500, 526, 535
Bath Additives, 53
Bathmotropic, Negatively, 460, 464, 621
Baummelonenblätter, **361**, 510, 519, 536
Beifußkraut, **352**, 509, 518, 535
Beifußwurzel, **352**, 509, 518, 535
Beinwellblätter, **115**, 503, 531, 548
Beinwellkraut, **115**, 503, 531, 548
Beinwellwurzel, **116**, 503, 531, 548
Belladonna
    leaf, 43, 73, 78, **87**, 374, 422, 430, 431, 436, 438, 440, 441, 442, 445, 447, 448, 449, 450, 462, 465, 466, 467, 475, 479, 480, 481, 491, 494, 497, 500, 518, 535, 593, 605-606
    root, 43, 73, **87**, 374, 397, **405**, 422, 430, 431, 436, 438, 440, 441, 442, 445, 447, 448, 449, 450, 462, 465, 466, 467, 475, 479, 480, 481, 491, 494, 497, 500, 518, 535, 605

Belladonnae
    folium, 43, **87**, 500, 504, 518, 535, 605, 606
    radix, 43, **87**, 500, 504, 518, 535, 605
Benediktenkraut, **92**, 500, 521, 537
benign prostatic hyperplasia (BPH), 22, 25 (see also Prostate)
Benzoic acid, 182, 491
Benzyl esters, 182, 491-492
Benzyl isothiocyanate, 241, 491
Berberidaceae, 500, 519, 535
Berberidiceae, 508, 528, 545
Berberidis
    cortex, **309**, 500, 519, 535
    fructus, **309**, 500, 519, 535
    radicis cortex, **309**, 500, 519, 535
    radix, **309**, 500, 519, 535
Berberine, 310, 491
Berberis vulgaris, **309-310**, 500, 519, 535, 593
Berberitze, **309**, 500, 519, 535
Berberitzenrinde, 500, 519, 535
Berichtigung, 59
Besenginsterblüten, **373**, 501, 512, 522, 530, 539
Besenginsterkraut, **203**, 501, 512, 522, 530, 539
Bestandteile des Arzneimittels, 58
Betula
    pendula, **89**, 500, 519, 535
    pubescens, **89**, 500, 519, 535
Betulaceae, **89**, 500, 519, 535
Betulae folium, **89**, 500, 519, 535, 594, 606, 613
Beurteilung, 58
Bibernellkraut, **366**, 510, 527, 544
Bibernellwurzel, **184**, 510, 527, 544
Bilberry, 11, 12
    fruit, 35, 49, 73, 76, **88**, 311, 425, 428, 431, 464, 483, 494, 500, 533, 543, 593-594
    leaf, 35, 49, 73, 76, **311**, 425, 428, 431, 455, 464, 483, 491, 494, 497, 500, 533, 543, 593-594
Bile Duct
    Inflammation, 434, 435, 623
    Obstruction, 45, 434-436
Biliary
    Dyskinesia, 233, 420, 422, 621
    Spasm, 420, 422
Bilirubinuria, 347, 452, 453, 621
Bilobalide, 136-137, 491
Birch leaf, 73, 75, **89**, 242, **259-260**, 428, 429, 430, 432, 440, 466, 468, 493, 494, 497, 500, 519, 535, 594, 606, 613
Birkenblätter, **89**, 500, 519, 535

Bisabolol, 107, 491, 575
  oxides, 491
Bishop's Weed fruit, 33, 35, 76, **312**, 374, 424, 429, 456, 494, 498, 500, 517, 534, 594, 609
Bitter Orange
  flower, **313**, 500, 520, 535, 594
    oil, 73, 76, 238, **313**, 423, 426, 427, 438, 449, 491, 500, 520, 535, 608
    peel, 50, 73, 75, 76, **89**, **247**, **282**, 422, 423, 425, 426, 427, 438, 442, 449, 464, 491, 493, 500, 520, 535, 594, 605, 608
Bitter principles, 44, 84, 89, 92, 93, 109, 117, 119, 130, 135, 148, 151, 160, 172, 177, 198, 233, 328, 491, 621
Bitterkleeblätter, **93**, 500, 526, 543
Bittersüßstengel, **232**, 516, 531, 539
Black Cohosh, 25, 26, 48
  root, xii, 48, 73, **90**, 425, 429, 430, 435, 441, 447, 466, 467, 498, 500, 520, 537, 594
Black Psyllium, 43
  (see Psyllium seed, Black)
Blackberry
  leaf, 36, 49, 73, 76, **91**, 374, 393, 395, 411, 425, 428, 431, 464, 483, 497, 500, 530, 546, 594
  root, 36, 49, 76, **314**, 374, 395, 425, 428, 431, 464, 497, 500, 530, 546, 594
Blackthorn
  berry, 73, **91**, 428, 431, 464, 498, 500, 529, 545, 594
  flower, 73, 76, **315**, 428, 431, 437, 439, 464, 498, 500, 529, 545, 594
Bladder Irritation, 35, 317, 319, 421, 423, 452
Bladderwrack, 35, 76, **315**, 453, 455, 500, 518, 523, 540, 594
Blasses Kegelblumenkraut, **327**, 504, 522, 539
Blauer
  Eisenhut, **351**, 500, 508, 516, 533
  Eisenhutkraut, **351**, 500, 509, 517, 533
  Eisenhutwurzel, **351**, 500, 509, 517, 533
Bleeding
  from the nose, lips, & eyelids, 371, 452, 453
  of the mucous membranes, 371, 452, 453, 632
  of the uterus, 329, 371, 379, 451, 453
Blessed Thistle herb, 73, **92**, 422, 425, 435, 466, 468, 491, 492, 500, 521, 537, 594
Blindness, 347, 452, 453
Bloating, Feeling of Abdominal Fullness, 420, 423
Blood
  sugar regulation, 459, 464

  superficial effusion of, 420, 423
  supply, increase, 459, 464
Blue
  Mallow flower, **164**, 500, 526, 543
  Monkshood
    herb, **351**, 500, 517, 533-534
    tuber, **351**, 500, 517, 533-534
Blueberry, 500, 533, 543
  leaf, **311**, 500, 533, 543
Bockshornsamen, **130**, 505, 532, 540
Bogbean, 73, **93**, 422, 425, 466, 468, 491, 500, 526, 543, 594
Boldine, 93, 488, 491
Boldo
  folium, **93**, 501, 527, 535, 594, 613
  leaf, 73, **93-94**, 425, 431, 435, 438, 440, 463, 465, 466, 488, 491, 494, 501, 527, 535, 594, 613
Boldoblätter, **93**, 501, 527, 535
Borage
  flower, 35, 42, 76, **316**, 455, 473, 496, 501, 519, 535
  herb, 42, 76, **316**, 455-456, 473, 474, 496, 501, 519, 535
Boraginaceae, 115-116, **316**, 338, 345, 501, 503, 506, 508, 519, 522, 529, 531, 535, 538-539, 546, 548
Boraginis
  flos, **316**, 501, 519, 535
  herba, **316**, 501, 519, 535
Borago officinalis, **316**, 501, 519, 535
Boretsch, **316**, 501, 519, 535
2-Bornanone, 101, 491
Bowel, Irritable (See Colon, Irritable), 420, 423
Bradycardia, 33, 35, 152, 293, 326, 351, 367, 400, 408, 410, 413, 415, 416, 433, 436, 451, 453, 476, 622
bradycardic arrhythmias, 63
Brassicaceae, 150, 193, 208, 228, 229, 506, 511, 513, 515, 518, 519, 521, 526, 529, 531, 534, 536, 543, 546, 548
Breast Pain, 420, 423, 632
Brechnußsamen, **355**, 509, 531, 548
Brennesselblätter, **216**, 509, 513, 532, 533, 549
Brennesselkraut, **216**, 509, 513, 532, 549
Brennesselwurzel, **217**, 509, 513, 514, 532, 533, 549
Brewer's Yeast, 75, **234, 235**, 236, 385, 394, 397, 477, 480, 494, 495, 498, 501, 516, 530, 540, 547, 594, 605
Brightening or Coloring Agent, 57
British Herbal Medicine Association, 65
Brombeerblätter, **91**, 500, 530, 546
Brombeerwurzel, **314**, 500, 530, 546

Bromelain, 25, 73, **94-95**, 431, 432, 435, 446, 447, 462, 475, 479, 480, 481, 483, 487, 501, 517, 536, 594
Bromelainum, **94**, 501, 517, 536, 594
Bromeliaceae, **94**, 501, 517, 536
Bronchial Secretion,
    excessive, 421, 423
    increased, 135, 461, 464
    reduced, 461, 464
Bronchitis, 21
Bronchoantispasmodic, 101, 218, 220, 260, 461, 464
Bronchodilator, 357, 472, 473
Bronchospasm increase, 444, 446
Broom, Scotch
    flower, **373-375**, 424, 501, 512, 522, 530, 539, 602
    herb, **203**, 501, 522, 530, 539, 602
Bruchkraut, **371**, 512, 524, 541
Bruises, Contusions, 240, 421, 423
Brunnenkressenkraut, **228**, 515, 523, 543
Bryonia, *Bryonia*, 35
    alba, **316**, 501, 519, 536
    cretica, **316**, 501, 519, 536
    root, 76, 242, **316-317**, 427, 431, 453, 454, 455, 456, 474, 501, 519, 536
Bryoniae radix, **316**, 501, 519, 536, 594
Buccoblätter, **317**, 501, 517-519, 535
Buchu leaf, 58, 76, **317**, 455, 501, 517, 519, 535, 594
Buckthorn
    bark, 39, 45, 47, 49, 73, **95**, 96, 425, 435, 436, 437, 440, 441, 445, 446, 447, 448, 449, 467, 475, 479, 480, 483, 490-494, 497, 501, 523, 529, 540, 546, 594, 614
    berry, 39, 45, 47, 49, 73, **96-97**, 375, 395, 425, 435, 436, 437, 440, 441, 445, 446, 447, 448, 449, 467, 475, 479, 480, 483, 491, 493, 494, 497, 501, 529, 546, 594
Bufenolide, 172, 492
Bugleweed, 73, **98-99**, 423, 430, 432, 442, 450, 463, 464, 468, 475, 480, 481, 492, 494, 495, 501, 525, 542, 594
Bundesanzeiger, 60
Bundesfachverband der Arzneimittel-Hersteller, 31
Bundesgesundheitsamt (BGA), 27
Bundesinstitut für Arzneimittel und Medizinprodukte (BfArM), 27
Bundesverband der Pharmazeutischen Industrie, 31
Burdock root, 36, 43, 76, **318**, 399, 501, 518, 535, 594
Burns, 101, 182, 215, 260, 321, 358, 359, 361, 380, 419, 423, 433, 436, 489

Bursae pastoris herba, **208**, 513, 519, 536, 603
Burseraceae, 173, 509, 521, 543
Butcher's Broom rhizome, **99**, 501, 530, 546
Cacao
    semen, **390**, 503, 532, 536, 595
    testes, **322-323**, 503, 532, 536, 595
Cactaceae, 353, 509, 531, 547
Cadinene, 155, 492
Caffeic acid, 83, 98, 489, 492, 556, 564
Caffeine, 113-114, 168, 414, 487, 492
Caffeoylquinic acid, 84, 492
Cajeput oil, 52, 75, **237-241**, 430, 431, 436, 447, 492, 493, 501, 526, 536, 594
Cajuputi aetheroleum, **237-241**, 501, 526, 536
Cajuputöl, **237-241**, 501, 526, 536
Calcium salts, 161, 216, 397, 492
Calendula, *Calendula*
    flower, 36, 73, 76, **100**, 428, 431, 432, 463, 466, 469, 490, 492, 493, 498, 501, 519, 536, 594, 613
    herb, 36, 73, 76, 242, **318**, 501, 519, 536, 594, 613
    officinalis, **100**, **318**, 501, 519, 536, 613
Calendulae
    flos, **100**, 501, 519, 536, 594
    herba, **318**, 501, 519, 536, 594
California poppy, 52, 77, **389**, 491, 492, 501, 523, 540, 594
Calluna vulgaris, **335**, 506, 519, 536
Callunae vulgaris
    flos, **335**, 506, 519, 536, 597
    herba, **335**, 506, 519, 536, 597
Callus formation, 459, 464
Campher, **101**, 501, 520, 536
Camphor, 51, 73, 75, **101**, 159, 198, **260**, 423, 424, 428, 429, 430, 435, 436, 440, 442, 447, 462, 464, 465, 466, 469, 490, 492, 501, 520, 536, 581, 594, 606
Camphora, **101**, 501, 520, 536, 594, 606
cancer treatment, 25
Candida utilis, **234**, 501, 516, 519, 540
Cape aloe, **80**, 501, 517, 534, 614
Caprifoliaceae, 124, 504, 530, 547
capsaicinarme Paprika-Arten, 502, 510, 519, 535
Capsaicinoids, 178, 492
Capsella bursa pastoris, **208**, 513, 519, 536
Capsicum, *Capsicum*, 502, 519, 536, 600
    frutescens, **178**, 502, 510, 519, 536
    spp., 502, 510, 519, 536
Caraway, 26
    oil, 73, 75, 76, **102**, 250, 261, 262, 286, 287, 288, 298, 423, 425, 426, 427, 430, 431, 435-441, 445-447, 449, 462-

465, 479, 492, 501, 519, 536, 594, 606-610, 614
  seed, 50, 73, 75, 76, **102, 245, 258, 263, 280, 281, 282, 283, 285,** 422, 423, 425, 426, 427, 430, 431, 435-441, 445-447, 449, 462-465, 492-493, 501, 519, 536, 594, 605-606, 608, 610, 614
Carcinogenic, 33, 35, 137, 143, 235, 311, 316, 324, 346, 348, 354, 365, 376, 388, 471, 473
Cardamom, 73, **103,** 425, 438, 464, 465, 492, 493, 498, 501, 523, 536, 594
Cardamomi fructus, **103,** 501, 523, 536, 594
Cardenolide glycosides, 226, 490, 492
Cardiac
  Arrest, 35, 313, 326, 367, 398, 451, 453
  Arrhythmia, 125, 334, 347, 354, 398, 416, 443, 446, 451, 453-454
  Arrhythmias (either tachycardia or bradycardia), 433, 436
  Glycosides, 45, 81, 96, 98, 105, 126, 195, 196, 205, 207, 208, 226, 292, 297, 298, 299, 335, 408, 409, 410, 411, 413, 414, 416, 475, 476, 477, 479, 480, 490, 492, 610
    Treatment with, 433, 436
  Insufficiency, 118, 142, 162, 175, 313, 334, 347, 375, 394, 397, 401, 413, 415, 419, 423, 433, 436-437, 451, 453-454
  Preparations, 25
  Symptoms, 101, 143, 239, 367, 408, 413, 415, 419, 423
cardiotonic, 26
cardiovascular, 26
  disorder, 21, 24
Cardui mariae
  fructus, 43, 56, **169,** 508, 531, 536, 553, **563-565,** 599, 608
  herba, 43, **350,** 508, 531, 536, 599, 608
Cardui marianum, 43
Carduus marianus, 43, **563-565**
Carex arenaria, **373,** 512, 519, 536
Carica papaya, **360-361,** 510, 519, 536, 544
Caricaceae, 360-361, 510, 519, 536, 544
Caricae
  fructus, **330,** 505, 510, 519, 523, 536, 596, 600
  papayae folium, **361,** 510, 519, 536, 600
Caricis rhizoma, **373,** 512, 519, 536, 602
Carminative, 161, 171, 181, 182, 245, 249, 261, 263, 272, 278, 280-290, 339, 460, 464, 623
Carnosol, 492
Carotenoids, 100, 492
Carum carvi, **102,** 501, 519, 536, 614
Carvacrol, 220, 492

Carvi
  aetheroleum, **102,** 501, 519, 536, 594, 606-610
  fructus, **102,** 501, 519, 536, 594, 605-606, 608, 610, 614
d-Carvone, 102, 492
Carvone, 121, 490, 492
Caryophyllaceae, 209-210, 371, 377, 512-513, 515, 524, 530, 541, 547
Caryophyllene, 155, 492, 562
Caryophylli flos, **112,** 503, 523, 525, 531, 536, 595
Cascara Sagrada, 12, 47, 49
  bark, 49, 73, **104,** 425, 435, 436, 437, 440, 441, 445, 446, 447, 448, 449, 467, 475, 479, 480, 483, 490, 491, 492, 494, 496, 502, 523, 529, 546, 595, 614
Cascaroside A, 105, 489, 492
Cassia
  acutifolia, **204, 206,** 512, 519, 547, 575, **577-579**
  angustifolia, **204, 206,** 512, 519, 547, 575, **579-581,** 615
  senna, **204, 206,** 512, 519, 547, **575-579,** 579, 614, 616
Castanea
  sativa, **321,** 502, 520, 536
  vesca, **321,** 502, 520, 536
  vulgaris, **321,** 502, 520, 536
Castaneae folium, **321,** 502, 520, 536, 595
Castin, 492
Cat's
  Claw, 12
  Ear flower, **319,** 502, 518, 534
  Foot flower, 36, 76, **319,** 502, 518, 534, 595
Catapol, 186, 492
Catarrh, Upper Respiratory Tract, 51, 129, 241, 275, 294, 399, 421, 423-424, 430
Catechin derivatives, 231, 492
Catechins, 142, 492
Cayenne (Paprika) species low in capsaicin, **178,** 502, 510, 519, 536, 600
Cayenne (Paprika), 12, 74, 178, 238, 401, 405, 502, 510, 519, 536
Celandine
  Greater, 25-26
  herb, 26, 73, 75, 76, **105, 271-272, 301-302,** 422, 426, 427, 431, 436, 437, 438, 439, 447, 463, 465, 466, 467, 469, 491-492, 502, 520, 537, 595, 607, 610
Celery, 35, 502, 518, 534
  herb, 76, **320,** 453, 456, 473, 474, 494, 502, 518, 534, 595

root, 76, **320**, 453, 473, 474, 494, 502, 518, 534
seed, **320**, 453, 473, 474, 502, 518, 534
Cellulose, 132, 487, 492
Centaurea cyanus, **325**, 503, 520, 538, 595
Centaurii herba, **106**, 502, 520, 522, 523, 536, 537, 595
Centaurium
minus, **106**, 502, 520, 536
umbellatum, **106**, 502, 520, 537
Centaury herb, 73, **106**, 422, 425, 466, 502, 520, 523, 536, 537, 595
Central Nervous System
disorders, 24
excitation, 452, 454
paralysis, 349, 367, 472-473
sensitivity, 452, 454
stimulant, 460, 465, 473, 618
central paralyzing and curare-like effect, 35
Cerebral circulation, impaired, 434, 436
Cetraria islandica, **151**, 507, 520, 542, 614
Ceylon Citronella grass, **341**, 502, 522, 538
Chamaemelum nobile, **320**, 502, 520, 537
Chamomile, 25, 53, 60
flowers, 26
German, viii, 42, 60, 73, 76, **107**, **273**, **274**, **285**, 321, 422, 427, 428, 429, 430, 431, 437, 439, 441, 442, 462, 463, 465, 467, 468, 469, 491, 493, 495, 502, 520, 526, 543, **573-575**, 595, 606, 608
Roman, 35, 77, **320-321**, 453, 456, 502, 518, 520, 537, 595
Chamomilla recutita, **107**, 401, 403, 502, 520, 543, **573-575**, 615
Chamomillae romanae flos, **320**, 502, 518, 520, 537, 595
Chaste Tree
fruit, 48, 73, **108**, 429, 430, 437, 441, 448, 465, 468, 475, 480, 489, 494, 498, 502, 534, 595
(Vitex), 25-26
Chelidonii herba, **105**, 502, 520, 537, 595, 607, 610
Chelidonine, 105-106, 492
Chelidonium majus, 105, 398, 403, 502, 520, 537
Chenopodiaceae, 513, 531, 548
Chestnut leaf, 77, **321-322**, 502, 506, 517, 520, 536, 542, 595
Chicory, 73, **109**, 422, 425, 435, 438, 446, 465, 487, 491, 495, 496, 502, 520, 537, 595
Children/Infants, 45, 128, 236, 251, 433, 436, 439
Chills, 172, 328, 365, 368, 392, 443, 446, 452, 454

Chinarinde, **109**, 502, 520, 537
Chinesischer Zimt, **111**, 503, 520, 537
Chlorogenic acid, 83, 489, 492
Cholagogue, 82, 103, 136, 171, 182, 460, 465, 623
Cholecystokinetic, 142, 222, 302, 358, 460, 465, 472, 473, 623
Cholelithiasis, 194, 321, 358, 398, 406, 420, 424, 623
Cholestatic Liver Disorders, 45, 161, 273, 274, 275, 434, 436-437
Cholesterol Lowering, 459, 465
Choloretic, 460, 465
Cholostatic Icterus/Jaundice, 313
Chronotropic
Negatively, 459, 465, 471, 473
Positively, 202, 459, 465
Chrysanthemi vulgaris
flos, **379**, 514, 520, 531, 532, 537
herba, **379**, 514, 520, 532, 537, 603
Chrysanthemum vulgare, **379**, 514, 520, 537
Chrysophanol, 47, 80, 95, 96, 104, 195, 489, 492
Chymopapain A & B, 360, 492
Cichorium intybus, *Cichorium intybus*, **109**, 502, 520, 537, 595
Cimicifuga racemosa, **90**, 398, 500, 519, 536
Cimicifugae racemosae rhizoma, **90**, 500, 520, 537, 594
Cimicifugawurzelstock, **90**, 500, 520, 537
Cinchona, *Cinchona*
bark, 55, 73, **109-110**, 422, 425, 435, 441, 446, 447, 449, 450, 466, 468, 476, 479, 488, 496, 502, 520, 537, 595
pubescens, **109**, 502, 520, 537
succirubra, **109**, 502, 520, 537
Cinchonae cortex, **109**, 502, 520, 537, 595
1,6-cineol, 492
1,8-cineol, 103, 126-127, 159, 487, 489, 492
Cineol, 174, 198, 241, 388, 476, 492
Cinnamic acid, 182, 492
Cinnamomi
cassiae cortex, **111**, 503, 520, 537, 595
ceylanici cortex, **110**, 502, 520, 537, 595
flos, **322**, 502-503, 520, 537, 595
Cinnamomum
aromaticum, **111**, 322, 502-503, 520, 536-537
camphora, **101**, 501, 520, 536
cassia, **111**, 322, 502-503, 520, 537, 615
verum, **110**, 502, 503, 520, 537, 615
zeylanicum, **110**, 502, 520, 537
Cinnamon, 502, 503, 520, 537, 615
bark, Chinese, 73, **111**, 422, 423, 425,

427, 431, 435, 445, 446, 462, 463, 467, 493, 503, 520, 537, 595
    flower, 35, 77, **322**, 453, 502, 503, 520, 537, 595
Circulatory
    circulatory/cognitive, 26
    disorders, 21, 84, 101, 160, 203, 239-241, 292, 313, 316, 331, 335, 351, 356, 364, 370, 375, 379, 396-398, 401, 415-416, 419, 424
    preparations, 25
    stimulant, 459, 465
    Circulatory/vascular tonic, 459, 465
Cirrhosis of the Liver (see also Liver Disease), 434, 437
Citral
    A, 160, 492, 561-562
    B, 160, 492
Citri sinensis pericarpium, **177**, 509, 520, 537, 600
Citronella, 35, 77, **341**, 453, 456, 502, 503, 507, 522, 538
Citronellal, 160, 492, 562
Citrullus colocynthis, **323**, 503, 520, 538
Citrus
    aurantium, **89**, 313, 500, 520, 535
    sinensis, **177**, 509, 520, 537
Clammy Skin, 370, 451, 454
Claviceps purpurea, **329**, 504, 521, 547
Clavicipitaceae, 329, 504, 521, 547
clinical studies, 30, 32
Cloves, 73, **112**, 422, 426, 428, 431, 448, 462, 463, 464, 489, 493, 503, 523, 525, 531, 536, 595
Cnici benedicti herba, **92**, 500, 521, 537, 594
Cnicin, 92, 490, 492
Cnicus benedictus, **92**, 500, 521, 537
Cochlearia armoracia, **150**, 506, 521, 534
Cocklebur, 79, 503, 517, 534
Cocoa, 35, 503, 532, 536
    seed, 78, **390**, 454, 455, 473, 474, 495, 503, 532, 536, 595
Coffea
    arabica, **112**, 503, 521, 537
    canephora, **112**, 503, 521, 537
    liberica, **112**, 503, 521, 537
    spp., 503, 521, 537
Coffeae carbo, **112**, 503, 521, 537
Coffee Charcoal, 73, **112-113**, 425, 428, 431, 462, 464, 476, 483, 503, 521, 537, 595
Cola, *Cola*
    nitida, **113**, 503, 521, 537
    nut, 73, **113**, 395, 411, 427, 442, 447, 449-450, 462-463, 465-467, 476, 479-480, 492, 495, 498, 503, 521, 537, 595
    spp., **113**, 503, 521, 537
Colae semen, **113**, 503, 521, 537, 595
Colchicine, 86, 492
Colchicum autumnale, **86**, 499, 508, 521, 537, 593
Colds, 21, 51
    and flu, 20-21, 26, 51, 421, 424
    cough & cold, 24
    cough remedy, 25
    symptoms, 21, 26
Colic, 317, 335, 352, 358, 365, 368, 383, 406, 452, 454
Colitis, Ulcerative, 433, 437, 624
Collagenosis, 123, 328, 392, 433, 437, 624
Colocynth, 35, 78, 323, 474, 492, 503, 520, 538, 595
Colocynthidis fructus, **323**, 503, 520, 538, 595
Colon, Irritable (Irritable Bowel Syndrome), 420, 425
coloring agent, 57
Coltsfoot
    flower, 35, 73, 77, **324**, 455, 456, 495, 496, 503, 532, 540, 595
    herb, xii, 73, 77, **324**, 455, 456, 496, 503, 532, 540, 595
    leaf, xii, 73, 77, **114**, 423, 425, 428, 431, 440, 441, 483, 495, 496, 498, 503, 532, 540, 595
    root, xii, 73, 77, **324**, 455, 456, 503, 532, 540, 595
Comfrey, 25
    herb, 49, 73, **115**, 423, 431, 441, 463, 483, 491, 496-497, 503, 531, 548, 595
    leaf, xii, 49, 73, **115**, 423, 431, 441, 463, 483, 491, 496-497, 503, 531, 548, 595
    root, 49, **116**, 423, 429, 431, 441, 442, 463, 464, 483, 491, 495, 496, 503, 531, 548, 595
Comminuted, 57
Commiphora molmol, **173**, 509, 521, 543
Commission on Dietary Supplement Labels (CDSL), 13, 15
Commission to 109a AMG, 76, 29, 39
Component Characteristics, 52
Concurrent Edema, 433, 440
Condurangin, 117, 492
Condurango
    bark, 59, 73, **116**, 422, 466, 468, 491, 492, 503, 526, 538, 595
    cortex, **116**, 503, 526, 538, 595
Condurangorinde, **116**, 503, 526, 538

Condyloma, 168, 420, 425, 624
Confusion, 44, 61, 347, 452, 454
Constipation, 80, 96, 104, 132, 165, 190, 191, 192, 195, 205, 207, 296, 298, 314, 321, 323, 339, 352, 358, 360, 420, 425, 451, 454, 621, 624
Consumer Use of Herbs, 10
contraction of smooth muscles, 35
Contraindications, 45, 53, 433-442
Convalescence, 124, 138, 315, 348, 361, 375, 377, 392, 415, 420, 425
Convallaria majalis, **162**, 507, 521, 538
Convallariae herba, **162**, 507, 521, 538, 598, 607, 609-610
Convallatoxin, 291-292, 408, 409, 490, 492
Convulsions, 198, 317, 347, 352, 355, 396, **444**, 446, 452, 454, 626
Cor pulmonale, 162, 408, 413, 415, 419, 425, 624
Coriander seed, 73, **117**, 422, 426, 493, 503, 521, 538, 595
Coriandri fructus, **117**, 503, 521, 538, 595
Coriandrum sativum, **117**, 503, 521, 538
Corn poppy, 77, **324-325**, 503, 527, 546, 595
Cornflower, 36, 57, 77, **325**, 503, 521, 538, 595
Coronary
    artery flow, increases, 459, 465
    dilator, 357, 471, 473
Corpus luteum-like effects, 459, 465
Corynanthe yohimbi, **383**, 516, 521, 550
Couch Grass, 73, **118**, 428, 429, 432, 437, 440, 463, 493, 497, 503, 517, 541, 596
Cough, 24, 25, 48, 51, 114, 131, 151, 152, 164, 165, 166, 167, 185, 218, 219, 239-241, 252, 254, 256, 257, 259, 267, 275, 276, 277, 294, 295, 300, 312, 319, 322, 324, 335, 340, 349, 359, 372, 377, 380, 388, 390, 399, 401, 406, 421, 425, 432, 434, 442, 476, 620, 622, 640
o-coumaric acid, 218, 492
Coumarin, 35, 81, 83, 161, 218, 219, 488, 492
    derivatives, 81, 124, 163, 180, 492
Cramps, 46, 97, 99, 149, 218, 239-240, 329, 352, 367, 420, 421, 429, 430, 444, 446, 451, 454
Cranberry, 11, 12
Crataegi
    extractum fluidum, **553-554**
    flos, **333**, 506, 521, 538, 597
    folium, **334**, 506, 521, 538, 597
        cum flore, 56, **142**, 506, 521, 538, 553, **555-557**, 597
    fructus, 56, **333**, 506, 521, 538, 553, 597

Crataegus
    laevigata, **142**, **333-334**, 506, 521, 538, **555-557**
    monogyna, 63, **142**, **333-334**, 506, 521, 538, **555-557**
Croci stigma, **371**, 512, 521, 537, 602
Crocus sativa, **371**, 512, 521, 538
Crohn's Disease, 80, 96, 97, 104, 195, 205, 207, 297, 298, 434, 437, 624
cross-sensitivities, 45
Cryptococcaeae, 516, 519, 540
Cryptopine, 389, 492
Cucurbita pepo, **193**, 511, 521, 538
Cucurbitaceae, 193, 316, 323, 501, 503, 508, 511, 513, 519, 520, 521, 525, 536, 538, 542
Cucurbitacin, 323, 492
Cucurbitae peponis semen, **193**, 511, 521, 538
Cucurbitin, 492
Cupressaceae, 155, 507, 525, 542
Curaçao aloe, **80**, 503, 517, 534
Curaçao-Aloe, **503**, 517, 534
Curcuma
    aromatica, **222**, 514, 521, 538
    domestica, **222**, 514, 521, 538
    longa, **222**, 514, 521, 538, 616
    xanthorrhiza, **222-223**, 514, 521, 538
    zedoaria, **383**, 516, 521, 550
Curcumae
    longae rhizoma, **222**, 514, 521, 538, 604, 610
    xanthorrhizae rhizoma, **222**, 514, 521, 538, 604, 610
Curcumawurzelstock, **222**, 514, 521, 538
Curcumin, 222, 492
Cyani flos, **325**, 503, 520, 538
Cymbopoginis
    citrati
        aetheroleum, **341**, 515, 522, 538
        herba, **341**, 515, 522, 538
    nardi herba, **341**, 502, 522, 538
    winteriani aetheroleum, **341**, 507, 522, 538
Cymbopogon
    citratus, **341**, 503, 515, 522, 538
    nardus, **341**, 502-503, 522, 538
    spp., **341**, 503, 515, 522, 538
    winterianus, 503, 507, 522, 538
Cymbopogon-Arten, **341**, 502, 503, 507, 515, 522, 538
Cynara scolymus, **84**, 499, 522, 538
Cynarae folium, **84**, 499, 522, 538, 593, 607
Cynarin, 83, 84, 493
Cynoglossi herba, **338**, 506, 522, 539, 598

Cynoglossum
   clandestinum, **338**, 506, 522, 538
   officinale, **338**, 506, 522, 539
Cyperaceae, 373, 512, 519, 536
Cytisi
   scoparii
      flos, **373**, 512, 522, 530, 539, 602
      herba, **203**, 512, 522, 539, 602-603
   scoparius
      flos, 501, 522, 530, 539
      herba, 501, 522, 530, 538, 539
Cytisus scoparius, **203**, **373**, 501, 512, 522, 539
Cytostatic, 106, 172, 392, 461, 465, 625
Cytotoxic, 209, 210, 317, 347, 460, 465
DAB, 55
Damiana
   herb, 36, 77, **325-326**, 504, 532, 549, 596
   leaf, 36, 77, **325-326**, 504, 532, 549, 596
Damianablätter, **325**, 504, 532, 549
Damianakraut, **325**, 504, 532, 549
Dandelion
   herb, 50, 73, 75, **118-119**, 422, 423, 426, 435, 437, 438, 439, 491, 497, 504, 532, 548, 596
   root with herb, 73, 75, **119-120**, 264-266, 422, 425, 426, 427, 435, 436, 437, 438, 439, 447, 464, 465, 466, 469, 491, 495, 496, 498, 504, 532, 548, 596, 607
Datura stramonium, **340**, 507, 522, 548
Deadly Nightshade, 43, **87**, 504, 518, 535
Debility, 124, 138, 383, 420, 425, 633
Delphinii flos, **326**, 504, 522, 539, 596
Delphinium, *Delphinium*
   consolida, **326**, 504, 522, 539
   flower, 35, 57, 77, **326**, 399, 455, 491, 504, 522, 539, 596
Demulcent, 164, 165, 461, 465, 625
Deodorant, 107, 240, 459, 465
Dependency, 125, 340, 444, 447
Depigmentation of skin, 348, 451, 454
Depression, xxi, 11, 19, 26, 69, 152, 156, 339, 351, 353, 355, 361, 396, 401, 406, 413, 416, 420, 425, 434, 437, 618, 626, 633, 636
depside ellagitannins, 493
Dermatitis (see Allergic Skin Reactions), 83, 311, 370,443, 447, 451, 454
dermatological, 25
Deutsche Gessellschaft für Phytotherapie, 31
Deutsches Arzneibuch (DAB), 55, 553-566
Devil's claw root, 73, **120**, 422, 426, 429, 438, 442, 462, 463, 464, 465, 491, 504, 524, 541, 596, 613

Diabetes Mellitus, 191, 192, 297, 311, 332, 376, 433, 437, 625
Diaphoresis/Diaphoretic, 124, 163, 230, 259, 308, 315-316, 318, 324, 328, 335, 342-343, 349, 359, 366, 372-373, 377, 379, 381, 390, 465, 625
Diarrhea, 35, 46, 49, 55, 79, 86, 88, 91, 94, 113, 127, 154, 158, 174, 175, 176, 188, 191, 192, 212, 214, 221, 226, 235-236, 255, 260, 267, 268, 293, 310, 315, 317, 323, 324, 329, 332, 335, 347, 349, 352, 354, 365, 367, 369, 371, 378, 390, 420, 425, 444, 447, 451, 454, 483, 484, 625
dicinnamoylmethane derivatives, 222, 223, 493
Dietary Supplement Health and Education Act of 1994 (DSHEA), 12
dietary supplements, 12
Digestive
   or intestinal complaints, 21, 50
   or intestinal upset, 20-21
digitalis glycosides, treatment with, 63, 433, 437
dihydrohelenalin, 83, 493
Dihydrosamidine, 493
1,8-dihydroxyanthracene derivatives, 97, 141, 493
Dill
   herb, 36, 73, 77, **327**, 504, 518, 534, 596
   seed, 36, 73, **121**, 426, 462, 463, 492, 493, 504, 518, 534, 596
   weed, 36
Dillfrüchte, **121**, 504, 518, 534
Dillkraut, **327**, 504, 518, 534
Diseases of
   digestive organs, 20
   heart and circulation, 20
   locomotor apparatus, 20
   respiratory tract, 20
   urogenital tract, 20
   (see also Use Index, 419-432)
Dislocations, bone, 370, 421, 425
Diterpenes, 493
Diuresis, 120, 293, 316, 372, 452, 454, 625
Diuretic, 19, 45, 58, 85, 89, 100, 114, 120, 140, 151, 155, 157, 168, 213, 260, 303, 307, 308, 309, 311, 315, 317, 318, 320, 323 324, 325, 326, 332, 335, 336, 337, 342, 348, 349, 357, 359, 361, 365, 366, 368, 369, 370, 372, 373, 377, 378, 390, 408, 415, 421, 425, 461, 466, 472, 473, 625, 630, 631, 639
Diverticulitis, 132, 420, 425
Dizziness, 137, 317, 319, 347, 351, 370-371, 375, 382, 394, 397, 402, 406, 413, 415, 452, 454, 632, 640

Dong quai, 12
Dosierung, 48
Dostenkraut, **358**, 510, 526, 543
droge, 57
Drogerien, 22
Dromotropic, Positively, 460, 466
Drosera
    intermedia, **217**, 514, 522, 539
    longifolia, **217**, 514, 522, 539
    ramentacea, **217**, 514, 522, 539
    rotundifolia, **217**, 514, 522, 539
Droseraceae, 218, 514, 522, 539
Droserae herba, **217-218**, 514, 522, 539, 603, 606, 610
Drug vs. Herb, 57
Dry Mouth, 404, 407, 444, 447
Dryopteris filix-mas, **346**, 508, 522, 540
Dulcamarae stipites, **232**, 516, 531, 539, 604
Duration of Administration, 49, 54
Dysmenorrhea, 90, 348, 392, 420, 625
Dyspepsia, 92, 93, 103, 109, 119, 121, 133, 136, 141, 148, 155, 233, 315, 321, 332, 398, 406, 420, 425-426, 626
Dyspnea, 142, 143, 144, 310, 347, 452, 454, 626
Dysuria, 20, 421, 426, 626
EAPC, 62
Ebereschenbeeren, **352**, 509, 531, 548
Echinacea, *Echinacea*, 12, 25, 26, 61
    Angustifolia, *angustifolia*
        herb, 36, 39, 77, **327**, 393, 412, 453, 454, 456, 504, 522, 539, 596
        root, 36, 39, 61, 77, **327**, 393, 412, 453, 454, 456, 504, 522, 539, 596
    Pallida, *pallida*
        herb, 36, 39, 61, 73, 77, 121, **327-328**, 453, 454, 456, 504, 522, 539, 596
        root, 61, 73, 77, **121**, 424, 428, 435, 437, 438, 440, 441, 442, 468, 483, 504, 522, 539, 596
    Purpurea, *purpurea*
        herb, 41, 42, 45, 61, 73, 78, **122-123**, 328, 424, 428, 430, 432, 435, 437, 440, 441, 442, 446, 447, 449, 450, 466, 468, 469, 483, 504, 511, 522, 539, 596
        leaf, 44
        root, 26, 41-42, 52, 61, 73, 78, **391-392**, 456, 504, 523, 539, 596
Echinaceae
    angustifoliae
        herba, **327**, 504, 522, 539, 596
        radix, **327**, 504, 522, 539, 596
    pallidae
        herba, **327**, 504, 522, 539, 596
        radix, **121**, 327, 504, 522, 539, 596
    purpureae
        herba, **122**, 504, 511, 523, 539, 596
        radix, **391**, 504, 511, 523, 539, 596
Echinacea-pallida-Wurzel, **121**, 504, 522, 539
Echtes Goldrutenkraut, 505, 531, 548
Eczema, 83, 101, 175, 232, 240, 260, 318, 337, 375, 394, 419, 426, 443, 447, 626
Edelkastanienblätter, 502, 520, 536
Edema, 433, 434, 437, 443, 447
    Post-traumatic, 421, 426
Editor's Notes, 60
EEC, 56
Efeublätter, **153**, 507, 524, 541
Efficacy-constituent relationship, 19
Ehrenpreiskraut, **380**, 513, 515, 533, 550
Eibischblätter, **166**, 508, 517, 534
Eibischwurzel, **167**, 508, 517, 534
Eichenrinde, **175**, 509, 529, 546
Eisenkraut, **380**, 514, 533, 550
Elder flower, 27, 73, **124**, 411, 424, 464, 465, 504, 530, 547, 596
Elecampane, 35, 44, 77, **328**, 390, 401, 411, 453, 454, 455, 456, 490, 491, 493, 497, 504, 525, 541, 596
Electrolyte Imbalance, 81, 105, 196, 206, 208, 443, 447
Electrolyte-like Reaction on Capillary Wall, 461, 466
Elemene, 155, 493
Elettaria cardamomum, **103**, 501, 523, 536
Eleuthero root, 61, 73, **124**, 391, 425, 427, 429, 432, 439, 466, 467, 492, 495, 504, 516, 522, 539, 596
Eleutherococci radix, **124**, 504, 513, 523, 539, 596
Eleutherococcus senticosus, 61, 68, **124**, 504, 513, 523, 539
Eleutherococcus-senticosus-Wurzel, **124**, 504, 513, 516, 523, 539
Ellagitannin, 231, 493
Emetic, 316-317, 349, 377, 420, 427, 471, 474, 626
Emodin, 47, 80, 96-97, 104, 195, 204-207, 489, 493
Emodin-physcion, 95, 493
Endurance, Increased, 125, 459, 466
English plantain, 504, 510, 511, 528, 544
Enzianwurzel, 135, 505, 524, 541
Ephedra
    shennungiana, **125**, 504, 523, 539
    sinica, **125**, 504, 523, 539, 616

Ephedraceae, 125, 504, 523, 539
Ephedrae herba, **125**, 504, 523, 539, 596
Ephedrakraut, **125**, 504, 523, 539
Ephedrine, 125-126, 399, 414, 476, 487, 493
Epicatechins, 142, 493
(-)-Epicatechol, 493
epidemiological studies, 30
Equisetaceae, 150, 506, 523, 539
Equiseti herba, **150**, 506, 523, 539, 598
Equisetum arvense, **150**, 506, 523, 539
Erdbeerblätter, **378**, 514, 523, 540
Erdrauchkraut, **133**, 505, 524, 540
Ergot, 35, 77, 329, 394, 488, 491, 504, 521, 547, 596
Ericaceae, 88, 224, 311, 335, 367, 500, 506, 519, 529, 533, 536, 543, 546
Ericaeae, 515, 518, 549
Erythraea centaurium, **106**, 502, 523, 537
Esche, **308**, 499, 523, 540
Eschscholzia californica, **389**, 501, 523, 540, 594
Eschscholziae, 389, 501, 523, 540
Escin, 17, 148-149, 493, 558
ESCOP, 18, 64-65, 613-614
Esophageal stenosis, 434, 437
Essential oil, 35, 43, 44, 47, 48, 51, 52, 81, 83, 89, 94, 102, 103, 107, 110, 111, 112, 117, 118, 121, 126, 128, 129, 130, 131, 133, 134, 136, 140, 147, 154, 155, 156, 159, 160, 163, 164, 169, 171, 174, 177, 179, 180, 181, 182, 184, 185, 188, 193, 197, 198, 199, 213, 215, 216, 220, 223, 226, 231, 233, 237, 238, 246, 249, 250, 251, 252, 253, 258, 261, 262, 263, 264, 267, 276, 281, 283, 284, 285, 286, 287, 288, 289, 290, 311, 317, 328, 338, 341, 347, 349, 354, 362-363, 379, 387, 493, 573, 581, 582, 627
Esters, 132, 170, 181, 182, 221, 303, 491, 492, 493, 495
Estragole, 35, 311, 388, 489, 493
Estragon, 128-129, 493
Estrogen Receptor Site Binding, 459, 466, 627
Eucalypti
    aetheroleum, **127**, 504, 523, 540, 596, 606, 607
    folium, **126**, 504, 523, 540, 596
Eucalyptus, *Eucalyptus*
    fructicetorum, **127**, 504, 523, 540
    globulus, **126-127**, 504, 523, 540
    leaf, 47, 51, 73, 75, **126-127**, 390, 405, 423, 424, 429, 430, 435, 436, 438, 439, 440, 447, 448, 449, 450, 463, 466, 468, 469, 476, 478, 492, 493, 498, 504, 523, 540, 596
    oil, 47, 51, 73, 75, **126-128**, 237, 238, 239, **254**, **255**, **260**, **267**, **268**, 387, **405**, 423, 424, 429, 430, 435, 436, 438, 439, 440, 441, 442, 445, 446, 447, 448, 449, 450, 463, 466, 468, 469, 476, 477, 478, 492, 504, 523, 540, 596, 606, 607
    polybractea, **127**, 504, 523, 540
    smithii, **127**, 504, 523, 540
Eucalyptusblätter, **126**, 504, 523, 540
Eucalyptusöl, **127**, 504, 523, 540
Eugenia caryophyllata, **112**, 503, 523, 536
Eupatorin, 154, 493
Euphrasia officinalis, **329**, 505, 523, 540, 596
Euphrasiae herba, **329**, 505, 523, 540
European Economic Community (EEC), 17, 56
European Pharmacopoeia, 18, 56
European Scientific Cooperative on Phytotherapy (see ESCOP)
European-American Phytomedicine Coalition (EAPC), 14, 62
Evaluation, 50, 58
Evaluation Criteria for Fixed Combinations, 51
Evaluation Methods and Criteria, 29
Evening Primrose oil, 11
Exanthemas, Urticarial, 433, 437
exhaustion, 21
Expectorant, 83, 127, 128, 153, 162, 173, 189, 190, 204, 209, 216, 220, 239, 251, 252, 253, 254, 255, 257, 259, 260, 267, 268, 270, 271, 276, 277, 278, 294, 295, 296, 300, 301, 316, 325, 338, 342, 358, 377, 390, 398, 399, 406, 461, 466, 627
Experimental, pharmacological, and toxicological studies, 30
Eye Irritation, 310, 452, 454
Eyebright herb, 36, 77, **329-330**, 393, 396, 505, 523, 540
Fabaceae, 130, 157, 161, 182, 204, 206, 210, 211, 213, 218, 221, 332, 372, 501, 505, 507, 510, 512, 513, 514, 519, 522, 524, 526, 527, 529, 530, 531, 532, 535, 539, 540, 541, 542, 543, 544, 547, 575, 577, 579
facial neuralgia, 57
Faex medicinalis, 234, 501, 516, 519, 530, 540
Fagaceae, 175, 322, 502, 509, 520, 529, 536, 546
Fainting, 370, 452, 454
Familial Mediterranean fever, 86, 420, 427, 627
Farfarae
    flos, **324**, 503, 532, 540, 595
    folium, **114**, 503, 532, 540, 595
    herba, **324**, 503, 532, 540, 595
    radix, **324**, 503, 532, 540, 595

Fatigue, 21, 113, 124, 138, 144, 152, 168, 337, 356, 377, 388, 392, 394, 420, 427, 623, 633
Fatty oil, 83, 132, 201, 238, 358, 362, 493, 563
Faulbaumrinde, **95**, 104, 501, 502, 505, 523, 529, 540, 546
FDA, 14
Federal Association of Pharmaceutical Manufacturers, 31
Federal Association of the Pharmaceutical Industry, 31
Federal Health Agency, 27
Federal Institute for Drugs and Medical Devices, 27
Feigen, **330**, 504, 523, 536
Fenchel, **129**, 505, 523, 540
Fenchelöl, **128**, 505, 523, 540
Fenchone, 128, 129, 493
Fennel
  oil, 45, 73, 75, 76, **128-129**, 238, **246**, **250**, **251**, **258**, **261**, **262**, **263**, **276**, **277**, **287**, **288**, **289**, **290**, 387, 400, 422, 423, 424, 426, 427, 436, 438, 441, 442, 445-449, 462-465, 467, 477, 483, 491, 493, 505, 523, 540, 596, 605, 606, 607, 608, 609
  seed, 50, 59, 73, 75-76, **128-129**, **253**, **254**, **258**, **262-264**, **276-277**, **280-281**, **283-285**, 390, 393, 396, **411**, 422, 423, 424, 426-427, 436-442, 445-449, 462-465, 467, 477-478, 484, 491, 493, 505, 523, 540, 596, 605, 606, 607, 608, 610, 613
Fenugreek seed, 73, **130**, 422, 446, 463, 466, 468, 505, 532, 540, 596
Fever, 420, 427, 447, 452, 454
  fever/hyperthermia, 444
Feverfew, 12
Fiber, 132, 237, 344, 493, 626
Fibrinolytic activity, increases, 460, 466
Ficthennadelöl, **130**, 505, 515-516, 527, 544
Ficus carica, **330**, 505, 523, 536
Figs, 36, 77, **330**, 505, 523, 536, 596
Filicis maris
  folium, **346**, 508, 522, 540, 599
  herba, **346**, 508, 522, 540, 599
  rhizoma, **346**, 508, 522, 540, 599
Filipendula ulmaria, *Filipendula ulmaria*, **169**, 508, 523, 531, 540, 599
Fir
  Needle oil, 73, **130**, 238, 239, 424, 429, 430, 435, 442, 446, 448, 449, 463, 466, 468, 505, 516, 527, 544, 596
  Shoots, Fresh, 73, **131**, 424, 430, 463, 466, 468, 493, 505, 516, 544, 596

Fixed Combinations, 50-51, 245-305, 403-416
Flatulence, 82, 102, 110-111, 119, 128-129, 135, 148, 165, 171, 234-235, 239-240, 245-250, 258, 261-264, 269, 280-290, 311, 348, 354, 358, 360, 382, 388, 399, 420, 427, 444, 447, 623, 627
Flavanone derivatives, 161, 493
Flavone derivatives, 107, 493
Flavones, 136, 142, 154, 198, 233, 488, 493
Flavonoid glycosides, 88, 133, 155, 198, 494
Flavonoids, 19, 39, 55, 63, 79, 83, 89, 93, 98, 133, 137, 139, 142, 143, 145, 150, 157, 158, 160, 161, 163, 169, 177, 180, 184, 188, 199, 213, 218, 231, 488, 494, 553, 554, 555, 557
Flavonols, 142, 488, 494
Flavor Corrigent, 58
Flaxseed, 47, 73, **132**, 425, 439, 467, 476, 487, 491, 492, 493, 494, 495, 505, 525, 542, 596
Flohsamen, **190**, 511, 528, 545
Flu, 20-21, 51
Flushed Face, 452, 454
Flüssigkeitszufuhr, 58
Foeniculi
  aetheroleum, **128**, 505, 523, 540, 596, 605, 606, 607, 608, 609
  fructus, **129**, 505, 523, 540, 596, 605, 606, 607, 608, 610, 613
Foeniculum vulgare, **128-129**, 505, 523, 540, 613
Foenugraeci semen, **130**, 505, 532, 540, 596
Foxglove leaf (*Digitalis purpurea*), 22
Fragaria
  vesca, **378**, 514, 523, 540
  viridis, **378**, 514, 523, 540
Fragariae folium, **378**, 514, 523, 540, 603
Frangula, *Frangula*, 397, 501, 502, 505, 523, 529, 540, 546, 614
  alnus, **95**, 501, 505, 523, 540
  purshiana, **104**, 502, 523, 529, 546
Frangulae cortex, **95**, 501, 505, 523, 529, 540, 594, 614
Frauenmantelkraut, **158**, 307, 499, 507, 517, 534
Fraxini
  cortex, **308**, 499, 523, 540
  folium, **308**, 499, 523, 540
Fraxinus
  excelsior, **308**, 499, 523, 540, 593
  ornus, **165**, 508, 523, 543
Free radical deactivation, 420, 427
French Pharmacopeia, 63
Frische Fichtenspitzen, **131**, 505, 516, 544
Frostbite, 188, 240, 241, 319, 321, 339, 347, 351, 419, 427, 628
Fucaceae, 315, 500, 518, 523, 540
Fuchskreuzkraut, **376**, 512, 531, 547

Fucus, 315, 500, 518, 523, 540, 594
Fucus vesiculosus, **315**, 500, 523, 540
Fumaria officinalis, **133**, 505, 524, 540
Fumariaceae, 133, 505, 524, 540
Fumariae herba, **133**, 505, 524, 540, 597
Fumitory, 73, **133**, 423, 427, 431, 463, 494, 495, 505, 524, 540, 597
Furanocoumarins, 36, 82, 282, 370, 488, 494
Furunculosis, 83, 234, 240, 419, 427, 628
Galangae rhizoma, **133**, 505, 517, 540, 597
Galangal, 73, **133**, 422, 426, 462, 463, 464, 493-494, 496, 505, 517, 540, 597
Galangtwurzelstock, **133**, 505, 517, 540
Galega officinalis, **332**, 505, 524, 540
Galegae officinalis herba, **332**, 505, 524, 540, 597
Galegin, 35, 332, 494
Galeopsidis herba, **145**, 506, 524, 541, 597
Galeopsis
    ochroleuca, **145**, 506, 524, 541
    segetum, **145**, 506, 524, 541
Galii odorati herba, **378**, 514, 524, 541, 603
Galium odoratum, **378**, 514, 524, 541
Gallbladder
    disorders, 21, 45, 171, 313-314, 331, 335, 369, 379, 380, 399, 416, 420, 434
    empyema, 120, 141, 265, 434, 437
    inflammation, 171, 181, 249, 282, 434, 437-438, 623, 628
Gallic acid, 188, 231, 488, 494, 572
Gallotannins, 231, 488-489, 494
Gallstones, 45, 84, 93, 103, 109, 119, 120, 136, 141, 180, 181, 200, 222, 223, 249, 265, 271, 272, 274, 278, 287, 298, 302, 344, 348, 358, 368, 369, 375, 392, 434, 438, 623
Gänsefingerkraut, **188**, 511, 513, 528, 545
Gargle/Mouthwash, 420, 427
Garlic, 11, 12, 13, 26, 32, 73, **134**, 238, 388, 395, 397, 427, 428, 446, 447, 448, 462, 463, 466, 467, 468, 491, 493, 505, 517, 534, 597, 614, 616
Gastric
    discomforts, 21
    irritation, 36, 64
    juices, stimulates, 460, 466
    mucosa, inflammation of, 420, 427
    ulcers, accelerate healing of, 460, 466
Gastroenteritis, 379, 401, 404, 406, 451, 454, 628
Gastrointestinal
    agent, 25
    disorders, 46, 80, 96, 171, 195, 205, 207, 240, 243, 257, 274, 298, 314, 317, 319, 327, 335, 348, 350, 351, 355, 358, 379, 382, 399, 420, 427, 432, 434
    disturbance, 46, 202, 205, 207, **444**, 447-448, 451, 454
    inflammation, 82, 107, 171, 181, 245, 249, 321, 366, 381, 420, 428, 432, 433, 434, 438, 628
    stenosis, 146, 202, 433-434, 438
    tract
        disturbance with nausea, 451, 454
        irritation, 349, 363, 381, 451, 454
Geißrautenkraut, **332**, 505, 524, 541
Gelsemii rhizoma, **400**, 516, 524, 541, 605
Gelsemium sempervirens, **400**, 403
Gelsemiumwurzelstock, **400**, 516, 524, 541
Gentian root, 27, 50, 73, 75, **135**, **245**, **246**, **247**, **248**, **249**, **269**, 422, 423, 426, 427, 431, 435, 437, 438, 440, 441, 442, 445, 446, 447, 448, 449, 464, 466, 468, 469, 491, 494, 505, 524, 541, 597, 605, 607, 614
Gentiana lutea, **135**, 505, 524, 541, 614
Gentianaceae, 106, 135, 502, 505, 520, 523, 524, 536, 537, 541
Gentianae radix, **135**, 505, 524, 541, 597, 605, 607, 614
Gentiobiose, 135, 494
Gentiopicroside, 135, 494
Gereinigtes Terpentinöl, **223**, 514, 527, 548
Geriatric vascular changes, 419, 427
German *Federal Gazette*, 60
German *Pharmacopoeia* (*DAB*), 37, 55, 59
German Society of Phytotherapy, 31
Geschmackskorrigenz, 58
Gesichtsneuralgie, 57
Gewürznelken, **112**, 503, 523, 525, 531, 536
gingerol, 62
Ginger root, 12, 26, 62, 73, 75, **135**, **269**, 422, 426, 429, 432, 438, 442, 462, 464, 465, 466, 467, 468, 469, 493, 495, 496, 505, 533, 550, 597, 607, 613
Ginkgo, *Ginkgo*, 11, 12, 26, 32, 62-63
    Biloba, *biloba*
        Blätter, **136**, 505, 524, 541
        extract, 62
        leaf, 36, 39, **331**, 505, 524, 541, 597
        Leaf Extract, 25, 36, 37, 44, 49, 62, 73, **136**, 422, 424, 425, 427, 429, 430, 432, 435, 446, 447, 448, 484, 491, 493, 494, 495, 496, 498, 505, 524, 541, 597
    flavonglycosides, 37
    folium, **136**, 331, 505, 524, 541, 597
Ginkgoaceae, 136, 505, 524, 541

Ginkgoblätter, **331**, 505, 524, 541
Ginkgolic acids, 37, 63, 136, 331, 494
Ginkgolides, 37, 136-137, 494
Ginseng, 11, 12, 26
    radix, **138**, 505, 516, 527, 541, 597
        root, 49, 61, 74, **138**, 425, 427, 429, 432, 466, 467, 469, 484, 492, 494, 505, 513, 527, 541, 597
Ginseng, Siberian (see Eleuthero)
Ginsengwurzel, **138**, 505, 527, 541
Ginsenosides, 138, 490, 494
Glaucoma, 87, 125, 146, 202, 404, 407, 434, 438, 444, 448, 628
Glockenbilsenkraut Wurzelstock, **202**, 512, 531, 547
Glucans, 234, 494
Glucofrangulin A, 98, 494
Glycine, *Glycine*
    antagonist, 471, 474
    max, 210-211, 513, 524, 542, 544
Glycogenolytic, 168, 460, 466, 628
Glycosides, 45, 47, 51, 64, 78, 80, 81, 88, 90, 96, 97, 98, 100, 104, 105, 126, 133, 136, 139, 148, 150, 152, 155, 161, 162, 169, 172, 184, 186, 188, 193, 195, 196, 198, 205, 207, 208, 214, 217, 226, 228, 229, 251, 254, 255, 256, 271, 273, 274, 275, 277, 291, 292, 293, 297, 298, 299, 335, 357, 372, 408-411, 413, 414, 416, 433, 436, 437, 475, 476, 477, 478, 479, 480, 487, 490, 492, 494, 495, 496, 498, 557, 559, 560, 561, 575, 577, 579, 583, 610
Glycyrrhiza glabra, **161**, 507, 524, 542, 616
Glycyrrhizic acid, 161-162, 273-274, 387, 494
Goat's Rue herb, 35, 77, **332**, 455, 494, 505, 524, 541, 597
Goldenrod, **139-140**, 259, 505, 531, 548
    European, 19, 139, 374, 505, 531, 548
Goldenseal, 12
Goldrute, **139**, 505, 531, 548
Gout, 86, 240, 308, 311, 314, 318, 319, 320, 335, 351, 364, 367, 369, 373, 378, 380, 381, 396, 406, 421, 427, 483, 628, 639
Graminis
    flos, **144**, 506, 517, 528, 541, 597
    rhizoma, **118**, 503, 528, 541, 596
Granulatory, 100, 459, 466, 628
Grapeseed extract, 11-12
Grayanotoxine, 36, 367, 494
Grindelia
    robusta, **140**, 505, 524, 541
    squarrosa, **140**, 505, 524, 541
Grindeliae herba, **140**, 505, 524, 541, 597, 607
Grindeliakraut, **140**, 505, 524, 541

Guaiac wood, 74, **140**, 393, 411, 430, 494, 497, 505, 524, 541, 597
Guaiaci lignum, **140**, 505, 524, 541
Guaiacum
    officinale, **140**, 505, 524, 541
    sanctum, **140**, 505, 524, 541
Guaiazulene, 242, 387, 415, 494, 562, 574-575
Guaiene, 494
Guajakholz, **140**, 505, 524, 541
Guidelines for the Assessment of Herbal Medicines, (WHO), 16
Gums, inflamed, 419, 427
Gumweed herb, 74-75, **140-141**, **269-270**, 424, 447, 449, 462, 493, 505, 524, 541, 597, 607
gynecological, 25
    disorders, 24
Gypsophila
    paniculata, **210**, 513, 515, 524, 541
    spp., **210**, 513, 515, 524, 541
Gypsophilae radix, **210**, 513, 515, 524, 541, 603
Haferfrüchte, **356**, 509, 518, 535
Haferkraut, **355**, 509, 516, 518, 535
Haferstroh, **176**, 509, 518, 535
Hagebutten, **368**, 512, 530, 546
Hagebuttenkerne, **369**, 512, 530, 546
Hagebuttenschalen, **368**, 511, 529, 546
Hallucination, 87, 444, 448, 452, 454, 628
Hamamelidaceae, 231, 516, 524, 541
Hamamelidis
    cortex, **231**, 516, 524, 541, 604
    folium, 56, **231**, 516, 524, 541, 567, **571-573**, 604
Hamamelis virginiana, **231**, 403, 516, 524, 541, **571-573**, 614
Hamamelisblätter, **231**, 516, 524, 541
Hamamelisrinde, **231**, 516, 524, 541
Hamamelitannins, 494
Haronga bark and leaf, 74, **141**, 426, 430, 436, 437, 438, 439, 441, 449, 465, 467, 493, 494, 505, 524, 541, 597
Harongarinde, **141**, 505, 524, 541
Harpagophyti radix, **120**, 504, 524, 541, 596, 613
Harpagophytum procumbens, **120**, 504, 524, 541, 613
Harungana madagascariensis, **141**, 505, 524, 541
Harunganae madagascariensis cortex et folium, **141**, 505, 524, 541, 597
Harunganin, 141, 494
Hauhechelwurzel, **213**, 513, 526, 543

Hawthorn, 26, 32, 33, 39, 63
　　berry, 33, 36, 39, 42, 63, 77, **333**, 506, 521, 538, 597
　　flower, viii, xiii, xx, 20, 28, 33, 36, 39, 42, 56, 60, 63, 77, **333**, 506, 521, 538, 551, 553, 555-556, 597
　　fluidextract, **553-554**
　　leaf, 36, 77, **334**
　　leaf with flower, viii, xx, 25, 28, 33, 36, 56, 60, 63, 74, **142-144**, 333-335, 423, 427, 464, 465, 466, 467, 484, 491, 492, 493, 494, 496, 497, 498, 506, 521, 538, 551, **555-557**, 597
Hay flower, 74, **144**, 422, 432, 446, 466, 506, 528, 541, 597
Headache, Migraine, 359, 401, 452, 455
headaches, 20, 21
Heart
　　& circulation, 24
　　　　Function, disorders of, 359, 401, 443, 448
　　　　Muscle stimulant, 394, 415, 471, 474
Heart's Ease herb, 74, **145**, 374, 401, 412, 429, 431, 494, 506, 533, 550, 597
Heather
　　flower, 36, 77, **335**, 506, 519, 536, 597
　　herb, 36, 77, **335**, 506, 519, 536, 597
Hedera helix, **153**, 507, 524, 541
Hederae helicis folium, **153**, 507, 524, 541, 598, 606-607
Heidekraut, **335**, 506, 519, 536
Heidekrautblüten, **335**, 506, 519, 536
Heidelbeerblätter, **311**, 500, 533, 543
Heidelbeeren, **88**, 500, 533, 543
Helenalin, 83, 494
Helenii radix, **328**, 504, 525, 541, 596
Helichrysi flos, **199**, 512, 524, 541, 602
Helichrysum arenarium, **199**, 512, 524, 541
Hematoma, 83, 239, 240, 337, 356, 361, 420, 427, 622, 628
Hematuria, 46, 81, 96, 98, 105, 195, 205, 207, 297, 298, 371, 444, 448, 452, 455, 629
Hemicellulose, 132, 494
Hemoglobinuria, 452, 455
Hemorrhoids, 99, 165, 182, 188, 191-192, 218, 231, 239, 311, 319, 321, 337, 344, 361, 364, 379, 392, 394, 396, 398, 403, 406, 413, 420, 428, 629
Hemostatic, 231, 365, 460, 466, 629
Hempnettle herb, 74, **145**, 424, 497, 498, 506, 524, 541, 597
Henbane leaf, 22, 32, 74, **146**, 405, 431, 436, 438, 441, 442, 445, 447, 450, 462, 467, 468, 476, 479, 480, 481, 491, 494, 497, 506, 525, 542, 597

Hepatica nobilis, **344**, 508, 524, 541
Hepatici nobilis herba, **344**, 508, 524, 541, 599
Hepatitis, 212, 344, 398, 420, 428, 629
Hepatoprotection, 25, 26, 211, 460, 466, 488
Hepatotoxic, 35-36, 49, 170, 316, 324, 338, 346, 376, 452, 455, 472, 474, 487, 629
Herb supplement sales in mass market retail outlets, 11
Herb supplement sales in natural food stores, 12
Herbs of Commerce, 41
Herbstzeitlose, **86**, 499, 508, 521, 537
Herniaria
　　glabra, **371**, 512, 524, 541
　　hirsuta, **371**, 512, 524, 541
Herniariae, 512, 524, 541
　　herba, **371**, 511, 524, 541
Herzgespannkraut, **172**, 509, 525, 542
Heublumen, **144**, 506, 528, 541
Hibisci flos, **336**, 506, 525, 541, 597
Hibiscus, *Hibiscus*
　　flower, 36, 42, 77, **336**, 389, 506, 525, 541, 597
　　sabdariffa, **336**, 506, 525, 541
Hibiscusblüten, **336**, 506, 525, 541
Himbeerblätter, **336**, 511, 530, 546
Hippocastanaceae, 148, 337, 393, 506, 517, 541, 542
Hippocastani
　　cortex, **393**, 506, 517, 541, 542, 597
　　flos, **393**, 506, 517, 541, 542
　　folium, 56, **337**, 506, 517, 541, 542, 553, 597
　　semen, 56, **148**, 506, 517, 542, 553, **557-559**, 597-598
　　　　extractum siccum normatum, **560-561**
Hirtentäschelkraut, **208**, 513, 519, 536
HIV, 122, 328, 392, 434, 438, 618, 629
Hives, 443, 448, 639
Hohlzahnkraut, **145**, 506, 524, 541
Hollyhock flower, 36, 77, **336**, 506, 517, 543, 597
Holunderblüten, **124**, 504, 530, 547
homeopathic drugs, 52
Hopfenzapfen, **147**, 506, 525, 542
Hops, 26, 51, 74, 76, **147**, **303-305**, 374, 389, 393, 395, 400, **412**, 422, 429, 430, 431, 468, 469, 491, 493, 495, 506, 525, 542, 597, 611, 614, 621, 638
Horehound herb, 74, **148**, 390, 393, 405, 422, 426, 427, 465, 491, 498, 506, 526, 543, 597
Horse Chestnut
　　bark, 78, **393-394**, 506, 517, 541, 597
　　flower, 64, 74, 78, **393-394**, 506, 517, 542, 551, 597

leaf, 36, 64, 77, **337**, 506, 517, 542, 551, 597
seed, viii, xx, 7, 25, 26, 32, 56, 63-64, 74, **148-149**, 428, 429, 430, 432, 447, 463, 465, 490, 493, 498, 506, 517, 542, 551, 553, **557-559**, 598
standardized extract, **560-561**
Horseradish, 74, **150**, 242, 424, 428, 432, 436, 442, 447, 463, 466, 495, 506, 518, 521, 534, 598, 620
Horsetail herb, 74, **150**, 242, 374-375, 387, 390, 394-396, 412, 426, 428-429, 432, 440, 466, 494, 497, 506, 523, 539, 598
Extract, 26, 37
Hound's Tongue herb, 35, 77, **338**, 455, 496, 506, 522, 538, 539, 598
Huflattichblätter, **114**, 503, 532, 540
Huflattichblüten, **324**, 503, 532, 540
Huflattichkraut, **324**, 503, 532, 540
Huflattichwurzel, **324**, 503, 532, 540
Humulus lupulus, **147**, 506, 525, 542, 614
Hundszungenkraut, **338**, 506, 522, 539
Hydrocinnamic acid, 98, 494
Hydroquinone derivatives, 225, 494
Hydroxyquinone, 35, 348, 494
Hyoscyami folium, **146**, 506, 525, 542, 597
Hyoscyamine, 87, 146, 202, 488, 494
Hyoscyamus niger, 32, **146-147**, 506, 525, 542
Hyoscyamusblätter, **146**, 506, 525, 542
Hypercalcemia, 293, 433, 439, 629
Hypercholesteremia, 419, 428
Hyperemia, 419, 428, 629
Hyperemic, 101, 128, 130, 131, 144, 150, 159, 178, 185, 224, 237, 240, 241, 267, 459, 466, 474, 629
Hypericaceae, 141, 215, 505, 513, 524, 525, 541, 542
Hyperici herba, **214**, 513, 525, 542, 603, 613
Hypericin, 48, 141, 215, 489, 494
Hypericum perforatum, **214**, 513, 525, 542, 613
Hyperoside, 89, 142-143, 397, 494, 553-557
Hypersensitivity (see Allergy/Hypersensitivity), 434, 438
Hypertension, 36, 61, 126, 152, 161, 331, 335, 419, 428, 433, 439, 443, 448, 451, 455, 476, 629
Hyperthyroidism, 35, 315, 341, 451, 455, 629
Hypertonia, 106, 161, 172, 175, 251, 253, 254, 255, 256, 270, 273, 274, 275, 277, 312, 313, 357, 367, 375, 434, 439, 629
hypocholesteremic, 25
Hypoglycemia, 451
Hypoglycemic, 35, 332, 357, 455, 471, 474

Hypokalemia, 161, 251, 253, 254, 255, 256, 270, 273, 274, 275, 277, 293, 433, 439, 630
Hypotension, 35, 333, 335, 451, 455, 634
Hypotensive, 357, 471, 474
Hypothermia, 351, 451, 455, 630
Hyssop
herb, 36, 42, 58, 77, **338-339**, 374, 456, 506, 525, 542
oil, **338-339**, 456, 506, 525, 542
Hyssopi
aetheroleum, **338**, 506, 525, 542
herba, **338**, 506, 525, 542
Hyssopus officinalis, **338**, 506, 525, 542, 598
Iceland Moss, 48, 74-76, **151**, **252**, **256**, **276**, 390, 422, 423, 424, 425, 428, 431, 439, 440, 441, 445, 446, 448, 449, 463, 465, 468, 478, 491, 495, 507, 520, 542, 598, 605, 607, 614
Ileus, 119-120, 132, 141, 191-192, 264-266, 434, 439, 630
Ilex paraguariensis, **167**, 508, 525, 543
Illiciaceae, 215, 513, 525, 534
Illicium verum, **215**, 513, 525, 534
Immergrünkraut, 364, 510, 533, 550
Immunology, AIDS, infectious diseases, 45, 420, 434, 444, 452, 460, 472
Immunomodulation, 460, 466
immunostimulant, 25-26
Impaired balance, 367, 452, 455
Indian Snakeroot, 32, 74, **152**, 422, 428, 432, 437, 440, 441, 442, 447, 476, 479, 480, 488, 497, 507, 513, 529, 546, 598, 616
Indication, 44
indigestion, 21
Indische,
Flohsamen, **191**, 511, 528, 545
Flohsamenschalen, **192**, 511, 528, 545
Infectious diseases, 28, 45, 175, 241, 242, 363, 368, 413, 415, 420, 434, 440, 444, 452, 460, 472
Inflammation,
gastrointestinal tract, 96, 104, 107, 126, 195, 205, 207, 324, 351, 420, 428, 444
oral or pharyngeal, 421, 428
Influenza, 239, 242, 319, 324, 328, 340, 366, 421, 428, 618
Ingwerwurzelstock, **135**, 505, 533, 550
Injuries, 22, 83, 144, 188, 208, 215, 231, 239-241, 337, 370, 421, 428
Inotropic, positively, 168, 459, 467, 472, 474
Insect bites, 83, 239-240, 388, 419, 428
Insomnia (see Sleep Disturbances), 20, 21, 51, 420, 428
Institute for Demoscopy in Allensbach, 20, 23

Interaction with
    psychopharmacological herbs, 36
    with conventional drugs, 54
    with other drugs, 47
Intestinal
    inflammation, 96, 104, 195, 205, 207, 348, 365, 434, 440, 448, 626
    obstruction, 80, 96, 104, 195, 205, 207, 434, 440
    sluggishness, 46, 55, 81, 96, 98, 105, 196, 206, 208, 240, 297, 299, 378, 444, 448, 483
Intoxication, 35, 142, 293, 311, 349, 351, 367, 379, 413, 416, 452, 455
Inula helenium, **328**, 504, 525, 541
Inulin, 109, 487, 495
Iodine, 35, 315-316, 341, 495
Iridaceae, **359**, 371, 510, 512, 521, 525, 538, 542
Iridis rhizoma, 359, 510, 525, 542, 600
Iridoid glycosides, 186, 495
Iris
    florentina [*Iris germanica* var. *florentina*], **359**, 510, 525, 542
    germanica, **359**, 510, 525, 542
    pallida, **359**, 510, 525, 542
Irrigation,
    mouth, 419, 428
    therapy, 58
        with concurrent edema, 433, 440
Irritability, 125, 353, 399-400, 444, 448, 621
Irritation, 35
    mucous membrane, 36, 452, 455
        or mucosa, 35
    skin, 35, 131, 185, 319, 349, 377, 381, 419, 443, 448, 449, 451-452, 455, 459, 468, 474, 625
Isländisches Moos, **151**, 507, 520, 542
Isoflavanone derivatives, 161, 495
Isoflavonoids, 213, 495
isolated
    compounds, 19
    plant substances, 17
Isoquercetin, 495
Isoquinoline, 488, 495
Isorhamnetin, 136, 488, 495
Itch, 630
Itching, 99, 108, 176, 199, 218, 235, 239, 344, 363, 367, 381, 396, 419, 428, 443, 448, 636
Ivy, 25
Ivy leaf, 51, 74-75, **153**, **253**, **270-271**, 374, **405**, 423, 424, 436, 437, 439, 440, 441, 445, 446, 448, 464, 466, 467, 468, 469, 478, 497, 507, 524, 541, 598, 606, 607

Jambolan
    bark, 49, 74, **154**, 425, 428, 429, 431, 464, 484, 498, 507, 531, 548, 598
    seed, 36, 49, 77, **339**, 425, 431, 464, 507, 531, 548, 598
Jambosa caryophyllus, **112**, 503, 525, 536
Jaundice/yellow skin, 444
Java
    citronella oil, **341**, 507, 522, 538
    tea, 74, 75, 76, **154**, **259-260**, **302-303**, 428, 429, 432, 440, 464, 466, 468, 479, 493, 496, 497, 507, 527, 544, 598, 606, 611, 613
Javanische Gelbwurzel, **222**, 514, 521, 538
Jimsonweed
    leaf, 77, **340**, 405, 456, 491, 494, 497, 507, 522, 548, 598
    seed, 77, **340**, 405, 456, 491, 494, 497, 507, 522, 548, 598
Johanniskraut, **214**, 513, 525, 542
Johnny Jump-Up, **145**, 507, 533, 550
Joint pain, 239-240, 359, 367, 421, 428-429, 620, 627
Juglandaceae, 227, 381, 515, 525, 542
Juglandis
    folium, **227**, 515, 525, 542, 604
    fructus cortex, **381**, 515, 525, 542, 604
Juglans regia, **227**, **381**, 515, 525, 541
Juglone, 36, 218, 381, 489, 495
Juniper berry, 45, 74, **155**, 237, 238, 239, 387, 396, 412, 426, 440, 442, 448, 466, 468, 492, 493, 494, 495, 496, 497, 498, 507, 525, 542, 598, 614
Juniperus communis, **155**, 507, 525, 542, 614
Juniperi fructus, **155**, 507, 525, 542, 598, 614
Kaempferol, 136, 489, 495
Kaffeekohle, **112**, 503, 521, 537
Kakaosamen, **390**, 503, 532, 536
Kakaoschalen, **322**, 503, 532, 536
Kalifornischer Goldmohn, **389**, 501, 523, 540
Kaliuretic, 162, 461, 467, 630
Kamilenblüten, 502, 520, 526, 543
Kansas Snake root, 61
Kap-Aloe, **80**, 499, 501, 517, 534
Kapuzinerkressenkraut, **241**, 509, 515, 532, 549
Kardamomen, **103**, 501, 523, 536
Kastanienblätter, **321**, 502, 520, 536
Katzenpfötchenblüten, **319**, 502, 518, 534
Kava Kava, xxi, 11, 12, 22, 25, 26, 32, 74, **156**, 242, 422, 429, 430, 431, 436, 437, 440, 442, 445, 446, 450, 462, 464, 468, 476, 479, 480, 484, 495, 507, 528, 544, 598
    pyrone, 495
Kava-Kava-Wurzelstock, **156**, 507, 528, 544

Keine bekannt, 58
Kelp, 35, 77, **340**, 375, 412, 453, 455, 495, 507, 525, 542, 598
Ketones, 171, 181, 495
Keuschlammfrüchte, **108**, 502, 533, 534
Khellin, 35, 312, 313, 488, 495
Kidney
    bean pods (without seeds), 74, **157**, 412, 426, 466, 507, 527, 544, 598
    capacity, diminished, 421, 429
    damage, 35-36, 155, 229, 317, 323, 370, 379, 413, 452, 455
    disease (inflammation), 434, 440
    inflammation, 163, 434, 440, 444, 448, 633
    insufficiency, 118, 161, 251, 253-254, 256, 270, 273-275, 277, 313, 408, 410, 415, 434, 440
    irritation, 35-36, 64, 310, 372, 377, 381, 421, 452, 455
    stones and gravel, 421, 429
kidney-bladder illness, 21
Kiefernnadelöl, **185**, 510, 528, 544
Kiefernsprossen, **185**, 511, 513, 528, 544
Klatschmohnblüten, **324**, 503, 527, 546
Klettenwurzel, **318**, 501, 518, 535
Knoblauch, **134**, 505, 517, 534
Knotweed, 74, **157**, 242, 374, 394, 424, 428, 431, 462, 464, 497, 498, 507, 528, 545, 598
Kolasamen, **113**, 503, 521, 537
Koloquinthen, **323**, 503, 520, 538
Königin der Nacht, **353**, 509, 531, 547
Kooperation Phytopharmaka, 29, 31, 62, 64
Koriander, **117**, 503, 521, 538
Kornblume, **325**, 503, 520, 538
Krameria triandra, **194**, 511, 525, 546
Krameriaceae, 511, 525, 546
Krappwurzel, **345**, 508, 530, 546
Kreuzdornbeeren, **93**, 501, 529, 546
Küchenschellenkraut, **363**, 510, 511, 529, 546
Kümmel, **102**, 501, 519, 536
Kümmelöl, **102**, 501, 519, 536
Kürbissamen, **193**, 511, 521, 538
lactation, 45, 46
Lactation, poor, 420, 429
Lactucopricin (taraxacin), 495
Lady's Mantle, 36, 49, 74, 76, **158**, 242, 425, 464, 484, 494, 498, 499, 507, 517, 534, 598
Lamiaceae, 98, 145, 148, 154, 159, 160, 170, 172, 180, 181, 197, 198, 219, 220, 229, 310, 338, 347, 349, 358, 382, 387, 500, 501, 506, 507, 508, 509, 510, 512, 514, 515, 524, 525, 526, 527, 530, 532, 535, 541, 542, 543, 544, 546, 547, 548

Lamii albi
    flos, **228**, 515, 525, 542, 604
    herba, **382**, 515, 525, 542, 604
Laminaria
    cloustonii, 340, 507, 525, 542
    hyperborea, 340, 507, 525, 542
Laminariaceae, 340, 507, 525, 542
Laminariae stipites, **340**, 507, 525, 542, 598
Laminariastiele, **340**, 507, 525, 542
Lamium album, **228-229**, 382, 515, 525, 542
Larch Turpentine, 74, **159**, 424, 427, 430, 435, 442, 446, 463, 466, 493, 507, 525, 548, 598, 606
Lärchenterpentin, **159**, 507, 525, 548
Larix decidua, **159**, 507, 515, 525, 548
Lauraceae, 101, 110, 111, 322, 501, 502, 503, 520, 535, 536, 537
Lavandula angustifolia, **159**, 507, 525, 542
Lavandulae flos, **159**, 507, 525, 542, 598
Lavendelblüten, **159**, 507, 525, 542
Lavender flower, 74, **159**, 424, 427, 429, 430, 431, 463, 468, 492, 495, 496, 498, 507, 525, 542, 598
Laxative, 22, 47, 53, 54, 80-81, 95-98, 104-105, 132, 166, 170, 195-196, 204-208, 296-299, 308, 315, 316, 317, 319, 323, 325, 330, 336, 352, 358, 369, 377, 406, 416, 419, 444, 448, 460, 467, 471, 474, 475, 483, 631
Leberblümchenkraut, **344**, 508, 524, 541
Lecithin ex soja, **210**, 513, 524, 542, 603
Lecithin, 37, **210** (see soy lecithin)
Ledi palustris herba, **349**, 508, 525, 542, 599
Ledum palustre, 349, 508, 525, 542
Leg cramps, 421, 429
Leinsamen, **132**, 505, 525, 542
Lemon Balm, viii, xx, 26, 51, 56, 74, 76, **160**, 237-238, **279**, **304**, 374, 389, 426, 430, 431, 465, 468, 469, 491, 492, 494, 495, 497, 498, 507, 526, 543, 551, 553, **561-563**, 598, 608, 611, 613
Lemongrass, Citronella oil, 35, **341**
Leonuri cardiacae herba, **172**, 509, 525, 542, 599
Leonurus cardiaca, **172**, 509, 525, 542
Lethargy, 310, 452, 455, 618
Leucocyte increase, 460, 467
Leukocytopenia, 365, 452, 455
Leukopenia, 86, 392, 444, 448, 631
Leukorrhea, 229, 420, 429, 627, 631
Leukosis, 122, 328, 392, 434, 440, 631
Levistici radix, **163**, 508, 525, 542, 599
Levisticum officinale, **163**, 508, 525, 542
L-Hyoscyamine, 87, 202, 340, 494
Lichen islandicus, **151**, 507, 520, 542, 598, 605, 607

Lichenic acid, 224, 495
Licorice root, 45, 49, 74, 75, 76, 81, 96, 98, 105, **161-162**, 196, 205, 208, **251**, **253-257**, **270-271**, **273-278**, **297**, **299**, 423, 424, 425, 430, 431, 432, 435, 436, 437, 438, 439, 440, 441, 442, 445, 446, 447, 448, 449, 450, 464, 466, 468, 469, 475, 476, 477, 478, 479, 480, 484, 492, 493, 494, 495, 496, 507, 524, 542, 598, 605, 607, 608
Liebstöckelwurzel, **163**, 508, 525, 542
Ligaments, pulled, 421, 429
Lignans, 124, 489, 495
Lignin, 132, 495
Ligustilide, 495
Liliaceae, 80, 85, 86, 99, 162, 176, 214, 309, 490, 499, 501, 503, 507, 508, 513, 517, 518, 521, 530, 532, 534, 535, 537, 538, 546, 547
Lily-of-the-valley herb, 45, 74, 78, **162**, **291**, **407-416**, 423, 425, 437, 439, 441, 446, 449, 450, 463, 465, 467, 469, 476, 480, 490, 492, 507, 521, 538, 598, 607, 609-610
Limonene, 155, 489-490, 495
Linaceae, 132, 505, 525, 542
Linalool, 159, 489-490, 495
Linalyl acetate, 159, 495
Linamarin, 132, 495
Linden
    Charcoal, 37, 77, **342**, 425, 507, 548, 598
    flower, 37, 74-75, 77, **163**, **258-259**, 423, 424, 425, 465, 494, 495, 498, 507, 508, 513, 532, 549, 599, 606
        Silver, 37, **342**, 512, 431, 549
    leaf, 37, 74, 75, 77, **343**, 507, 508, 513, 532, 549, 599
    wood, 37, 77, 342-343, 507, 508, 532, 549, 599
Lindenblätter, **343**, 507, 532, 549
Lindenblüten, **163**, 507, 532, 549
Lindenholz, **343**, 507, 508, 532, 549
Lindenholzkohle, **342**, 507, 532, 548
Lini semen, **132**, 505, 525, 542, 596, 613
Linolenic acid esters, 132, 495
Linum usitatissimum, **132**, 505, 525, 542, 613
Linustatin, 132, 495
Lipid-lowering, 134, 211, 459, 467, 631
Lipolytic, 114, 168, 460, 467, 631
Liquiritiae radix, **161**, 507, 524, 542, 598, 605, 606, 607, 608
Lithospermic acid, 98, 495
Liver
    and gallbladder diseases, 21
    and gallbladder, 45
    and kidney damage associated with furanocoumarins, 36
    cirrhosis, 45, 161, 170, 251, 253, 254, 256, 270, 273, 274, 275, 277, 344, 420, 429, 434
    disease, 45, 170, 174, 212, 286, 360, 378, 413, 420, 429, 434, 437, 440, 488
Liverwort herb, 35, 77, **344**, 453, 455, 457, 496, 508, 524, 541, 599
Loasaceae, 349, 508, 526, 543
Locomotor system, degenerative disorders of, 420, 429
Loganiaceae, 355, 400, 509, 516, 524, 531, 541, 548
Loofa, 37, 77, **344**, 508, 525, 542, 599
Lovage root, 45, 74, **163-164**, 242, 374, 393, 412, 428, 429, 432, 440, 442, 464, 492, 493, 495, 508, 525, 542, 599
Löwenzahnkraut, **118**, 504, 532, 548
Löwenzahnwurzel-mit Kraut, **119**, 504, 532, 548
L-Scopolamine, 340, 497
Lucidin, 33, 35, 47, 346, 495
Luffa aegyptiaca, *Luffa aegyptiaca*, **344**, 508, 513, 525, 542, 599
Luffaschwamm, **344**, 508, 513, 525, 542
Lungenkraut, **345**, 508, 529, 546
Lungwort, 37, 77, **345**, 399, 508, 529, 546, 599
Lupuli strobulus, **147**, 506, 525, 542, 597, 611
Luteinizing hormone suppression, 90, 460, 467
Luteolin-7-glucoside, 83, 495
Lycopi herba, **98**, 501, 525, 542, 594
Lycopus
    europaeus, **98**, 501, 525, 542
    virginicus, **98**, 403, 501, 525, 542
Lymphocyte increase, 460, 467
Lymphocytopenia, 365, 452, 455
Mace, **354**, 508, 526, 543
Madagascin, 141, 495
Madder root, 33, 35, 77, **345-346**, 455, 473, 495, 508, 530, 546, 599
Mädesüß, **169**, 508, 523, 531, 540
Maiglöckchenkraut, **162**, 507, 521, 538
Majoran, 347, 508, 526, 543
Majorana hortensis, **347**, 508, 526, 543
Majoranae
    aetheroleum, **347**, 508, 526, 542, 543
    herba, **347**, 508, 526, 543
Majoranöl, 508, 526, 542, 543
Male Fern, 32, 35
    herb, 77, **346-347**, 453, 454, 455, 456, 457, 508, 522, 540
    leaf, 77, **346**, 453, 455, 456, 508, 522, 540, 599
    rhizome, 346-347, 508, 522, 540
Malignant tumors, 171, 360, 420, 429

Mallow
  flower, 74, **164**, 238, 425, 428, 429, 431, 465, 495, 500, 508, 526, 543, 599
  leaf, 74, **165**, 425, 428, 429, 431, 465, 467, 495, 500, 508, 526, 543, 599
Maltol, 180, 495
Malva sylvestris, **164-165**, 500, 508, 526, 543
Malvaceae, 164, 165, 166, 167, 336, 500, 506, 508, 517, 525, 526, 534, 541, 543
Malvae
  arboreae flos, **336**, 506, 517, 543
  flos, **164**, 336, 500, 506, 508, 517, 526, 543, 597, 599
  folium, **165**, 500, 506, 508, 517, 526, 543, 599
Malvenblätter, **165**, 508, 526, 543
Malvenblüten, **164**, 500, 508, 526, 543
Manna, *Manna*, 74, **165**, 422, 425, 428, 430, 447, 449, 467, 484, 495, 508, 523, 543, 599
Mannans, 234, 495
Mannitol, 165, 495
MAO
  inhibitor, 460, 467, 472, 474, 632
  therapy and hypertension, 36
Marian thistle, 43
Mariendistelfrüchte, **169**, 508, 531, 536
Mariendistelkraut, **350**, 508, 531, 536
Marjoram, 35
  herb, 77, **347-348**, 396, 412, 454, 508, 526, 543
  oil, 77, 238, **347-348**, 454, 494, 508, 526, 543
Market
  for herbs and phytomedicines in Germany, 20
  statistics, 11
Märkte, 22
Marrubii herba, **148**, 506, 526, 543, 597
Marrubium vulgare, **148**, 506, 526, 543
Marsdenia condurango, **116**, 503, 526, 538
Marsh Tea, 35, 77, **349**, 374, 453, 454, 455, 456, 457, 473, 474, 493, 508, 525, 542, 599
Marshmallow
  leaf, 74, 75, 76, **166**, 423, 424, 425, 427, 428, 429, 431, 435, 437, 438, 439, 440, 441, 445, 446, 448, 449, 463, 465, 468, 476, 479, 495, 508, 517, 534, 599, 606, 608, 610, 613
  root, 47, 74, 75, 76, **167**, **254-257**, **275-277**, **294**, 423, 424, 425, 427, 428, 429, 431, 435, 437, 438, 439, 440, 441, 442, 445, 446, 448, 449, 463, 465, 468, 469, 476, 477, 478, 479, 495, 508, 517, 534, 599, 606, 607, 608, 610, 613

Mary's thistle, 43
Märzveilchen/blüten, **398-399**, 513, 532, 549
Maté, 74, **167**, 395, 412, 427, 462, 465, 466, 467, 492, 508, 525, 543, 599
Mate folium, **167**, 508, 525, 543, 599
Mateblätter, **167**, 508, 525, 543
Matricaria recutita, 70, **107**, 502, 526, 543, **573-575**
Matricariae flos, 56, **107**, 502, 520, 526, 543, 567, **573-575**, 595, 606, 607, 608, 609
Matricin, 107, 495, 574-575
Mäusedornwurzelstock, **99**, 501, 530, 546
Mayapple
  resin, 74, **168**, 425, 442, 508, 528, 545, 599
  root, 74, **168**, 425, 442, 496, 508, 528, 545, 599
Meadow Saffron, **86**, 508, 521, 537
Meadowsweet, 74, **169**, 242, 374, 394-395, 412, 424, 435, 493-494, 496, 508, 523, 531, 540, 599
Medizinische Hefe, **234**, 501, 516, 519, 530, 540, 547
Meerrettich, **150**, 506, 518, 521, 534
Meerzwiebel, **214**, 513, 532, 547
Megacolon, 87, 146, 202, 404, 407, 434, 441, 632
Melaleuca leucodendra, **237**, 501, 526, 536
Melaleuca viridiflora, **174**, 237, 509, 526, 543
Melancholic moods, 370, 452, 455
Meliloti herba, **218**, 514, 526, 543, 603, 614
Melilotin, 218, 495
Melilotoside, 218, 495
Melilotus
  altissimus, **218**, 514, 526, 543
  officinalis, **218**, 514, 526, 543, 614
Melissa officinalis, **160**, 507, 526, 543, **561-563**, 613
Melissae folium, 56, **160**, 507, 526, 543, 553, **561-563**, 598, 608, 611
Melissenblätter, **160**, 507, 526, 543
Memory, 137, 364, 420, 429
Menopausal symptoms, 344, 397, 420, 429
Menopause, 26
Menorrhagia, 208, 329, 420, 429, 632
Menstrual disorders, 325, 348, 370, 382, 396, 420, 429
Menstruation, early post-partum return of, 443, 448
Mental concentration, 331, 420, 429
Mentha
  arvensis, 170, 508, 526, 543
  x *piperita*, 42, **180**, 510, 526, 543, 614
Menthae
  arvensis aetheroleum, 170, 508, 526, 543, 599

piperitae
   aetheroleum, 42-43, **181**, 510, 526, 543, 600, 601, 605, 607, 608, 609, 610
   folium, 42, **180**, 510, 526, 543, 600, 607, 608, 610, 614
   herba, 42
Menthol, 170, 171, 181, 237-239, 242, 387, 495
Menthone, 171, 181, 495
Menthyl acetate, 171, 181, 495
Mentzelia, *Mentzelia*, 37
   cordifolia, 41, **349**, 508, 526, 543, 599
Mentzeliae cordifoliae, **349**, 508, 526, 543
Menyanthaceae, 93, 500, 526, 543
Menyanthes trifoliata, **93**, 500, 526, 543
Menyanthis folium, 93, 500, 526, 543, 594
Methemoglobinuria, 452, 455, 632
2-Methyl-3-butanol, 147, 495
Methyl xanthines, 495
Metrorrhagia, 208, 329, 420, 429, 632
migraine, 35
Milk
   Scall, 145, 419, 429, 632
   Thistle, 11, 25, 26, 43
      fruit, 20, 26, 56, 59, 74, 76, **169**, **278**, 424, 426, 429, 438, 448, 464, 465, 466, 497, 508, 531, 536, 551, 553, **563-565**, 599, 608
      herb, 11, 26, 37, 43, 74, 77, **350**, 508, 531, 536, 599
Millefolii
   flos, **233**, 516, 517, 543
   herba, **233**, 516, 517, 543
Mineral salts, 216, 495
Mineralocorticoid effects, 161, 251, 253, 255-256, 270, 273-275, 277, 443, 448
Mint oil, 42, 74, **170**, 424, 427, 430, 436, 438, 441, 447, 462, 463, 464, 465, 468, 493, 495, 508, 526, 543, 599
Minzöl, **170**, 508, 526, 543
Mistelfrüchte, **395**, 508, 533, 550
Mistelkraut, **171**, 509, 533, 550
Mistelstengel, **397**, 509, 533, 550
Mistletoe, 25
   berry, 52, 78, **395-396**, 456, 466, 508, 509, 533, 550, 599
   herb, 74, 78, **171**, 422, 426, 428, 429, 435, 438, 439, 442, 446, 447, 448, 449, 466, 509, 533, 550, 599
   stem, 52, 78, **397-398**, 509, 533, 550, 599
Mitosis inhibitor, 460, 467
Mode of Administration, 48
Monimiaceae, 93, 501, 527, 535

Monkshood, 32, 35, 77, **351**, 430, 453, 454, 455, 456, 488, 490, 500, 509, 517, 533, 534, 599
Monograph format, 40
Monoterpenes, 226, 495
Mood disturbance, 420, 429
Moraceae, 147, 330, 505, 506, 523-525, 536, 542
morning sickness, 62
Motherwort herb, 74, **172**, 423, 432, 491, 492, 494, 497, 509, 525, 542, 599
Motility,
   inhibiting, 95, 97, 104, 195, 204, 206, 460, 467, 471, 474
   stimulating, 95, 97, 104, 195, 204, 206, 460, 467
Motion sickness, 26, 62, 136, 420, 429
Mountain Ash berry, 37, 77, **352**, 455, 496, 509, 531, 548, 599
Mucilage, 47, 114, 130, 132, 151, 163, 164, 165, 166, 186, 229, 336, 476, 495, 632
Mucociliary activity, increases, 461, 467
Mucopolysaccharides, 149, 173, 495
Mucosal irritation, 472, 474
Mucous membrane,
   irritant, 461, 467
   irritation, 36, 421, 429, 444, 448, 452, 455
Mugwort,
   herb, 35, 43, 77, 238, 321, **352**, 398, 453, 473, 509, 518, 535, 600
   root, 43, 77, **352**, 398, 453, 509, 518, 535, 600
Muira Puama, 37, 77, **353**, 509, 529, 546, 600
Mullein flower, 74, **173**, 424, 463, 466, 495, 497, 509, 533, 550, 600
Multiple sclerosis, 122, 123, 328, 392, 434, 441, 633
Muscarine-like, 88, 202, 209, 460, 467, 619, 633
Muscle
   pain, 239, 240, 241, 341, 347, 358, 359, 367, 388, 421, 429, 444, 452, 624, 630, 633, 639
   spasm, 421, 429, 430, 444, 448, 452, 455, 639
Musculotropic, 107, 460, 467, 633
Muskatnußbaum, **354**, 508, 509, 526, 543
Mustard oil glycosides, 150, 193, 229, 487, 495
Mutagenic, 33, 35, 36, 62, 69, 80, 137, 143, 205, 207, 212, 235, 311, 346, 354, 370, 388, 471, 474
   activity, 62
   effect, 35

Mutterkorn, **329**, 504, 521, 547
Mydriasis, 379, 452, 455, 621, 633
Myocardial circulation, increases, 459, 467
Myoglobinuria, 161, 251, 253, 255, 256, 270, 273, 274, 275, 277, 444, 449, 633
Myopathy, 86, 444, 449, 633
Myrcene, 155, 496
Myristica
    aril, **354**, 508, 526, 543
    fragrans, **354**, 508, 509, 526, 543
Myristicaceae, 354, 508-509, 526, 543
Myristicin, 55, 363, 487-489, 496
Myroxylon balsamum, **182**, 220, 510, 514, 526, 535
Myrrh, 74, **173-174**, 238, 242, 428, 464, 509, 521, 543, 600
Myrrha, **173**, 509, 521, 543, 600
Myrrhe, **173**, 509, 521, 543
Myrtaceae, 112, 126, 127, 154, 174, 237, 339, 501, 503, 504, 507, 509, 523, 525, 526, 531, 536, 540, 543, 548
Myrtilli
    folium, **311**, 500, 533, 543, 594
    fructus, **88**, 500, 533, 543, 593
Myrtle (*Myrtus communis*), 25
Naphthoquinone derivatives, 218, 496
Nasturtii herba, **228**, 515, 526, 543, 604
Nasturtium, 75, 241, 424, 429, 432, 436, 442, 509, 515, 526, 532, 543, 549, 600
Nasturtium herb, 52
Nasturtium officinale, **228**, 515, 526, 543
Natriuretic, 162, 461, 467, 633
Nausea, 36, 46, 54, 62, 86, 99, 123, 125, 127, 149, 162, 165, 174, 184, 189, 190, 199, 214, 225, 240, 253, 255, 257, 260, 267, 268, 270, 275, 277, 293, 294, 295, 296, 302, 310, 318, 328, 347, 383, 392, 406, 408, 410, 413, 416, 444, 449, 451, 454, 456, 628, 633
Negative (Unapproved) monographs, 34
Negative-Null (Unapproved) monographs, 36
Neoruscogenin, 100, 496
Nephritis, 310, 375, 416, 452, 456, 629, 633
Nerium oleander, **356**, 509, 526, 543
Nerve
    damage, 229, 444, 449
    damaging, 460, 467
Nervous
    excitation, 383, 452, 454, 456
    stomach, 24, 159, 239, 273, 350, 401, 420, 430
    system disorder, 420, 430, 444, 452, 617
nervousness, 21, 36

Nettle
    herb and leaf, 41, 74, 77, **216**, 242, 428, 429, 432, 440, 492, 494, 495, 496, 497, 498, 509, 513, 514, 515, 525, 532, 533, 542, 549, 603, 614
    root, 25, 27, 41, 75, 77, **217**, 242, 424, 429, 431, 432, 447, 468, 469, 497, 509, 513, 514, 515, 525, 532, 533, 542, 549, 603
Neuralgia, 57, 181, 186, 239-241, 314, 337-338, 341, 347, 351, 356, 359, 363-364, 367, 379, 386, 388, 406, 413, 415, 420, 430, 633, 639
New Drug Application (NDA), 13
new drugs, 13
New York Heart Association (NYHA), 63
Niauli
    aetheroleum, **174**, 237, 509, 526, 543, 600
    oil, 74, **174**, 237, 238, 239, 424, 438, 440, 441, 447, 449, 450, 476, 492, 509, 526, 543, 600
Niauliöl, **174**, 509, 526, 543
Night-blooming Cereus, 37
    flower, 77, **353**, 473, 509, 531, 547
    herb, 37, 52, 77, 242, **353**, 473, 509, 531, 547, 600
None known, 58
Nose bleed, 310, 421, 430, 452, 456
Numbness, 371, 452, 456
Nutmeg, 35, 55, 77, 238, **354**, 453, 454, 456, 473, 474, 487, 489, 493, 509, 526, 543, 600
Nutrition Labeling and Education Act of 1990, (NLEA), 13
Nux Vomica, 35, 57, 77, **355**, 454, 456, 474, 491, 497, 509, 531, 548, 600
Oak bark, 74, **175**, 238, 422, 425, 428, 431, 436, 439, 440, 442, 464, 476, 479, 484, 498, 509, 529, 546, 600
Oat
    herb, 37, 77, **355-356**, 509, 516, 519, 535, 600
    straw, 74, **176**, 242, 428, 431, 497, 509, 518, 535, 600
Oats, 77, **356**, 453, 490, 509, 518, 535, 600
Ocimene, 159, 496
Ocimum basilicum, **310**, 500, 526, 535
Odermennigkraut, **79**, 499, 503, 517, 534
Olacaceae, 353, 509, 529, 546
Old drugs, 13-14
Olea europaea, **357-358**, 509, 526, 543
Oleaceae, 165, 308, 357-358, 499, 508, 509, 523, 526, 540, 543

Oleae folium, **357**, 509, 526, 543, 600
Oleander leaf, 35, 51, 76, 77, 78, **291-292, 356-357, 411, 414**, 436, 439, 456, 473, 474, 479, 509, 526, 543, 588, 600, 609, 610
Oleanderblätter, **356**, 509, 526, 543
Oleandri folium, **356**, 509, 526, 543, 600, 609-610
Oligomeric procyanidins, 142, 496
Olivae oleum, **358**, 509, 526, 543, 600
Olive
    leaf, 37, 77, **357**, 453, 473, 474, 509, 526, 543, 600
    oil, 37, 77, **358**, 453, 473, 474, 509, 526, 543, 600
Olivenblätter, **357**, 509, 526, 543
Olivenöl, **358**, 509, 526, 543
Onion, 74, **176-177**, 422, 427, 462, 463, 467, 469, 484, 493, 509, 517, 534, 600, 616, 623
Ononidis radix, **213**, 513, 526, 543, 603, 614
Ononin, 213, 496
Ononis spinosa, 213, 513, 526, 543, 614
Oral-pharyngeal anti-irritant, 461, 467
Orange peel, 50, 74, **177**, 238, 247, 282-283, 387, 399, 405, 422-423, 425-427, 438, 442, 449, 464, 491, 493, 500, 509, 520, 535, 537, 594, 600, 605, 608
Orange peel, Bitter (see Bitter Orange peel)
Orangenschalen, **177**, 509, 520, 537
Oregano, 36-37, 77, **358-359**, 395-396, 510, 526, 543, 600
Organotoxic, 316, 324, 376, 452, 456
Origani vulgaris herba, **358**, 510, 526, 543, 600
Origanum
    majorana, **347**, 508, 526, 543, 599
    vulgare, **358**, 510, 526, 543
Orris root, 37, 58, 77, **359**, 510, 525, 542, 600
Orthosiphon
    spicatus, **154**, 507, 527, 544, 613
    stamineus, **154**, 507, 527, 544
Orthosiphonblätter, **154**, 507, 527, 544
Orthosiphonis folium, **154**, 507, 527, 544, 598, 606, 611, 613
Orthostatic circulatory disturbance, 443, 449, 634
OTC Drug Review, 13
Paeonia
    mascula, **364**, 510, 527, 544
    officinalis, **364**, 510, 527, 544, 616
Paeoniaceae, 364, 510, 527, 544
Paeoniae
    flos, **364**, 510, 527, 544
    radix, **364**, 510, 527, 544
Pain,
    gastrointestinal, 80, 87, 96, 104, 195, 205, 207, 298, 351, 407, 420, 430, 433, **444**, 445, 451, 623
    in muscles and joints, 240, 260, 452, 456
Panax ginseng, 62, **138**, 505, 527, 541, 616
Pancreas, exocrine insufficiency, 420
Pancreatic exocrine secretion, stimulates, 460, 467
Pancreatitis, 141, 394, 433, 441, 634
Papain, *Papain*, 35, 77, **360-361**, 453, 492, 496, 510, 519, 544, 600
Papainum crudum, **360**, 510, 519, 544, 600
Papaver rhoeas, **324**, 503, 527, 546
Papaveraceae, 105, 324, 389, 501, 502, 503, 520, 523, 527, 537, 540, 546
Papaverine-like, 106, 265, 266, 272, 302, 460, 467, 634
Papaya leaf, 37, 77, **361**, 510, 519, 536, 600
Papayapeptidase A, 496
Pappelblätter, **385**, 499, 528, 545
Pappelknospen, **187**, 511, 528, 545
Pappelrinde, **385**, 499, 528, 545
Paprika, *Paprika*, 12, 74, 77, **178**, 238, 362, 401, 405, 430, 431, 435, 442, 448, 457, 466, 467, 468, 484, 490, 492, 502, 510, 519, 536, 600
Paralysis, 452, 456
    Respiratory system, 310, 351, 452, 456, 472, 625
Parasorbic acid, 352, 496
Parasympatholytic, 88, 146-147, 202, 460, 467, 635
Parmeliaceae, 151, 507, 520, 542
Parsley
    herb and root, 39, 45, 58, 74, **179**, 429, 432, 440, 442, 446, 510, 527, 544, 600
    seed, 35, 39, 55, 59, 77, **362-363**, 453, 454, 455, 457, 491, 496, 510, 527, 544, 600
Parthenium integrifolium, 61
Pasque flower, 35, 40, 77, **363**, 453, 455, 457, 473, 474, 496, 497, 510, 529, 546, 600
Passiflora incarnata, **179**, 401, 510, 527, 544
Passifloraceae, 180, 510, 527, 544
Passiflorae herba, **179**, 510, 527, 544, 600, 608, 611, 614
Passionflower herb, 26, 41, 51, 74, 76, **179**, **279**, **305**, 389, **412**, 422, 430, 431, 467, 468, 469, 492, 493, 494, 495, 498, 510, 527, 544, 600, 608, 611, 614
Passionsblumenkraut, **179**, 510, 527, 544
Pausinystalia johimbe, **382**, 516, 527, 550
Pedaliaceae, 120, 504, 524, 541
Pelvic cramps, 420, 430
Pentosan, 496

Peony, 37
    flower, 77, **364**, 394, 510, 527, 544, 600
    root, 77, **364**, 394, 510, 527, 544, 600
Peppermint,
    leaf, 26, 42, 50, 74, 75, 76, **180**, 237, 242, **266**, **272**, **274**, **278**, **280-286**, 422, 423, 425-432, 435-442, 445-447, 449, 462-465, 468-469, 478, 493, 495, 498, 510, 526, 543, 600-601, 607-608, 610, 614
    oil, 42, 74-76, **181**, 237-239, **249**, **286-290**, **298**, 422-430, 435-442, 445-447, 449, 462-465, 468-469, 479, 493, 495, 510, 526, 543, 600-601, 605, 607-610, 614
Peptides, 177, 496
Peristalsis, Regulation of, 460, 468
Periwinkle, 35, 77, 364-365, 455, 488, 498, 510, 533, 550, 601
Perspiration, 451, 456
    dcreased, 443, 449
    excessive, 420, 430
Perubalsam, **182**, 510, 526, 535
Peruvian balsam, 74, **182**, 238, 423, 427, 428, 430, 432, 435, 446, 462, 463, 466, 484, 491, 492, 493, 510, 526, 535, 601
Pestwurzblätter, **365**, 510, 527, 544
Pestwurzwurzelstock, **183**, 510, 527, 544
Petasin, 183, 496
Petasites, *Petasites*
    hybridus, **183**, 365, 510, 527, 544, 601
    leaf, 36, 77, **365**, 455, 456, 474, 510, 527, 544, 601
    root, 36, 49, 74, 77, **183**, 424, 429, 431, 440, 442, 464, 484, 496-497, 510, 527, 544, 601
    spp., **365**, 510, 527, 544
Petasitidis
    folium, **365**, 510, 527, 544
    rhizoma, **183**, 510, 527, 544, 601
Petersilienfrüchte, **362**, 510, 527, 544
Petersilienkraut/wurzel, **179**, 510, 527, 544
Petroselini
    fructus, **362**, 510, 527, 544, 600
    herba/radix, **179**, 510, 527, 544, 600
Petroselinum crispum, **179**, 362, 510, 527, 544
Peumus boldus, **93**, 501, 527, 535, 613
Pfefferminzblätter, **180**, 510, 526, 543
Pfefferminzöl, 42, **181**, 510, 526, 543
Pfingstrosenblüten, **364**, 510, 527, 544
Pfingstrosenwurzel, **364**, 510, 527, 544
Phagocytosis, stimulates, 460, 468
pharmacokinetics, 63
pharmacological actions, 50, 54
Pharmacopeia/Pharmacopoeia, 59

Pharmacopeial Names, 42
Pharmacopoeia of the People's Republic of China, 62
Phaseoli fructus sine semine, **157**, 507, 527, 544, 598
Phaseolus vulgaris, **157**, 507, 527, 544
Pheasant's Eye herb, 45, 74, 78, **183**, **291-292**, **409-416**, 423, 424, 437, 439, 441, 467, 469, 476, 479, 480, 490, 492, 494, 510, 517, 534, 601, 609-610
Phenol
    carbonic acid, 83, 496
    glycosides, 139, 169, 188, 496
Phenols, 219, 489, 496
Pheochromocytoma, 125, 152, 433-434, 441, 635
Phlebitis, 83, 240, 314, 316, 337, 419, 430, 635
Phosphalipide aus Sojabohnen, **211**, 513, 524, 544
3-sn-phosphatidylcholine, 211-212, 496
Phosphatidylethanolamine, 211, 496
Phosphatidylinositic acid, 211, 496
Phosphatidylinositol, 496
Phosphoglycerides, 211-212, 496
Phospholipide ex soja cum 73-79% (3-Sn Phosphatidyl)-cholin, **211**, 513, 524, 544
Phospholipids, 210-212, 496, 631
photosensitivity, 35
Photosensitization, 46, 90, 215, 443, 449, 451, 456, 635
Phototoxic, 35-36, 320, 370, 471, 474, 488
Physcion, 47, 96, 104, 195, 489, 496
Phytoalexins, 157, 496
Phytosterols, 161, 188, 201, 496
Picea
    abies, **130-131**, 505, 515, 527, 544
    excelsa, **130**, 505, 515, 527, 544
Piceae aetheroleum, **130**, 505, 515-516, 527, 544, 596
Piceae turiones recentes, 505, 516, 544
Pimpinella, *Pimpinella*, 37
    anisum, **82**, 499, 527, 534, 614
    herb, 37, 77, **366**, 510, 527, 544, 601
    major, **184**, 366, 510, 527, 544
    root, 74, 77, **184**, 411, 424, 493, 497, 510, 527, 544, 601, 614
    saxifraga, **184**, 366, 510, 527, 544
Pimpinellae
    herba, 366, 510, 527, 544, 601
    radix, **184**, 510, 527, 544, 601
Pinaceae, 130, 131, 159, 185, 223, 505, 507, 510, 511, 513-516, 525, 527, 528, 544, 548
Pine
    Needle oil, 74, 75, **185**, 237, 238, 239, **267**, 424, 430, 431, 435, 442, 446, 448-449, 463, 466, 468, 469, 510, 527, 528, 544, 601

Sprouts, 74, **185-186**, 238, 239, 429, 430, 463, 465, 468, 493, 497, 510, 528, 544, 601
Pini
    aetheroleum, **185**, 510, 527, 528, 544, 601, 607
    turiones, **185**, 510, 513, 528, 544, 601
Pinus
    australis, **223**, 514, 527, 548
    mugo, **185**, 510, 527, 544
    nigra, **185**, 510, 527, 544
    palustris, **223**, 514, 527, 548
    pinaster, **185**, **223**, 510, 514, 527, 544, 548
    spp., 511, 514, 527, 528, 548
    sylvestris, **185**, 510, 513, 527, 544
Piper methysticum, **156**, 507, 528, 544
Piperaceae, 156, 507, 528, 544
Piperis methystici rhizoma, **156**, 507, 528, 544, 598
Plant family, 44
Plantaginaceae, 186, 190-192, 504, 511, 528, 544-545
Plantaginis
    lanceolatae herba, **186**, 504, 510, 527, 544, 601
    ovatae semen, **191**, 511, 528, 545
    ovatae testa, **192**, 511, 528, 545, 601, 610, 613
Plantago, 43
    afra, **190**, 511, 528, 544
    arenaria, **190**, 511, 528, 545
    indica, **190**, 511, 528, 545, 616
    isphagula, **191-192**, 511, 528, 545
    lanceolata, **186**, 504, 511, 528, 544, 545
    ovata, **191-192**, 511, 528, 545, 616
    psyllium, 43, **190**, 511, 528, 545, 613-614, 616
Plantain, 74, **186**, 242, 390, 424, 428, 429, 431, 462, 463, 464, 491, 492, 495, 498, 504, 511, 528, 544, 545, 601
Platelet aggregation, inhibits, 460, 468
Poaceae, *Poaceae*, 118, 144, 176, 341, 355, 356, 394, 502, 503, 506, 507, 509, 515, 516, 517, 518, 519, 522, 528, 535, 538, 541
    spp., 506, 528, 541
Podophylli peltati
    resina, **168**, 508, 528, 545, 599
    rhizoma, **168**, 508, 528, 545, 599
Podophyllotoxin, 168, 489, 496
Podophyllum peltatum, **168**, 508, 528, 545
Podophyllumharz, **168**, 508, 528, 545
Podophyllumwurzelstock, **168**, 508, 528, 545

Poisoning, 35, 36, 310, 317, 332, 339, 340, 347, 349, 357, 367, 396, 402, 407, 451, 456
    central nervous system, 223, 260, 367, 444, 449, 451
    renal, 444, 449
Polygala
    senega, **203**, 512, 513, 528, 545, 614
    spp., **203**, 512, 513, 528, 545
Polygalaceae, 203, 512, 513, 528, 545
Polygalae radix, **203**, 512, 513, 528, 545, 603, 614
Polygonaceae, 157, 195, 507, 511, 528, 529, 545-546
Polygoni avicularis herba, **157**, 507, 528, 545, 598
Polygonum aviculare, 157, 507, 528, 545
Polysaccharides, 116, 201, 487, 496
Pomeranzenblüten, 313, 500, 520, 535
Pomeranzenblütenöl, 500, 520, 535
Pomeranzenschale, 89, 500, 520, 535
Poplar bud, 74, **187**, 427, 428, 431, 435, 446, 449, 462, 466, 469, 493, 494, 496, 511, 528, 545, 601
Populi
    cortex, **385**, 499, 528, 545, 593, 601
    folium, **385**, 499, 528, 545
    gemma, **187**, 511, 528, 545, 601
Populus
    spp., **187**, **385**, 499, 511, 528, 545
    tremula, **385**, 499, 528, 545
    tremuloides, **385**, 499, 528, 545
Positive (Approved) monographs, 33
Posology, 48
Post-thrombic syndrome, 419, 430
Potassium
    deficiency, 81, 96, 98, 105, 162, 184, 195, 196, 205, 207, 208, 214, 293, 297, 298, 299, 408, 410, 413, 415, 416, 433, 441, 443, 449, 475, 476, 477, 479
    salts, 154, 161, 216, 496
Potentilla, *Potentilla*, 74, **188**, 425, 428, 447, 464, 469, 491, 494, 496, 498, 511, 513, 514, 528, 529, 545, 601
    anserina, **188**, 511, 513, 528, 545
    erecta, **221**, 514, 529, 549
    tormentilla, **221**, 514, 529, 549
Potentillae anserinae herba, **188**, 511, 513, 528, 545, 601
Potenzholz, 353, 509, 529, 546
Pregnancy, 45, 46, 62, 66, 68, 81, 86, 96, 97, 98, 104, 105, 108, 110, 114, 115, 116, 123, 128, 129, 136, 152, 155, 156, 161, 168, 179, 183, 191, 192, 195, 196, 198, 205, 207, 225,

246, 250, 251, 253, 254, 256, 258, 261, 262, 263, 264, 270, 273, 274, 275, 276, 277, 281, 283, 284, 285, 288, 289, 290, 297, 298, 311, 313, 322, 323, 344, 349, 358, 363, 388, 389, 390, 392, 433, 441-442
Premenstrual syndrome (PMS), 26, 420, 430
Prescribed herbal drugs (semi-ethical), 24
Prescriptions, 22
Primelwurzel, **189**, 511, 529, 545
Primrose
    flower, 27, 74-75, **189**, 424, 425, 435, 449, 466, 468, 497, 511, 529, 545, 601, 607
    root, 27, 51, 74-76, **189**, **252-253**, 257, **268**, **269**, **275**, **277**, **294-296**, 423, 424, 425, 435, 437, 438, 439, 440, 441, 442, 445, 446, 447, 448, 449, 450, 466, 468, 469, 478, 479, 497, 511, 529, 545, 601, 605, 606, 607, 608, 610
Primula
    elatior, **189**, 511, 529, 545
    veris, **189**, 511, 529, 545, 614
Primulaceae, 189, 511, 529, 545
Primulae
    flos, **189**, 511, 529, 545, 601, 607, 614
    radix, **189**, 511, 529, 545, 601, 605, 606, 607, 608, 610, 614
proanthocyanidins, 63
Proazulene, 233, 496
Progressive, systemic diseases, 122-123, 392, 433, 442
Prolactin level, decreases, 460, 468
Promoting resistance to diseases, 24
proof of efficacy, 16
Proscillaridin A, 214, 291-292, 408, 496
Prostaglandin synthesis, inhibits, 471, 474
Prostate
    adenoma, 87, 202, 432, 433, 442
    (BPH), 26-27
Prostatitis, 242, 319, 392, 406, 413, 420, 430
Prostheses, bruises caused by, 421, 430
Prothrombin time, increases, 460, 468
Protoanemonin, 35, 344, 363, 496
Pruni spinosae
    flos, **315**, 500, 529, 545, 594
    fructus, **91**, 500, 513, 529, 545, 594
Prunus spinosa, **91**, **315**, 500, 513, 529, 545
Pseudoallergic reaction, 452, 456
Pseudoephedrine, 125, 496
Pseudohypericin, 141, 496
Psychic disturbances, 354, 452, 456
psychoactive, 35
psychoactive herbal drugs, 22
Psychovegetative syndrome, 20
Psyllii semen, **190**, 511, 528, 545, 601

Psyllium seed,
    Black, 42, 74, **190**, 425, 437, 438, 446, 468, 511, 528, 545, 601
    Blonde, 42, 74, **191**, **422**, 425, 428, 430, 437, 438, 439, 446, 465, 468, 476, 484, 511, 528, 545, 602
    husk, Blonde, 49, 74, 190, **192**, **296**, 422, 425, 428, 437, 438, 439, 440, 446, 464, 465, 476, 484, 511, 528, 545, 602
Pterocarpus santalinus, **372**, 512, 529, 547
Ptychopetali lignum, **353**, 509, 529, 546, 600
Ptychopetalum
    olacoides, **353**, 509, 529, 546
    unicatum, **353**, 509, 529, 546
Pulmonaria officinalis, **345**, 508, 529, 546
Pulmonariae herba, **345**, 508, 529, 546, 599
Pulmonary edema, 146, 433, 434, 442, 636
Pulsatilla, *Pulsatilla*, 77, 511, 529, 546, 510
    pratensis, **363**, 511, 529, 546, 510
    vulgaris, **363**, 511, 529, 546, 510
Pulsatillae herba, **363**, 510, 511, 529, 546, 600
Pulse irregularity, 443, 449
Pumpkin seed, 52, 74, **193**, 423, 432, 492, 496, 497, 498, 511, 521, 538, 602
Pungent principles, 133, 136, 496, 636
Pupillary rigidity, 379, 452, 456
Purgative, 420, 430, 489
Purple Coneflower
    herb, 42, **122**, 511, 523, 539
    root, 42, 52, **391-392**, 511, 523, 539
Purpursonnenhutkraut, 42, **122**, 504, 511, 523, 539
Purpursonnenhutwurzel, 42, **391**, 504, 511, 523, 539
Pyranocoumarins, 496
Pyretic, 460, 468, 636
Pyrones, 156, 312, 496
Pyrrolizidine alkaloids, 35, 36, 49, 114, 115, 116, 183, 316, 324, 338, 365, 376, 488, 496
Quality standards and phytoequivalence, 37
Queckenwurzelstock, **118**, 503, 517, 541
Quendelkraut, **220**, 514, 532, 547
Quercetin, 496
    glycosides, 136, 496
Quercus, *Quercus*
    cortex, 175, 509, 529, 546, 600
    petraea, 175, 509, 529, 546
    robur, 175, 509, 529, 546
Quinidine, 55, 87, 109-110, 146, 162, 184, 202, 214, 293, 404, 407-408, 410, 414, 416, 475-477, 479-480, 496
Quinine, ix, 55, 109-110, 398, 488, 496
Radish, 74, **193**, 422, 424, 426, 438, 463, 467, 468, 487, 493, 495, 511, 529, 546, 602

Rainfarnblüten, **379,** 514, 520, 531, 537
Rainfarnkraut, **379,** 514, 520, 532, 537
Ranunculaceae, 90, 183, 326, 344, 351, 363, 488, 499, 500, 504, 508, 509, 510, 511, 517, 520, 522, 524, 529, 533, 534, 537, 539, 541, 546
Ranunculin, 363, 497
Raphani sativi radix, **193,** 511, 529, 546, 602
Raphanus sativus, **193,** 511, 529, 546
Raspberry leaf, 36-37, 77, **366,** 511, 530, 546, 602
Ratanhiae radix, **194,** 511, 525, 546, 602
Ratanhiawurzel, **194,** 511, 525, 546
Rational Phytotherapy, 19
Rautenblätter, **370,** 512, 530, 546
Rautenkraut, **370,** 512, 530, 546
Rauvolfia serpentina, 32, **152,** 507, 513, 529, 546, 616
Rauwolfiae radix, **152,** 507, 513, 529, 546, 598
Rauwolfiawurzel, **152,** 507, 513, 529, 546
Rectum, post-surgical care of, 420, 430
Red Sandalwood, 37
Reformhäusern, 22
Renal inflammation or disease, 434, 442
Reserpine, 152, 497
Residual urine, reduces, 461, 468
Resin, 74, 140, 168, 173, 174, 185, 238, 425, 442, 497, 508, 527, 544, 581, 599, 636
Respiratory
    disorders, 24
    catarrh (see Catarrh, upper respiratory tract), 421, 430
    infection, chronic, 421, 430
    inflammation, 107, 114, 126, 159, 171, 181, 229, 246, 324, 366, 399, 421, 434, 442, 444, 625
    insufficiency, 161, 251, 256, 270, 275, 277, 347, 360, 434, 452, 456
Restlessness, 113, 125, 147, 156, 159, 180, 227, 240, 335, 353, 363, 365, 420, 430, 434, 442, 444, 449, 452, 456, 618, 620
Retail Outlets, 22
Rettich, **193,** 511, 529, 546
Revisions
    and corrections, 41, 59
Rhabarber, **195,** 511, 529, 546
Rhamnaceae, 95, 97, 104, 501-502, 505, 523, 529, 540, 546
Rhamni
    cathartici fructus, **97,** 501, 529, 546, 594
    purshianae cortex, **104,** 502, 523, 529, 546, 595

Rhamnus
    catharticus, **97,** 501, 529, 546
    frangula, **95,** 104, 501, 502, 505, 529, 540, 546, 614
    purshiana, **104,** 502, 529, 546
Rhatany root, 74, **194,** 394, 428, 445, 446, 464, 484, 498, 511, 525, 546, 602
Rhei radix, **195,** 511, 529, 546, 602
Rhein Anthrone, 497
Rheum
    officinale, **195,** 511, 529, 546, 616
    palmatum, **195,** 511, 529, 546, 616
Rheumatism, 101, 239-240, 242, 319, 337, 347, 367, 369, 371, 379, 421, 430, 637
Rhinitis, 321, 348, 452, 456, 637
Rhododendri ferruginei folium, **367,** 511, 529, 546, 602
Rhododendron, *Rhododendron,*
    ferrugineum, **367,** 511, 529, 546
    Rusty-leaved, 36, 77, **367,** 453, 454, 456, 491, 494, 511, 529, 546, 602
Rhoeados flos, **324,** 503, 527, 546, 595
Rhubarb root, 49, 74, **195,** 425, 435, 436, 437, 440, 442, 445, 446, 447, 448, 449, 467, 475-476, 484, 490, 491, 493, 494, 511, 529, 546, 602
Ringelblumenblüten, **100,** 501, 519, 536
Ringelblumenkraut, **318,** 501, 519, 536
Risk assessment, 16
Risks, 49
Ritterspornblüten, **326,** 504, 522, 539
Roborant, 135, 187, 339, 355, 431, 459, 468, 637
Roman Chamomile, 57, **320,** 502, 517, 519, 536
Römishe Kamillenblüten, **320,** 502, 518, 520, 537
Rosa
    centifolia, **196,** 511, 529, 546
    gallica, **196,** 511, 529, 546
    spp., 511, 512, 529, 530, 546
Rosaceae, 79, 91, 142, 158, 169, 188, 196, 221, 307, 314, 315, 333, 334, 352, 366, 368, 369, 378, 499, 500, 503, 506, 507, 508, 509, 511, 512, 513, 514, 517, 521, 523, 528, 529, 530, 531, 534, 538, 540, 545, 546, 548, 549
Rosae
    flos, **196,** 511, 512, 529, 530, 546, 602
    fructus, **369,** 512, 530, 546, 602
    pseudofructus cum fructibus, **368,** 512, 530, 546, 602
Rose
    flower, 74, **196,** 428, 464, 498, 511, 512, 529, 546, 602

hip, 36-37, 58, **368**, 511, 512, 529, 530, 546, 602
    and seed, 37, 58, 77, **368**, 498, 512, 530, 546, 602
        seed, 37, 58, 77, **369**, 498, 511, 512, 530, 546, 602
Rosemary, 48
    leaf, 74, **197**, 237, 238, 239, 242, 424, 426, 431, 464-465, 467-468, 493, 497, 512, 530, 546, 602, 614
    oil, 48
Rosenblüten, **196**, 511, 529, 546
Rosmarinblätter, **197**, 512, 530, 546
Rosmarini folium, **197**, 512, 530, 546, 602, 614
Rosmarinic acid, 115, 497
Rosmarinus officinalis, **197**, 512, 530, 546, 614
Roßkastanienblätter, **337**, 506, 517, 542
Roßkastanienblüten, **393**, 506, 517, 542
Roßkastanienrinde, **393**, 506, 517, 541
Roßkastiensamen, **148**, 506, 517, 542
Rostrote Alpenrosenblätter, **367**, 511, 529, 546
Rote Seifenwurzel, **209**, 513, 530, 547
Rotes Sandelholz, **372**, 512, 529, 547
Rubefacient, 241, 419, 431, 637
Rubi
    fruticosi
        folium, **91**, 500, 530, 546, 594
        radix, **314**, 500, 530, 546, 594
        idaei folium, **366**, 511, 530, 546, 602
Rubia tinctorum, **345**, 508, 530, 546
Rubiaceae, 109, 112, 345, 378, 383, 502, 503, 508, 514, 516, 520, 521, 524, 527, 530, 537, 541, 546, 550
Rubiae tinctorum radix, **345**, 508, 530, 546, 599
Rubus
    fruticosus, **91**, 314, 500, 530, 546
    idaeus, **366**, 511, 530, 546
Rue
    herb, 36, 77, **370**, 453, 454, 455, 456, 457, 473, 474, 494, 497, 505, 512, 524, 530, 541, 546, 597
    leaf, 77, **370**, 453, 456, 473, 494, 497, 505, 512, 524, 530, 541, 546, 602
Ruhrkrautblüten, **199**, 512, 524, 541
Rupturewort, 37, 77, **371**, 473, 512, 524, 541, 602
Rusci aculeati rhizoma, 99, 501, 530, 546, 594
Ruscin, 99, 497
Ruscocide, 497
Ruscogenin, 100, 490, 497
Ruscus aculeatus, **99**, 501, 530, 546
Ruta graveolens, **370**, 395, 511, 530, 546

Rutaceae, 89, 177, 313, 317, 370, 488, 500, 501, 509, 512, 517, 519, 520, 530, 535, 537, 546
Rutae
    folium, **370**, 512, 530, 546
    herba, **370**, 512, 529, 546
Rutin, 142, 397, 489, 497
Sabal, *Sabal*
    fructus, **201**, 512, 530, 531, 546, 547, 602
    serrulata, **201**, 512, 530, 546
Sabalfrüchte, **201**, 512, 530, 531, 547
Sabinene, 155, 497
Saccharomyces, *Saccharomyces*
    cerevisiae, *cerevisiae*, **234-235**, 501, 516, 530, 540, 547, 594, 605
Saccharomycetaceae, 234-235, 501, 516, 530, 540, 547
safety, 16
Saffron, 36, 40, 77, **371**, 453, 454, 455, 456, 457, 508, 512, 521, 537, 538, 602, 641
Safran, **371**, 512, 521, 538
Sage leaf, 74, **198**, 238, 239, 426, 428, 430, 442, 446, 462, 463, 464, 468, 491, 492, 493, 494, 497, 498, 512, 530, 547, 602, 613
Salbeiblätter, **198**, 512, 530, 547
Salicaceae, 188, 230, 385, 499, 511, 515, 516, 528, 530, 545, 547
Salicin, 230, 385, 489, 497
Salicis cortex, **230**, 515, 516, 530, 547, 604, 614
Salivation, increases, 460, 468
Salix
    alba, **230**, 515, 530, 547
    fragilis, **230**, 515, 530, 547
    purpurea, **230**, 515, 530, 547
    spp., **230**, 516, 530, 547, 614
Salvia officinalis, **198**, 512, 530, 547, 613
Salviae folium, **198**, 512, 530, 547, 602, 613
Sambuci flos, **124**, 504, 530, 547, 596
Sambucus nigra, **124**, 504, 530, 547
Samenfreie Gartenbohnenhülsen, **157**, 507, 527, 544
Samidine, 497
Sandalwood,
    Red, 42, 74, 77, **372**, 412, 512, 529, 530, 547, 602
    White, 37, 42, 74, 77, **199**, 432, 440, 442, 448, 449, 462, 469, 484, 493, 512, 515, 530, 547, 602
Sandriedgraswurzelstock, **373**, 512, 519, 536
Sandy Everlasting, 74, **199**, 426, 436, 465, 494, 512, 524, 541, 602
Sanicle herb, 74, **200**, 424, 497, 512, 516, 530, 547, 602

Sanicula europaea, **200**, 512, 516, 530, 547
Saniculae herba, **200**, 512, 516, 530, 547, 602
Sanikelkraut, **200**, 512, 516, 530, 547
Santalaceae, 199, 512, 515, 530, 547
Santali
    albi lignum, **199**, 512, 515, 530, 547
    lignum rubrum, **372**, 512, 529, 547, 602
Santalum album, **199**, 512, 515, 530, 547
Saponaria officinalis, **209**, 375, 377, 513, 530, 547
Saponariae rubrae
    herba, **377**, 513, 530, 547
    radix, **209**, 513, 530, 547, 603
Sarothamnus scoparius, **373**, 501, 512, 530, 539
Sarsaparilla root, 36, 64, **372**, 512, 519, 531, 547, 602
    German, 77, **373**, 512, 519, 536, 602
Sarsaparillae radix, **372**, 512, 531, 547, 602
Sarsaparillewurzel, **372**, 512, 531, 547
Saw Palmetto, 11, 12, 25, 26, 27
    berry, 74, **201**, 405, 412, 432, 447, 462, 463, 493, 496, 512, 530, 531, 546, 547, 602
Schachtelhalmkraut, **150**, 506, 523, 539
Schafgarbe, **233**, 516, 517, 543
Schafgarbenkraut, 516, 517, 543
Schlehdornblüten, **315**, 500, 529, 545
Schlehdornfrüchte, **91**, 500, 513, 529, 545
Schlüsselblumenblüten, **189**, 511, 529, 545
schmalblättriges
    Sonnenhutkraut, **327**, 504, 522, 539
    Sonnenhutwurzel, **327**, 504, 522, 539
Schmuckdroge, 57
Schöllkraut, **105**, 502, 520, 537
Schwertlilienwurzelstock, **359**, 510, 525, 542
Scillae bulbus, **214**, 513, 532, 547, 603, 607, 609-610
Scillaren A, 214, 497
Scopolamine, 87, 146, 202, 497
Scopoletin, 83, 217, 497
Scopolia, Scopolia
    carniolica, **202**, 512, 531, 547
    rhizoma, **202**, 512, 531, 547, 602
    root, 74, **202**, 423, 431, 432, 436, 438, 445, 447, 448, 449, 450, 462, 465, 466, 477, 479-481, 491, 494, 497, 512, 531, 547, 602
Scotch Broom
    flower, 36, 78, **373-375**, 424, 497, 498, 501, 512, 522, 530, 539, 602
    herb, 36, 74, 78, **203**, 242, 424, 477, 497, 501, 512, 522, 530, 539, 602-603
Scrophulariaceae, 173, 330, 381, 490, 505, 509, 513, 515, 523, 533, 540, 549, 550

Scutellarein tetramethyl ether, 497
Seborrhea, 392, 419, 431, 632, 637
Secale cornutum, **329**, 504, 521, 547, 596
Second Medicines Act, 22-23, 27-28, 46, 65
Secretion of gastric juices, 82, 92-93, 117, 136, 460, 468
Secretolytic, 57, 129, 130, 131, 162, 171, 182, 185, 186, 189, 190, 204, 251, 253, 254, 255, 257, 260, 267, 268, 270, 276, 278, 294, 295, 296, 380, 460, 468, 472, 474, 637
Secretomotory, 127, 128, 255, 460, 468, 637
Sedation & sleep, 24
Sedative, 18, 26, 27, 60, 64, 147, 160, 161, 227, 279, 303, 304, 305, 314, 316, 325, 326, 344, 352, 359, 361, 365, 371, 375, 379, 401, 406, 416, 460, 468, 472, 474, 637
Seed vs. Fruit, 59
Seifenkraut, **377**, 513, 530, 547
Seifenwurzel
    Rote, **209**, 513, 530, 547
    Weiße, **210**, 513, 515, 524, 541
sekretolytisch, 57
Selenicerei grandiflori
    flos, **353**, 509, 531, 547
    herba, **353**, 509, 531, 547
Selenicereus grandiflorus, **353**, 397, 509, 531, 547, 600
Selenium, 193, 497
Sellerie, **320**, 502, 518, 534
Selleriefrüchte, 502, 518, 534
Selleriekraut, 502, 518, 534
Selleriewurzel, 502, 518, 534
semi-ethical drugs, 22
Senecio, Senecio
    herb, 36, 77, **376**, 455, 456, 473, 474, 496, 512, 531, 547, 603
    nemorensis, **376**, 512, 531, 547
Senecionis herba, **376**, 512, 531, 547, 603
Senega Snakeroot, 74, **203**, 424, 447, 466, 468, 490, 497, 512, 513, 528, 545, 603
Senegawurzel, **203**, 512, 513, 528, 545
Senna, *Senna*, 47
    alexandrina, **204**, 206, 512, 513, 531, 547
    leaf, viii, xx, 22, 28, 39, 45, 47, 49, 56, 74, 76, **204-205**, 207, 296, **298-299**, 425, 428, 430, 435, 436, 437, 438, 439, 440, 441, 442, 445, 447, 448, 449, 467, 475, 477, 479, 480, 484, 490, 491, 493, 494, 497, 512, 513, 519, 531, 547, 551, 567, **576**, 603, 610, 614, 616
    pod, 39, 47, 49, 74, **206-207**, 425, 435, 436, 437, 440, 445, 447, 448, 449, 467, 477, 479, 480, 484, 490, 491, 493, 494, 497, 512, 513, 519, 531, 547, **577**, 579, 603, 616

Alexandrian, **577-579**
Tinnevelly, **579-581**
Sennae
folium, 56, **204**, 512, 519, 531, 547, 567, **575-576**, 583, 603, 610, 614
fructus, 56, **206**, 512, 513, 519, 531, 547, 567, **577-580**, 603, 610, 614
Acutifoliae, **577-579**
Angustifoliae, **579-581**
Sennesblätter, **204**, 512, 519, 531, 547
Sennesfrüchte, **206**, 513, 531, 547
Sennosides, 204, 205, 206, 207, 296, 298, 497, 576, 578, 580
sensitive individuals, 46
Serenoa repens, **201**, 512, 531, 547
Serpylli herba, **220**, 514, 532, 547, 604
Sesquiterpene lactones, helenaloid, 497
Sesquiterpenes, 160, 183, 226, 497
Severe irritation of skin and mucosa, 35
Shepherd's Purse, 74, **208**, 393, 395, 429, 430, 431, 465, 467, 469, 513, 519, 536, 603
Siberian Ginseng, 7, 12, 61, 68, 73, **124**, 425, 427, 429, 432, 466, 467, 492, 513, 516, 523, 539, 596
Side Effects, 46, 54, 443-457
Silberlindenblüten, **342**, 513, 532, 549
Silicic acid, 150, 157, 176, 216, 497
Silver Linden flower, **342**, 513, 532, 549
Silverweed, **188**, 393, 400, 411, 513, 528, 545
Silybin, 497, 563-564
Silybinin, 497
Silybum marianum, *Silybum marianum*, 43, **169**, 350, 401, 508, 531, 536, **563-565**
Silychristin, 169, 497, 564
Silydianine, 497
Sinapis, *Sinapis*
alba, **229**, 515, 531, 548
albae semen, **229**, 515, 531, 548, 604
Sinensetin, 154, 497
sinus, 27
Sinusitis, 321, 345, 421, 431
Sitosterol, 52, 217, 391, 497
Skin,
and connective tissue disorders, 24
allergy, 110, 443, 449
alteration, 443, 449, 626
bacterial infections, 419, 431
damage, 35, 175, 229, 240, 260, 370, 443, 444, 449, 455
discoloration, 381, 451, 456
diseases, 21
dryness, 443, 449
injury or irritation, 419, 431

irritation,
decreases, 459, 468
stimulates, 310, 451, 456, 459, 468
metabolism, stimulates, 459, 468
reddening of the, 443, 450
vesicles and necrosis of the, 443, 449, 450
Sleep
disorder, 420, 444, 450, 452, 456
disturbances, 147, 347, 348, 359, 420, 428, 431, 452, 627
sleeplessness, 36
Sloe berry, **91**, 513, 529, 545
Smilacaceae, 372, 512, 531, 547
Smilax
aristolochiaefolii, **372**, 512, 531, 547
febrifuga, **372**, 512, 531, 547
regelii, **372**, 512, 531, 547
Smooth muscle contraction, 156, 460, 468
Snakeroot,
Indian, **152**, 432, 476, 479, 480, 512, 529, 546
Senega, **203**, 447, 497, 512, 513, 528, 545, 603
Soapwort
herb, Red, 36, 77, **377**, 474, 497, 513, 530, 547, 603
root,
Red, 74, **209**, 424, 447, 466, 497, 513, 530, 547, 603
White, 74, **210**, **301**, **406**, 424, 447, 465, 467, 497, 513, 515, 524, 541, 603
Sodium retention, 161, 251, 253, 255-256, 270, 273-275, 277, 443, 450
Sojalecithin, **210**, 513, 524, 542
Solanaceae, 87, 146, 178, 202, 232, 340, 362, 403, 488, 500, 502, 504, 506, 507, 510, 512, 516, 518, 519, 522, 525, 531, 535, 536, 539, 542, 547, 548
Solanum dulcamara, **232**, 516, 531, 539
Solidago, *Solidago*
canadensis, 44, **139**, 505, 531, 548
gigantea, 44, **139**, 505, 531, 548
serotina, **139**, 505, 531, 548
virgaurea, 19, 44, **139**, 505, 531, 548, 613
virgaureae herba, **139**, 505, 530, 547
Sonnentaukraut, **217**, 514, 522, 539
Soporific, 460, 468, 637
Sorbi aucupariae fructus, **352**, 509, 531, 548, 599
Sorbus aucuparia, **352**, 509, 531, 548
Sorrel, 27

Soy
  Lecithin, 74, **210-211**, 428, 467, 496, 513, 524, 542, 603
    Phospholipid, 74, **211-212**, 422, 428, 429, 447, 466, 496, 513, 524, 544, 603
Spargelkraut, **309**, 499, 518, 535
Spargelwurzelstock, **85**, 499, 518, 535
Sparteine, 203, 373-374, 497
Spasmolytic, 199, 246, 249, 250, 252, 254, 255, 257, 258, 259, 261-268, 271, 272, 278, 280-290, 302, 313, 460, 469
Spasms, clonic-tonic, 452, 456
spastic CNS, 35
Speedwell, **380**, 513, 533, 550
Spinach leaf, 36, 37, 77, **377**, 513, 531, 548, 603
Spinacia oleracea, **377**, 513, 531, 548
Spinaciae folium, **377**, 513, 531, 548, 603
Spinatblätter, **377**, 513, 531, 548
Spiny Restharrow root, 74, **213**, 411, 428, 429, 432, 440, 466, 493, 494, 495, 496, 513, 526, 543, 603
Spiraea ulmaria, **169**, 508, 531, 540
Spitzwegerichkraut, **186**, 504, 511, 528, 545
Spleen cell increase, 460, 469
Sponge cucumber, **344**, 513, 525, 542
Squill, 32, 45, 51, 74, 76, 78, **214**, 242, **291-292**, **411**, **414**, 423, 429, 436, 437, 439, 441, 446, 447, 449, 450, 463, 465, 467, 469, 477, 479, 480, 490, 491, 492, 494, 496, 497, 513, 532, 547, 588, 603, 607, 609-610
St. John's Wort, xxi, 11, 12, 19, 20, 22, 25, 26, 27, 32, 48, 74, **214-215**, 237, 238, 242, 374, 389, 393, 422, 423, 425, 426, 428, 429, 449, 462, 463, 467, 489, 494, 513, 525, 542, 603, 613
Stachydrine, 172, 497
Standards for Quality of Herbal Remedies, 56
Star Anise, 74, 76, **215**, 237, 238, **299-300**, 424, 426, 464, 466, 493, 513, 525, 534, 603, 610
Steinkleekraut, **218**, 514, 526, 543
Sterculiaceae, 113, 322, 390, 503, 521, 532, 536, 537
Sternanis, **215**, 513, 525, 534
Steroid
  alkaloids, 232, 497
  saponins, 99, 232, 490, 497
Steroids, 81, 98, 195, 196, 198, 205, 297, 298, 299, 477, 490, 497, 632
Stiefmütterchenkraut, **145**, 506, 507, 533, 550
stimulant laxative, 47, 49
Stinging Nettle
  herb and leaf, 41, 74, **216**, 428, 429, 431, 432, 440, 447, 468, 469, 492, 494, 495, 496, 497, 513, 514, 532, 533, 549, 603
  root, 25, 27, 41, 74-75, **217**, 429, 431, 432, 440, 447, 468, 469, 492, 494, 495, 496, 497, 513, 514, 533, 549, 603
Stockrosenblüten, **336**, 506, 517, 543
Stomach,
  & digestion, 24
  bowel, liver, or biliary tract disorders, 24
  disorders, 26
  ulcer, 21
Stramonii
  folium, **340**, 507, 522, 548, 598
  semen, **340**, 507, 522, 548
Stramoniumblätter, **340**, 507, 522, 548
Stramoniumsamen, **340**, 507, 522, 548
Strawberry leaf, 37, 77, **378**, 453, 514, 523, 540, 603
Strychni semen, **355**, 509, 531, 548, 600
Strychnine, 35, 355, 497
Strychnos nux-vomica, **355**, 509, 531, 548
Südafrikanische Teufelskrallenwurzel, **120**, 504, 524, 541
Summary of product characteristics (SPCs), 40
Sumpfporstkraut, **349**, 508, 525, 542
Sundew, 75-76, **217**, **257**, **295**, **300**, 423, 424, 425, 445, 446, 447, 449, 464, 468, 495, 496, 514, 522, 539, 603, 606, 610
Süßholzwurzel, **161**, 507, 523, 542
Sweet
  Clover, 75, **218-219**, 423, 427, 428, 429, 430, 432, 448, 462, 469, 492, 494, 495, 514, 526, 543, 603
  Violet root and herb, 78, **398-399**, 497, 514, 533, 550, 603
  Woodruff, 37, 77, **378-379**, 514, 524, 541, 603
Swelling of tongue, 370, 451, 457
Swiss Pharmacopoeia, 59
Sympathalgie, 57
Sympathomimetic, 126, 373, 460, 469, 476, 638
Symphyti
  folium, **115**, 503, 531, 548
  herba, **115**, 503, 531, 548, 595
  radix, **116**, 503, 531, 548, 595
Symphytum officinale, **115-116**, 503, 531, 548
Syzygii cumini
  cortex, **154**, 507, 531, 548, 598
  semen, **339**, 507, 531, 548, 598
Syzygium
  aromaticum, **112**, 503, 531, 536
  cumini, **154**, **339**, 507, 531, 548
  jambolana, **154**, **339**, 507, 531, 548

Syzygiumrinde, **154**, 507, 531, 548
Syzygiumsamen, **339**, 507, 531, 548
Tachycardia, 36, 87, 125, 146, 152, 202, 293, 312, 383, 419, 432, 433, 436, 443, 450, 451, 457, 621, 638, 640
Tanacetum vulgare, **379**, 514, 532, 537
Tang, **315**, 500, 518, 523, 540
Tannins, 44, 55, 79, 88, 89, 91, 114, 126, 148, 154, 155, 158, 159, 160, 163, 175, 180, 188, 194, 196, 198, 227, 231, 232, 233, 487-489, 497, 498, 571, 573
Tansy
    flower, 36, **379**, 453, 455, 456, 473, 498, 514, 520, 531, 532, 537
    herb, 36, 77, **379-380**, 453, 454, 455, 456, 473, 474, 493, 498, 514, 520, 532, 537
Taraxaci
    herba, **118-119**, 504, 532, 548, 596, 607
    radix cum herba, **119**, 504, 532, 548, 596, 607
Taraxacum officinale, **118-119**, 504, 532, 548, 614
Taraxagin, 498
Tausendgüldenkraut, **106**, 502, 520, 523, 537
T-cell production, 460, 469
Teas or infusions, 59
Temperature elevation, 460, 469
Tendency to bleed, 35
Teratogenic effects, 94, 363, 471, 474
Terebinthina laricina, **159**, 507, 525, 548, 598
Terebinthina veneta, **159**, 515, 525, 548
Terebinthinae aetheroleum rectificatum, **223**, 514, 527, 528, 548, 604, 606
Terpene
    alcohols, 155, 498
    lactones, 136, 498
Terpineol, 103, 155, 388, 489, 489
4-Terpineol, 155, 498
Terpinyl acetate, 103, 498
Theobroma cacao, **322**, 390, 503, 532, 536
Theobromine, 113, 390, 487, 498
Thrombocyte aggregation, inhibits, 460, 469
Thrombocytopenia, 110, 371, 444, 450, 639
Thujone, 36, 155, 198, 233, 379, 498
Thyme, 75, 76, **219**, **251**, **252-253**, **258**, **268**, **269**, **270**, **276**, **277**, **295**, **300**, **301**, **406**, 423, 424, 432, 436 437, 438, 439, 440, 441, 445, 446, 447, 448, 449, 450, 462, 464, 466, 469, 477, 478, 496, 498, 514, 532, 547, 548, 603, 604, 607, 616
    Wild, 75, **220**, 424, 463, 464, 492, 493, 498, 514, 532, 547, 604
Thymi herba, **219**, 514, 532, 548, 603-608, 610, 613

Thymiankraut, **219**, 514, 532, 548
Thymol, 83, 219-220, 498
Thymus
    serphyllum, **220**, 514, 532, 547
    vulgaris, **219**, 514, 532, 548, 613, 616
    zygis, **219**, 514, 532, 548, 616
Thyroid,
    enlargement, 99, 433, 442, 444, 450, 628
    low-functioning, 433, 442
Thyrotoxicosis, 125, 415, 433, 442, 639
Tilia
    argentea, **342**, 513, 532, 549
    cordata, **163**, **342-343**, 507, 532, 548, 549
    platyphyllos, **163**, **342-343**, 507, 508, 532, 549
    tomentosa, **342**, 513, 532, 549
Tiliaceae, 163, 342-343, 507, 508, 513, 532, 548, 549
Tiliae
    carbo, **342**, 507, 532, 548, 598
    flos, **163**, 507, 508, 513, 532, 549, 598-599, 606
    folium, **343**, 507, 508, 513, 532, 549, 599
    lignum, **343**, 507, 508, 532, 549, 599
    tomentosae flos, **342**, 513, 532, 549, 598-599
Tinnevelly-Sennesfrüchte, **206**, 512, 519, 547
Tocopherol, 52, 193, 391, 498
Tollkirsche, **87**, 500, 504, 518, 535
Tolu Balsam, 75, **220-221**, 424, 491, 492, 493, 514, 526, 534, 604
Tolubalsam, **220**, 514, 526, 535
Tonics & geriatric, 24, 26
Tonus, increases, 460, 469
Tormentil root, 75, **221**, 412, 425, 428, 448, 514, 529, 549, 604
Tormentillae rhizoma, **221**, 514, 529, 549, 604
Tormentillwurzelstock, **221**, 514, 529, 549
Tormentoside, 188, 498
toxic alveolitis, 35
Traditional medicine, 16, 19, 22, 29
Traditional use, 16, 30
Tranquilizer, 25
Tremor, 36, 88, 142, 347, 383, 402, 452, 457
Trigonella foenum-graecum, **130**, 505, 532, 540
Triterpene glycosides, 64, 90, 100, 148, 498, 557, 559-561
Triterpenes, 198, 498
Triterpenoids, 119, 489-490, 498
Triterpenylic acid, 160, 498
Trokenhefe aus Saccharomyces cerevisiae, **235**, 501, 516, 530, 547
Tropaeolaceae, 241, 509, 532, 549
Tropaeolum majus, *Tropaeolum majus*, **241**, 509, 532, 549

Tuberculosis, 123, 172, 324, 328, 392, 406, 434, 442, 639
Turmeric,
    Javanese, 75, **222**, **271-272**, 426, 436, 438, 447-448, 464, 465, 469, 493, 514, 521, 538, 604, 610
    root, 75-76, **222**, **301-302**, 426, 436, 438, 448, 463, 465, 489, 492, 493, 498, 514, 521, 538, 604, 610
Turnera diffusa, **325**, 504, 532, 549, 596
Turneraceae, 325-326, 504, 532, 549
Turnerae diffusae
    folium, **325**, 504, 532, 549
    herba, **325**, 504, 532, 549
Turpentine oil, Purified, 75, **223**, 238, **260**, 423, 424, 429, 430, 431, 435, 442, 449, 463, 464, 466, 514, 527, 528, 548, 604
Tussilago farfara, **114**, 324, 503, 532, 540
Tyramine, 203, 373, 375, 477, 498
Tyrosinase inhibiting, 460, 469
Ulcers, gastric and duodenal, 401, 434, 442
Umbelliferone, 83, 488, 498
Unapproved Monographs with
    Documented or suspected risk, 35
    No documented risk, 36
United States Pharmacopeia — *USP*, 16, 48
unrest, 51
Urginea maritima, *Urginea maritima*, 32, **214**, 513, 532, 547
Urinary
    Flow, increases, 461, 469
    Tract
        disorders, 24
        irritation, 317, 363, 381, 421, 452, 457
Urination,
    Difficulties in, **444**, 450
    Diminished, associated with BPH stages 1 and 2, 420, 432
urologic, 25
Urtica
    dioica, **216-217**, 509, 513, 532, 549, 614
    urens, **216-217**, 509, 514, 533, 549
Urticaceae, 216-217, 509, 514, 533, 549
Urticae
    folium, **216**, 509, 514, 533, 549, 603, 614
    herba, **216**, 509, 514, 533, 549, 603, 614
    radix, **217**, 509, 514, 533, 549, 603, 614
Urticaria, 178, 235, 362, 451, 457, 639
Uses/Indications, 44, 53
Usnea, *Usnea*, 75, 224, 428, 463, 495, 515, 533, 549, 604
    barbata, **224**, 515, 533, 549
    florida, **224**, 515, 533, 549
    hirta, **224**, 515, 533, 549
    plicata, **224**, 515, 533, 549
    spp., **224**, 515, 533, 549
Usneaceae, 224, 515, 533, 549
Uterine contraction, stimulates, 451, 457, 460, 469
Uva Ursi, 49
    leaf, 49, 75, 76, **224-225**, **302-303**, 432, 440, 442, 450, 462, 469, 477, 479, 481, 491, 494, 498, 515, 518, 549, 604, 611
Uvae ursi folium, **224**, 515, 518, 549, 604, 611, 614
Uzara root, 75, **226**, 406, 425, 436, 467, 484, 492, 494, 515, 533, 549, 604
Uzarae radix, **226**, 515, 533, 549, 604
Uzarawurzel, **226**, 515, 533, 549
Vaccinium myrtillus, **88**, **311**, 500, 533, 543
Valerenic acid, 498, 582
Valerian root, viii, xx, 11-12, 14, 20, 26, 27, 32, 51, 53, 56, 64, 75-76, **226**, 242, **279**, **303-305**, 422, 430, 431, 468, 469, 493, 495, 497, 498, 515, 533, 549, 551, 567, **581-582**, 604, 608, 611, 614
Valeriana officinalis, **226**, 515, 533, 549, **581-582**, 614, 616
Valerianaceae, 226, 394, 515, 533, 549, 581
Valerianae radix, 56, **226**, 515, 533, 549, 567, **581-582**, 604, 608, 611
Vascular congestion, 35, 362, 451, 457
Vasodilator, 390, 471, 474, 639
Vegetable drugs, 17
vein preparations, 25
Venezianischer Terpentin, 515, 525, 548
Venous
    Pressure, lowers, 459, 469
    Tonic, 26, 162, 459, 469
Verband der Reformwaren-Hersteller, 31
Verbasci flos, **173**, 509, 533, 549, 600
Verbascum
    densiflorum, **173**, 509, 533, 549
    thapsus, **173**, 509, 533, 549
Verbena, *Verbena*
    herb, 37, 77, **380**, 515, 533, 550, 604
    officinalis, **380**, 515, 533, 550
Verbenaceae, 108, 380, 502, 515, 533, 534, 550
Verbenae herba, **380**, 515, 533, 550, 604
Veronica, *Veronica*
    herb, 37, 77, **380-381**, 515, 533, 550, 604
    officinalis, **380**, 513, 515, 533, 550
Veronicae herba, **380**, 513, 515, 533, 550, 604
Vertigo, 137, 331, 371, 396, 432, 452, 457, 484, 632, 640
Vervain, 27

Vinca minor, **364**, 510, 533, 550
Vincae minoris herba, **364**, 510, 533, 550, 601
Vincamine, 365, 498
Viola
    odorata, **398**, 513, 532, 549
    tricolor, **145**, 506, 507, 532-533, 549
Violaceae, 145, 398, 506-507, 514, 533, 550
Violae
    odoratae rhizoma and herba, 514, 533, 550
    tricoloris herba, **145**, 506-507, 533, 550, 597
Viscaceae, 171, 395, 397, 508, 509, 533, 550
Visci albi
    fructus, **395**, 508, 509, 533, 550, 599
    herba, **171**, 509, 533, 550, 599
    stipitis, 509, 533, 550
Viscum album, **171**, **395**, **397**, 508, 509, 533, 550
Visnadin, 312, 498
Visnagin, 312, 498
Visual disturbances, 347, 402, 452, 457
Vitamin
    B complex, 498, 623
    C, 352, 368-369, 498
Vitex agnus castus, **108**, 399, 502, 533, 534
Vitexin, 489, 498
    rhamnose, 498
Vogelknöterichkraut, **157**, 507, 528, 545
Volatile oils, 487, 498, 620
Vomiting, 36, 46, 54, 62, 86, 96, 104, 123, 125, 127, 162, 174, 184, 214, 225, 260, 267-268, 293, 302, 310, 317, 328-329, 349, 351-352, 367, 379, 383, 392, 406, 408, 410, 413, 416, 443-444, 450, 619, 626, 628, 632
VRH, 31
Wacholderbeeren, **155**, 507, 525, 542
Waldmeisterkraut, **378**, 514, 524, 541
Walnußfrüchtschalen, **381**, 515, 525, 542
Walnußblätter, **227**, 515, 525, 542
Walnut
    hull, 36, 77, **381**, 456, 473, 495, 515, 525, 542, 604
    leaf, 75, 77, **227**, 430, 431, 464, 473, 489, 495, 498, 515, 525, 542, 604
Water retention, 161, 251, 253, 255-256, 270, 273-275, 277, 444, 450, 621
Watercress, 45, 75, **228**, 242, 375, 393, 396, 424, 436, 440, 442, 448, 487, 495, 515, 526, 543, 604
Wax, 498
Wegwarte, **109**, 502, 520, 537
Weidenrinde, **230**, 515, 516, 530, 547

Weight loss, 212, 320, 378, 451, 457, 561, 622, 629
Weißdornblätter mit Blüten, **142**, 506, 521, 538
Weißdornfrüchte, **333**, 506, 521, 538
Weiße
    Seifenwurzel, **210**, 513, 515, 524, 541
    Senfsamen, **229**, 515, 531, 548
    Taubnesselbüten, **228**, 515, 525, 542
Weißes
    Sandelholz, **199**, 512, 515, 530, 547
    Taubnesselkraut, **382**, 515, 525, 542
Wermutkraut, **232**, 516, 518, 533
West Indian lemongrass oil, **341**, 515, 522, 538
White
    Dead Nettle
        flower, 75, 77, **228**, 242, 424, 428, 429, 431, 432, 495, 497, 498, 515, 525, 542, 604
        herb, 37, 77, 242, **382**, 424, 515, 525, 542, 604
    Mustard seed, 75, **228-229**, 422, 424, 449, 462, 468, 484, 487, 495, 515, 531, 548, 604
    Sandalwood, 42, 45, **199**, 515, 530, 547
    Soapwort root, 74, 76, **210**, **301**, **406**, 424, 497, 513, 515, 524, 530, 541, 547, 610
    Spruce oil, **130**, 515, 516, 527, 544
    Willow bark, 75, **230**, 427, 431, 462, 463, 477, 497, 515, 516, 530, 547, 604
WHO (World Health Organization), 16, 615-616
Whooping Cough, 131, 185, 219, 267, 312, 322, 349, 380, 399, 406, 432, 434, 442, 640
Wild
    candytuft (*Iberis amara*), 26
    Indigo root (*Baptisia tinctoria*), 26
    Oat herb, **355**, 516, 519, 535
Wirkungen, 50
Witch Hazel
    bark, 39, 75, **231**, 428, 429, 431, 432, 463, 464, 466, 492, 493, 494, 498, 516, 524, 541, 604, 614
    leaf, viii, xx, 39, 56, 75, **231**, 238, 242, 428, 429, 431, 432, 463, 464, 466, 492, 493, 494, 498, 516, 524, 541, 551, 567, **571-573**, 604, 614
Wolfstrappkraut, **98**, 501, 525, 542
Wollblumen, **173**, 509, 533, 549, 550
Wood Sanicle, **200**, 497, 516, 530, 547
Woody Nightshade, 75, **232**, 426, 435, 437, 438, 440, 441, 442, 462, 463, 464, 467, 497, 498, 516, 531, 539, 604

World Health Organization (WHO), 16, 615-616
Wormwood, 50, 75-76, **232**, **248-249**, **265-266**, 269, **271-272**, 278, 422, 426, 427, 435, 436, 437, 438, 439, 440, 442, 447, 449, 464, 465, 469, 490, 491, 493, 497, 498, 516, 518, 533, 604, 605, 607, 608, 610, 614
Wound Healing, 100, 107, 188, 273, 365, 381, 459, 469
Wurmfarmblätter, **346**, 508, 522, 540
Wurmfarmkraut, **346**, 508, 522, 540
Wurmfarmwurzelstock, **346**, 508, 522, 540
Xysmalobium undulatum, **226**, 515, 533, 549
Yarrow
　　flower, 39, **233**, 422, 426, 430, 464, 465, 496, 516, 517, 543
　　herb, 39, **233-234**, 242, 422, 426, 430, 462, 464, 465, 493, 496, 516, 517, 543
Yeast, 25
Yeast Brewer's/Hansen CBS 5926, 75, **234-236**, 477, 480, 494, 495, 498, 501, 516, 519, 530, 540, 547, 605
Yellow Jessamine, 78, **400-402**, 455, 473, 474, 516, 524, 541, 605
Yohimbe bark, 36, 77, **382-383**, 453, 455, 498, 516, 521, 527, 550, 605

Yohimbehe cortex, **382**, 516, 521, 527, 550, 605
Yohimberinde, **382**, 516, 521, 527, 550
Yohimbine, 36, 383, 498
Ysopkraut, **338**, 506, 525, 542
Ysopöl, **338**, 506, 525, 542
Zaunrübenwurzel, **316**, 501, 519, 536
Zedoariae rhizoma, **383**, 516, 521, 550, 605
Zedoary rhizome, 37, 77, **383**, 516, 521, 550, 605
Zerkleinerte, 57
Zimtblüten, **322**, 502, 520, 537
Zimtrinde, **110**, 502, 520, 537
Zingiber officinale, 69, **135**, 505, 533, 550, 613, 616
Zingiberaceae, 103, 136, 222-223, 383, 501, 505, 514, 516, 517, 521, 523, 533, 536, 538, 540, 550
Zingiberis rhizoma, **135**, 505, 533, 550, 597, 607, 613
Zitwerwurzelstock, **383**, 516, 521, 550
Zweigspitzen, Stengel-und-Wurzel, **349**, 508, 526, 543
Zwiebel, **176**, 509, 517, 534
Zygophyllaceae, 505, 524, 541

Addendum
Contraindications of Unapproved Herbs

The editors initially decided to exclude listing the contraindications of herbs that were negatively evaluated by Commission E. This decision was based on the presumption that since the herbs were not approved, there would be no need to show their contraindications, as they would not normally be used in clinical practice by physicians and other qualified practitioners. However, it is also quite likely that practitioners will encounter the use of some of these herbs by consumers in the general population who may have self-selected these herbs. It is also possible that practitioners may want to use the herbs for specific indications, and thus, they should be aware of potential risks (e.g., pregnancy) as noted by Commission E. Unfortunately, the decision to include the following index was made after this book was already formatted, paginated, and indexed. Thus, it is added here as a last-minute addendum. The reader should note that Commission E did not always specify contraindications for herbs that were negatively evaluated; thus, although some of the herbs in the Unapproved Herbs section pose potential health risks, detailed contraindications are not always provided, as is the case with the Approved Herbs.

As with the other therapeutic indexes in this book, the reader should always refer to the original monograph before making a therapeutic judgment. For a complete set of risks of Unapproved Herbs, please see Table 13 in the Introduction, pages 35-36. For a list of Unapproved Herbs without documented risk, please see Table 14 on pages 36-37.

AIDS
Echinacea Angustifolia herb and root/Pallida herb
Echinacea Purpurea root

Allergy to Aster/Composite Family
Echinacea Angustifolia herb and root/Pallida herb (parenteral use only)
Echinacea Purpurea root
Roman Chamomile (rare)

Allergy to Cocoa Products
Cocoa seed

Autoimmune Diseases
Echinacea Angustifolia herb and root/Pallida herb
Echinacea Purpurea root

Bradycardia
F.C. of Lily-of-the-valley herb and Squill
F.C. of Pheasant's Eye herb and Lily-of-the-valley herb

F.C. of Pheasant's Eye herb and/or
Lily-of-the-valley herb, and/or
Squill and/or Oleander leaf with
herbs that do not contain cardiac
glycosides

F.C. of Pheasant's Eye herb and/or
Lily-of-the-valley herb, and/or
Squill and/or Oleander leaf with
chemically defined drugs

CARDIAC INSUFFICIENCY
Yellow Jessamine root

CHILDREN
F.C. of Lily-of-the-valley herb and Squill
F.C. of Pheasant's Eye herb and
Lily-of-the-valley herb
F.C. of Pheasant's Eye herb and/or
Lily-of-the-valley herb, and/or
Squill and/or Oleander leaf with
herbs that do not contain cardiac
glycosides
F.C. of Pheasant's Eye herb and/or
Lily-of-the-valley herb, and/or
Squill and/or Oleander leaf with
chemically defined drugs

COLLAGENOSIS
Echinacea Angustifolia herb and
root/Pallida herb
Echinacea Purpurea root

DIGITALIS GLYCOSIDE THERAPY
F.C. of Lily-of-the-valley herb and Squill
F.C. of Pheasant's Eye herb and
Lily-of-the-valley herb
F.C. of Pheasant's Eye herb and/or
Lily-of-the-valley herb, and/or
Squill and/or Oleander leaf with
herbs that do not contain cardiac
glycosides

F.C. of Pheasant's Eye herb and/or
Lily-of-the-valley herb, and/or Squill
and/or Oleander leaf with chemically defined drugs

DIGITALIS INTOXICATION
F.C. of Lily-of-the-valley herb and Squill
F.C. of Pheasant's Eye herb and
Lily-of-the-valley herb
F.C. of Pheasant's Eye herb and/or
Lily-of-the-valley herb, and/or
Squill and/or Oleander leaf with
herbs that do not contain cardiac
glycosides
F.C. of Pheasant's Eye herb and/or
Lily-of-the-valley herb, and/or
Squill and/or Oleander leaf with
chemically defined drugs

GLAUCOMA, NARROW ANGLE
F.C. of Belladonna with drugs in
homeopathic preparations
F.C. of Belladonna with other drugs

HIV
Echinacea Angustifolia herb and
root/Pallida herb
Echinacea Purpurea root

HYPERCALCEMIA
F.C. of Lily-of-the-valley herb and Squill
F.C. of Pheasant's Eye herb and
Lily-of-the-valley herb
F.C. of Pheasant's Eye herb and/or
Lily-of-the-valley herb, and/or
Squill and/or Oleander leaf with
herbs that do not contain cardiac
glycosides
F.C. of Pheasant's Eye herb and/or
Lily-of-the-valley herb, and/or
Squill and/or Oleander leaf with
chemically defined drugs

HYPERTENSION
Scotch Broom flower

HYPERTHYROIDISM
Bladderwrack (containing doses of iodine over 150 mcg per day)
Kelp (containing doses of iodine over 150 mcg per day)

INFANTS AND TODDLERS
Basil oil (due to high estragole content)
Marjoram (extracts contraindicated in ointments for children)

LACTATION
Basil oil

LEUKOSIS
Echinacea Angustifolia herb and root/Pallida herb
Echinacea Purpurea root

LUNGS, ACUTE EDEMA OF
F.C. of Belladonna with drugs in homeopathic preparations
F.C. of Belladonna with other drugs

MAO-INHIBITOR THERAPY
Scotch Broom flower

MECHANICAL STENOSIS OF THE GASTROINTESTINAL TRACT
F.C. of Belladonna with drugs in homeopathic preparations
F.C. of Belladonna with other drugs

MEGACOLON
F.C. of Belladonna with drugs in homeopathic preparations
F.C. of Belladonna with other drugs

MULTIPLE SCLEROSIS
Echinacea Angustifolia herb and root/Pallida herb
Echinacea Purpurea root

POTASSIUM DEFICIENCY
F.C. of Lily-of-the-valley herb and Squill
F.C. of Pheasant's Eye herb and Lily-of-the-valley herb
F.C. of Pheasant's Eye herb and/or Lily-of-the-valley herb, and/or Squill and/or Oleander leaf with herbs that do not contain cardiac glycosides
F.C. of Pheasant's Eye herb and/or Lily-of-the-valley herb, and/or Squill and/or Oleander leaf with chemically defined drugs

PREGNANCY
[Ed. Note: It should be noted that with respect to pregnancy, Commission E sometimes contraindicated a particular herb (e.g., California Poppy) because experimental information was not available and also due to the known activity of the herb. Thus, some contraindications are made as a measure of caution, without direct evidence of risk.]
Basil oil
California Poppy
Cinnamon flower
Echinacea Angustifolia herb and root/Pallida herb
Liverwort herb
Marsh Tea
Pasque flower (use is "absolutely" contraindicated)

Prostate Edema with Residual Urine
    F.C. of Belladonna with drugs in homeopathic preparations
    F.C. of Belladonna with other drugs

Salicylate Hypersensitivity
    Aspen bark and leaf

Sensitivity to Cinnamon or Peruvian Balsam
    Cinnamon flower

Sunlight, Long Exposure
    Bishop's Weed fruit

Tachycardia, Ventricular
    F.C. of Lily-of-the-valley herb and Squill
    F.C. of Pheasant's Eye herb and Lily-of-the-valley herb
    F.C. of Pheasant's Eye herb and/or Lily-of-the-valley herb, and/or Squill and/or Oleander leaf with herbs that do not contain cardiac glycosides
    F.C. of Pheasant's Eye herb and/or Lily-of-the-valley herb, and/or Squill and/or Oleander leaf with chemically defined drugs

Tachycardiac Arrhythmia
    F.C. of Belladonna with drugs in homeopathic preparations
    F.C. of Belladonna with other drugs

Tuberculosis
    Echinacea Angustifolia herb and root/Pallida herb
    Echinacea Purpurea root

Errata

The editors regret that in the editing and preparation of this book at least one error was discovered just prior to press time at a critical point after the book had been completely paginated and the General Index had been completed. The monograph for Scotch Broom flower was inadvertently placed in Chapter 5, Unapproved Herbs, on page 373. It is actually an Unapproved Component Characteristic, belonging in Chapter 6. This placement is only of technical importance with respect to the actual intricacies of the German Commission E monograph system; otherwise, it has no real therapeutic relevance. That is, whether as an Unapproved Herb (i.e., negatively evaluated by Commission E) or as an Unapproved Component Characteristic within combinations of herbal drug ingredients, the net difference is the same: the herb is not approved by Commission E and is not generally recommended in clinical practice, due to lack of scientific documentation of the benefits.